POCKET GUIDE TO UROLOGY

Third Edition

Jeff A. Wieder, M. D.

IMPORTANT NOTICE

- This book is intended for use by health care professionals.
- During our rigorous attempts to make *Pocket Guide to Urology* accurate, we have depended on references that are presumed to be true and correct. Typographical errors, printing errors, omissions, and inaccuracies may be present despite our meticulous efforts to make the contents of this book error-free. The information in this book may be inaccurate, incomplete, and out of date. Health care professionals should verify the information contained within this text before applying it to any circumstance.
- This book provides methods of working up, diagnosing, and treating various medical conditions. There may be alternatives that are not listed. This book is not meant to serve as a strict guideline, but rather to provide suggestions to consider when making *your* decision regarding the work up and treatment of a patient. Appropriate work up and treatment must be determined by the health care professional based on each patient's unique circumstance.
- This book is not a substitute for appropriate medical training and education.
- Some medications and medical devices listed in this book are not approved by the Food and Drug Administration (FDA) for the indication given herein. Furthermore, this book does not provide complete or current prescribing information. Before prescribing any medication or medical device (including the ones listed within this book), the health care provider should completely read a product's label, package insert, instructions, and prescribing information and should be aware of a product's appropriate use, including (but not limited to) its FDA status, its FDA approved indications, contraindications, dose, route of administration, adverse reactions, drug interactions, and duration of therapy.
- The information in this book is subject to change at any time.
- This book comes without warranties and guarantees expressed or implied. The author, publisher, editors, and sponsors disclaim any and all liability, injury, loss, damage, expense, and any other consequences caused by the use, misuse, or application of the information in *Pocket Guide to Urology.*
- If you do not want to be bound by the conditions, stipulations, and warnings listed above, other reference books are available for your use.

ISBN # 978-0-9672845-3-8
Printed in the United States of America

Produced by J. Wieder Medical in association with
    Griffith Publishing
    www.hodi.com

POCKET GUIDE TO UROLOGY

Third Edition

"If I have been able to see farther than others, it was because I stood on the shoulders of giants."
—Sir Isaac Newton

In the references, consensus statements, guidelines, and best practice policies are in bold print. I encourage you to read these publications on your own. With your support, I hope to continue improving and updating the *Pocket Guide to Urology*. Thanks to all the professors, residents and co-workers who contributed to my education and helped make this book a reality.

Jeff A. Wieder, M.D.

To order additional copies of this book and for more information, please visit my website:

www.pocketguidetourology.com

CONTENTS

CONTENTS

RENAL TUMORS

Presentation
1. Symptoms
   a. Many tumors are found incidentally during the evaluation of unrelated medical issues; therefore, many tumors are asymptomatic.
   b. Symptoms include pain, hematuria, weight loss, flank mass, fever, night sweats, hypertension, varicocele (especially rapid onset), and paraneoplastic syndromes (see page 10).
2. The classic triad (flank mass, hematuria, and pain) occurs in 10% of patients.
3. 25-33% of patients with renal tumors have metastasis at initial presentation. Only 1-3% present with solitary metastasis.

Work Up

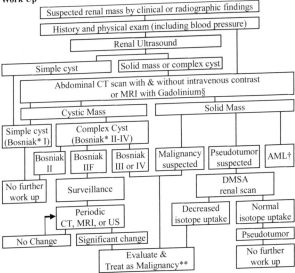

AML = Angiomyolipoma, CT = Computerized Tomography,
MRI = Magnetic Resonance Imaging, US= Ultrasound
§ On CT/MRI note: size of tumor, location of tumor within kidney (is it amenable to renal sparing surgery?), contralateral kidney (is it normal?), enlarged lymph nodes, metastases, and renal vein or vena cava extension.
* See Imaging of Renal Cysts, page 163.
† See Angiomyolipoma, page 6.
** See Evaluation of Suspected Malignancy, page 2 and Summary of Treatment for RCC, page 15.

Evaluation of Suspected Renal Malignancy
1. Physical exam including blood pressure and lymph node exam. Hypertension may be caused by a paraneoplastic syndrome from RCC (see page 10) or by a juxtaglomerular tumor.
2. If neurologic exam is abnormal or neurologic symptoms are present, obtain a brain CT or MRI to look for metastasis and for lesions associated with von Hippel Lindau and tuberous sclerosis.
3. In women at risk for breast cancer, consider performing a breast exam and a mammogram (breast cancer may metastasize to the kidney).
4. Skin lesions associated with renal tumors (see page 3)
   a. Tuberous sclerosis
      i. Adenoma sebaceum—pink or red colored papules usually overlying the cheek bones or the nasolabial folds.
      ii. Ash-leaf spots—hypopigmented macules on the trunk or buttocks.
      iii. Shagreen patches—orange-peel textured plaques on the lower back.
      iv. Periungual fibromas—flesh-colored papules near the nail bed.
   b. Birt-Hogg-Dubé—fibrofolliculomas are small white or flesh-colored papules on the face, neck, back, or upper trunk.
5. BUN, creatinine, CBC, alkaline phosphatase, serum calcium, liver function tests, LDH ± ESR (see Paraneoplastic Syndromes, page 10).
6. On CT/MRI note: size of tumor, location of tumor within kidney (is it amenable to renal sparing surgery?), contralateral kidney (is it normal?), enlarged lymph nodes, metastases, and renal vein or vena cava extension.
7. If CT suggests vena cava invasion, obtain an abdominal and chest MRI.
8. Chest x-ray (if the chest x-ray is abnormal, obtain a chest CT).
9. If the patient has bone pain, bone fracture, hypercalcemia, or elevated alkaline phosphatase, obtain a bone scan (correlate with plain x-rays if indicated). Hypercalcemia and elevated alkaline phosphatase may be caused by bone metastases or by a paraneoplastic syndrome (see page 10).
10. Biopsy of a renal lesion is usually unnecessary (see below).

Biopsy of Renal Masses
1. Biopsy often fails to determine whether a mass is benign or malignant. Biopsy is not recommended unless the there is a suspicion that the lesion may be lymphoma, angiomyolipoma, infectious, inflammatory, or a tumor that has metastasized to the kidney. Reasons for this include
   a. Most primary solid renal masses are malignant (85%-95%).
   b. The biopsy is nondiagnostic in up to 20% of cases. Reasons for this include tissue necrosis or an insufficient amount of tissue.
   c. Studies suggest that false negatives occur in 2-10% of biopsies when adequate tissue is obtained. Causes for false negatives include
      i. The biopsy missed the lesion and hit normal surrounding tissue.
      ii. Benign tumors can coexist with cancer (oncocytoma coexists with RCC in up to 10% of cases). Thus, a biopsy may sample the benign component, but miss the malignant component.
      iii. Solid tissue may be difficult to obtain from a cystic mass.
   d. There have been reports of tumor spreading along the biopsy tract. Biopsy of cystic masses may cause tumor spillage.
   e. Biopsy may change the appearance of the mass—if surveillance is chosen, it is difficult to determine if a change in the lesion represents tumor progression or effects from the biopsy.
   f. Biopsy side effects—include hematoma, hemorrhage, and infection.
2. If a biopsy stains positive for HMB-45, it is probably an AML. AML is the only primary renal tumor that stains positive for HMB-45. Metastatic melanoma in the kidney will also stain positive for HMB-45.

<u>General Information About Renal Masses</u>

Primary Renal Masses
1. Benign examples
   a. Pseudotumors
   b. Simple renal cyst—the most common benign renal mass.
   c. Papillary adenoma—the most common benign *solid* renal mass.
   d. Angiomyolipoma (AML)
   e. Oncocytoma
   f. Juxtaglomerular tumor
   g. Multilocular cystic nephroma
   h. Mesoblastic nephroma
2. Malignant examples
   a. Renal cell carcinoma (RCC)—the most common malignant primary renal mass in adults.
   b. Wilms' tumor—most common malignant primary renal mass in children.
   c. Clear cell sarcoma of kidney
   d. Rhabdoid tumor of kidney
   e. Sarcoma—usually hypovascular without arteriovenous (AV) fistulas. Leiomyosarcoma is the most common type.

Secondary Renal Masses (Metastases to Kidney)
Metastases to kidney (listed most common to least common):
1. Lymphoma/leukemia
2. Lung
3. Breast
4. Other less common sites include stomach, colon, cervix, and melanoma.

Pseudotumors
1. These appear to be solid renal masses on some radiographic studies, but are actually *normal* renal parenchyma. Examples include column of Bertin, fetal lobation, dromedary hump, hilar lip or uncus, and nodular compensatory hypertrophy.
2. To differentiate pseudotumors from true tumors, obtain a DMSA renal scan. Pseudotumors demonstrate normal isotope uptake. True tumors show decreased isotope uptake.
3. Dromedary hump—a focal bulge at mid-lateral kidney thought to be from downward pressure from the spleen or liver during development. It is more common on the left.

Relative Frequency of Renal Neoplasms

Clear cell RCC	66-75%
Papillary RCC	10-15%
Chromophobe RCC	5%
Oncocytoma	5%
Angiomyolipoma	1-2%
Collecting duct carcinoma	< 1%

<u>Hereditary Syndromes Associated with Renal Tumors</u>

Summary of Hereditary Syndromes
1. Hereditary clear cell RCC
2. Hereditary papillary RCC
3. Familial oncocytoma
4. von Hippel Lindau (clear cell RCC)
5. Birt-Hogg Dubé Syndrome (clear cell, chromophobe, oncocytoma)
6. Tuberous sclerosis (RCC and angiomyolipoma)

Birt-Hogg-Dubé Syndrome (BHD)

1. Affected people may have skin fibrofolliculomas, air filled pulmonary cysts, spontaneous pneumothorax, and renal tumors.
2. Fibrofolliculomas are benign small white or flesh-colored papules on the face, neck, back, or upper trunk and usually appear after age 20.
3. Approximately 25% of people with BHD develop renal tumors. Most develop bilateral renal tumors and multiple tumors per kidney.
4. Renal tumors that develop include clear cell RCC, chromophobe RCC, oncocytoma, and mixture of oncocytoma and RCC.
5. BHD is autosomal dominant. The BHD gene is on chromosome 17.

Tuberous Sclerosis

1. The classic triad of tuberous sclerosis (*mental retardation, seizures, and adenoma sebaceum*) is seen in only 30% of cases.
2. Tuberous sclerosis is an autosomal dominant disease caused by a mutation of the TSC1 gene (chromosome 9) or the TSC2 gene (chromosome 16).
3. Tuberous sclerosis causes hamartomas, which usually occur in the retina, brain (cerebral cortex tubers, subependymal nodules, subependymal giant cell astrocytomas), skin (adenoma sebaceum), kidney (AML), lung (lymphangioleiomyomatosis), and heart (cardiac rhabdomyomas).
4. Renal cysts, angiomyolipoma (AML), or RCC may develop.
   a. Renal cysts usually develop in childhood.
   b. Approximately 60% of adults with tuberous sclerosis develop AML, usually multiple and bilateral.
   c. There is an increased risk for renal cell carcinoma (2% develop RCC).
5. Adenoma sebaceum are pink or red colored papules usually on the skin overlying the nasolabial folds or the cheek bones. They appear between age 4 and puberty and may be mistaken for acne. Other skin manifestations include hypopigmented macules on the trunk or buttocks (ash-leaf spots), orange-peel textured plaques on the lower back (shagreen patches), and flesh-colored papules near the nail bed (ungual or periungual fibromas).

von Hippel Lindau (VHL)

1. VHL is an autosomal dominant disorder caused by mutation of the VHL gene on chromosome 3p, with manifestations that may include
   a. Non-urologic—cerebellar hemangioblastomas, spinal hemangioblastomas, and retinal angiomas.
   b. Urologic—renal cysts (75%), clear cell RCC (50%), pheochromocytomas (15%), epididymal cystadenomas (10%), and epididymal cysts (7%).
2. Renal cell carcinoma
   a. Clear cell RCC occurs in 50% of patients with VHL.
   b. VHL is associated with mutation of chromosome 3p; therefore, *clear cell RCC is the most common renal cancer in VHL.*
   c. RCC is often multi-focal and bilateral.
   d. RCC develops at an earlier age in VHL (age 20-40) than in sporadic RCC (age 40-60).
   e. In patients with VHL, all renal cysts (including simple cysts) have malignant potential.
3. In patients with VHL and a renal neoplasm, renal sparing surgery is the treatment of choice when possible. If extensive bilateral RCC is present and renal sparing surgery is not possible, treatment usually consists of bilateral nephrectomy and dialysis.

Benign Renal Tumors

Papillary Adenoma

1. Adenomas are the most common solid renal mass.
2. They are usually found incidentally during autopsy.
3. Adenomas are lesions < 5 mm whose microscopic appearance is similar to low grade papillary renal cell carcinoma. Microscopically, papillary adenoma and papillary RCC are indistinguishable. However, the benign nature of lesions < 5 mm is inferred based on the frequency of adenomas and the rarity of metastasis.
4. Adenomas arise from the proximal tubule and have similar cytogenetic abnormalities as papillary RCC.

Oncocytoma

1. A benign renal tumor composed of oncocytes (cells with an *eosinophilic* granular cytoplasm) that probably derives from the collecting duct. "Malignant" oncocytomas have been reported, but these were probably chromophobe RCC or oncocytoma mixed with RCC that were misdiagnosed as pure oncocytoma.
2. Presentation—most common in males age 40-60. They may be asymptomatic or symptomatic.
3. Radiography
   a. Oncocytoma cannot be distinguished from RCC radiographically; therefore, it is often treated as RCC.
   b. A *"spoke wheel"* pattern of tumor arterioles with a lucent rim around the tumor (from the avascular capsule) is often seen on arteriography. However, this is not specific for oncocytoma and can occur with RCC.
4. Pathology
   a. Gross—mahogany or tan mass with a fibrous capsule and often with a *central scar*. Necrosis and hemorrhage are rare.
   b. Microscopic—*nests* of polygonal cells with a granular *eosinophilic* cytoplasm. Mitoses and necrosis are rare.
   c. Electron microscopy—the *cytoplasm is packed with mitochondria.*
   d. It may be difficult to distinguish between chromophobe RCC and oncocytoma (see Chromophobe RCC, page 7).
   e. RCC may be present in approximately 10% of oncocytomas, although the range reported in the literature is 2-32%.
5. Treatment—surgical excision is the treatment of choice because
   a. Radiographs cannot distinguish between RCC and oncocytoma.
   b. RCC may coexist with oncocytoma.
   c. Renal biopsy cannot rule out coexisting malignant elements.

Juxtaglomerular Tumor

1. A rare benign renin secreting tumor derived from the juxtaglomerular apparatus. They are usually < 3 cm in diameter.
2. Presentation—young (average age is 25 years old), diastolic hypertension, headaches, elevated renin, and hyperaldosteronism with hypokalemia.
3. Treatment—nephron sparing excision is the treatment of choice.

Mesoblastic Nephroma—see page 26.

Multilocular Cystic Nephroma—see page 26.

Metanephric Adenoma/Metanephric Adenofibroma

1. Since there are only a few reports of these lesions, their classification as benign is provisional pending further information.
2. They consist of small uniform tubules lined with cuboidal epithelium.

Angiomyolipoma (AML)

1. AML is a benign renal mass composed of blood vessels (angio), smooth muscle (myo) and fat (lipo).

2. Presentation

   a. AML occurs most often in the following populations.
      i. Females age 40-60.
      ii. Tuberous sclerosis—up to 60% of patients with tuberous sclerosis develop AML, usually multiple and bilateral. However, most patients with AML do not have tuberous sclerosis. See page 4.

   b. AML is often asymptomatic. If symptoms develop, they may include flank pain, hematuria, anemia, and hemorrhage with hypotension.

   c. Lesions ≥ 4 cm are more likely to be symptomatic and more likely to hemorrhage.

Size of AML	Symptomatic	Hemorrhage
< 4 cm	0-24%	0-13%
> 4 cm	46-82%	33-51%

3. Radiographic characteristics

   a. AML rarely contains calcification. If calcium and fat are present in a renal mass, renal cell carcinoma must be considered likely.

   b. CT scan—AML enhances (indicating vascularity) and *Hounsfield units are usually -20 to -80 on noncontrast CT images* (indicating fat content).

   c. Ultrasound—AML is hyperechoic on ultrasound.

4. Diagnosis

   a. AML is usually diagnosed by CT scan based on the classic features listed above. AML cannot be diagnosed using only ultrasound because ultrasound cannot distinguish AML from RCC.

   b. *AML is the only primary renal tumor that expresses HMB-45.* If a primary renal tumor stains positive for HMB-45, it is an AML.

   c. If AML cannot be diagnosed definitively by CT scan, options include surgical extirpation or percutaneous biopsy of the lesion. If the biopsy is inconclusive or not consistent with AML (especially if it is HMB-45 negative), surgical removal of the mass should be performed.

5. Treatment

   a. Unstable patients presenting with acute life-threatening hemorrhage should have immediate surgical exploration. Stable patients with acute hemorrhage may undergo arterial embolization. If this fails, open surgery may be required.

   b. Observation is recommended if *all* of the following criteria exist:
      • AML < 4 cm in greatest dimension (AML < 4 cm has a low risk of hemorrhage).
      • Asymptomatic
      • The tumor has all the classic features of AML (not calcified, no cysts, homogenous, and Hounsfield units = -20 to -80).
   In these patients, follow up should include a yearly renal ultrasound (check for growth > 4 cm, new renal lesions, and/or hemorrhage).

   c. For patients with asymptomatic AML ≥ 4 cm, options include observation, embolization (see post-infarction syndrome, page 397), and surgical removal. Observation in these patients is problematic because AML may grow (making nephron sparing surgery in the future more difficult) and the risk of hemorrhage is high. If these patients elect to undergo observation, perform a renal ultrasound every 6-12 months.

   d. Patients with persistent symptoms should be treated. The preferred management is either arterial embolization or partial nephrectomy. Large or centrally located lesions may require radical nephrectomy.

Renal Cell Carcinoma (RCC)

Etiology of RCC (Risk Factors for RCC)

1. Tobacco smoking
2. von Hippel Lindau (VHL) disease—50% develop RCC (see page 4).
3. Tuberous sclerosis—2% develop RCC (see page 4).
4. Birt-Hogg-Dubé—25% develop RCC (see page 4).
5. Family history
6. Horseshoe kidney
7. Adult polycystic kidney disease—less than 1% develop RCC.
8. Acquired cystic renal disease from chronic renal failure—1-3% develop RCC.
9. Obesity
10. Hypertension

Note: The incidence of RCC in the general population is 0.04%.

Classification of RCC

1. Sarcomatoid elements may be present in any of these tumor types; therefore, sarcomatoid is not a unique type of RCC. The presence of sarcomatoid elements indicates a high grade tumor and a worse prognosis.
2. "Granular cell RCC" is no longer used to designate a specific type of RCC because many renal tumor types have a granular cytoplasm.
3. Clear cell (conventional) RCC—*this is the most common renal malignancy.* Microscopically, it demonstrates a low nuclear/cytoplasmic ratio and has a *clear cytoplasm*. The cytoplasm is filled with glycogen and lipids (these substances dissolve during tissue processing, resulting in a clear cytoplasm). Clear cell RCC arises from the *proximal tubule* and is associated with the loss of 3p (the short arm of chromosome 3). This tumor and chromosome abnormality are associated with VHL and hereditary clear cell RCC.
4. Chromophobe RCC—this tumor has abundant cytoplasm and distinct cell borders. It usually has two cells types based on the appearance of the cytoplasm: granular eosinophilic cells (often with a perinuclear halo) and pale, almost transparent cells. It arises from the *collecting duct* and is associated with multiple chromosomal losses. Chromophobe RCC and oncocytoma may have a similar microscopic appearance. In oncocytoma, Hale's colloidal iron stains the cell border blue, but *not* the cytoplasm (negative stain). In chromophobe RCC, it stains the entire cytoplasm blue (positive stain). Seen with electron microscopy, the cytoplasm of oncocytoma is filled with mitochondria (microvesicles are rare), while the cytoplasm of chromophobe RCC is filled mainly with *microvesicles* (although some mitochondria are seen).

Feature	Oncocytoma	Chromophobe RCC
Cell Cytoplasm Types	One (granular eosinophilic)	Two (granular eosinophilic or pale)
Electron microscopy of cytoplasm shows	Rare microvesicles, *Many mitochondria*	*Many microvesicles,* Some mitochondria
Hale's colloidal iron stain	Negative	Positive
Binucleate	Rare	Common
Nucleus outline	Smooth	Irregular
Cell origin	Collecting duct	Collecting duct

5. Chromophil (papillary) RCC—the characteristic pathologic feature is the *papillary architecture*. The cytoplasm may be eosinophilic or basophilic. Papillary RCC arises from the *proximal tubule* and is associated with polysomy (especially of chromosome 7 and 17), c-met gene mutations on chromosome 7, and loss of the Y chromosome. This is the most common renal cancer in patients with acquired cystic kidney disease from *chronic renal failure*; therefore, it is the most common renal neoplasm in patients on *dialysis*. Hereditary papillary RCC is a familial form of this cancer.

6. Collecting duct carcinoma (Bellini duct carcinoma)—this rare, highly malignant cancer derives from the collecting duct (of Bellini) and is usually located in the renal medulla or papilla. Approximately 40% of these tumors present with metastasis. Microscopic appearance often demonstrates hobnail cells lining the tubular spaces and pronounced stromal desmoplasia. 5-year survival is rare.

7. Renal medullary carcinoma—this rare tumor may be a form of collecting duct carcinoma. They occur primarily in young African American adults with *sickle cell trait* (age range approximately 10-39). The tumors have a poor prognosis (mean survival time from surgery is approximately 15 weeks and the longest time of survival from diagnosis was 17 months). These tumors are rarely confined to the kidney at surgery and rarely respond to chemotherapy or radiation. This is the only renal tumor with a racial predilection.

8. When comparing clear cell, papillary, and chromophobe tumors of similar stage and grade, *tumor type is not an independent predictor of prognosis*. However, when comparing these tumor types without regard to stage and grade, chromophobe has a better prognosis because most chromophobe tumors are low stage and low grade.

Comparison of Types of RCC

Feature	Clear Cell RCC	Chromophil RCC	Chromophobe RCC	Collecting duct RCC
Cytoplasm	Clear	Eosinophilic or basophilic	Eosinophilic or pale	Eosinophilic or basophilic
Hale's colloidal iron stain	−	−	+	−
Microvesicles*	No	No	Yes	No
Characteristic pathologic features	Clear cytoplasm	Papillary architecture	Distinct cell borders, Perinuclear halo	Hobnail cells, Tumor located in medulla
Common cytogenetics	Loss of 3p	Polysomy 7 & 17, Loss of Y, c-met mutation	Multiple deletions	Unclear
Cell origin	Proximal tubule	Proximal tubule	Collecting duct	Collecting duct
Disease association	VHL, BHD†	Chronic renal failure	BHD	Sickle cell**
Malignant potential	Moderate	Moderate	Low	High

− = negative, + = positive,
VHL = von Hippel Lindau disease, BHD = Birt-Hogg-Dubé
* Cytoplasmic microvesicles seen by electron microscopy
** Sickle cell trait is associated with renal medullary carcinoma, which is thought to be a variant of collecting duct carcinoma.
† RCC rarely occurs in tuberous sclerosis. VHL and BHD have a much higher risk of clear cell RCC.

Comparison of Renal Masses

	Clear Cell RCC	AML	Oncocytoma
Potential	Malignant	Benign	Benign*
Origin	Proximal tubule	?	Collecting duct
Sex §	M > F	F > M	M > F
Average Age §	40-60	40-60	40-60
Side §	Left = Right	Right > Left	Left = Right
Gross Color	Golden yellow	Yellow or gray	Mahogany or tan
Capsule	Pseudo-capsule	None	Fibrous capsule
Necrosis	Often	Rare	Rare
Hemorrhage	Common	Occasionally	Rare
Common macroscopic features §	Solitary, Unilateral	Solitary, Unilateral	*Central scar,* Solitary, Unilateral
Mitosis	Common	Rare	Rare
Common microscopic features	Clear cytoplasm	Fat, Smooth muscle, Blood vessels, HMB-45 positive	Nests of eosinophilic polygonal cells
Hypervascular	Most	Most	Few
Disease association**	VHL, BHD ‡	Tuberous sclerosis	BHD
Paraneoplastic	Up to 30%	No	No
Ultrasound	Hyperechoic	Hyperechoic	Hyperechoic
CT Scan	Enhances	Enhances, *HU -20 To -80*	Enhances
Arteriogram	Venous pooling, AV fistula, Neovascularity, Accentuation of capsular vessels	Hypervascular	*Spoke wheel* pattern of tumor arterioles, Lucent rim of tumor capsule†
Metastasis	Lung, bone, etc.	None	None
Usual Treatment	Surgery	Observe, surgery, or embolize.	Surgery
Diagnosis	Pathologic	Radiographic or pathologic	Pathologic

VHL = von Hippel Lindau, HU = Hounsfield Units, BHD = Birt-Hogg-Dubé

§ Refers to sporadic tumors, not those associated with a genetic disease.

* Some reports of "malignant" oncocytomas have been published, but these were probably chromophobe RCC or oncocytoma mixed with RCC. Oncocytoma may coexist with RCC in up to 10% of cases.

** Tumors tend to be multiple and bilateral in these diseases.

† Angiographic spoke wheel pattern and lucent rim of capsule are not specific to oncocytoma and have been seen in RCC.

‡ RCC rarely occurs in tuberous sclerosis. VHL and BHD have a much higher risk of clear cell RCC.

Paraneoplastic Syndromes Associated with RCC

Up to 30% of patients with RCC have a paraneoplastic syndrome. These syndromes are reversible with tumor resection. When paraneoplastic syndromes persist after tumor resection, metastatic disease is probably present and these patients have a poor prognosis. Paraneoplastic syndromes (listed from most to least common):

1. Elevated erythrocyte sedimentation rate (ESR)
2. Weight loss, cachexia
3. Fever
4. Anemia
5. Hypertension (from increased renin)
6. Hypercalcemia (from release of PTH-like substance)
7. Stauffer's syndrome (hepatic dysfunction)—a reversible hepatitis associated with RCC that has *not* metastasized to the liver.
8. Elevated alkaline phosphatase
9. Polycythemia (from increased erythropoietin)

Metastatic RCC

1. 25-33% of patients present with metastatic disease.
2. Approximately 1% present with a renal mass and a solitary metastasis. Approximately 1% present with solitary metastasis after nephrectomy. Thus, metastases usually involve multiple sites rather than a single site.
3. The lymphatic drainage of kidney varies tremendously. Furthermore, metastases occur by lymphatic spread and hematogenous spread with equal frequency. Also, 50% of those with positive regional lymph nodes have distant metastatic disease.
4. Metastatic sites (most to least common)
   a. Lung
   b. Bone—the most common site of bone metastasis is the spine.
   c. Regional lymph nodes
   d. Liver
   e. Ipsilateral adrenal
   f. Contralateral kidney
   g. Brain
5. Elevated alkaline phosphatase, calcium, or liver function tests (LFTs) may indicate a paraneoplastic syndrome or metastatic disease. Persistence of a paraneoplastic syndrome after nephrectomy indicates unrecognized or micrometastatic disease.
6. If metastases develop after nephrectomy for an M0 lesion, they usually occur within one year of surgery.

Integrated Staging for Renal Cancer

The UCLA Integrated Staging System (UISS) uses the TNM stage, Fuhrman grade, and the Eastern Cooperative Oncology Group performance status (ECOG PS) to stratify patients into categories that predict survival after treatment. For survival based on UISS, see page 17.

ECOG PS	Activity
0	Normal Activity
1	Symptomatic but ambulatory
2	Bedridden < 50% of the time
3	Bedridden > 50% of the time
4	Completely bedridden

Stage (AJCC 2002)

The following TNM classification refers to both clinical and pathological staging. Higher stage implies a worse prognosis. This staging system applies only to renal cell carcinomas (and not to other renal tumors).

Primary Tumor (T)

Tx	Primary tumor cannot be assessed
T0	No evidence of primary tumor
T1	Tumor 7 cm or less in greatest dimension, limited to the kidney
T1a	Tumor 4 cm or less in greatest dimension, limited to the kidney
T1b	Tumor more than 4 cm but not more than 7 cm in greatest dimension, limited to the kidney
T2	Tumor more than 7 cm in greatest dimension limited to the kidney
T3	Tumor extends into major veins or invades the adrenal gland or perinephric tissue, but not beyond Gerota's fascia
T3a	Tumor directly invades the adrenal gland or perirenal and/or renal sinus fat but not beyond Gerota's fascia
T3b	Tumor grossly extends into the renal vein or its segmental (muscle containing) branches or vena cava below the diaphragm
T3c	Tumor grossly extends into vena cava above the diaphragm or invades the wall of the vena cava
T4	Tumor invades beyond Gerota's fascia

Regional Lymph Nodes (N)*

Nx	Regional lymph nodes cannot be assessed
N0	No regional lymph node metastases
N1	Metastasis in a single regional lymph node
N2	Metastasis in more than one regional lymph node

Distant Metastasis (M)

Mx	Distant metastasis cannot be assessed
M0	No distant metastasis
M1	Distant metastasis

> * Note: Laterality does not affect the N classification. If a lymph node dissection is performed, then pathologic evaluation would ordinarily include at least 8 lymph nodes.

Grade

Fuhrman nuclear grading is based on nuclear characteristics (size, contour, and nucleoli). Mitotic activity is *not* considered. The tumor is assigned the highest identified grade. If spindle shaped (sarcomatoid) cells are present, nuclear grade IV is assigned. Higher grade implies a worse prognosis.

Fuhrman Nuclear Grade	Nuclear Size	Nuclear Contour	Prominent Nucleoli at x100†
I	Small (~10μ)	Round, smooth, uniform	No
II	Medium (~15μ)	Minor irregularities	No*
III	Large (~20μ)	Major irregularities	Yes
IV	Large (~20μ)	Major irregularities (often multi-lobulated, pleomorphic)	Yes

† Low power magnification (x100).

* Nucleoli may be seen with high power magnification (x400).

Treatment of RCC

Radical Nephrectomy (RN)

RN is removal of Gerota's fascia and its contents (kidney, perirenal fat, and adrenal gland). When present, tumor thrombus in the renal vein, vena cava, and the heart should be removed. Lymph node dissection is controversial (see page 13). In some cases, the adrenal gland may be spared (see page 13).

Renal Sparing Surgery (Nephron Sparing Surgery)

1. Renal sparing surgery may be indicated in the following situations:
   a. Solitary kidney
   b. Bilateral renal tumors
   c. Poor renal function
   d. Contralateral kidney is threatened by a disease that may cause renal damage (tuberous sclerosis, VHL, diabetes, hypertension, etc.)
   e. Definitive diagnosis of a benign tumor
   f. When none of the above indications exist, but the patient wants renal sparing surgery ("elective indication").
2. Renal sparing surgery may be performed if complete tumor removal is possible based on the tumor size and its location within the kidney. Small peripheral tumors are more amenable to renal sparing surgery.
3. "Elective indication" renal sparing surgery is usually limited to a solitary clinical stage T1 tumor (i.e. < 7 cm in largest diameter) because
   a. Partial nephrectomy has a higher local recurrence rate for T2-T4 tumors than for T1 tumors (5-10% versus 0-4%, respectively).
   b. For clinical stage T3 and T4 tumors, radical nephrectomy achieves longer survival than partial nephrectomy.
   c. Favorable prognostic factors for partial nephrectomy include stage T1, tumor < 4 cm, solitary tumor, unilateral tumor, and incidental tumor.
4. Renal sparing can be performed in situ or extracorporeal (nephrectomy with bench surgery and autotransplantation). In situ surgery is preferred.
5. Renal sparing surgery can be achieved by
   a. Enucleation—the tumor is removed by dissecting between the tumor capsule and the normal kidney; therefore, there is no margin of normal renal tissue around the tumor. Enucleation is thought to have a higher recurrence rate than partial nephrectomy.
   b. Partial nephrectomy—partial nephrectomy is the preferred method of renal sparing surgery. The tumor is removed with a margin of normal renal tissue. Some urologists recommend obtaining a 1 cm margin (i.e. 1 cm of normal tissue between the tumor and the surgical margin). *However, the size of a negative margin does not impact prognosis. In other words, a close margin achieves the same cure rate as an ample margin; therefore a close margin should be considered as truly negative.*
   c. Tumor ablation—tumor destruction without removal of the tumor (e.g. cryoablation, radiofrequency ablation). Long-term data are lacking.
6. A randomized trial comparing nephron sparing surgery and radical nephrectomy has not been performed. *Retrospective studies show that partial nephrectomy and radical nephrectomy result in equivalent disease-free survival,* but local recurrence (3-6% versus < 1%) and complications (4% versus 2%) may be slightly higher for renal sparing surgery.
7. *Compared to radical nephrectomy, nephron sparing surgery has a lower risk of chronic renal insufficiency and proteinuria with long-term follow up.*

8. Minimizing ischemic renal damage during partial nephrectomy
   a. Give mannitol 12.5 grams IV 5 minutes and 10 minutes prior to clamping the renal artery. Mannitol reduces ischemic injury by scavenging free radicals and by reducing oxidative cellular damage.
   b. Clamp the renal artery only once (avoid unclamping and re-clamping). Leaving the renal vein unclamped may permit retrograde renal perfusion; however, it may result in more bleeding.
   c. If renal ischemia time is > 30 minutes, cool the kidney with an ice bath for 15 minutes (until the kidney is 15° C) after clamping the artery. Re-cool the kidney every 30 minutes. *Cooling the kidney provides up to 3 hours of ischemia time without permanent renal damage.*
   d. Minimize renal ischemia time.
   e. Avoid hypotension and hypovolemia.

Adrenal Sparing Surgery
1. Direct invasion or metastasis to the adrenal occurs in 2%-10% of cases.
2. Some advocate sparing the adrenal gland when all of the following criteria are present: stage T1 or T2 tumor, no tumor in the upper pole of the kidney, and no tumor in the adrenal gland. Adrenal metastases are rare when these criteria are present.
3. Consider adrenal sparing if only one adrenal gland is present.

Regional Lymph Node Dissection (LND)
The need for LND is controversial. Non-randomized studies reveal that LND does not improve survival in clinical stage N0. For clinical stage N1-2, LND may provide prognostic information. Thus, LND is done for staging rather than for therapeutic effect. Results of the EORTC 30881 are pending (a randomized trial comparing RN with and without LND for clinical stage T1-3 N0M0 tumors; Eur Urol 36: 570, 1999).

Renal Tumor with No Metastasis
1. Radical nephrectomy is recommended for all renal tumors except
   a. Some angiomyolipomas (see Angiomyolipoma, page 6).
   b. Bosniak category I, II, or IIF cysts (see Renal Cysts, page 163).
   c. Tumors metastatic to kidney (e.g. lymphoma)—these are usually treated with the indicated systemic treatment. Nephrectomy is seldom indicated.
   d. Renal sparing surgery is indicated (see Renal Sparing Surgery, page 12).
   e. Unresectable tumor.
2. Adjuvant therapy after nephrectomy is not recommended when the tumor is completely resected.

RCC with Multiple Metastases
1. For metastatic RCC with a resectable primary tumor, the standard treatment is RN followed by systemic therapy. Systemic therapy options include
   a. High dose interleukin-2 (IL-2)—radical nephrectomy followed by immunotherapy (RN+IMT) improves time to progression and overall survival compared to immunotherapy alone. RN + IMT is best suited for patients who are candidates for *both* nephrectomy and immunotherapy and who have ECOG performance status = 0-1 and clear cell carcinoma.
   b. Kinase inhibitor—tyrosine kinase inhibitors (sunitinib and sorafenib) or mTOR kinase inhibitors (temsirolimus).
2. If the patient is not a candidate for RN and systemic therapy, treatment options include surveillance, immunotherapy alone, tyrosine kinase inhibitor alone, and palliative embolization (see post-infarction syndrome, page 397). Debulking (i.e. partial resection) is usually not indicated.
3. Radiation may be used for palliation of bone and brain metastasis; however, radiation is not effective against the primary tumor.
4. Chemotherapy and hormone therapy are ineffective.

RCC with a Solitary Metastasis
1. When a solitary metastasis presents at the same time as the primary RCC, the preferred treatment usually consists of RN and metastasis resection.
2. When a solitary metastasis develops after RN (even years later), the metastasis should be treated (e.g. excision, ablation).
3. Prognosis is better for lung metastases than for other metastatic sites.

Bilateral RCC
1. When possible, renal sparing surgery is preferred.
2. When planning radical nephrectomy on one side and partial nephrectomy on the other side, do the partial nephrectomy first and remove the other kidney at a later date. While the kidney that underwent partial nephrectomy recovers from postoperative acute tubular necrosis (ATN), the contralateral kidney sustains enough renal function to avoid dialysis.
3. When renal sparing surgery is not feasible, treatment consists of bilateral RN and dialysis. If the patient satisfies the criteria (e.g. being cancer-free for a long enough interval), renal transplant may be performed.

Tyrosine Kinase Inhibitors
1. Sunitinib (Sutent®) and sorafenib (Nexavar®) are *tyrosine kinase inhibitors* that decrease angiogenesis and tumor growth. They inhibit multiple tyrosine kinases including vascular endothelial growth factor receptor (VEGFR), platelet derived growth factor receptor (PDGFR), stem cell factor receptor (KIT), and Fms-like tyrosine kinase-3 (FLT3).
2. Sunitinib and sorafenib are FDA approved for the treatment of advanced RCC. Trials included mainly patients who underwent nephrectomy and then failed post-operative immunotherapy for metastatic clear cell RCC.
3. Sorafenib improves overall survival by 3 months compared to placebo. Sunitinib achieves a 30% partial response rate with a median response duration of 27-54 weeks. Sunitinib prolongs progression free survival compared to subcutaneous interferon. However, neither agent has been compared to high dose IL-2 (the most effective immunotherapy regimen).
4. Side effects—gastrointestinal (nausea, vomiting, diarrhea, increased lipase and amylase), rash, alopecia, fatigue, hypertension, bleeding (from any site, including tumor hemorrhage), neutropenia, and hypophosphatemia.
5. Sunitinib decreases ejection fraction in 15% of patients. Sorafenib had a higher incidence of cardiac ischemia versus placebo (2.9% vs. 0.4%). Patients who had recent cardiovascular events were excluded from the trials. Discontinue these agents in patients who develop a cardiac event.
6. Dose
   a. Sunitinib 50 mg po q day with or without food. Sunitinib is administered in cycles, with each cycle consisting of 4 weeks on treatment, followed by 2 weeks off treatment [Capsules: 12.5, 25, 50 mg].
   b. Sorafenib 400 mg po BID without food (at least one hour before or 2 hours after eating) [Tabs: 200 mg].
7. During therapy, check complete blood count and serum chemistries (e.g. sodium, potassium, phosphate, creatinine, liver function tests, amylase, and lipase). Evaluation of ejection fraction should be considered.

mTOR Kinase Inhibitor
1. Temsirolimus inhibits mammalian target of rapamycin (mTOR) kinase.
2. Temsirolimus (Torisel™) is FDA approved for the treatment of advanced RCC in patients with predictors of short survival (see page 15).
3. Dose—temsirolimus 25 mg intravenously q week.
4. Side effects—include rash, edema, hyperglycemia, and hyperlipidemia.
5. Temsirolimus improves overall survival by 3 months.

Immunotherapy

1. Interleukin-2 (IL-2)—a cytokine that stimulates cell mediated immunity. It is FDA approved for treatment of advanced RCC.
   a. To be a candidate for IL-2, the patient must have no brain metastasis and have adequate cardiac, renal, and pulmonary function.
   b. The most effective regimen is "high dose bolus IL-2". Each cycle consists of intravenous IL-2 (600,000 or 720,000 IU/kg) q 8 hours x 14 doses. 2 cycles are given with 5-9 days of rest in between cycles. In responding patients, this 2 cycle course is repeated every 6-12 weeks.
   c. Toxicity— includes fever, chills, weight gain, fluid retention, reversible renal and hepatic insufficiency, and hypotension.
   d. Response rate = 16% (5% complete response; 11% partial response).
   e. These criteria predict better response to IL-2: ECOG PS of 0, absence of metastases in multiple organs, no bone metastasis, lung only metastasis, prior nephrectomy, and no sarcomatoid features in the primary tumor.
2. Interferon is less effective than IL-2.
3. Combining interferon and IL-2 allows a reduction in the IL-2 dose, which reduces toxicity, but it may decrease efficacy.
4. Immunotherapy is most effective for clear cell RCC.

Summary of Treatment for RCC

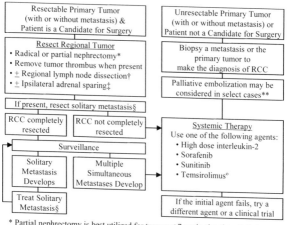

* Partial nephrectomy is best utilized for tumors < 7 cm in size (i.e. clinical stage T1) without tumor thrombus in the vena cava.

** Embolization may be considered for patients with significant bleeding, pain, or other tumor related symptoms.

† Regional lymph node dissection does not improve survival, but may provide prognostic information. Grossly enlarged nodes should probably be removed.

‡ Adrenal sparing may be attempted when the tumor is not in the upper pole of the kidney, the tumor is stage T1-T2, and the adrenal gland appears uninvolved. It may also be considered in patients with a solitary adrenal gland.

§ When a solitary metastasis is resectable, surgical excision is preferred. Other options for treating a solitary metastasis include cryotherapy and radiation.

° Reserved for patients with ≥ 3 predictors of short survival: ≥ 2 metastatic sites, Karnofsky performance status ≤ 70, < 1 year from diagnosis to metastasis, serum calcium >10, low hemoglobin, or LDH elevated more than 1.5 times normal.

Hyperfiltration Renal Injury
1. When functional renal tissue is removed, glomerular hyperfiltration occurs in the remaining tissue to restore filtration capacity.
2. Prolonged glomerular hyperfiltration may cause renal injury. This injury leads to *focal segmental glomerulosclerosis* and progressive renal failure. Hyperfiltration injury may take more than 10 years to develop.
3. *Proteinuria is the harbinger of hyperfiltration renal injury*; therefore, it precedes pathologic and clinical evidence of renal damage.
4. If *more than 75%* of the functional renal mass is removed, hyperfiltration renal injury is more likely to occur. When ≤ 50% of functional renal mass is removed, hyperfiltration may occur without clinical signs of renal injury. For example, after nephrectomy in kidney donors, glomerular filtration rate (GFR) does not decline significantly with 20 years of follow up.
5. Characteristics that increase the risk of hyperfiltration injury: removal of more than 75% of functional renal mass, high protein diet, obesity, steroid use, hypertension, hyperlipidemia, and poorly controlled diabetes mellitus.
6. Ways of reducing the risk of hyperfiltration renal injury
   a. Angiotensin converting enzyme inhibitors (ACEI)—may help prevent hyperfiltration injury by lowering intraglomerular pressure. Some suggest beginning an ACEI if 24 hour urine protein is >150 mg.
   b. Weight loss in obese patients
   c. Low protein, low sodium diet
   d. Strict control of diabetes, hypertension, and hyperlipidemia.
   e. Avoid steroid use
   f. Avoid nephrotoxins (e.g. NSAIDS)

Follow up after Radical/Partial Nephrectomy for RCC
1. History, physical, blood pressure, liver function tests, alkaline phosphatase, serum calcium, BUN, creatinine, and chest x-ray (and tests for paraneoplastic syndromes that were present pre-operatively) every 6 months for 2-3 years, then each year.
2. Abdominal CT/MRI at 4-6 months postoperatively, then every 1-2 years.
3. For low stage, low grade tumors, consider less frequent follow up.
4. Bone scan when clinically indicated.
5. In patients with less than one whole kidney, periodically obtain a 24 hour urine for creatinine, protein, and volume to assess for hyperfiltration injury.
6. Patients with a solitary kidney should be advised that participation in contact/collision sports places the kidney at risk for traumatic injury. Need to avoid contact/collision sports is determined on an individual basis.

Survival with RCC

Poor Prognostic Factors of RCC
1. Symptomatic tumor
2. High tumor grade—higher grade tumors are usually higher stage.
3. Sarcomatoid features
4. High tumor stage
5. Large tumor size
6. Tumor type—collecting duct and medullary RCC have worse prognosis.
7. Tumor necrosis
8. Incomplete resection or positive margins
9. Tumor thrombus invading the vena cava wall.
10. It is unclear if the level tumor thrombus extension influences survival.
11. Metastasis (including to lymph nodes)

Survival Based on TNM Stage

Pathologic Stage (AJCC 2002)	Procedure (complete resection)	5-Year *Disease Specific* Survival
T1N0M0	Radical or partial nephrectomy	95-100%
T2N0M0	Radical Nephrectomy	88%

Pathologic Stage (AJCC 2002)	Procedure (complete resection)	5-Year *Overall* Survival
T3aN0M0	Radical nephrectomy	47-68% §
T3bN0M0 or T3cN0M0 ‖	Radical nephrectomy & thrombectomy	43-72% §
T4	Radical nephrectomy	28%
T4 (into contiguous organs)	Radical nephrectomy	< 5%
N+M0	Radical nephrectomy	0-33%
Solitary metastasis develops after nephrectomy for M0 tumor	Treatment† of metastasis	13-54*
Solitary metastasis present at initial diagnosis	Radical nephrectomy & treatment† of metastasis	0-20%**
Multiple unresectable metastases	Any therapy	0%‡

§ Note that survival is similar between these two groups. Thus, tumor thrombus in a tumor confined to Gerota's fascia does not impact survival.
‖ It is unclear if level tumor thrombus influences survival. Tumor thrombus invading the caval wall has a worse prognosis than free floating thrombus.
* Survival is from time of metastasis resection. Pulmonary metastasis probably have better prognosis than other metastatic locations. A longer interval between RN and the development of metastasis (especially >2 years) is associated with a longer survival from the time of metastasis.
** Most die within 2 years of diagnosis. These patients have a worse survival than patients who develop a solitary metastasis after RN.
† Treatments may include resection, cryotherapy, and radiotherapy.
‡ Most die within one year of diagnosis.

Survival Based on Integrated Stage (UISS)

2002 TNM Stage	ECOG PS	Fuhrman Grade	5-Year Disease-Specific Survival	Treatment
T1 N0M0	0	1-2	91%	Radical Nephrectomy*
	0	3-4	80%	
	≥1	Any		
T2 N0M0	Any	Any		
T3 N0M0	0	Any		
	≥1	1		
	≥1	≥2	55%	
T4 N0M0	Any	Any		
N1M0	Any	Any	32%	Radical Nephrectomy* ± Immunotherapy
N2M0 or M1	0	1-2		
	0	3-4	20%	
	≥1	1-3		
	≥1	4	0%	

* Tumor thrombectomy was performed as indicated.
ECOG PS = ECOG performance status (see page 10)

REFERENCES

General

Greene FL, Page DL, Fleming ID, et al. AJCC Cancer Staging Manual, Sixth Edition. New York: Springer, 2002. (effective January 1, 2003)

deKernion JB, Belldegrun A: Renal Tumors. Campbell's Urology. 6th Edition. Ed. PC Walsh, AB Retik, TA Stamey, et al. Philadelphia: W. B. Sanders Company, 1992, pp 1053-1093.

Israel GM, Bosniak MA: An update of the Bosniak renal cyst classification system. Urology, 66(3): 484, 2005.

Modlin CS, Novick AC: Hyperfiltration renal injury: urologic implications. AUA Update Series, Vol. 20, Lesson 6, 2001.

Renal Biopsy

Dechet CB, Bostwick DG, Blute ML, et al. Renal Oncocytoma: multifocality, bilateralism, metachronous tumor development and coexistent renal cell carcinoma. J Urol, 162: 140, 1999.

Dechet CB, et al: Prospective analysis of computerized tomography and needle biopsy with permanent sectioning to determine the nature of solid renal masses in adults. J Urol, 169: 71, 2003.

Herts BR, Remer EM. The role of percutaneous biopsy in the evaluation of renal and adrenal mass. AUA Update Series, Vol. 19, Lesson 36, 2000.

Lechevallier E, Andre M, Barriol D, et al. Fine needle percutaneous biopsy of renal masses with helical CT guidance. Radiology, 216: 506, 2000.

Neuzillet Y, et al: Accuracy and clinical role of fine needle percutaneous biopsy with computerized tomography guidance of small (less than 4.0 cm) renal masses. J Urol, 171:1802, 2004.

Wood BJ, et al. Imaging guided biopsy of renal masses: indications, accuracy and impact on clinical management. J Urol, 161: 1470, 1999.

Hereditary Disorders Associated with Renal Tumors

Klein EA, Novick AC: Urologic manifestations of von Hippel Lindau disease. AUA Update Series, Vol. 19, Lesson 33, 1990.

Lendvay TS, Marshall FF: The tuberous sclerosis complex and its highly variable manifestations. J Urol, 169: 1635, 2003.

Pavlovich CP, et al: Evaluation and management of renal tumors in the Birt-Hogg-Dubé syndrome. J Urol, 173: 1482, 2005.

Benign Tumors

Dechet CB, et al: Renal oncocytoma: multifocality, bilateralism, metachronous tumor development and coexistent renal cell carcinoma. J Urol, 162: 40, 1999.

Feldman AE, Pollack HM, Perri Jr AJ, et al: Renal pseudotumors: an anatomic-radiographic classification. J Urol, 120: 133, 1978.

Minor LD, et al: Benign renal tumors. AUA Update Series, Vol. 22, Lesson 22, 2003.

Nelson CP, Sanda M: Contemporary diagnosis and management of renal angiomyolipoma. J Urol, 168: 1315, 2002.

Steiner MS, Goldman SM, Fishman EK, et al: The natural history of renal angiomyolipoma. J Urol, 150: 1782, 1993.

Lymph Node Dissection

Blom JHM, van Poppel H, Marechal JM, et al: Radical nephrectomy with and without lymph node dissection: preliminary results of the EORTC randomized trial phase III protocol 30881. Eur Urol 36: 570, 1999.

Minervini A, Lilas L, Morelli G, et al: Regional lymph node dissection in the treatment of renal cell carcinoma: is it useful in patients with no suspected adenopathy before or during surgery? BJU Int 88: 16, 2001.

Vasselli JR, et al: Lack of retroperitoneal lymphadenopathy predicts survival of patients with metastatic renal cell carcinoma. J Urol 166: 68, 2001.

Renal Cell Carcinoma

Bonsib SM: Risk and prognosis in renal neoplasms. Urol Clin North Am, 26: 643, 1999.

Bostwick DG, Eble JN: Diagnosis and classification of renal cell carcinoma. Urol Clin North Am, 26: 627, 1999.

Cindolo L, et al: Chromophobe renal cell carcinoma: comprehensive analysis of 104 cases from multicenter European database. Urology, 65: 681, 2005.

Crotty TB, Farrow GM, Lieber MM: Chromophobe cell renal carcinoma: clinicopathological features of 50 cases. J Urol, 154: 964, 1995.

Davis CJ Jr., Mostofi FK, Sesterhen IA: Renal medullary carcinoma. The seventh sickle cell nephropathy. Am J of Surg Pathol, 19: 1, 1995.

Eggener S, Reiher FK, et al: Surveillance for renal cell carcinoma after surgical management. AUA Update Series, Vol. 20, Lesson 26, 2001.

Fuhrman SA, Lasky LC, Limas C: Prognostic significance of morphologic parameters in renal cell carcinoma. Am J Surg Pathol, 6: 655, 1982.

National Comprehensive Cancer Network (NCCN) clinical practice guidelines in oncology: Kidney cancer. 2007. (http:\\www.nccn.org)

Patard JJ, et al: Prognostic value of histologic subtypes in renal cell carcinoma: a multicenter experience. J Clin Oncol, 23(12): 2763, 2005.

Pirich LM, et al: Prolonged survival of a patient with sickle cell trait and metastatic renal medullary carcinoma. J Pediatr Hematol Oncol, 21: 67, 1999

Storkel S, et al: Classification of renal cell carcinoma. Cancer, 80: 987, 1997.

Tsui KH, Shvarts O, Smith RB, et al: Prognostic indicators for renal cell carcinoma: a multivariate analysis of 643 patients using the revised 1997 TNM staging criteria. J Urol, 163: 1090, 2000.

Zambrano NR, et al: Histopathology and molecular genetics of renal tumors: toward unification of a classification system. J Urol, 162: 1246, 1999.

Zisman A, Pantuck AJ, et al: Improved prognostication using of RCC using an integrated staging system (UISS). J Clin Oncol, 19: 1649, 2001.

Zisman A, Pantuck AJ, Wieder J, et al: Risk group assessment and clinical outcome algorithm to predict the natural history of patients with surgically resected renal cell carcinoma. J Clin Oncol, 20: 4559, 2002.

Nephron Sparing Surgery

Castilla EA, et al: Prognostic importance of resection margin width after nephron sparing surgery for renal cell carcinoma. Urology, 60(6): 993, 2002.

Herr HW: Partial nephrectomy for unilateral renal carcinoma and a normal contralateral kidney: 10 year follow up. J Urol, 161: 33, 1999.

Huang WC, et al: Chronic kidney disease after nephrectomy in patients with renal cortical tumours: a retrospective study. Lancet Oncol, 7(9): 735, 2006.

Lau WK, et al: Matched comparison of radical nephrectomy vs. nephron sparing surgery in patients with unilateral renal cell carcinoma and a normal contralateral kidney. Mayo Clin Proc, 75(12): 1236, 2000.

McKiernan J, et al: Natural history of chronic renal insufficiency after partial and radical nephrectomy. Urology, 59(6): 816, 2002.

Pahernik, S, et al: Nephron sparing surgery for renal cell carcinoma with normal contralateral kidney: 25 years of experience. J Urol, 175: 2027, 2006.

Piper NY, et al: Is a 1 cm margin necessary during nephron sparing surgery for renal cell carcinoma? Urology, 58(6): 849, 2001.

Sutherland SE, et al: Does the size of the surgical margin in partial nephrectomy for renal cell cancer really matter? J Urol, 167: 61, 2002.

Timsit MO, et al: Prospective study of safety margins in partial nephrectomy. Urology, 67(5): 923, 2006.

Uzzo RG, Novick AC: Nephron sparing surgery for renal tumors: indications, techniques, and outcomes. J Urol, 166: 6, 2001.

van Ophoven A, Tsui KH, Shvarts O, et al: Current status of partial nephrectomy in the management of kidney cancer. Cancer Control, 6: 560, 1999.

Renal Vein and Vena Caval Invasion

Glazer AA, Novick AC: Long-term follow up after surgical treatment for renal cell carcinoma extending into the right atrium. J Urol, 155: 448, 1996.

Hatcher PA, Anderson EE, et al: Surgical management and prognosis of renal cell carcinoma invading the vena cava. J Urol, 145: 20, 1991.

Libertino JA, Zinman L, Watkins, E: Long-term results of resection of renal cell carcinoma with extension into inferior vena cava. J Urol, 137: 21, 1987.

Nesbitt JC, Soltero ER, et al: Surgical management of renal cell carcinoma with inferior vena cava tumor thrombus. Ann Thorac Surg, 63: 1592, 1997.

Polascik TJ, et al: Frequent occurrence of metastatic disease in patients with renal cell carcinoma and intrahepatic or supradiaphragmatic intracaval extension treated with surgery: an outcome analysis. Urology, 52: 995, 1998.

Skinner DG, Pritchett TR, Lieskovsky G, et al: Vena caval involvement by renal cell carcinoma. Ann Surg, 210: 387, 1989.

Suggs WD, Smith RB III, Dodson TF, et al: Renal cell carcinoma with inferior vena cava involvement. J Vasc Surg, 14: 413, 1991.

Swierzewski DJ, et al: Radical nephrectomy in patients with renal cell carcinoma with venous, vena caval and atrial extension. Am J Surg, 168: 205, 1994.

Tongaonkar HB, Dandekar NP, Dalal AV, et al: Renal cell carcinoma extending to the renal vein and inferior vena cava: results of surgical treatment and prognostic factors. J Surg Oncol, 59: 94, 1995.

Wieder JA, et al: Renal cell carcinoma with tumor thrombus extension into the pulmonary artery. J Urol, 169: 2296, 2003.

Zisman A, Wieder JA, et al: Renal cell carcinoma with tumor thrombus extension: biology, role of nephrectomy and response to immunotherapy. J Urol, 169: 909, 2003.

Metastatic Renal Cell Carcinoma - Nephrectomy Before Immunotherapy

Flanigan RC, Salmon SE, Blumenstein BA, et al: Nephrectomy followed by interferon alfa-2b compared with interferon alfa-2b alone for metastatic renal-cell carcinoma. N Engl J Med 345: 1655, 2001.

Mickisch GH, Garin A, van Poppel H, et al: Radical nephrectomy plus interferon-alfa-based immunotherapy compared with interferon alfa alone in metastatic renal-cell carcinoma: a randomized trial. Lancet 358: 966, 2001.

Pantuck AJ, Zisman A, Belldegrun AS: The changing history of renal cell carcinoma. J Urol 166: 1611, 2001.

Metastatic Renal Cell Carcinoma - General

Dineen MK, Patore RD, Emrich LJ, et al: Results of surgical treatment of renal cell carcinoma with solitary metastasis. J Urol, 140: 277, 1988.

Durr HR, Maier M, Pfahler M, et al: Surgical treatment of osseous metastasis in patients with renal cell carcinoma. Clin Orthop, 367: 283, 1999.

Escudier B, et al: Sorafenib in advanced clear cell renal cell carcinoma. N Engl J Med, 356(2) 185, 2007.

Friedel G, Hurtgen M, Penzenstadler M, et al: Resection of pulmonary metastasis from renal cell carcinoma. Anticancer Res, 19: 1593, 1999.

Giehl JP, Kluba T: Metastatic spine disease in renal cell carcinoma - indication and results of surgery. Anticancer Res, 19: 1619, 1999.

Hudes G, et al: Temsirolimus, interferon alfa, or both for advanced renal cell carcinoma. N Engl J Med, 356(22): 2271, 2007.

Middleton R: Surgery for metastatic renal cell carcinoma. J Urol, 97: 973, 1967.

Motzer RJ, et al: Sunitinib in patients with metastatic renal cell carcinoma. JAMA, 295(21): 2516, 2006.

O'Dea MJ, Zincke H, Utz DC, et al: The treatment of renal cell carcinoma with solitary metastasis. J Urol, 120: 540, 1978.

Tolia BM and Whitmore Jr. WF: Solitary metastasis from renal cell carcinoma. J Urol, 114: 836, 1975.

WILMS' TUMOR & OTHER PEDIATRIC RENAL TUMORS

Wilms' Tumor

Presentation

1. *Wilms' tumor is the most common primary malignant renal tumor in children.*
2. Mean age of presentation is 3.5-4.0 years old. Bilateral cases usually present earlier at a mean age of 2.5 years old. Bilateral tumor occurs in approximately 5% of patients.
3. The most common presenting symptom is an *abdominal mass*. Hypertension occurs in up to 65%. Microscopic hematuria may be seen, but gross hematuria is rare.
4. Physical examination often reveals a large, smooth, firm flank mass that *rarely crosses the midline*.
5. Congenital anomalies occur with 15% of Wilms' tumors.
   a. Genitourinary anomalies (5% of cases)—including renal anomalies (ectopia, fusion, hypoplasia), ureteral duplications, hypospadias, cryptorchidism, and ambiguous genitalia.
   b. Hemihypertrophy (3% of cases)—may be ipsilateral or contralateral to the tumor. Isolated hemihypertrophy (i.e. not accompanied by other congenital abnormalities) is associated with chromosome 11p disorders.
   c. Aniridia (1% of cases)—abnormal development of the iris of the eye. Isolated aniridia is associated with chromosome 11p disorders. Up to 33% of patients with aniridia develop Wilms' tumor.
6. Gross renal vein invasion may occur in up to 20% of cases.

Etiology

1. Wilms' tumor is thought to arise from an abnormal proliferation of metanephric blastema. It may arise from nephrogenic rests and nephroblastomatosis.
2. Premalignant lesions
   a. Nephrogenic rest—a focus of abnormally persistent nephrogenic cells. Microscopically, Wilms' tumor and nephrogenic rests are indistinguishable. The only way to differentiate them is by following their clinical course. Most nephrogenic rests do *not* develop into Wilms' tumor. Nevertheless, patients with nephrogenic rests must be followed closely.
   b. Nephroblastomatosis—diffuse or multi-focal nephrogenic rests.
3. Wilms' tumor genes (WT)
   a. WT1—tumor suppressor gene on chromosome 11p13. Inactivation of WT1 results in Wilms' tumor.
   b. WT2—on chromosome 11p15. Inactivation of WT2 results in Wilms' tumor.
   c. 16q—Loss of heterozygosity at this site results in Wilms' tumor.

Metastasis

Location of metastasis (from most to least common):
   1. Pulmonary
   2. Hepatic
   3. Other sites: include bone and rarely brain

Disease Associations

1. WAGR syndrome (*W*ilms' tumor, *A*niridia, *G*enitourinary abnormalities, mental *R*etardation)—associated with WT1. Up to 30% develop Wilms' tumor.
2. Denys-Drash syndrome (Wilms' tumor, ambiguous genitalia, glomerulopathy)—associated with WT1.
3. Beckwith-Wiedemann syndrome (multiple growth abnormalities which may include visceromegaly, gigantism, hemihypertrophy, omphalocele, and macroglossia)—associated with WT2. Up to 5% with this syndrome develop Wilms' tumor.
4. Mixed gonadal dysgenesis
5. Trisomy 18
6. Perlman syndrome
7. Congenital syndromes such as aniridia (see Presentation, page 21)

Bilateral Wilms' Tumor

1. Approximately 5% of patients present with bilateral tumors.
2. Bilateral cases usually present earlier (at a mean age of 2.5 years) than unilateral Wilms' tumor.
3. *Nephrogenic rests are always present in bilateral Wilms' tumor.* Thus, the presence of nephrogenic rests should raise the suspicion of bilateral Wilms' tumor.
4. Bilateral tumors are generally treated with preoperative chemotherapy followed by renal sparing surgery.
5. Patients with a unilateral Wilms' tumor and nephrogenic rests or nephroblastomatosis may be at higher risk for metachronous Wilms' tumor in the contralateral kidney. Therefore, these patients are followed more frequently regardless of histology and stage.

Work Up

1. History and physical (including search for aniridia, hemihypertrophy, hypospadias, cryptorchidism, etc.)
2. Blood pressure measurement
3. CBC with platelets, BUN, serum creatinine, liver function tests, serum calcium, and urinalysis. Obtain urinary catecholamines if neuroblastoma is suspected.
4. Abdominal ultrasound is often the initial imaging study. It can visualize the liver as well as tumor thrombus in the vena cava. Wilms' tumor usually has a heterogeneous echo texture. CT scan may be obtained if a solid renal mass is suspected based on ultrasound.
5. Chest x-ray to look for pulmonary metastasis.
6. Bone scan if the patient has bone pain, elevated alkaline phosphatase, or elevated serum calcium.

Initial Exploratory Surgery

1. After a complete work up, the initial therapy for a suspected Wilms' tumor is usually surgical exploration. However, preoperative chemotherapy is indicated in certain circumstances (see #8 below).
2. In general, a transverse supra-umbilical abdominal incision is made.
3. Peritoneal exploration is performed to rule out metastasis. Biopsies should be taken of suspicious lesions and resectability is determined. If the tumor is unresectable, close and administer chemotherapy.
4. Palpate the renal vein for tumor thrombus.

5. When the preoperative CT or MRI shows a normal contralateral kidney, exploration of the contralateral kidney is unnecessary. When preoperative imaging shows an abnormal contralateral kidney, the *entire* surface of the contralateral kidney is exposed and inspected. Biopsy any suspicious lesions (a cleft or discoloration suggests a nephrogenic rest). If the contralateral kidney was abnormal on preoperative imaging but appears grossly normal, intraoperative ultrasound may localize lesions for biopsy. After inspection of the contralateral kidney, close Gerota's fascia. If bilateral Wilms' tumor is present, close the patient and treat accordingly.

6. Inspect the retroperitoneal lymph nodes. Biopsy abnormal nodes and obtain random node biopsies. Regional lymph node dissection does not improve survival but may provide prognostic information.

7. If the tumor is unilateral, perform a nephrectomy (and tumor thrombectomy if indicated). Resect the adrenal gland if it is grossly involved, the tumor is in the upper pole of the kidney, or the adrenal is adherent to the kidney.

8. Preoperative chemotherapy has not improved survival, but may reduce the morbidity of surgery by shrinking the tumor. It is administered when the mass has any of the following characteristics:
   a. Unresectable at initial presentation
   b. Bilateral renal involvement
   c. Extensive intracaval involvement

Stage

I   Tumor limited to the kidney and completely excised (margins negative and no tumor spillage either before or during tumor removal)

II   Tumor beyond the kidney (into perinephric tissues and/or into the renal vein or vena cava) but completely excised (margins negative and tumor thrombus completely removed) or tumor completely excised with local tumor spillage confined to flank.

III   Residual non-hematogenous tumor confined to abdomen (positive abdominal lymph nodes, peritoneal invasion, peritoneal implants, tumor spillage beyond flank either before or during tumor removal, positive margins, or incomplete resection)

IV   Hematogenous metastasis

V   Bilateral tumor at diagnosis (an attempt should be made to stage each side by the above criteria before biopsy)

Pathology and Histology

1. Gross features—fleshy tan tumor with a pseudocapsule. Cysts may be present.

2. Microscopic features—three tissue elements must be present: *stroma, epithelial cells,* and *blastema.*

3. Histology—favorable histology is most common.
   a. Unfavorable (anaplastic) histology (5% of cases)—nuclear enlargement (≥ 3 fold larger than adjacent cells), nuclear hyperchromasia, and abnormal mitoses. This histology is rare when Wilms' is diagnosed at < 2 years of age. *Unfavorable histology has a worse prognosis.* Clear cell sarcoma and rhabdoid tumor are no longer classified as unfavorable histology Wilms' tumor. They are classified as non-Wilms' tumors.
   b. Favorable histology (95% of cases)—no characteristics of unfavorable histology.

Treatment

Treatment After Removal of Wilms' Tumor (based on NWTS V)

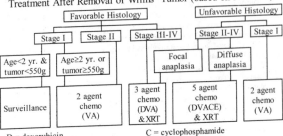

D = doxorubicin
V = vincristine
A = actinomycin D (dactinomycin)
C = cyclophosphamide
E = etoposide
XRT = external beam radiation therapy
NTWS V = National Wilms' Tumor Study 5

Survival

Tumor	Stage & Histology	4-Year Relapse-Free Survival*	4-Year Overall Survival*
Wilms'	I FH	90%	97%
Wilms'	II FH	88%	92%
Wilms'	III FH	79%	87%
Wilms'	IV FH	75%	83%
Wilms'	V	-	56-87%**
Wilms'	I-IV UH	60%	62%
Clear cell sarcoma	Any	65%	75%
Rhabdoid sarcoma	Any	25%	26%

FH = favorable histology; UH = unfavorable histology
* Data is from National Wilms' Tumor Study 3 (Cancer, 64: 349, 1989)
** Survival is better in those with negative lymph nodes, favorable histology, younger age, and lower tumor stage of each kidney. This data is from selected studies, not from NWTS 3.

Follow Up

1. Initially, obtain follow up tests at least every 3 months.
   a. History and physical (especially abdominal exam).
   b. Serum BUN, creatinine, liver function tests, and urinalysis.
   c. Abdominal ultrasound—every 3 months for any stage with unfavorable histology, stage III-IV with favorable histology, and any stage with nephrogenic rests. Favorable histology stage I-II without nephrogenic rests may be imaged less often.
   d. Chest x-ray—every 3 months.
2. Patients with a unilateral Wilms' tumor with nephrogenic rests or nephroblastomatosis may be at higher risk for metachronous Wilms' tumor in the contralateral kidney. Therefore, these patients are followed more frequently regardless of histology and stage.
3. If metastases were present, the metastatic locations should be monitored with routine imaging.
4. In patients receiving radiation to bones, imaging studies of these areas should be conducted at least each year until bone growth is complete, and then at least every 5 years thereafter. Secondary malignancies (such as osteosarcomas) have been reported after radiation for Wilms' tumor.

5. Side effects of doxorubicin include a 4-17% long-term risk of congestive heart failure. Consider monitoring the patient for heart disease.
6. Most recurrences occur within 2 years of diagnosis. Therefore, follow up should be intensive during this interval and may be less frequent thereafter.
7. Patients with a solitary kidney should be advised that participation in contact/collision sports places the kidney at risk for traumatic injury. Need to avoid contact/collision sports is determined on an individual basis.

Relapse

1. *The most common site of relapse is pulmonary.*
2. Relapses usually occur within 2 years of diagnosis.
3. Treatment of relapse often consists of a combination of surgery, radiation, and chemotherapy. Patients that have not had doxorubicin (i.e. patients who have not had chemotherapy or who have had chemotherapy without doxorubicin) are given doxorubicin based chemotherapy. There is no consensus regarding a chemotherapy regimen for patients that relapse after receiving doxorubicin.
4. Factors that increase the risk of relapse
   a. Age > 2 years
   b. Higher stage
   c. Unfavorable histology—*histology is the most important prognostic factor.*
   d. Lymph node metastasis
   e. Hematogenous metastasis
5. No apparent influence on survival
   a. Level of caval involvement
   b. Lymph node dissection
6. Factors that increase local recurrence
   a. Unfavorable histology
   b. Tumor spill
   c. Positive surgical margins
   d. Incomplete tumor resection
   e. Lymph node metastasis

Other Malignant Pediatric Renal Tumors

Relative Frequency of Malignant Pediatric Renal Tumors

Wilms' Favorable Histology	89%
Wilms' Unfavorable Histology	5%
Rhabdoid Tumor	4%
Clear Cell Sarcoma	2%

Clear Cell Sarcoma of the Kidney

1. This tumor is *not* classified as a Wilms' tumor. It is a sarcoma.
2. Mean age of diagnosis = 3-4 years of age
3. This tumor been called the "bone-metastasizing renal tumor of childhood" because *bone is the most common metastatic location and bone metastases occur frequently.* 50% of patients present with bone metastases. If this tumor is discovered, a bone scan must be performed.
4. This tumor has a worse prognosis than Wilms' tumor.
5. Treatment—nephrectomy followed by chemotherapy and external beam radiation. In NWTS 5, these patients (regardless of pathologic stage) are treated the same as stage II-IV Wilms' tumor with unfavorable histology and diffuse anaplasia (5 agent chemotherapy and radiation).
6. The 4-year relapse-free and overall survival with treatment is 65% and 75%, respectively (see Survival table, page 24).

Rhabdoid Tumor of the Kidney
1. This tumor is *not* classified as a Wilms' tumor. It is a sarcoma.
2. Mean age of diagnosis is 13 months.
3. *The most common metastatic site is the brain.* All patients that have this tumor should undergo a brain CT or MRI.
4. This tumor has the *worst prognosis of all childhood renal masses.*
5. Treatment is nephrectomy followed by chemotherapy and external beam radiation. In NWTS 5, the chemotherapy regimen consists of carboplatin, etoposide, and cyclophosphamide.
6. The 4-year relapse-free and overall survival with treatment is 25% and 26%, respectively (see Survival table, page 24).

Benign Pediatric Renal Tumors

Multilocular Cystic Nephroma
1. A benign cystic renal mass.
2. Presentation
   a. It is virtually always *unilateral.*
   b. Incidence is highest in two populations
      i. Male child (usually age <2)—presents with painless abdominal mass.
      ii. Female adult (usually age >40)—presents with pain or hematuria.
3. Pathology
   a. Gross—well-circumscribed non-calcified mass with fibrous capsule surrounding non-communicating cysts.
   b. Microscopic—cysts separated by fibrous septa.
4. Imaging—imaging cannot differentiate between multilocular cystic nephroma and malignant cystic masses (e.g. cystic Wilms'). Renal scan usually shows that the *kidney functions.*
5. Treatment—nephrectomy is curative. If nephron sparing surgery is performed, consider intraoperative frozen sections to rule out malignancy.

Mesoblastic Nephroma
1. The *most common renal tumor in the newborn* (i.e. the most common congenital renal tumor). It is benign, but may be locally invasive. Metastases are rare and are usually associated with the cellular variant.
2. Presentation
   a. Mean age of presentation = 3.5 months. It is uncommon after the age of 6 months. It is more common in males.
   b. Usually discovered as a unilateral abdominal mass.
   c. It is associated with *polyhydramnios* in utero.
   d. 14% of patients have associated congenital anomalies.
3. Pathology
   a. Gross—*resembles a leiomyoma* (firm, rubbery, light colored).
      i. It interdigitates with surrounding kidney.
      ii. There is no capsule and calcifications are absent.
      iii. These tumors may be friable and *prone to rupture.*
   b. Microscopic—*spindle cells that infiltrate the renal parenchyma.*
      i. Classic variant—rare mitotic figures.
      ii. Cellular variant—densely cellular mass with many mitotic figures.
4. Imaging—imaging studies cannot reliably differentiate this mass from other solid renal masses.
5. Treatment—nephrectomy with wide local excision is usually curative. Complete resection and avoiding tumor spillage are imperative to prevent local recurrence. Patients diagnosed at < 3 months of age may have a lower recurrence rate. Although local recurrence is uncommon, it does occur; therefore, surveillance after nephrectomy is recommended.

Multicystic Dysplastic Kidney (MCDK)

1. MCDK is a congenital benign cystic dysplasia of the kidney.
2. Presentation
   a. Usually presents as a childhood abdominal mass or is found incidentally on prenatal ultrasound.
   b. MCDK is associated with contralateral vesicoureteral reflex (VUR) in 20-40% of cases and contralateral ureteropelvic junction (UPJ) obstruction in 3-12% of cases. *VUR is the most common defect associated with MCDK; therefore, patients with MCDK should undergo voiding cystourethrogram.*
3. Gross appearance—cysts with minimal renal parenchyma ("bunch of grapes" appearance). *The ureter is usually atretic.*
4. Histologic appearance—primitive tubules that are not organized into nephrons (disorganized architecture). *Ectopic cartilage is often present.*
5. Imaging
   a. Ultrasound shows non-communicating cysts and minimal parenchyma (small communications may exist, but they are not visible on ultrasound), whereas hydronephrosis usually shows fluid filled areas that have visible communications.
   b. Renal scan usually reveals *no kidney function*, whereas other cystic lesions will usually show renal function
6. Sometimes MCDK may involute into a "nubbin" or disappear completely.
7. Hypertension can develop in up to 8% of patients with MCDK.
8. Treatment
   a. Patients with UPJ obstruction and VUR should be treated accordingly.
   b. Patients with MCDK should be observed with yearly blood pressure measurement. A repeat renal ultrasound can be performed at age 1 year (and perhaps another ultrasound around age 6).
   c. If the kidney enlarges or becomes symptomatic (e.g. the patient develops hypertension), nephrectomy should be performed.

Differentiating Cystic Renal Masses

Cystic Mass	Grossly Visible Communication Between Fluid Spaces	Functioning Kidney on Renal Scan
MCDK	No	No
CMN	No	Yes
Cystic Wilms'	No	Yes
Hydronephrosis	Yes	Sometimes

MCDK = multicystic dysplastic kidney
CMN = congenital mesoblastic nephroma

Survival Pediatric Renal Tumors

Tumor	2-Year Relapse-Free Survival (all stages combined)
Multilocular cystic nephroma	100%
Mesoblastic nephroma	98%
Wilms' tumor FH	84%
Clear cell sarcoma	75%
Wilms' tumor UH	63%
Rhabdoid sarcoma	25%

FH = favorable histology; UH = unfavorable histology

REFERENCES

Argani P, Perlman EJ, Breslow NE, et al: Clear cell sarcoma of the kidney. Am J Surg Pathol, 24: 4, 2000.

Clericuzio CL, Johnson C: Screening for Wilms' tumor in high-risk individuals. Hematol Oncol Clin North Am, 9: 1253, 1995.

D'Angio GJ, Breslow N, Beckwith JB, et al: Treatment of Wilms' tumor - results of the Third National Wilms' Tumor Society. Cancer, 64: 349, 1989.

Green DM, D'Angio GJ, et al: Wilms' tumor. CA Cancer J Clin, 46: 46, 1996.

Howell CG, Othersen HB, Kiviat NE, et al: Therapy and outcome in 51 children with mesoblastic nephroma: a report of the National Wilms' Tumor Study. J Pediatr Surg, 17: 826, 1982.

Kirsch AJ, Snyder III HM: What's new and important in pediatric urologic oncology. AUA Update Series, Vol. 17, Lesson 11, 1998.

Metzger ML, Dome JS: Current therapy for Wilms' tumor. The Oncologist, 10: 815, 2005.

Peters CA, Badwan K: The multicystic dysplastic kidney. AUA Update Series, Vol. 24, Lesson 37, 2005.

Ross JH: Wilms' tumor: updated strategies for evaluation and management. Contemporary Urology, 18(11): 18, 2006.

Shamberger RC, et al: Surgery-related factors and local recurrence of Wilms' tumor in National Wilms' Tumor Study 4. Ann Surg, 229: 292, 1999.

Snyder III HM, D'Angio GJ, Evans AE, et al: Pediatric Oncology. Campbell's Urology. 7th Edition. Ed. PC Walsh, AB Retik, ED Vaughan Jr., et al. Philadelphia: W. B. Sanders Company, 1998, pp 2210-2256.

Wilimas JA, Greenwald CA, Rao BN: Wilms' tumor. Genitourinary Oncology. 2nd Edition. Ed. NJ Vogelzang, PT Scardino, WU Shipley, et al. Philadelphia: Lippincott Williams and Wilkins, 2000, pp 65-72.

BLADDER TUMORS

General Information
1. Bladder is the most common site of cancer in the urinary system.
2. Bladder cancer is the fourth leading cause of cancer death in males (lung, prostate, colon, bladder).
3. Most patients with bladder cancer die from other causes.
4. Urothelial carcinoma (UC) is the most common histology of bladder cancer in the United States.

Epidemiology
1. Bladder cancer is more common in males.
2. The average age of diagnosis is 65. Approximately 80% of cases are diagnosed after the age of 50, but bladder cancer can occur at any age.

Types of Bladder Cancer
1. Primary tumors
   a. Urothelial carcinoma (UC)— more than 90% of cases in the U.S.
   b. Non-urothelial cancers
      i. Squamous cell carcinoma (SCC)—5% of cases in the U.S.
      ii. Adenocarcinoma—2% of cases in the U.S.
      iii. Other—small cell carcinoma, rhabdomyosarcoma (most commonly seen in children), bladder pheochromocytoma, bladder lymphoma.
2. Secondary (metastatic to bladder)—from most to least common: melanoma, colon, prostate, lung, breast.

Etiology
1. Smoking—*smoking is the most common cause of bladder cancer.* Smoking increases the risk of bladder cancer 2 to 4 fold. The risk increases with higher frequency and longer duration of smoking. Smoking cessation slowly reduces the risk, which returns to baseline 20-30 years later.
2. Chronic cystitis—associated with an increased risk of SCC.
   a. Chronic urinary tract infection.
   b. Indwelling bladder catheter—SCC is the most common type of bladder cancer in patients with long-term indwelling catheters.
   c. Schistosoma haematobium (bilharzial) infection.
   d. Chronic bladder stones
3. Chemical exposure—*most bladder carcinogens are aromatic amines.* Exposure to dye (especially aniline dye) may increase the risk of bladder cancer. Occupations with an increased risk for bladder cancer include

Textile workers	Dye workers	Drill press operators
Tire/rubber workers	Leather workers	Petroleum workers
Bootblacks	Painters	Dry cleaners
Truck drivers	Hairdressers (hair dye)	Chemical workers

4. Phenacetin—an analgesic with a chemical structure similar to aniline dyes. Phenacetin has been removed from the market.
5. Cyclophosphamide—acrolein, a urinary metabolite of cyclophosphamide, causes hemorrhagic cystitis and an increased risk of bladder cancer. The latency period for acrolein induced bladder cancer is 6-13 years. *Mesna, which binds to acrolein in the urine, is often administered with cyclophosphamide to reduce the risk of hemorrhagic cystitis. Mesna may also reduce the risk of bladder cancer.*
6. Radiation (bladder exposure)

Presentation/Symptoms
1. Painless hematuria (microscopic or gross)—occurs in 80%.
2. Irritative symptoms (e.g. frequency, urgency, dysuria)—usually associated with invasive or higher grade tumors (including CIS).
3. Other symptoms
   a. Flank pain from ureteral obstruction or retroperitoneal metastasis.
   b. Bone pain from metastasis
   c. Pelvic mass

Work Up
1. History and physical exam
2. Cystoscopy with biopsy
3. Bimanual examination
4. Urine cytology
5. Intravenous pyelogram (IVP), CT urogram, or retrograde pyelograms.
6. Metastatic work up—usually reserved for patients who have a significant risk of metastases.
   a. Abdominal/pelvic CT scan
   b. Liver function tests
   c. Chest x-ray
   d. Bone scan—recommended in patients with bone pain, elevated calcium, or elevated alkaline phosphatase.

Diagnosis

Transurethral Resection of Bladder Tumors (TURBT)
1. Perform bimanual exam before *and* after TURBT. Include a prostate exam in males. *Clinical stage is based on the bimanual exam after TURBT.*
2. If surgically feasible and if the patient's medical condition permits, all visible tumor should be completely eradicated, except when
   a. Extensive CIS is present—extensive resection or fulguration may cause a contracted bladder. CIS may be treated with intravesical therapy.
   b. The tumor appears to be unresectable by the transurethral approach.
3. TURBT completely excises invasive bladder tumors in approximately 10% of cases (based on the fact that 10% of cystectomy specimens are pT0 when pre-cystectomy TURBT revealed invasive bladder cancer).
4. Obturator reflex—resection of tumors on the lateral wall can stimulate the obturator nerve, resulting in a sudden adduction of the leg. This abrupt movement can force the resectoscope into the bladder wall and cause bladder perforation. Methods to avoid the obturator reflex include
   a. General anesthesia with neuromuscular blockade—the obturator nerve can still be stimulated, but the impulse is not transmitted to the muscles.
   b. Avoid bladder over-distention—bladder over-distension may move the bladder wall closer to the obturator nerve.
   c. Lower the resection current.
   d. Obturator nerve block with local anesthesia.
5. *Bladder perforation should be avoided because it increases the risk of bleeding, urinary tract infection, sepsis, and death from bladder cancer.* Methods to decrease the risk of bladder perforation include
   a. Use caution when resecting tumors in a diverticulum—the diverticulum lacks muscularis propria and is thinner than the normal bladder.
   b. Avoid the obturator reflex.
   c. Avoid bladder over-distention—over-distention can thin the bladder wall and can increase intravesical pressure.
   d. Avoid deep resection of tumors that appear low grade and superficial.

6. Tumors at the ureteral orifice
   a. *Extensive cauterization of the ureteral orifice should be avoided because it causes distal ureteral stenosis. When only cutting current is used to resect the ureteral orifice, stenosis is unlikely.* When bleeding at the resection site is encountered, a minimal amount of focal "pin-point" low current coagulation may be used.
   b. After resection of the ureteral orifice, placing a temporary ureteral stent may maintain drainage while it is indwelling, but it is unclear if it reduces the long-term risk of stenosis compared to not placing a stent. Consider placing a temporary stent in patients with a solitary kidney or poor renal function.
   c. Perform a urogram or renal scan 3-6 weeks after resection of the ureteral orifice to check for ureteral obstruction.
   d. Resection of the ureteral orifice can cause vesicoureteral reflux (VUR). VUR increases the risk of upper tract UC by 15 to 22 fold. Therefore, surveillance of the upper tracts should be performed more frequently in patients with VUR and a history of bladder cancer.
7. *A repeat TURBT 1-4 weeks later should be performed in patients with high grade Ta or any grade T1 tumor* because the second TURBT finds residual tumor in at least 25% of cases and upstages at least 30% of cases (especially when muscularis propria was absent in the initial TURBT specimen). Up to 50% of "pT1" bladder tumors without muscularis propria in the specimen are upstaged to pT2 after a repeat TURBT.
8. Treatment beyond transurethral resection should not be instituted unless there is a histologic diagnosis of bladder cancer.

Prostatic Urethra Biopsies
1. Routine prostatic urethra biopsies are not recommended.
2. Prostatic urethra biopsies are indicated in any of these circumstances:
   a. Multifocal UC of the bladder.
   b. CIS of the bladder.
   c. A visible abnormality suspicious for tumor in the prostatic urethra.
3. Prostatic urethra biopsies should include
   a. Electrocautery loop resection at 5 and 7 o'clock just cephalad to the verumontanum. The diagnostic yield is lower when biopsies are taken from other areas of the prostatic urethra or when obtaining cold cup biopsies.
   b. Resection of visible tumors.

Random Bladder Biopsies
1. Routine random bladder biopsies are not recommended.
2. Random bladder biopsies are indicated in any of these circumstances:
   a. Partial cystectomy is planned.
   b. Abnormal tumor marker without visible tumor in the bladder. See Positive Tumor Marker Without Visible Tumor In the Bladder, page 48.
   c. High grade cells are seen on urine cytology, but TURBT reveals only low grade tumor.
   d. After intravesical therapy to evaluate for complete response.

Grade
Higher grade lesions progress more often, recur more often, and have a worse prognosis. Grade may accompany the stage designation and is abbreviated as "G". For example, T1G2 is tumor stage T1 and grade 2.

Grade 1	Well differentiated
Grade 2	Moderately differentiated
Grade 3-4	Poorly differentiated or undifferentiated

Stage (AJCC 2002)

This TNM classification refers to both clinical and pathological staging. Bimanual exam under anesthesia should be performed before and after transurethral resection/biopsy. Bimanual exam *after* transurethral resection is used to determine clinical stage. Higher stage lesions progress more often, recur more often, and have a worse prognosis.

Primary Tumor (T)

Tx	Primary tumor cannot be assessed
T0	No evidence of primary tumor
Ta	Noninvasive papillary carcinoma
Tis	Carcinoma in situ: "flat tumor"
T1*	Tumor invades subepithelial connective tissue
T2	Tumor invades muscle (muscularis propria)
T2a	Tumor invades superficial muscle (inner half)
T2b	Tumor invades deep muscle (outer half)
T3	Tumor invades perivesical tissue
T3a	Microscopically
T3b	Macroscopically (extravesical mass)
T4	Tumor invades any of the following: prostate, uterus, vagina, pelvic wall, abdominal wall
T4a	Tumor invades prostate, uterus, vagina
T4b	Tumor invades pelvic wall, abdominal wall

Regional Lymph Nodes (N)

Laterality does not affect the N classification. Regional lymph nodes are nodes in the true pelvis; all others are distant lymph nodes.

Nx	Regional lymph nodes cannot be assessed
N0	No regional lymph node metastasis
N1	Metastasis in a single lymph node, 2 cm or less in greatest dimension
N2	Metastasis in a single lymph node, more than 2 cm but not more than 5 cm in greatest dimension; or multiple lymph nodes, none more than 5 cm in greatest dimension
N3	Metastasis in a lymph node more than 5 cm in greatest dimension

Distant Metastasis (M)

Mx	Distant metastasis cannot be assessed
M0	No distant metastasis
M1	Distant metastasis

Used with the permission of the American Joint Committee on Cancer (AJCC), Chicago, Illinois. The original source for this material is the *AJCC Cancer Staging Manual, Sixth Edition* (2002) published by Springer Science and Business Media LLC, www.springerlink.com.

* Several studies suggest that a greater depth of invasion with T1 UC results in a higher progression rate. Subclassification of T1 tumors is currently not recommended, but noting the depth of invasion may provide useful prognostic information.

p53 Mutation

1. *p53*, a gene on chromosome 17, encodes a protein that halts the cell cycle in the G1 phase. The gene is designated in italics (*p53=gene*), whereas the protein encoded by this gene is designated in plain text (p53=protein).
2. Normal (also called wild type) p53 halts the cell cycle in the G1 phase, which creates time to repair damaged DNA. Mutant p53 cannot halt the cell cycle; therefore, replication occurs even in the presence of damaged DNA, which may ultimately lead to cancer.
3. Normal p53 is essentially undetectable by standard immunohistochemical stains because it has a short half-life. Most *p53* mutations are missense mutations (i.e. the amino acid sequence of its protein is changed). These mutations increase the protein's half-life. Mutant p53 accumulates in the cell because of its longer half-life, allowing its detection by special stains.
4. For clinical purposes, p53 overexpression is often defined as positive p53 staining in > 20% of cancer cells. Patients with p53 overexpression are *more likely to progress* and are *less likely to respond to chemotherapy.*
5. Since p53 overexpression is associated with a higher rate of progression, it may help guide treatment recommendations (although its use is still considered experimental). For example:
   a. In pT1G3 UC with p53 overexpression, cystectomy may be considered over intravesical therapy.
   b. After cystectomy for bladder UC with p53 overexpression, adjuvant therapy may be considered.

Non-Urothelial Cancer of the Bladder

Squamous Cell Carcinoma (SCC) of Bladder

1. SCC is associated with chronic inflammation and cigarette smoking.
2. SCC often presents at a higher stage than UC.
3. SCC is more common in Egypt than the U.S. because of a higher incidence of Bilharzial (Schistosoma haematobium) infections.
4. SCC has a worse prognosis than UC, except Bilharzial SCC, which is usually well differentiated and has a low incidence of metastasis. The average age of diagnosis is 45-55 for Bilharzial bladder SCC and 65 for UC.
5. SCC is less responsive to chemotherapy and radiation than UC.
6. Intravesical therapy is generally not effective.
7. Treatment–radical cystectomy, pelvic lymphadenectomy, ± urethrectomy.

Adenocarcinoma of Bladder

1. Classification of bladder adenocarcinoma
   a. Primary—arises from the bladder.
   b. Urachal—arises from the urachus (see Urachal Tumors, pages 34).
   c. Metastatic—adenocarcinoma that has metastasized to bladder.
2. Patients must be evaluated for a site of origin other than the bladder (e.g. colon, stomach, breast, prostate, lung, endometrium, and ovary).
3. Adenocarcinoma is the most common tumor in exstrophic bladders.
4. Adenocarcinoma usually presents at a higher stage than UC and may elevate serum carcinoembryonic antigen (CEA).
5. Adenocarcinoma has a worse prognosis than UC.
6. It is less responsive to chemotherapy and radiation than UC.
7. Intravesical therapy is generally not effective.
8. Treatment—radical cystectomy (with en block removal of the urachus), pelvic lymphadenectomy, ± urethrectomy. Urachal adenocarcinoma may be treated differently.

Urachal Tumors

1. Gross hematuria is the most common presenting symptom. Mucin is seen in the urine of only 15-33% of patients.
2. Pathology—adenocarcinoma is the most common type of urachal tumor. These tumors are usually high grade and cystic.
3. Patients with urachal adenocarcinoma may have an elevated serum CEA.
4. Most cases involve the lower third of the urachus and extend through the bladder wall. *Tumors usually occur at the bladder dome*, but may also occur on the anterior bladder wall.
5. Chemotherapy and radiation are *not* effective for urachal adenocarcinoma.
6. Treatment—wide local excision (partial or radical cystectomy) with en block removal of the urachus and umbilicus, pelvic lymphadenectomy.
7. Mean 5-year cancer free survival is 55% (range 33-88%).
8. After excision, local recurrence occurs in 20-50% of patients.

Urothelial Carcinoma (UC) of Bladder

General Information

1. Urothelial carcinoma was previously called transitional cell carcinoma.
2. At presentation, 75% of UC are low grade and stage Ta or T1.
3. In patients with muscle invasive UC, 60% have muscle invasive tumors at initial presentation, while 40% have progressed from non-invasive tumors.
4. The majority of patients develop recurrences after endoscopic resection.
5. Higher tumor grade and stage increases recurrence and progression.

Metastasis From Bladder

1. Sites of bladder cancer metastasis (from most to least common):
   pelvic lymph nodes, liver, lung, bone, adrenal gland.
2. Most patients with metastatic UC die within 2 years.

Nephrogenic Adenoma

1. Nephrogenic adenoma is a rare benign lesion. It is a metaplastic urothelial response to trauma, inflammation, or radiation.
2. Histologically it has a *single layer of cuboidal epithelium* (which resembles primitive renal collecting tubules) with few mitosis and minimal nuclear atypia. The classic microscopic finding is *hobnail* epithelial cells.
3. It is often associated with dysuria and urinary frequency.
4. Treatment—transurethral resection and long-term antibiotics (antifungus medications may also be used when indicated).

Carcinoma In Situ (CIS)

1. *CIS is a urothelial cancer that is flat, high grade, and non-invasive.*
2. CIS often appears as a velvety patch of erythematous urothelium, but may look like normal urothelium.
3. CIS is more common in patients with multiple or high grade tumors.
4. *CIS often produces irritative voiding symptoms.*
5. *Urine cytology is positive in approximately 95% of patients with CIS* because of the poor cohesiveness of the cells.
6. CIS has a propensity for recurrence and progression.
   a. Progression occurs in 20% after a complete response to BCG
   b. Recurrence occurs in 80% after TURBT alone, but in 30% after BCG.
7. The first line of treatment for CIS is BCG (see Intravesical Therapy, page 37 and Intravesical Immunotherapy with BCG, page 39). External beam radiation and systemic chemotherapy for CIS are not effective.
8. Up to 20% of patients undergoing cystectomy for CIS will have metastases to the lymph nodes.

Treatment of Urothelial Carcinoma (UC)

Stage Tis (Carcinoma in Situ)
1. Recurrence—80% after TURBT, but in only 30% after BCG.
2. Progression—20% after a complete response to BCG.
3. Treatment
   a. Fulguration of focal areas that appear suspicious. When CIS is diffuse, extensive fulguration or resection should be avoided because it can cause bladder contracture.
   b. *A 6 week course of intravesical BCG is recommended* (beginning at least 2 weeks after TURBT). See Intravesical Therapy, page 37.
      i. If CIS is not eradicated after a 6 week course of BCG, options include cystectomy or a second course of BCG. If 2 courses of BCG fail to eradicate CIS, cystectomy should be strongly considered.
      ii. *If CIS is eradicated after 1 or 2 six week courses of BCG, maintenance BCG is recommended.*
4. Follow up
   a. Perform bladder biopsy and bladder wash for cytology or FISH within 6 weeks after finishing BCG to rule out persistent tumor.
   b. In the absence of recurrent UC, perform cystoscopy and a urine tumor marker every 3 months for 2 years, every 6 months for 2 years, then every year, and—
   c. IVP, CT urogram, or retrograde pyelograms every 1-2 years. Patients with CIS have a higher risk (up to 21%) of developing upper tract UC.

Stage Ta
1. Recurrence—5% progress to muscle invasion after TURBT.
2. Progression—50% recur, most within one year of TURBT.
3. High grade increases the risk of recurrence and progression.
4. Treatment
   a. TURBT—for high grade tumors, perform a second TURBT within 1-4 weeks to ensure complete tumor resection and to confirm the stage.
   b. Fulguration—only used for patients with a history of pathologically confirmed low grade stage Ta UC. Fulguration may be used when urine cytology is negative and the recurrence is small and appears to be low grade and stage Ta.
   c. *A single dose of intravesical chemotherapy within 24 hours of TURBT (ideally within 6 hours) is recommended in the absence of bladder perforation because it decreases the recurrence rate by 40%.*
   d. Low grade Ta tumors—administer a 6 week course of intravesical chemotherapy when risk factors for recurrence are present. Maintenance intravesical chemotherapy is not useful. When intravesical chemotherapy fails to prevent recurrences, BCG may be used.

Risk Factors for Recurrence
Multiple or diffuse bladder tumors
Recurrence < 1 year of resection
Incomplete tumor resection
Large tumor (e.g. > 2 cm)

   e. High grade Ta tumors—administer a 6 week course of intravesical BCG followed by maintenance BCG.
5. Follow up
   a. Cystoscopy in 3 months, then 9 months later, then every 12 months. Tumor markers may be considered, especially for high grade tumors. High grade tumors require more intensive follow up.
   b. Consider IVP, CT urogram, or retrograde pyelograms in the following situations:
      i. When there are frequent recurrences.
      ii. Every 1-2 years when the tumor is high grade.

Stage T1

1. Recurrence—50-70% recur after treatment.
2. Progression—30-40% progress to muscle invasion after TURBT, often within the first year after treatment.
3. High grade increases the risk of recurrence and progression.
4. Treatment
   a. TURBT—perform a second TURBT within 1-4 weeks to ensure complete tumor resection and to confirm the stage.
   b. *A single dose of intravesical chemotherapy within 24 hours (ideally within 6 hours) of TURBT is recommended in the absence of bladder perforation because it decreases the recurrence rate by 40%.*
   c. An initial T1 tumor is usually treated with intravesical BCG. Cystectomy (partial or radical) is an option for high grade or bulky T1 tumors.
   d. When cystectomy is not performed, *a 6 week course of intravesical BCG is recommended* (beginning at least 2 weeks after TURBT).
      i. If UC is not eradicated after a 6 week course of BCG, options include cystectomy or a second course of BCG. If 2 courses of BCG fail to eradicate UC, cystectomy should be strongly considered.
      ii. *If UC is eradicated after 1 or 2 six week courses of BCG, maintenance BCG is recommended.*
5. Follow up
   a. Perform bladder biopsy and bladder wash for cytology or FISH within 6 weeks of finishing BCG to rule out persistent tumor.
   b. Cystoscopy and urine tumor markers every 3 months for 2 years, every 6 months for 2 years, then every year, and—
   c. Consider IVP, CT urogram, or retrograde pyelograms every 1-2 years or when recurrences are frequent.

Stage T2-T4a

1. *Intravesical therapy is not effective for stages T2-T4.*
2. Treatment
   a. The gold standard is radical cystectomy, urinary diversion, and pelvic lymphadenectomy, with or without urethrectomy.
      i. Neoadjuvant chemotherapy before cystectomy has not consistently improved survival; however, a recent meta-analysis showed that it offers a 5% absolute improvement in survival at 5 years after treatment (Lancet, 361: 1927, 2003). This benefit must be balanced with the potential toxicity of neoadjuvant chemotherapy.
      ii. Limited data suggests that adjuvant chemotherapy may improve survival. More definitive data will be available when EORTC 30994 is completed (a randomized comparison of immediate versus deferred chemotherapy after cystectomy in M0 patients with pT3-T4 or pN+).
   b. Bladder preservation is another option (see Bladder Sparing Therapies for Muscle Invasive UC, page 44).
3. Follow up
   a. Chest x-ray, LFTs, electrolytes, BUN, creatinine, and urine cytology every 6-12 months.
   b. Abdominal CT or CT urogram every 6 months.
   c. After cystectomy
      i. If the urinary diversion contains a significant length of ileum, obtain a vitamin B12 level each year.
      ii. For patients with a retained urethra, perform a urethral wash cytology and/or urethroscopy every 6-12 months.
      iii. Consider imaging the urinary diversion (e.g. endoscopy or pouchogram) every 6-12 months.
   d. After bladder sparing–cystoscopy and tumor markers every 3 months.

Stage T4b, N1-N3, or M1
1. Treatment consists of chemotherapy.
2. *Platinum is the most effective agent against UC*. Combination chemotherapy is more effective than a single agent.
3. The standard of care is either MVAC (methotrexate, vinblastine, adriamycin, cisplatin) or GC (gemcitabine and cisplatin). GC and MVAC have a similar response rate and survival rate, but GC is less toxic. GC has higher rate of thrombocytopenia and anemia, whereas MVAC has a higher rate of neutropenia, sepsis, mucositis, alopecia, and fatigue.
4. For patients who cannot tolerate full dose chemotherapy, less aggressive chemotherapy or radiation may be appropriate.

Tumors Arising in a Bladder Diverticulum
1. Transurethral resection of these tumors has a higher risk of bladder perforation because diverticula typically have no muscularis propria.
2. For CIS or low grade papillary UC, intravesical therapy may be tried. However, recurrent, high grade, or stage T1 to T4 tumors are probably best treated with diverticulectomy or cystectomy (partial or radical).

Tumors in the Prostatic Urethra or Prostatic Ducts
1. UC in the prostatic urethra or prostatic ducts (without prostate stroma invasion), is treated by TURBT ± TURP, followed by intravesical BCG.
   a. TURP removes tumor and may improve penetration of BCG into the prostate. See Response Rate To Intravesical BCG (table), page 41.
   b. If the tumor recurs in the prostate (especially high grade or invasive tumor), consider radical cystectomy and urethrectomy.
   c. Simultaneous TURBT and TURP does not appear to increase recurrence of UC in the prostatic urethra compared to TURBT alone.
2. For UC invading the prostatic stroma, radical cystectomy and urethrectomy should probably be performed (see Urethrectomy, page 44).

Intravesical Therapy

General Information
1. *Intravesical therapy is indicated for stage Ta, T1, or CIS urothelial carcinoma of the bladder.* Intravesical therapy is not effective for stage T2-T4 or for non-urothelial tumors.
2. There are two types of intravesical therapy: chemotherapy (mitomycin, thiotepa, doxorubicin, etc.) and immunotherapy (BCG, interferon, etc.).
3. The optimal dose and regimen for intravesical therapy is unknown.
4. The three main indications for intravesical therapy are
   a. Eradication of CIS with or without associated papillary tumor.
   b. Eradication of residual tumor after incomplete resection.
   c. To reduce recurrence and progression in completely resected tumors.

Comparison of Intravesical Chemotherapy and BCG
1. BCG reduces tumor recurrence and progression. Intravesical chemotherapy reduces recurrence, but does *not* alter progression.
2. Maintenance BCG improves long-term results, whereas maintenance chemotherapy offers no advantage.
3. *BCG is superior to intravesical chemotherapy for treating CIS and high grade tumors.*
4. One dose of intravesical chemotherapy may be used within 24 hours (ideally within 6 hours) of TURBT in the absence of bladder perforation. *BCG should never be given intravesically within 2 weeks of TURBT.*
5. BCG can be more toxic than intravesical chemotherapy.

6. Comparison of intravesical therapy

	Intravesical BCG	Intravesical Chemotherapy
Used for single dose after TURBT	–	+
Mean reduction in recurrence	–	40%
6-8 week course reduces recurrence	+	+
Mean reduction in recurrence	43%	14-17%
Maintenance therapy improves response	+	–
Reduces progression	+	–
Side effects/toxicity	Moderate-High	Low-Moderate

+ = yes; – = no; TURBT = transurethral resection of bladder tumor.

Intravesical Chemotherapy
1. Intravesical chemotherapy agents have a direct cytotoxic effect.
2. Studies have shown that each of the chemotherapy agents achieve similar benefit. In other words, one agent is not superior to another.
3. 6 weeks of intravesical chemotherapy does not change progression, time to metastasis, or overall survival. It does reduce recurrences by an average 14% at 1-3 years after treatment compared to TURBT alone. A 6 week course is used for low grade Ta tumors when risk factors for recurrence are present. BCG is reserved for low grade Ta tumors that fail to respond to intravesical chemotherapy, high grade tumors, and stage T1 tumors.
4. Maintenance intravesical chemotherapy offers no advantage.
5. Single dose of intravesical chemotherapy after TURBT
   a. A single dose of mitomycin C, doxorubicin, or epirubicin may be used within 24 hours (ideally within 6 hours) of TURBT when bladder perforation is absent. Valrubicin is not used is this setting.
   b. When used in this fashion, these agents decrease recurrence by 40%.
6. Side effects of intravesical chemotherapy tend to be less severe than BCG.
7. When urothelial integrity is disrupted, systemic absorption of an intravesical agent is more likely. Thus, these agents should probably not be administered when any of the following are present: urinary infection, gross hematuria, bladder perforation, or traumatic catheterization.
8. Before starting a course of therapy
   a. Ensure that the patient does not have a urinary infection.
   b. Advise the patient to limit fluid intake before each instillation to avoid rapid dilution of the chemotherapy agent.
   c. When using mitomycin, consider using oral methods to alkalinize the urine before each instillation (mitomycin is more effective at pH > 6).
9. Instillation technique
   a. Preparing the agent—see the individual agents for recommendations.
   b. Before each instillation
      i. The patient voids before each instillation. Perform a urinalysis to check for gross hematuria and urinary infection.
      ii. When the catheter is placed, a post void residual is measured. Patients with a high post void residual may be catheterized 2 hours after instillation to prevent excessive exposure to chemotherapy.
      iii. The bladder should be emptied completely before each instillation.
   c. Instillation—infused through a catheter and into the bladder.
   d. After each instillation
      i. Patients should attempt to hold the agent in their bladder for at least 2 hours. The body position may be varied to insure thorough distribution within the bladder. If the patient has a high post void residual, consider catheterizing the patient 2 hours after instillation.
      ii. Patients should wash their hands and genitals after voiding.

10. Mitomycin C (not FDA approved for intravesical use)
   a. Mitomycin C is more effective when urine pH > 6 (consider alkalinization of the urine during therapy) and when its concentration is high (mix mitomycin C in 20 ml of water rather than 40 ml).
   b. Mechanism of action—alkylating agent (inhibits DNA synthesis).
   c. Therapeutic course—40 mg in 20 ml sterile water intravesically every week for 6-8 weeks.
   d. Immediate adjuvant therapy after TURBT—40 mg in 20 ml sterile water intravesically.
   e. *Systemic absorption usually does not occur when mitomycin C is given intravesically because of its high molecular weight.*
   f. Side effects include
      i. Irritative voiding symptoms
      ii. Contact dermatitis on the hands and genitals—it is minimized by washing the hands and genitals after instillation and after voiding.
11. Thiotepa (FDA approved for Ta, T1, and CIS bladder cancer)
   a. Mechanism of action—alkylating agent (inhibits DNA synthesis).
   b. Therapeutic course—60 mg in 30-60 ml of sodium chloride instilled intravesically each week for 6 weeks. Therapy is often continued with a single instillation each month for one year.
   c. *Systemic absorption may occur when thiotepa is given intravesically because of its low molecular weight.* Systemic absorption can cause myelosuppression (especially leukopenia and thrombocytopenia).
   d. Side effects include
      i. Myelosuppression—occurs in 10% in of patients.
      ii. Irritative voiding symptoms
12. Doxorubicin (not FDA approved for intravesical use)
   a. Mechanism of action—intercalating agent and inhibits topoisomerase.
   b. Therapeutic course—30-100 mg in 30-100 ml of sterile water instilled intravesically each week for 6 weeks.
   c. *Systemic absorption usually does not occur when doxorubicin is given intravesically because of its high molecular weight.* Systemic absorption can cause myelosuppression.
   d. Side effects include—irritative voiding symptoms.
13. Valrubicin—indicated in patients who have CIS that is refractory to BCG and who are not candidates for radical cystectomy. Response rate in this group is 15-18%. Valrubicin is an analogue of doxorubicin. It was taken off the market, but it may be available again soon.

Intravesical Immunotherapy with Bacillus Calmette-Guerin (BCG)

1. BCG is an attenuated live bacillus vaccine (Mycobacterium bovis).
2. The three main indications for intravesical BCG are
   a. Eradication of CIS with or without associated papillary tumor.*
   b. Eradication of residual tumor because of incomplete resection.
   c. To reduce recurrence in completely resected stage Ta or T1 bladder tumors (prophylactic therapy).*
   * BCG is FDA approved for these indications.
3. Intravesical BCG decreases tumor recurrence and progression. It may also reduce cystectomy rate and cancer related deaths.
4. Mechanism of action—stimulates the body's immune system to destroy tumor cells. By binding to fibronectin sites, the bacillus organism activates T-cells. Since anti-clotting drugs or fibrinolysins will inhibit fibronectin binding, consider discontinuing these drugs during BCG treatment. BCG may also have a direct inhibitory effect on tumor cell invasion.
5. BCG immune response peaks during the sixth instillation of the initial course and during the third instillation of subsequent courses.

6. BCG is superior to intravesical chemotherapy for CIS and high grade UC. 70% of patients with CIS have a complete initial response to BCG. Of those with a complete response, 52-71% are disease free at 5 years.
7. Complications
   a. Low-grade symptoms
      i. Common side effects—cystitis, dysuria, hematuria, malaise, fatigue, and low grade fever (usually resolve in 24-48 hours).
      ii. Treatment—NSAIDS, Pyridium®, anticholinergics. If symptoms are intense or last more than 24 hours, consider the following:
         • Delay additional instillations until symptoms improve or abate.
         • Reduce BCG dose—it is unknown if this reduces efficacy.
         • Isoniazid (INH)* 300 mg po the day before, the day of, and the day after each BCG instillation. Alternatively, administer INH* 300 mg po q day starting the day before BCG instillation and continue it until symptoms abate. INH does not appear to affect the efficacy of BCG. Some studies have shown that routine use of INH with BCG does not reduce symptoms.
   b. Fever—if a patient has fever >101.5° for > 12-24 hours without signs of sepsis, stop the BCG instillations, obtain a urine culture for bacteria and acid fast bacilli, start broad spectrum antibiotics and isoniazid* 300 mg po q day. Continue isoniazid for 3 months. Resume BCG when the patient is asymptomatic.
   c. BCG sepsis (0.4%)—admit patients with fever ≥102° or signs of sepsis. Obtain urine and blood cultures for bacteria and acid fast bacilli. Administer prednisolone 40 mg IV q day (start immediately), broad spectrum antibiotics, and anti-tuberculosis drugs (INH* 300 mg po q day, rifampin 600 mg po q day, ethambutol 1200 mg po q day, adjust medications based on sensitivity from cultures). Type IV hypersensitivity plays an important role in severe acute reactions to BCG; therefore, the prednisolone may be life saving. Consider giving cycloserine* 250-500 mg po BID in very ill patients. Cycloserine works faster (within 24 hours) than other anti-tuberculosis drugs (which may take up to one week to work). Do not use cycloserine in patients with renal failure. Cycloserine's major toxicity is neurologic (seizures, psychosis, headache, confusion, etc.). Blood cycloserine levels may be monitored (at least weekly) in patients with side effects or those taking more than 500 mg per day (adjust the dose to keep blood levels less than 30 ug/ml). Continue prednisolone 40 mg IV q day and then taper when sepsis has resolved. Antituberculosis drugs should be continued for 6 months. After BCG sepsis, the patient should not receive BCG again.
   d. Other rare side effects—granulomatous prostatitis, contracted bladder, hepatitis, arthritis, pneumonia, myelosuppression, skin rash, ureteral obstruction, and epididymitis/orchitis. Symptomatic BCG epididymitis, orchitis, or granulomatous prostatitis may be treated with INH* 300 mg po q day and rifampin 600 mg po q day for 3-6 months. Asymptomatic BCG granulomatous prostatitis requires no therapy.
   e. Most patients convert to a positive protein purified derivation (PPD). This does not require treatment. Patients that convert to positive PPD have a higher chance of complete response to BCG.
   f. There are no known reports mycobacterial infection caused by close contact with patients receiving BCG.

* When giving isoniazid or cycloserine, administer pyridoxine (vitamin B6) 50 mg po q day to prevent neurotoxicity. When giving isoniazid, check liver function tests periodically.

8. Contraindications to BCG therapy
   a. Gross hematuria (BCG may be given during microscopic hematuria)
   b. Within 2 weeks after TURBT
   c. Recent traumatic catheterization
   d. Urinary tract infection, sepsis, or high fever
   e. Immunosuppressed (lymphoma, leukemia, steroids, HIV, etc.)
   f. Previous severe BCG reaction (such as BCG sepsis)
9. Before starting a course of therapy
   a. Ensure that the patient does not have a urinary infection.
   b. Advise the patient to limit fluid intake before each instillation to avoid rapid dilution of BCG and the need to void too soon after instillation.
10. Instillation technique
    a. Dose—the optimal dose is unknown. Recommended dose: 1 vial Tice® BCG in 50 ml normal saline or 1 vial (81 mg) Theracys® BCG in 50 ml normal saline infused intravesically.
    b. Before each instillation
       i.   Check the patient's temperature (BCG is contraindicated with fever).
       ii. The patient voids before each instillation. Perform a urinalysis to check for gross hematuria and urinary infection.
       iii. When the catheter is placed, a post void residual is measured. Patients with a high post void residual may be catheterized 2 hours after instillation to prevent excessive exposure to BCG.
       iv. If traumatic catheterization is suspected, do not give BCG. Consider waiting at least 1 week before attempting the next instillation.
       v.   The bladder should be emptied completely before each instillation.
    c. Instillation—infused through a catheter and into the bladder.
    d. After instillation
       i. Attempt to hold the BCG in the bladder for at least 2 hours. The body position may be varied to thoroughly distribute BCG in the bladder.
       ii. Some urologists suggest that the patient void the BCG into dilute bleach to safely dispose of the mycobacteria, void into a single toilet for 24 hours after BCG then clean it with bleach, wash their hands and genitals after voiding, and refrain from sex for 48 hours.
11. Cytology may be positive for up to 3 months after BCG.
12. Duration of therapy–individualize to each patient. General principles are
    a. BCG intravesically once a week for 6 weeks, followed by at least 6 weeks of rest, then re-evaluate the bladder.
    b. If T1, high grade Ta, or CIS recurs after the initial 6 weeks of BCG, consider another 6 week course of BCG versus radical cystectomy.
    c. If BCG eradicates UC, consider maintenance therapy (see page 42).
13. Two 6 week courses of BCG have a higher response rate than one 6 week course.

Reason for Intravesical BCG	CR at 1 Year		CR at 4-5 Years	
	Mean	Range	Mean	Range
Eradication of residual papillary tumor	60%	35-73%	-	-
Eradication of CIS (bladder only)	70%	46-100%	64%	52-71%
Eradication of CIS (prostatic urethra)*				
Response in prostate only	83%	70-100%	-	-
Response in bladder & prostate	68%	47-80%	-	-
Prophylaxis for tumor recurrence	80%	35-91%	58%	28-86%

CR = Complete response to 1 or 2 six-week courses of BCG.

  * Some urologists recommend performing TURP before instilling BCG to remove tumor and to facilitate contact between BCG and the prostatic ducts.

14. Maintenance therapy—in patients with CIS and/or completely resected recurrent Ta or T1 bladder UC who where disease free 3 months after a 6 week induction course of BCG (one intravesical BCG instillation each week for 6 weeks), the Southwest Oncology Group (SWOG) studied periodic courses of maintenance BCG (J Urol, 163: 1124, 2000). Maintenance therapy consisted of one intravesical BCG instillation each week for 3 weeks at 3 months, 6 months, and then every 6 months thereafter for a total of three years from the initial course of BCG. *Maintenance BCG improved complete response rate, improved disease-free survival, and decreased recurrence rate compared to the 6 week induction therapy alone.* A trend toward improved overall survival was seen, but this was not statistically significant. Only 16% of patients completed the 3 year maintenance regimen because of BCG toxicity.

Patients with CIS and/or Completely Resected Ta or T1 Bladder UC	6 Week Induction Course of BCG	6 Week Induction Course of BCG + Maintenance BCG
Complete response rate (CIS only)*	57%	84%
5-year recurrence-free survival*	41%	60%
5-year overall survival	78%	83%

* Statistically significant difference.

Intravesical Immunotherapy with Interferon
1. Interferon is not FDA approved for intravesical use.
2. Mechanism of action—stimulates the immune system to destroy tumor.
3. Response appears to be better when at least 50 million units of interferon are used and when interferon is combined with BCG.
4. Interferon alone to treat residual tumor
   a. For stage Ta, T1, and Tis, complete response at 1-2 years is 20-40%.
   b. For BCG refractory CIS, complete response at 1-2 years is 10-20%.
5. Combination of interferon and BCG to treat residual tumor—after intravesical interferon + BCG for stage Ta, T1, and Tis (6 week induction followed by maintenance therapy), the cancer free rate at 24 months was 57% in BCG naive patients and 42% in patients who failed BCG.
6. Dose: 50-100 million units interferon α-2b in 50 ml normal saline. For combination therapy, mix BCG (one tenth dose up to full dose) directly into the interferon. Instillation schedule is similar to BCG alone.
7. Side effects include flu like symptoms.

Radical Cystectomy

General Information
1. Radical cystectomy is the treatment of choice for muscle invasive UC.
2. Radical cystectomy involves removal of the bladder and pelvic lymph nodes. In men, the prostate and seminal vesicles are usually removed. In women, the uterus, fallopian tubes, ovaries, and anterior vagina are usually removed. In some cases, the reproductive organs and nerves can be spared in patients wishing to preserve sexual or reproductive function.
3. Delaying radical cystectomy more than 12 weeks (from the time of diagnosis of muscle invasion) is associated with lower survival.
4. Radical cystectomy reveals incidental prostate cancer in 28-61% of men.
5. 10% of cystectomy specimens are pT0. In other words, TURBT completely excises invasive tumors 10% of the time.
6. The worst prognostic finding in the primary bladder tumor is prostatic stromal invasion. The 5-year survival is 22-36%.

7. Pelvic lymph node dissection (PLND)
    a. A bilateral pelvic lymph node dissection should be performed during radical cystectomy and should include at least 10 lymph nodes.
    b. The limits of a standard PLND are the common iliac vessels superiorly, the inguinal ligament inferiorly, the bladder medially, the pelvic side wall and genitofemoral nerve laterally.
    c. It is not clear whether extending the lymph node dissection above the common iliac vessels is beneficial.
    d. Recent evidence suggests that an adequate lymph node dissection improves survival.
    e. PLND during radical cystectomy is rarely associated with a lymphocele because the surgery is performed intraperitoneal (the lymph fluid is absorbed by the peritoneum).
8. Recurrence after cystectomy
    a. Local (pelvic) recurrence occurs in ≤ 12% of cases.
    b. When the urethra is not removed, urethral recurrence rate is 10%.
    c. Upper tract UC develops in 2-4% of cases when CIS was absent and up to 17% of cases when CIS was present in the bladder.
    d. Recurrence usually occurs within 2 years after cystectomy.

Urinary Diversion

1. Urinary diversion options include conduit, orthotopic neobladder, catheterizable continent diversion, and ureterosigmoidostomy. See Use of Intestine in the Urinary Tract, page 414.
2. Ureteral anastomosis to the diversion
    a. For conduits and neobladders, an anti-refluxing anastomosis has a higher stricture rate and offers no significant benefit compared to a refluxing anastomosis. Thus, a refluxing anastomosis is recommended.
    b. For catheterizable continent diversions and for ureterosigmoidostomy variations, an anti-refluxing ureteral anastomosis is recommended.
3. For conduits, the risk of hydronephrosis and renal dysfunction increases with time. Renal deterioration is less common with orthotopic neobladder. *Life long follow up of the upper tracts is mandatory, and may include urography or renal scan.*
4. Published evidence shows no advantage of one type of urinary diversion over the others in terms of quality of life. The risks and benefits of each type of diversion must be considered.

Survival After Radical Cystectomy for UC

Pathologic Stage (AJCC 2002)	5-Year Disease-Free Survival*		10-Year Disease-Free Survival*	
	Mean†	Range	Mean†	Range
pT0N0	92%	—	86%	—
pTaN0	79%	79-100%	74%	74-80%
pTcisN0	91%	85-92%	89%	—
pT1N0	83%	80-93%	78%	72-78%
pT2aN0	89%	62-89%	87%	82-87%
pT2bN0	78%	74-78%	76%	—
pT3N0	62%	57-62%	61%	—
pT4N0	50%	50-62%	45%	41-45%
N+	35%	28-48%	34%	21-34%
All stages	68%	55-79%	66%	65-69%

* Without adjuvant or neoadjuvant therapy.

† Mean values are weighted toward studies with more patients.

Urethrectomy

1. An orthotopic neobladder cannot be performed after urethrectomy.
2. After cystectomy without urethrectomy, urethral tumor recurrence occurs in approximately 10% of patients, usually within 2 years postoperatively.
   a. In females, the risk of urethral recurrence is highest in patients with tumor at the bladder neck.
   b. In males, the risk of urethral recurrence is highest in patients with prostatic stroma invasion (approximately 23%) and prostatic ductal invasion (approximately 15%)

Degree of Prostate Involvement with UC	Anterior Urethral Recurrence	
	Mean	Range
Prostatic Urethral Mucosa	5%	0-8%
Prostatic Ducts	15%	0-25%
Prostatic Stroma	23%	0-64%

3. Consider performing urethrectomy if any of the following criteria exist:
   a. In a female, UC in any part of the urethra.
   b. In a male, UC in the anterior urethra.
   c. UC at the urethral margin during cystectomy (based on frozen section).
   d. In patients with a high risk of urethral recurrence (especially those who are not candidates for orthotopic neobladder).
      i. Males with ductal or stromal invasion of the prostate.
      ii. Females with tumors involving the bladder neck.
4. In patients with a grossly normal urethra, some urologists advocate performing an intraoperative urethral margin frozen section. If this margin has no tumor, orthotopic neobladder is constructed.
5. In females, a urethrectomy should be performed when a neobladder is not created because it adds minimal morbidity to cystectomy.
6. After cystectomy without urethrectomy, perform urethral wash cytology every 6-12 months. Place a catheter or cystoscope all the way into the urethra. Flush at least 20 ml of normal saline through the catheter/scope. The saline is collected as it drains out the meatus. Urethroscopy may be useful in patients with urethral symptoms or at risk for urethral recurrence. However, urethral wash cytology is more sensitive than urethroscopy.
7. For a resectable urethral recurrence, perform a total urethrectomy.
8. Urethrectomy decreases the potency rate of nerve sparing cystectomy.

Bladder Sparing Therapies for Muscle Invasive UC

General Information

1. Bladder sparing therapy for muscle invasive tumors usually consists of one of the following treatments:
   a. Partial cystectomy with bilateral pelvic lymph node dissection.
   b. TURBT (to decrease the tumor burden) followed by chemoradiation.
   c. Single modality therapy with TURBT, chemotherapy, or radiation.
2. Single modality therapy (TURBT, chemotherapy, or radiation alone) is not as effective as combined therapy (TURBT with chemoradiation).

TURBT With Chemoradiation

1. *Patients with hydronephrosis are poor candidates for this approach.*
2. A small bladder capacity may limit the benefits of bladder sparing.
3. Candidates for this approach usually undergo another TURBT 4-6 weeks after the initial TURBT to attempt to completely resect the tumor.
4. Multiple modalities result in greater survival compared to radiation, chemotherapy or TURBT alone.
5. External beam radiation is administered with a radiosensitizing systemic chemotherapy agent such as cisplatin or 5-fluorouracil (chemoradiation).
6. An additional course of systemic chemotherapy may be administered after the chemoradiation.

7. This therapy commits the patient to a long treatment regimen and may and expose the patient to severe side effects.

8. 22-47% of patients that undergo this therapy will require cystectomy. Most of these patients undergo cystectomy for incomplete response to chemoradiation. Some patients undergo cystectomy for tumor recurrence. The delay in cystectomy (compared to cystectomy as the initial treatment) may increase the risk of disease progression (although this point is controversial). After incomplete response to induction therapy, the patient may not be healthy enough to undergo cystectomy. Furthermore, cystectomy after radiation may have a higher complication rate and may limit the options for urinary reconstruction.

9. The 5-year overall survival for patients undergoing TURBT and chemoradiation (including those who eventually undergo delayed cystectomy) is approximately 55%, which is similar to immediate cystectomy. The 5-year overall survival with an intact bladder is 41%.

10. This multimodal approach is more expensive than primary cystectomy.

11. After this therapy, cystoscopy and bladder biopsy should be performed. If bladder cancer is still present, radical cystectomy is recommended.

Partial Cystectomy

1. Partial cystectomy is an attractive option because it preserves the bladder and maintains potency.

2. Partial cystectomy and pelvic lymphadenectomy may be performed for primary bladder cancer if all of the following criteria are met:
   - Ability to achieve negative margins—tumors at the bladder dome or in a diverticulum are good candidates. Resection of the ureteral orifice with ureteral reimplant may be performed when necessary.
   - Tumor stage T1 or higher—for stage T1, partial cystectomy is often reserved for T1G3 tumors. T1G1 or T1G2 tumors are usually treated with TURBT and intravesical therapy.
   - Negative random bladder biopsies
   - No prior history of bladder tumors
   - No prostate invasion
   - Ability to maintain adequate bladder capacity after resection.

3. Retrospective data shows that survival is similar for partial and radical cystectomy. A randomized prospective study comparing radical and partial cystectomy has not been performed.

4. Tumor implantation along the incision or suprapubic tube tract is a potential risk, and has been reported in 0-18% of cases. However, most of these recurrences were reported in older studies. With current surgical techniques, tumor recurrence in the incision is rare. Some surgeons recommend leaving only a urethral catheter postoperatively, to avoid tumor implantation along a suprapubic tube tract.

5. After partial cystectomy, tumor recurrence in the bladder ranges from 29-78%. Up to 17% require radical cystectomy for tumor recurrence after partial cystectomy.

6. 5-year overall survival rate for all stages is 35-80%.

7. Neoadjuvant or adjuvant treatments such as chemotherapy and radiation have not altered survival.

8. Partial cystectomy for non-UC bladder tumors—partial cystectomy is the treatment of choice for bladder pheochromocytoma. It may be indicated in some urachal adenocarcinomas and non-urologic cancers that invade the bladder by local extension (e.g. colon cancer).

Comparison of Therapies for Muscle Invasive UC

	Radical Cystectomy	Partial Cystectomy	TURBT with Chemo & XRT
		Mean (range)	
5-Year overall survival All Stages	55% (30-67%)	49% (35-80%)	55% (47-63%)
5-year overall survival with intact bladder	—	?	41% (36-46%)
Mortality	2-3%	< 5%	4%
Require cystectomy after therapy	—	8% (0-17%)	34% (22-47%)
Local recurrence rate	≤ 12%	53% (29-78%)	43% (29-57%)

TURBT = transurethral resection of bladder tumor; XRT = external beam radiation

Recurrence

1. Factors that increase the risk of recurrence
   a. Larger tumor size (especially > 3 cm)
   b. Higher tumor stage
   c. Higher tumor grade
   d. Multiple tumors
   e. Prior history of tumors
   f. Associated CIS
   g. Tumor aneuploidy
   h. Loss of marker chromosomes or ABO antigen expression
   i. Vascular or lymphatic invasion
   j. Positive urine cytology after treatment
   k. Visible bladder tumor within 6 months after treatment
2. Bladder recurrence after TURBT
   a. CIS—80% will recur after TURBT, only 30% recur after BCG.
   b. Ta—50% will recur after TURBT, most within one year.
   c. T1—more than 70% recur after TURBT.
3. After Cystectomy
   a. Local recurrence after cystectomy ≤ 12%.
   b. After radical cystectomy for an invasive bladder tumor, development of upper tract urothelial tumor occurs in 2-4% of patients. If the patient had CIS in the cystectomy specimen, the rate of upper tract tumor recurrence may be as high as 17%
   c. Recurrence usually occurs within 2 years after cystectomy.
   d. After cystectomy without urethrectomy, urethral recurrence occurs in approximately 10% of cases and usually occurs within 2 years.
4. Upper tract recurrence
   a. If bladder tumors continue to recur, re-evaluate upper urinary tracts with urogram and/or retrograde pyelogram.
   b. *Patients with CIS in the bladder are more likely to have an upper tract recurrence than those without CIS.* Up to 6% of those with Ta or T1 bladder UC develop upper tract UC later in life. Up to 21% with bladder CIS develop upper tract UC.
   c. 30%-75% of those with upper tract tumors eventually develop bladder tumors.

Tumor Markers For Urothelial Cancer

Indications for Performing Urinary Tumor Markers

1. Irritative voiding symptoms (dysuria, frequency, etc.).
2. Hematuria (microscopic or gross)
3. Preoperative evaluation of urothelial tumors
4. Post-treatment surveillance of urothelial tumors
   a. After endoscopic resection
   b. After cystectomy
      i. From the urinary diversion.
      ii. Lavage cytology of urethral stump (see Urethrectomy, page 44).
5. Screening in high risk groups (for conditions that increase risk of urothelial tumors, see Bladder Cancer, Etiology, page 29)

Urine Cytology

1. Urine cytology detects abnormal appearing exfoliated urothelial cells.
2. The higher the tumor grade, the more likely urine cytology will detect the tumor (i.e. the sensitivity of urine cytology is greater for high grade tumors). This is because the more poorly differentiated the tumor, the less cohesive the cells.

Urothelial Carcinoma Grade	Approximate Sensitivity of Urine Cytology
Grade I	< 50%
Grade II	65-80%
Grade III and CIS	> 90%

3. The diagnostic yield of urine cytology is increased when at least 3 urine samples are analyzed.
4. For bladder cancers, bladder washings provide better diagnostic yield than voided urine.
5. Urine cytology can remain positive for up to 3 months following BCG therapy.
6. Patients that have a positive cytology and no history of UC should undergo a cystoscopy and urogram (IVP or CTU) because these patients have a risk of both lower tract and upper tract tumors. Patients with positive urine cytology within 6 months of treatment for bladder cancer almost always recur in the bladder; therefore, these patients probably do not need a repeat urogram, but should have a cystoscopy.

History of Patient with Positive Urine Cytology	Approximate % that Develop UC	Location UC Develops (%)		
		Bladder	Prostate	Upper Tract
No history of UC (asymptomatic)	94%	74%	7%	5%
No history of UC (symptomatic)*	70%	77%	9%	5%
< 6 months after TURBT	84-100%	100%	-	-
< 6 months after intravesical therapy	58-88%	100%	-	-

UC = Urothelial carcinoma; TURBT = Transurethral resection of bladder tumor
* Symptoms include hematuria and prostatism.

Other Tumor Markers
1. Bladder cancer detection is highest when urine cytology is combined with another tumor marker.
2. Most markers have a higher sensitivity and lower specificity than cytology.
   a. Sensitivity—the chance cancer is present when the test is positive.
   b. Specificity—the chance that cancer is absent when the test is negative.
3. BTA (bladder tumor antigen)—detects a complement factor H-related protein in the urine.
   a. BTA TRAK®—a quantitative test performed in a lab.
   b. BTA stat®—a qualitative test performed in the office.
   c. False positive results are more common in patients with gross hematuria during the test, genitourinary inflammation (e.g. infection, recent intravesical therapy), urolithiasis, urinary foreign bodies (e.g. stents, nephrostomy tubes), bowel interposition (e.g. conduit, neobladder), non-urothelial genitourinary cancer, and recent urinary tract instrumentation.
4. NMP22®—detects nuclear matrix protein in the urine.
   a. NMP22® test—a quantitative test performed in a lab.
   b. NMP22® bladderchek®—a qualitative test performed in the office.
   c. False positive results are more common in patients with genitourinary inflammation, urolithiasis, urinary foreign bodies, bowel interposition, non-urothelial genitourinary cancer, and recent urinary tract instrumentation.
5. ImmunoCyt™—detects two antigens (carcinoembryonic antigen and mucin glycoprotein) in exfoliated urothelial cells. For low grade tumors, ImmunoCyt™ has a higher sensitivity than cytology and FISH (i.e. it is better at detecting low grade tumors). ImmunoCyt™ is performed in a lab.
6. Urovysion™—uses fluorescence in situ hybridization (FISH) to detect chromosomal abnormalities in exfoliated urothelial cells. FISH is performed in a lab.
   a. Urovysion™ detects extra copies of chromosome 3, 7, and 17 and the loss of the 9p21 locus.
   b. FISH and urine cytology have a higher specificity than ImmunoCyt™, NMP22®, and BTA (i.e. FISH and cytology are more reliable at predicting the absence of cancer when the test is negative).
   c. FISH has a low rate of false positive results with infection and inflammation. *Urovysion™ is rarely affected by intravesical therapy.*

Positive Tumor Marker Without Visible Tumor In the Bladder
1. Urothelial tumor markers can be positive before a grossly visible tumor develops (microscopic cancer). False positive tests are also a possibility.
2. The source of the positive urinary tumor marker may be the upper tracts, bladder, prostate, or urethra. Work up should include evaluation of these regions. One method of evaluation is as follows:
   a. Upper tract imaging (IVP, CT urogram, or retrograde pyelograms) and cystoscopy with bladder wash cytology and random bladder biopsies. If this fails to reveal the source of the positive marker then:
   b. Cystoscopy, bladder wash cytology, differential ureteral wash cytology, repeat random bladder biopsies, and biopsy of the prostatic urethra (transurethral loop resection of the verumontanum at 5 and/or 7 o'clock has the highest yield in detecting UC in the prostatic ducts and acini). If this fails to reveal the source of the positive marker then:
   c. Consider evaluating the gastrointestinal tract and female reproductive organs. If this fails to reveal the source of the positive cytology then:
   d. Cystoscopy and urine tumor marker in 3 months. Consider repeating the above process in 6 months.

REFERENCES

General

Bladder Tumors: 1st International Consultation on Bladder Tumors. Ed. M Soloway, et al. Plymouth, United Kingdom: Health Publication Ltd., 2006.

Delnay KM, Stonehill WH, Goldman H, et al: Bladder histological changes associated with chronic indwelling urinary catheter. J Urol, 161: 1106, 1999.

DeWolf WC: p53–an important key to understanding urologic cancer. AUA Update Series, Vol. 14, Lesson 32, 1995.

Greene FL, Page DL, Fleming ID, et al. AJCC Cancer Staging Manual, Sixth Edition. New York: Springer, 2002. (effective January 1, 2003)

National Comprehensive Cancer Network (NCCN) clinical practice guidelines in oncology: Bladder cancer. 2007. (http:\\www.nccn.org)

Superficial Bladder UC and Intravesical Therapy

Au JL, et al: Methods to improve efficacy of intravesical mitomycin C: results of a randomized phase III trial. J Natl Cancer Inst, 93: 597, 2001.

Bohle A, et al: Intravesical bacillus calmette-guerin versus mitomycin C for superficial bladder cancer: a formal meta-analysis of comparative studies on recurrence and toxicity. J Urol, 169: 90, 2003.

Lamm DL, et al: Maintenance bacillus Calmette-Guerin immunotherapy for recurrent Ta, T1 and carcinoma in situ transitional cell carcinoma of the bladder: a randomized SWOG study. J Urol, 163: 1124, 2000.

Pawinski A, et al: A combined analysis of European Organization for Research and Treatment of Cancer, and Medical Research Council randomized clinical trials for the prophylactic treatment of stage TaT1 bladder cancer. J Urol, 156: 1934, 1996.

Smith J Jr., et al: Bladder cancer clinical guidelines panel summary report on the management of nonmuscle invasive bladder cancer (stages Ta, T1, and TIS). J Urol, 162: 1697, 1999.

Sylvester RJ, et al: A single immediate postoperative instillation of chemotherapy decreases the risk of recurrence in patients with stage Ta T1 bladder cancer: a meta-analysis of published results of randomized clinical trials. J Urol, 171: 2186, 2004.

Sylvester RJ, et al: Intravesical bacillus Calmette-Guerin reduces the risk of progression in patients with superficial bladder cancer: a meta-analysis of the published results of randomized clinical trials. J Urol, 168: 1964, 2002.

Sylvester RJ, et al: Bacillus Calmette-Guerin versus chemotherapy for the intravesical treatment of patients with carcinoma in situ of the bladder: a meta-analysis of the published results of randomized clinical trials. J Urol, 174: 86, 2005.

van der Meijden APM, et al: Intravesical Bacillus Calmette-Guerin treatment for superficial bladder cancer: results after 15 years of experience. Anticancer Res, 11: 1253, 1991.

Vegt P, et al: Does isoniazid reduce side effects of intravesical bacillus calmette-guerin therapy in superficial bladder cancer? J Urol, 157: 1246, 1997.

Urothelial Cancer Markers

Friedrich MG, et al: Comparison of multitarget fluorescence in situ hybridization in urine with other non-invasive tests for detecting bladder cancer. BJU Int, 92(9), 911, 2003.

Schwalb DM, et al: The management of positive urinary cytology in the absence of visible disease. AUA Update Series, Vol. 13, Lesson 36, 1994.

Sharma S, et al: Exclusion criteria enhance the specificity and positive predictive value of NMP22 and BTA stat. J Urol, 162(1): 53, 1999.

Muscle Invasive and Advanced UC

Abbas F, et al: Incidental prostatic adenocarcinoma in patients undergoing radical cystoprostatectomy for bladder cancer. Eur Urol, 30: 322, 1996.

Advanced Bladder Cancer (ABC) Meta-analysis Collaboration: Neoadjuvant chemotherapy in invasive bladder cancer: a systematic review and meta-analysis. Lancet, 361: 1927, 2003.

Advanced Bladder Cancer (ABC) Meta-analysis Collaboration: Adjuvant chemotherapy for invasive bladder cancer: Cochrane Database Syst Rev, Issue 2: CD006018, 2006.

Kim HL, Steinberg GD: The current status of bladder preservation in the treatment of muscle invasive bladder cancer. J Urol, 164: 627, 2000.

Shipley WU, et al: Selective bladder preservation by combined modality protocol treatment: long term outcomes of 190 patients with invasive bladder cancer. Urology, 60: 62, 2002.

Vaidya A, Soloway MS: De novo muscle invasive bladder cancer: is there a change in trend? J Urol, 165: 47, 2001.

von der Maase H, et al: Long term survival results of a randomized trial comparing gemcitabine plus cisplatin with methotrexate, vinblastine, doxorubicin, plus cisplatin in patients with bladder cancer. J Clin Oncol, 23(21): 4602, 2005 [update of J Clin Oncol, 17(17): 3068, 2000].

Radical and Partial Cystectomy

Gschwend JE, et al: Radical cystectomy for invasive bladder cancer: contemporary results and remaining controversies. Eur Urol, 38: 121, 2000.

Kassouf W, et al: Partial cystectomy for muscle invasive urothelial carcinoma of the bladder: a contemporary review of the M.D. Anderson Cancer Center experience. J Urol, 175: 2058, 2006.

Lerner SP, Skinner DG: Radical cystectomy for bladder cancer. Genitourinary Oncology. 2nd Edition. Ed. NJ Vogelzang, PT Scardino, WU Shipley, et al. Philadelphia: Lippincott Williams and Wilkins, 2000, pp 425-447.

Sanchez-Ortiz RF, Huang WC, et al: An interval longer than 12 weeks between the diagnosis of muscle invasion and cystectomy is associated with worse outcome in bladder carcinoma. J Urol, 169: 110, 2003.

Stein JP, et al: Radical cystectomy in the treatment of invasive bladder cancer: Long-term results in 1,054 patients. J Clin Oncol, 19(3): 666, 2001.

Sweeney P, et al: Partial cystectomy. Urol Clin North Am, 19(4): 701, 1992.

Urethral and Prostatic Involvement

Freeman JA, Esrig D, Stein JP, et al: Management of the patient with bladder cancer: urethral recurrence. Urol Clin North Am, 21: 645, 1994.

Hardeman SW, Soloway MS: Urethral recurrence following radical cystectomy. J Urol, 144: 666, 1990.

Laor E, et al: The influence of simultaneous resection of bladder tumors and prostate on the occurrence of prostatic urethral tumors. J Urol, 126: 171, 1981.

Lebret T, Herve JM, Barre P, et al: Urethral recurrence of transitional cell carcinoma of the bladder. Eur Urol, 33: 170, 1998.

Sakamoto N, et al: An adequate sampling of the prostate to identify prostatic involvement by urothelial carcinoma in bladder cancer patients. J Urol, 149: 318, 1993.

Stenzl A, Draxl H, Posch B, et al: The risk of urethral tumors in female bladder cancer: can the urethra be used for orthotopic reconstruction of the lower urinary tract? J Urol, 153: 950, 1995.

Urachal Cancer

Herr, HW, et al: Urachal carcinoma: contemporary surgical outcomes. J Urol, 178: 74, 2007.

Weiss RE, Fair WR: Urachal anomalies and urachal carcinoma. AUA Update Series, Vol. 17, Lesson 38, 1998.

PENILE TUMORS

Benign Penile Lesions

Papilloma (Pearly Penile Papules, Hirsute Papilloma)
1. These benign lesions consist of rows of 1 to 2 mm white/yellow papules on the corona of the glans.
2. These lesions do not contain human papilloma virus (HPV).
3. Treatment is usually unnecessary. Laser ablation has been reported.

Condyloma Acuminatum (Genital Warts)
1. Nontender wart-like lesions or papillary frondular lesions.
2. Condyloma acuminatum is a sexually transmitted disease caused by HPV.
3. *90% of visible genital warts are caused by HPV types 6 and 11, which have an extremely low oncogenic potential.*
4. HPV rarely leads to cervical carcinoma, penile carcinoma, and anal cancer.
5. For details, see Condyloma Acuminatum, page 385.

Buschke-Lowenstein Tumor (Giant Condyloma, Verrucous Carcinoma)
1. An exophytic cauliflower-like mass in the genital or anorectal region.
2. It is benign (i.e. it does not metastasize), but it is *locally invasive*.
3. HPV has been found in these tumors (especially HPV 6 and HPV 11).
4. Treatment—complete excision (tends to recur after inadequate excision). Radiation therapy is not recommended because it may induce anaplasia.

Zoon's (Plasma Cell) Balanitis
1. Zoon's balanitis is seen on the glans or prepuce of uncircumcised men.
2. Exam reveals an asymptomatic, well-circumscribed, red, flat lesion that contains pinpoint redder spots ("cayenne pepper spots"). It may look similar to carcinoma in situ. Diagnosis requires biopsy. Histology shows plasma cells in the dermis.
3. Treatment—topical steroids, circumcision, or CO_2 laser ablation.

Premalignant Penile Lesions

Bowenoid Papulosis
1. Presentation—red-brown papules on the glans or shaft. The average age of diagnosis is 20-30 and it usually occurs in circumcised men.
2. HPV is usually identified in these lesions (especially HPV 16).
3. Bowenoid papulosis has a similar histologic appearance to carcinoma in situ (CIS), but it is much less likely to develop into malignancy than CIS.
4. Treatment options—surveillance, topical 5-fluorouracil (for dose see Carcinoma in Situ, page 52), or ablation (laser, cryotherapy, cautery).
5. Comparison of bowenoid papulosis and CIS

Characteristic	Bowenoid Papulosis	CIS
Age at diagnosis	20-30	50-60
Usual foreskin status	Circumcised	Uncircumcised
HPV has been detected	Yes	Yes
Risk of Developing SCC	Rare	10%

Carcinoma in Situ (CIS, Erythroplasia of Queyrat, Bowen's disease)
1. 10% of men with CIS eventually develop invasive SCC of the penis.
2. HPV has been detected in CIS, especially types 16, 18, 31, and 33.
3. Presentation
   a. Red, velvety, well-marginated papules or plaques. It may ulcerate.
   b. Symptoms—often asymptomatic, rarely painful.
   c. Age of presentation = 50-60.
   d. Rare in circumcised men.
4. Work up—biopsy.
5. Treatment
   a. 5% 5-fluorouracil (5-FU) topically BID for 3-4 weeks [5% Cream: 25 grams]. Several courses may be required. 5-FU can cause dermatitis (which may simulate worsening of CIS). If 5-FU fails, consider penile sparing therapies or penectomy.
   b. Penile sparing therapies or penectomy may be the initial treatment choice, especially for extensive or ulcerated lesions.

Balanitis Xerotica Obliterans (BXO, Lichen Sclerosus et Atrophicus)
1. Inflammatory lesion from chronic infection, trauma, or inflammation.
2. BXO rarely undergoes malignant degeneration.
3. Presentation
   a. Flat white patches (often a mosaic pattern) on the glans and prepuce. It may involve the meatus and fossa navicularis. It may feel fibrotic.
   b. Occurs in females and males (circumcised and uncircumcised).
   c. BXO is usually *asymptomatic*. Symptoms may include pruritus, burning, painful erections in males, and dyspareunia in females.
   d. *BXO is associated with meatal and urethral strictures.*
4. Work up—if BXO is atypical or progresses rapidly, perform a biopsy to rule out malignancy. Men with perimeatal/meatal BXO or obstructive voiding symptoms should be evaluated for urethral strictures.
5. Treatment
   a. Asymptomatic BXO—no therapy required.
   b. Symptomatic BXO—topical steroids relieve itching and burning (2% testosterone cream in petrolatum or 0.1% triamcinolone BID).
   c. Consider meatotomy/meatoplasty for meatal stenosis and circumcision for phimosis. Treat urethral strictures accordingly.
   d. When there is a poor response to any of these therapies, consider biopsy.
   e. Excision is discouraged because of high recurrence rates.
6. Long-term follow up is required because of the risk of malignancy.

Leukoplakia
1. Usually associated with chronic irritation or inflammation.
2. Malignant transformation occurs in 10-20% of cases.
3. Leukoplakia is often detected concurrently with SCC of the penis.
4. Presentation—sharply marginated white scaly plaques, often involving the meatus. Symptoms are irritative in nature.
5. Work up—biopsy.
6. Treatment—complete excision and long-term follow up.

Cutaneous Horn
1. A mound of hyperkeratosis usually on the glans.
2. The cutaneous horn is benign, but up to 33% of these horns arise from underlying malignancy (i.e. SCC is at the base of the horn).
3. Treatment—complete excision with long-term follow up. If pathology shows penile cancer, then treat accordingly.

Squamous Cell Carcinoma (SCC)

General Information
1. Squamous cell carcinoma (SCC) accounts for $\geq$ 95% of penile cancers.
2. SCC of the penis is rare in the United States. In some locations in Asia and Africa, penile cancer is the most common malignant tumor in men.

Etiology
1. Uncircumcised—circumcision in newborns virtually eliminates the risk of penile cancer. Circumcision before puberty may lower the risk of penile SCC. Men circumcised after puberty have the same risk of penile SCC as uncircumcised men.
2. Premalignant lesions (see Premalignant Penile Lesions, page 51)
3. Psoralen and ultra violet light type A (PUVA), which is used to treat psoriasis, increases the risk of penile SCC when the penis is not shielded.
4. Tobacco smoking
5. Possible causes of penile cancer may include
   a. Smegma—may cause chronic irritation or it may be a carcinogen.
   b. Phimosis—it is unknown if this is a cause or an effect or unrelated.
   c. Human papilloma virus (HPV)—HPV is found in some penile cancers, (especially types 16, 18).
6. No increased risk of penile SCC
   a. Carcinogens (topical contact)—these increase the risk of scrotal cancer.
   b. Sexually transmitted diseases other than HPV.
   c. Balanoposthitis

Presentation
1. Mean age = 50-60. Delay in seeking treatment is common.
2. The presence of the penile lesion is usually the reason for presentation. Pain is usually *not* a presenting complaint.
3. The lesion may be nodular, ulcerative, fungating, or obscured by phimosis.
4. Presenting location—most to least common: glans, prepuce, shaft. Multiple penile sites may be involved in up to 30% of cases.
5. Most penile cancers are superficial and low grade.
6. Paraneoplastic syndromes may be present, most commonly *hypercalcemia*.
7. 50% of men have palpable inguinal lymph nodes at presentation (caused by inflammation or tumor. See Inguinal Lymph Node Dissection, page 55).
8. Less than 10% present with distant metastasis.

Metastasis
1. The most common site of metastasis is the inguinal lymph nodes.
2. Spread occurs in a stepwise fashion (sentinel node, to other superficial inguinal nodes, to deep inguinal nodes, to pelvic nodes, to distant metastasis). Spread to the inguinal lymph nodes can be bilateral because the penile lymphatics usually drain to both sides.
3. Distant metastasis—most to least common: lung, liver, bone, brain. Less than 10% of men present with distant metastasis.

Work Up
1. History and physical exam (especially genitals and inguinal lymph nodes)
2. Biopsy
3. Patients with cancer in the regional lymph nodes should undergo:
   a. Chest x-ray
   b. CT scan of the abdomen and pelvis.
   c. Blood tests including serum calcium (check for paraneoplastic syndrome) and liver function tests (check for liver metastasis).
4. Bone scan when the patient has bone pain, elevated calcium, or elevated alkaline phosphatase.

Stage (AJCC 2002)

This TNM classification refers to both clinical and pathological staging.
Higher stage implies worse prognosis.

Primary Tumor (T)

Tx	Primary tumor cannot be assessed
T0	No evidence of primary tumor
Tis	Carcinoma in situ
Ta	Noninvasive verrucous carcinoma
T1	Tumor invades subepithelial connective tissue
T2	Tumor invades corpus spongiosum or cavernosum
T3	Tumor invades urethra or prostate
T4	Tumor invades other adjacent structures

Regional Lymph Nodes (N)

Nx	Regional lymph nodes cannot be assessed
N0	No regional lymph node metastasis
N1	Metastasis in a single superficial inguinal lymph node
N2	Metastasis in multiple or bilateral superficial inguinal lymph nodes
N3	Metastasis in deep inguinal or pelvic lymph node(s) unilateral or bilateral

Distant Metastasis (M)

Mx	Distant metastasis cannot be assessed
M0	No distant metastasis
M1	Distant metastasis

Used with the permission of the American Joint Committee on Cancer (AJCC), Chicago,
Illinois. The original source for this material is the *AJCC Cancer Staging Manual, Sixth
Edition* (2002) published by Springer Science and Business Media LLC,
www.springerlink.com.

Grade

Higher grade implies worse prognosis.

Grade 1	Well differentiated
Grade 2	Moderately differentiated
Grade 3-4	Poorly differentiated or undifferentiated

Treatment of Penile SCC

General Information

1. Penile cancer is mainly treated by surgical excision of the primary lesion
   and the involved lymph nodes.
2. Systemic chemotherapy has not been well studied and is often reserved for
   men with advanced cancer (e.g. T4 or N3 or M1). Common regimens:
   a. 5-FU and cisplatin
   b. Bleomycin, methotrexate, and cisplatin.

Penectomy

1. A 2 cm negative margin should be excised proximal to the tumor.
2. Partial penectomy
   a. Indicated for tumors confined to the glans, prepuce, or distal shaft.
   b. Try to leave 2-3 cm of penile length because this permits the patient to
      • Maintain some degree of sexual function.
      • Void in a standing position.
3. Total penectomy
   a. Indicated for tumors of the proximal shaft.
   b. Requires a perineal urethrostomy (allows voiding in a sitting position).
4. Advanced disease may require more extensive resection including removal
   of the scrotum and the perineum.

Penile Sparing Therapies

1. The gold standard for all invasive penile tumors is partial or total penectomy with a 2 cm negative margin. Penile sparing therapies may be indicated in patients that
   a. Refuse penectomy or who are medically unfit for penectomy.
   b. Desire to maintain sexual function or preserve penile anatomy.
   c. Have carcinoma in situ or low stage, low grade invasive tumors.
2. Penile sparing therapies have a higher recurrence rate than penectomy.
3. Penile sparing therapies include
   a. Circumcision—reserved for lesions confined to the prepuce.
   b. Laser ablation
   c. Radiation (external beam or interstitial)
   d. Cryosurgery
   e. Mohs' surgery—removal of tumor layer by layer under microscopic control until negative margins are obtained. This is best utilized for lesions < 1 cm in diameter.
   f. Topical chemotherapy (topical 5-FU, see page 52)—used only for CIS.
   g. Wedge resection—has an unacceptably high recurrence rate and is *not* a recommended therapy.

Inguinal Lymph Node Dissection (ILND)

1. Of those with palpable inguinal lymph nodes at presentation, 50% are palpable because of inflammation and 50% because of tumor. Of those that still have palpable inguinal nodes after 6 weeks of postoperative antibiotics, 85% have tumor in these palpable nodes.
2. Only 20% of men with non-palpable inguinal nodes at presentation have metastasis to these nodes. Therefore, prophylactic ILND in these patients may treat up to 80% unnecessarily.
3. ILND is recommended in men with any of the characteristics listed below. These characteristics increase the risk for tumor in the inguinal nodes.
   a. High stage tumor (i.e. T2 or greater)
   b. High grade tumor
   c. Palpable nodes after 6 weeks of postoperative antibiotics (85% chance of having tumor in these nodes).
   d. Positive sentinel node biopsy.
4. The superficial and deep inguinal lymph nodes are separated by the *fascia lata*. The superficial nodes are superficial to the fascia lata, whereas the deep inguinal nodes are deep to the fascia lata.
5. During ILND, inguinal skin flaps are developed *deep to Scarpa's fascia*.
6. *The femoral vessels are found in the femoral triangle*, which is bounded by the sartorius laterally, the inguinal ligament superiorly, and the adductor longus medially.
7. Progressing lateral to medial (toward the navel), structures in the femoral triangle are represented by "N(AVEL)". N = femoral nerve; A = femoral artery; V = femoral vein; E = empty space; L = lymph nodes. The structures in parenthesis are within the femoral sheath.
8. Do not dissect lateral to the femoral artery because there are no nodes in this region and dissection in this region may injure the femoral nerve.
9. A *sartorius muscle* flap may be needed to cover the femoral vessels after ILND. The sartorius is mobilized from its origin at the anterior superior iliac spine and moved medial to cover the femoral vessels. Its origin is then sutured to the ilioinguinal ligament. This *reduces the incidence of femoral vessel hemorrhage*.

Treatment of Penile Cancer

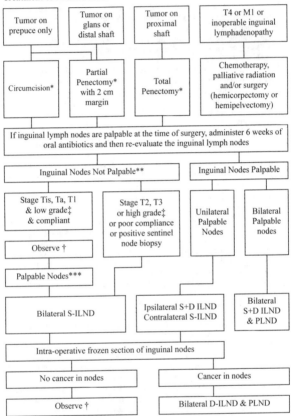

ILND = Inguinal Lymph Node Dissection; S-ILND = Superficial ILND
D-ILND = Deep ILND; S+D ILND = Superficial and Deep ILND
PLND = Pelvic Lymph Node Dissection

* Other treatment modalities that may be considered are listed under Penile
Sparing Therapies, page 55. Penile sparing therapies tend to have a higher
recurrence rate than penectomy. For treatment of Tis, see Premalignant
Penile Lesions, page 51.

** Some urologists consider performing a sentinel node biopsy when the
patient is at risk for metastasis to the inguinal lymph nodes.

***Lymph node metastases usually develop within 2-3 years postoperatively.

† Follow with genital examination and node examination every 1-2 months for
at least 3 years, then less often thereafter.

‡ Patients with moderate grade may be observed or undergo ILND.

Survival

1. Without treatment of penile carcinoma, 5-year survival is rare.
2. The following factors are poor prognostic indicators:
   a. Higher tumor stage
   b. Higher tumor grade
   c. More extensive lymph node involvement

Node Status	Approximate Mean 5-year Survival (range)	
pN0	80%	(74-100%)
pN1	81%	(75-82%)
pN2	50%	(17-80%)
pN3 (deep inguinal)	29%	(17-40%)
pN3 (pelvic)	0%	(0-38%)
pN+ (unilateral)	83%	(79-96%)
pN+ (bilateral)	30%	(12-60%)

REFERENCES

Akporiaye LE, Jordan GH, Devine Jr CJ: Balanitis xerotica obliterans (BXO). AUA Update Series, Vol. 16, Lesson 12, 1997.

Solsona E, et al: Guidelines on penile cancer. European Association of Urology, 2004. (http://www.uroweb.org/nc/professional-resources/ guidelines/online/) [accessed September 2007].

Greene FL, Page DL, Fleming ID, et al. AJCC Cancer Staging Manual, Sixth Edition. New York: Springer 2002. (effective January 1, 2003)

Herr HW: Surgery of penile and urethral carcinoma. Campbell's Urology. 6th Edition. Ed. PC Walsh, AB Retik, TA Stamey, et al. Philadelphia: W. B. Sanders Company, 1992, pp 3073-3089.

Kulaylat MN, Satchidanand SK, Doerr RJ: Buschke-Lowenstein tumor. Surgical Rounds, April 1997: 125.

Lynch DF, Schellhammer PF: Contemporary concepts in ilioinguinal lymphadenectomy for squamous cell carcinoma of the penis. AUA Update Series, Vol. 16, Lesson 33, 1997.

Mukamel E, deKernion JB: Early versus delayed lymph node dissection versus no lymph node dissection for carcinoma of the penis. AUA Update Series, Vol. 9, Lesson 2, 1990.

Schellhammer PF, Jordan GH, Schlossberg SM: Tumors of the penis. Campbell's Urology. 6th Edition. Ed. PC Walsh, AB Retik, TA Stamey, et al. Philadelphia: W. B. Sanders Company, 1992, pp 1264-1294.

Srinivas V, Morse MJ, Herr HW, et al: Penile cancer: relation of extent of nodal metastasis to survival. J Urol, 137: 880, 1987.

Sufrin G, Huben R: Benign and malignant lesions of the penis. Adult and Pediatric Urology. 3rd Edition. Ed. JY Gillenwater, JT Grayhack, SS Howards, et al. Saint Louis: Mosby-Year Book, Inc., 1996, pp 1997-2037.

Thompson IM, Fair WR: Penile carcinoma. AUA Update Series, Vol. 9, Lesson 1, 1990.

TESTICULAR TUMORS

General Information

Primary Testicular Tumors

Germ Cell Tumors (90-95%)	Non-germ Cell Tumors (5-10%)
Seminoma	Leydig Cell Tumor
Non-seminoma	Sertoli Cell Tumor

1. Typical/classic seminoma is the most common type of seminoma.
2. Seminoma
   a. The most common testis tumor in adults.
   b. The most common *bilateral primary* testis tumor.
   c. The most common tumor in an undescended testis.
3. Malignant lymphoma
   a. It is the most common *bilateral* testis tumor (including metastases).
   b. *Lymphoma is the most common metastatic tumor of the testis.*
   c. It is the most common testis tumor in men > 50 years old.
4. Yolk sac tumor—the most common testis cancer in infants and children.
5. Leydig cell tumor—the most common non-germ cell tumor.
6. Mixed tumors are more common than pure tumors.
7. Only 1% of testis tumors are benign.

Etiology

1. Cryptorchidism—the higher the testis location, the higher the risk of cancer. The highest risk occurs with an intra-abdominal testes. Cryptorchidism is more common on the right; thus, testis tumors are more common on the right. In males with unilateral cryptorchidism, the contralateral descended testis has an increased risk of tumor.
2. HIV infection
3. Gonadal dysgenesis with Y chromosome—20-30% develop testicular tumors. These patients should undergo prophylactic gonadectomy.
4. Testicular feminization > 30 years of age—the testes are removed after secondary sexual characteristics develop.
5. Presence of intratubular germ cell neoplasia (see below).
6. Conditions that probably do not increase the risk of testicular cancer
   a. Testis atrophy (nonspecific or mumps induced atrophy) has been suggested as a cause of testis cancer, but is still speculative.
   b. Diethylstilbestrol and oral contraceptives during pregnancy probably do *not* increase the risk of testicular tumors.
   c. Testis tumors usually do not have a genetic predisposition.
   d. Trauma is *not* a cause of tumor, but often prompts medical evaluation.

Intratubular Germ Cell Neoplasia (IGCN)/Carcinoma in Situ

1. IGCN is a pre-malignant non-invasive precursor of germ cell tumors.
2. Risks for IGCN include a history of testicular cancer, atrophic testis, cryptorchidism, extragonadal germ cell cancer, intersex, and infertility.
3. The chance of developing clinical testis cancer from IGCN is unknown.
4. There is controversy regarding several key aspects of IGCN: its clinical significance, the necessity of diagnosis, and the optimal management.
5. Currently, testicle biopsy is the only method to diagnose IGCN.
6. Treatment—see page 64.

Presentation

1. Testis tumors are more common on the right because cryptorchidism is more common on the right.
2. 1-3% of tumors are bilateral (including synchronous and metachronous tumors).
3. Symptoms
   a. *Painless mass or swelling in the testis.*
   b. Back pain from retroperitoneal metastases.
4. Signs
   a. Firm, usually non-tender testis mass.
   b. Abdominal mass—may be present with retroperitoneal metastases.
   c. Gynecomastia—seen in 5% of patients with germ cell tumors, but up to 30-50% of Sertoli or Leydig tumors.
5. Differential diagnosis includes epididymo-orchitis (10% of tumors present with epididymo-orchitis), hydrocele (5-10% of tumors present with hydrocele), testicular torsion, hematoma, and spermatocele.

Age	Most Common Testicular Tumor
0-10	Yolk sac tumor
20-30	Choriocarcinoma
25-35	Embryonal & teratoma
30-40	Classic Seminoma
>50	Malignant lymphoma

Metastasis From Testis Tumors

1. Testis tumors usually metastasize by lymphatic spread. Choriocarcinoma and yolk sac tumor may also metastasize hematogenously.
2. *Retroperitoneal lymph nodes are the most common site of metastasis.*
3. When the normal lymphatic flow has not been altered, lymphatic spread occurs in a predictable and stepwise fashion.
   a. Right testis tumors spread to the *interaortal caval* retroperitoneal nodes.
   b. Left testis tumors spread to the *left para-aortic* retroperitoneal nodes.
   c. *Lymphatic metastases in the retroperitoneum often spread from the right to the left side, but they usually do not spread from left to right.*
4. When lymphatic flow has been altered by tumor invasion or prior surgery
   a. Inguinal nodes may be involved if
      i. The tumor invades beyond the tunica albuginea or into the scrotum.
      ii. There was previous scrotal or inguinal surgery (e.g. inguinal hernia repair, orchiopexy, trans-scrotal orchiectomy, trans-scrotal biopsy).
   b. Pelvic nodes may be involved if the tumor invades into the epididymis or spermatic cord.
5. Distant non-node metastasis (most to least common)—lung, liver, brain, bone, kidney, adrenal, gastrointestinal tract, and spleen.
6. In men with pure seminoma, approximately 20% present with metastasis. In men with non-seminoma, 60-70% present with metastasis.
7. Spermatocytic seminoma has a very low metastatic potential.
8. Choriocarcinoma can present with distant metastasis in the presence of a small (sometimes clinically inapparent) primary testis tumor.

Work Up

1. See Management of Testicular Mass in Adults - Part 1, page 65.
2. History and physical exam including genitals, lymph nodes, abdomen, neurological, and breasts (for gynecomastia).
3. Scrotal ultrasound—if tumor is suspected, obtain the following tests:
   a. Blood tests—serum tumor markers (AFP, HCG, LDH), CBC, creatinine (retroperitoneal metastases can obstruct the ureters), and liver function tests (check for liver metastasis and hepatic causes of elevated AFP).
   b. Chest x-ray—if abnormal, obtain chest CT.
   c. CT abdomen and pelvis—performed after the orchiectomy confirms cancer. If the abdominal CT or chest-ray is abnormal, obtain a chest CT.
   d. Brain MRI or bone scan when clinically indicated.
   e. *Offer sperm banking prior to cancer treatment.*

Stage

TNMS Staging System (AJCC 2002)

<u>Primary Tumor (T)</u> - The extent of the primary tumor is usually classified after radical orchiectomy, and for this reason, a pathologic stage is assigned.

pTx Primary tumor cannot be assessed

pT0 No evidence of primary tumor (e.g. histologic scar in testis)

pTis Intratubular germ cell neoplasia (carcinoma in situ)

pT1 Tumor limited to the testis and epididymis without vascular/lymphatic invasion; tumor may invade into the tunica albuginea but not the tunica vaginalis

pT2 Tumor limited to the testis and epididymis with vascular/lymphatic invasion, or tumor extending through the tunica albuginea with involvement of the tunica vaginalis

pT3 Tumor invades the spermatic cord with or without vascular/lymphatic invasion

pT4 Tumor invades the scrotum with or without vascular/lymphatic invasion

<u>Regional Lymph Nodes (N) - Clinical Stage</u>

Nx Regional lymph nodes cannot be assessed

N0 No regional lymph node metastasis

N1 Metastasis with a lymph node mass 2 cm or less in greatest dimension; or multiple lymph nodes, none more than 2 cm in greatest dimension

N2 Metastasis with a lymph node mass more than 2 cm but not more than 5 cm in greatest dimension; or multiple lymph nodes, any one mass greater than 2 cm but not more than 5 cm in greatest dimension

N3 Metastasis with a lymph node mass more than 5 cm in greatest dimension

<u>Regional Lymph Nodes (N) - Pathologic Stage</u>

pNx Regional lymph nodes cannot be assessed

pN0 No regional lymph node metastasis

pN1 Metastasis with a lymph node mass 2 cm or less in greatest dimension and less than or equal to 5 nodes positive, none more than 2 cm in greatest dimension

pN2 Metastasis with a lymph node mass more than 2 cm but not more than 5 cm in greatest dimension; or more than 5 nodes positive, none more than 5 cm; or evidence of extranodal extension of tumor

pN3 Metastasis with a lymph node mass more than 5 cm in greatest dimension

<u>Distant Metastasis (M)</u>

Mx Distant metastasis cannot be assessed

M0 No distant metastasis

M1 Distant metastasis

M1a Nonregional nodal or pulmonary metastasis

M1b Distant metastasis other than to nonregional nodes and lungs

<u>Serum Tumor Markers (S)</u> - S stage is determined using the nadir value of the post-orchiectomy tumor markers. N = upper limit of normal for LDH.

	LDH		HCG (mIu/ml)		AFP (ng/ml)
S0	Normal	&	Normal	&	Normal
S1	< 1.5 x N	&	< 5,000	&	< 1,000
S2	1.5-10 x N	or	5,000-50,000	or	1,000-10,000
S3	> 10 x N	or	> 50,000	or	> 10,000
Sx	Marker studies not available or not performed				

Stage Grouping

Stage 0	pTis	N0	M0	S0
Stage I	pT1-4	N0	M0	Sx
IA	pT1	N0	M0	S0
IB	pT2	N0	M0	S0
	pT3	N0	M0	S0
	pT4	N0	M0	S0
IS	Any pT/Tx	N0	M0	S1-3
Stage II	Any pT/Tx	N1-3	M0	Sx
IIA	Any pT/Tx	N1	M0	S0
	Any pT/Tx	N1	M0	S1
IIB	Any pT/Tx	N2	M0	S0
	Any pT/Tx	N2	M0	S1
IIC	Any pT/Tx	N3	M0	S0
	Any pT/Tx	N3	M0	S1
Stage III	Any pT/Tx	Any N	M1	Sx
	Any pT/Tx	Any N	M1a	S0
	Any pT/Tx	Any N	M1a	S1
	Any pT/Tx	N1-3	M0	S2
	Any pT/Tx	Any N	M1a	S2
	Any pT/Tx	N1-3	M0	S3
	Any pT/Tx	Any N	M1a	S3
	Any pT/Tx	Any N	M1b	Any S

Used with the permission of the American Joint Committee on Cancer (AJCC), Chicago, Illinois. The original source for this material is the *AJCC Cancer Staging Manual, Sixth Edition* (2002) published by Springer Science and Business Media LLC, www.springerlink.com.

Tumor Markers
1. Beta-human chorionic gonadotropin (HCG)
   a. HCG is produced by syncytiotrophoblasts.
   b. Half life = 24-36 hours.
   c. HCG has the same alpha subunit found in LH, FSH, and TSH.
   d. *HCG is always elevated when choriocarcinoma is present.*
   e. Elevation of HCG can also occur with
      i. Marijuana use.
      ii. Elevation of LH (from bilateral orchiectomy, orchiectomy with atrophy of the contralateral testis, etc.; see Hypergonadotropic Hypogonadism, page 274)—high levels of LH can cross react with some assays for HCG, resulting in a falsely high HCG.
2. Alpha-fetoprotein (AFP)
   a. Half life = 5-7 days.
   b. *AFP is never elevated in pure choriocarcinoma or in pure seminoma.*
   c. Elevation of AFP can also occur with
      i. Liver dysfunction—e.g. post chemotherapy hepatitis.
      ii. Infants less than one year of age—it is normal for newborns to have elevated AFP, which usually declines to the low adult levels by one year of age.
3. Lactate dehydrogenase (LDH)—LDH may be elevated in seminoma and nonseminoma, and can indicate the presence of bulky metastasis.

CT Scan of Abdomen
1. CT cannot differentiate between tumor, teratoma, necrosis, or fibrosis.
2. Abdominal CT has a 25-30% false negative rate (i.e. up to 30% of men with a normal abdominal CT will have tumor in the retroperitoneal nodes). Therefore, CT accurately stages approximately 70% of patients.
3. If the abdominal CT shows tumor, obtain a chest CT.

Risk Categories for Stage IIC and Stage III Germ Cell Tumors

Risk Status	Nonseminoma	Seminoma
Good Risk	All of the following: • Testicular or retroperitoneal primary tumor • M0 or M1a • S0 or S1	All of the following: • Any primary site • M0 or M1a • Normal AFP
Intermediate Risk	All of the following: • Testicular or retroperitoneal primary tumor • M0 or M1a • S2	All of the following: • Any primary site • M1b • Normal AFP
Poor Risk	Any of the following: • Mediastinal primary tumor • M1b • S3	No patients are classified as poor risk

Based on the International Germ Cell Consensus Collaborative Group, J Clin Oncol, 1997. For survival based on these risk groups, see page 75.

Seminoma

Types of Seminoma

1. Classic or typical seminoma (85% of seminomas)
   a. Gross pathology—lobulated and pale color.
   b. Histology—large cells of *uniform size* with *clear cytoplasm and distinct cell borders*. The nuclei may look like a "fried egg" and may contain 2 nucleoli. Syncytiotrophoblasts are seen in 10-15% (parallels the rate of HCG production). Lymphocytic infiltration occurs in 20%.
2. Anaplastic seminoma (10% of seminomas)
   a. Same histology as typical seminoma except it has a high mitotic activity (diagnosis requires ≥ 3 mitosis per high power field).
   b. *Not* more aggressive than typical seminoma (cure rates are similar to typical seminoma); therefore, most experts believe that this is not a distinct form of seminoma. It is usually classified as typical seminoma.
3. Spermatocytic seminoma (5% of seminomas)
   a. Histology—cells of *varying size* that resemble maturing spermatogonia.
   b. Most men have pure spermatocytic seminomas (i.e. not mixed with non-seminoma elements).
   c. The risk of spermatocytic seminoma is not higher in the undescended testicle.
   d. Presents at an older age than classic seminoma (see below).
   e. These tumors are usually treated with radical inguinal orchiectomy and surveillance because of their *low metastatic potential*.

General Information on Seminoma

1. *The diagnosis of pure seminoma requires a normal AFP and orchiectomy histology demonstrating only seminoma (no nonseminoma elements).*
2. *Seminoma is the most common germ cell tumor (65% of germ cell tumors).*
3. Age of presentation—spermatocytic seminoma presents at an older age than classic seminoma (peak age > 50 versus 35-39 years, respectively).
4. At presentation, 75% of tumors are confined to the testis, while 25% present with metastasis. Most metastases are in the retroperitoneal lymph nodes. See Metastasis from Testis, page 59.
5. *Pure seminoma never secretes AFP*, but it secretes HCG in 10% of cases.
6. *Seminoma is radiosensitive.*

Nonseminoma

Mixed Tumor—a combination of seminoma and nonseminoma elements.

Embryonal Carcinoma
1. Presenting age = 25-35.
2. Gross pathology—grey/white fleshy mass with poorly defined capsule. Necrosis and hemorrhage are often present.
3. Histology—epithelial-like cells that form *papillary projections*.
4. Tumor markers—may secrete both AFP and HCG.

Yolk Sac Tumor
1. Presenting age = infants and children
2. Gross pathology—yellow or pale grey.
3. Histology—epithelial-like cells that form cystic spaces. *Schiller-Duvall bodies*, embryoid bodies, and hyaline globules may be seen.
4. Tumor markers—may secrete both AFP and HCG.
5. Metastasis—often metastasizes hematogenously.

Choriocarcinoma
1. Presenting age = 20-30.
2. Gross pathology—grey white mass that tends to be peripheral in testis, often has central region of hemorrhage.
3. Histology—*syncytiotrophoblasts* (multinucleated cells with vacuolated eosinophilic cytoplasm and hyperchromatic nuclei; these cells secrete HCG) and *cytotrophoblasts* (closely packed uniform cells with distinct cell border, clear cytoplasm, and single nucleus).
4. Tumor markers—*never* secretes AFP and *always* secretes HCG.
5. Metastasis—early hematogenous spread especially to lungs. Bizarre metastatic locations such as spleen may be seen. There may be a small primary testis tumor, but a large volume of metastasis.
6. Choriocarcinoma has the worst prognosis of all testis tumors.

Teratoma
1. Presenting age usually = 25-35.
2. Histology—*more than one germ cell layer in different stages of maturation*: endoderm (gastrointestinal, respiratory), mesoderm (bone, cartilage, muscle), and/or ectoderm (squamous epithelium, neural tissue). Teratoma is often cystic (the cyst lining stains positive for CEA).
3. Tumor markers—pure teratoma should not secrete AFP or HCG.
4. Teratoma is resistant to chemotherapy and radiation; therefore, it requires surgical resection.
5. Prepubertal teratoma is usually benign.
6. Teratocarcinoma is mixture of teratoma and embryonal cell carcinoma.

Non-germ Cell Tumors

1. 10% of Leydig cell and Sertoli cell tumors are malignant. The only reliable indicator of malignancy is the presence of metastasis.
2. Leydig cell tumors
   a. Histology—eosinophilic cells, extracellular *Reinke's crystals* (cigar shaped or lobular shaped red crystals).
   b. Leydig cell tumors may produce testosterone and 17-ketosteroid.
   c. Children may present with precocious puberty. Adults may present with gynecomastia, impotence, and low libido. Klinefelter's, adrenal cancer, and congenital adrenal hyperplasia may cause similar symptoms.
3. Sertoli cell tumors may be capable of secreting estrogen or testosterone and may present with virilization or gynecomastia.
4. Non-metastatic tumors are treated with radical inguinal orchiectomy followed by surveillance.

Treatment

Intratubular Germ Cell Neoplasia (IGCN)/Carcinoma in Situ
1. Testicular biopsy may be offered to patients at high risk for IGCN.
2. Management of IGCN may include surveillance, orchiectomy, testis radiation, and chemotherapy. Surveillance is recommended because
   a. Treatment can cause infertility and hypogonadism.
   b. The risk of developing clinical testis cancer from IGCN is unknown.
3. Surveillance includes serial self testis exams and testis exams by a doctor.

General Treatment Concepts
1. See Management of Testicular Mass in Adults - Part 1, page 65.
2. If a solid intratesticular mass is suspected, obtain preoperative tumor markers and perform a *radical inguinal orchiectomy*. Avoid trans-scrotal biopsy and trans-scrotal orchiectomy. Offer a testicular prosthesis.
3. If orchiectomy reveals a testis malignancy, stage the patient.
   a. Post-orchiectomy markers—elimination of markers from the circulation takes ≥ 5 half lives. Postoperatively, wait at least *5 weeks before measuring AFP* (half life = 5-7 days) and at least *1 week before measuring HCG* (half life = 24-36 hours). Measure markers until the nadir is reached. S stage is determined using the nadir value of the post-orchiectomy markers.
   b. CT abdomen and pelvis
   c. If the abdominal CT or chest-ray is abnormal, obtain a chest CT.
   d. Brain MRI or bone scan when clinically indicated.
4. Lymphoma—usually treated with the appropriate systemic therapy.
5. Non-metastatic spermatocytic seminoma, Leydig cell tumor, and Sertoli cell tumor are treated with radical inguinal orchiectomy and surveillance.
6. For adult testis masses without scrotal violation, see pages 65-68.

Scrotal Violation
1. Scrotal violation is present if there is pT4 tumor, previous inguinal surgery, or previous scrotal surgery (including trans-scrotal orchiectomy or biopsy).
2. Men with scrotal violation are not good candidates for surveillance.
3. Trans-scrotal biopsy and trans-scrotal orchiectomy increase the risk of local recurrence, but they do not alter prognosis.
4. Treatment of scrotal violation
   a. After a trans-scrotal biopsy, perform a radical inguinal orchiectomy and excision of the ipsilateral hemiscrotum including the scrotal scar.
   b. After a trans-scrotal orchiectomy, excise the ipsilateral spermatic cord, hemiscrotum, and scrotal scar (may be done during RPLND).
   c. Biopsy the inguinal lymph nodes if they are palpable or enlarged on CT.
   d. For seminoma stage I, IIA, IIB, or M1a in the inguinal nodes, treatment options include chemotherapy or XRT. For XRT, the radiation field should include the bilateral pelvic and bilateral inguinal lymph nodes. If trans-scrotal surgery was performed and scrotectomy did not completely remove the local tumor (i.e. gross tumor spillage, unresectable, positive margins), include the ipsilateral hemiscrotum in the radiation field.
   e. For nonseminoma stage I, IIA, or IIB (no cancer in the inguinal nodes) options include chemotherapy or RPLND. If trans-scrotal surgery was performed and scrotectomy did not completely remove the local tumor, chemotherapy may be preferred.
   f. For nonseminoma with cancer in the inguinal nodes (M1a), consider administering chemotherapy.
   g. Follow up—include inguinal lymph node palpation in the physical examination and include inguinal imaging on CT scan.

Management of Testicular Mass in Adults - Part 1

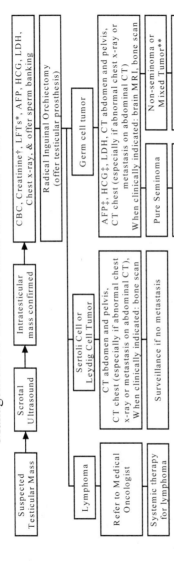

CBC = complete blood count; LFTs = liver function tests; AFP = alpha-fetoprotein; HCG = beta-human chorionic gonadotropin

LDH = lactate dehydrogenase, CT = computerized tomography

* Liver dysfunction can elevate AFP. Liver dysfunction may indicate the presence of liver metastasis.

† Creatinine may be elevated when bulky retroperitoneal metastases obstruct the ureter.

‡ Postoperatively, wait at least 5 *weeks before measuring AFP* (half life = 5–7 days) and at least *1 week before measuring HCG* (half life = 24–36 hours).

Several measurements may be required before the nadir values are reached. S stage is determined using the nadir value of the post-orchiectomy markers.

** A mixed tumor has both seminoma and non-seminoma elements.

Management of Testicular Mass in Adults - Part 2 (PURE SEMINOMA)

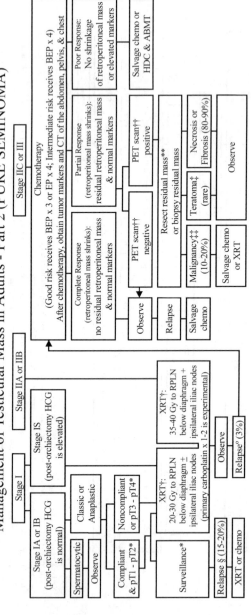

EP = Etoposide and cisplatin; BEP = Bleomycin and EP; CT = Computerized tomography scan; RPLN = Retroperitoneal lymph nodes

XRT = External beam radiation; HDC & ABMT = High dose chemotherapy & autologous bone marrow transplant; HCG = Human chorionic gonadotropin

† Shield the contralateral testis if it is not involved. With scrotal violation (pT4, prior inguinal/scrotal surgery, trans-scrotal orchiectomy or biopsy), include the bilateral pelvic and bilateral inguinal lymph nodes in the radiation field. If trans-scrotal surgery was performed and scrotectomy did not completely remove the local tumor (i.e. gross tumor spillage, unresectable, positive margins), include the ipsilateral hemiscrotum in the radiation field. For men with prior abdominal radiation, inflammatory bowel disease, or the kidney in the radiation field (e.g. horseshoe kidney, ectopic kidney, adenopathy near the kidney), XRT is usually avoided (surveillance is recommend for stage I and chemotherapy is recommended for stage II).

†† When PET is not available, observation is suggested for residual masses ≤ 3 cm (malignancy is rare in these cases), while biopsy/resection is recommended for residual masses > 3 cm (malignancy present in 10-20% of these cases).

§ Approximately 90% of relapses occur in the retroperitoneal lymph nodes. If recurrence occurs only in the retroperitoneal nodes, XRT may be administered. If relapse occurs at other sites, chemotherapy is administered.

○ Relapse after XRT usually occurs outside the retroperitoneum; therefore, chemotherapy is offered to these patients.

* Surveillance is usually recommended for stage I men with prior abdominal radiation, inflammatory bowel disease, or their kidney is in the radiation field (e.g. horseshoe kidney, ectopic kidney). Relapse is more likely in patients with tumors > 4-6 cm in size, rete testis invasion, and age > 34 years; therefore, patients with any of these characteristics should probably be treated with XRT. Men with scrotal violation are not good candidates for surveillance. Example surveillance protocol: chest X-ray, CT abdomen and pelvis, and tumor markers every 3-4 months for 1-3 years, then every 6 months for 4-7 years, then every 12 months thereafter.

** Template RPLND is difficult in these patients because chemotherapy for seminoma causes a desmoplastic reaction that makes it difficult to discern the tissue planes. Resection or biopsy of the residual mass is performed instead.

‡ Rational for resection of teratoma includes 1) it may grow rapidly and cause local complications, 2) after chemotherapy, teratoma can undergo malignant transformation into sarcoma or carcinoma, and 3) teratoma can lead to late recurrences (of both teratoma and other nonseminomatous germ cell tumors).

‡‡ Malignancy occurs in 10-20% of residual retroperitoneal masses > 3 cm in size, but is rare in masses ≤ 3 cm.

Management of Testicular Mass in Adults - Part 3 (NONSEMINOMA & MIXED)

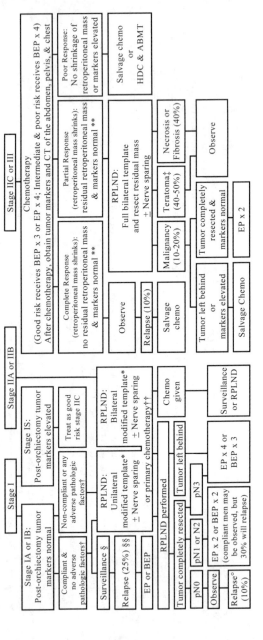

EP = Etoposide and cisplatin; BEP = Bleomycin and EP; CT = Computerized tomography scan; RPLND = retroperitoneal lymph node dissection

HDC & ABMT = High dose chemotherapy and autologous bone marrow transplant;

† Adverse pathologic factors: vascular invasion, lymphatic invasion, stage pT2 or higher, and predominance of embryonal cell carcinoma.

†† For stage I, primary chemotherapy consists of BEP x 2 cycles. For stage IIA and IIB, primary chemotherapy consists of BEP x 3 or EP x 4 cycles.

For stage IIA or IIB, primary chemotherapy is often recommended when post-orchiectomy markers are elevated.

§ Men with scrotal violation or adverse pathologic factors are not good candidates for surveillance. Example surveillance protocol: chest x-ray and tumor markers every 1-2 months for the first year, every 2 months for the second year, every 3 months for the third year, every 4 months for the fourth year, every 6 months for the fifth year, and every 12 months thereafter. Abdominal/pelvic CT scan every 2-3 months for the first year, every 3-4 months for the second year, every 4 months for the third year, every 6 months for the fourth year, and every 12 months thereafter.

§§ 60% of relapses occur in the retroperitoneum, while 40% occur outside the retroperitoneum. 80% of relapses occur within the first year.

° Most relapses occur outside the retroperitoneum, primarily in the lungs.

* If palpable nodal metastases are discovered during a modified template, a full bilateral template should be performed.

** Some will observe patients after chemotherapy if all of the following markers are present: negative post-chemotherapy markers, > 90% reduction in the volume of the retroperitoneal mass after chemotherapy, and no teratomatous elements in the primary tumor.

‡ Rational for resection of teratoma includes 1) it may grow rapidly and cause local complications, 2) after chemotherapy, teratoma can undergo malignant transformation into sarcoma or carcinoma, and 3) teratoma can lead to late recurrences (of teratoma and other nonseminoma tumors).

Children

1. Nonseminoma (except pure teratoma)—boys with stage IA or IB cancer (i.e. stage I with normal post-orchiectomy markers) are treated with radical orchiectomy and surveillance. Boys with stage IS, II or III are treated with radical orchiectomy and chemotherapy.
2. Pure teratoma—teratoma is almost always benign in prepubertal children and is treated with radical orchiectomy and surveillance.
3. Seminoma—usually does not occur in this age group.

Seminoma Stage I—Surveillance, Radiation, or Chemotherapy?

1. Surveillance
   a. Rationale—over 80% with clinical stage N0 (no adenopathy on CT) will have pathologic stage N0 (no cancer in retroperitoneal nodes). If all stage I men receive treatment, over 80% will be treated unnecessarily.
   b. Disadvantages—surveillance has a higher relapse rate than treatment. Strict compliance and intensive follow up are required. Patients may have more psychological stress (worry about the higher recurrence rate).
   c. Indicated for *compliant* stage I with normal post-orchiectomy markers.
   d. Relapse appears to be more likely with tumors > 4-6 cm in size, rete testis invasion, and age > 34 years. Relapses usually occur in the retroperitoneal lymph nodes. 20% of relapses occur more than 4 years after orchiectomy.
   e. Treatment of relapse—restage and treat (XRT or chemotherapy).
2. Abdominal external beam radiation (XRT)—see page 72.
   a. Rationale—very low morbidity and mortality. Men with clinical stage N0 but pathologic stage N1 will be treated.
   b. Disadvantages—recent data suggests that XRT increases the risk of death (by 2-fold) from cardiac disease and secondary cancer starting 15 years after XRT. The risk of secondary malignancy increases with time and may be as high as 18% at 25 years after XRT.
   c. Indicated for stage I men with normal post-orchiectomy tumor markers.
   d. Relapses usually occur outside the retroperitoneum.
   e. Treatment of relapse—chemotherapy.
3. Chemotherapy—still considered experimental.
   a. Rational—may have a lower mortality than XRT (less risk of death from cardiac disease and secondary malignancy). Men with clinical stage N0 but pathologic stage N1 will be treated.
   b. Disadvantages—myelosuppression, nausea, fatigue, and possibly infertility. The long-term effects of chemotherapy are unknown.
   c. 1 or 2 doses of carboplatin appear to be as effective as abdominal XRT.
   d. Relapses usually occur in the retroperitoneal lymph nodes. Optimal treatment of relapse is unknown.

Stage I Seminoma	Surveillance	XRT	Chemotherapy† (Carbo x 1 or 2)
Morbidity	Low	Low	Low
Overall long-term survival	98%	99%	99%
Relapse rate	15-20%	3%	3%
Usual location of relapse	Retroperitoneal Nodes	Outside Retroperitoneum	Retroperitoneal Nodes
Treatment of relapse	XRT or Chemo	Chemo	?

† Chemotherapy is still considered experimental.

Nonseminoma Stage I—RPLND, Surveillance, or Chemotherapy?

1. Surveillance
   a. Rational—70% with clinical stage N0 (no adenopathy seen on CT) will have pathologic stage N0 (no cancer in retroperitoneal nodes). If all stage I patients received treatment, 70% would be treated unnecessarily.
   b. Disadvantages–surveillance has a higher relapse rate than treatment. Strict compliance and intensive follow up are required. Patients may have more psychological stress (worry about the higher recurrence rate).
   c. Relapse is more likely when any of the following are present: lymphatic invasion, vascular invasion, stage pT2 or higher, predominance of embryonal cell carcinoma, and absence of yolk sac elements.
   d. Indicated for *compliant* stage I men with normal post-orchiectomy tumor markers and absence of the following adverse pathologic factors: lymphatic invasion, vascular invasion, pT2 or higher, and predominance of embryonal cell carcinoma.
   e. 60% of relapses occur in the retroperitoneum, while 40% occur outside the retroperitoneum. 80% of relapses develop within 1 year.
   f. Treatment of relapse—chemotherapy.

2. Retroperitoneal lymph node dissection (RPLND)—see page 72.
   a. Rationale—RPLND treats retroperitoneal metastases, permits more accurate staging, and requires less intensive follow up than surveillance.
   b. Disadvantages—RPLND is invasive, it may treat up to 70% of men unnecessarily, can cause ejaculatory dysfunction, and has a small long-term risk of bowel obstruction if performed intraperitoneal. With nerve sparing surgery, ejaculation can be preserved in 99% of men.
   c. Indicated for stage I men with normal post-orchiectomy tumor markers.
   d. Relapses occur in 10% of men who are pN0. Relapses usually occur outside the retroperitoneum. *Relapses in the retroperitoneum are rare.*
   e. Treatment of relapse—chemotherapy.

3. Chemotherapy
   a. Rational—chemotherapy treats metastases (inside or outside the retroperitoneum), is less invasive than RPLND, requires less intensive follow up than surveillance, and has a lower relapse rate than either surveillance or RPLND.
   b. Disadvantages—chemotherapy treats up to 70% of men unnecessarily, it will not adequately treat teratoma if present (see page 72), it may cause infertility, the long-term effects of chemotherapy are unknown, and there is a small risk of secondary malignancy with etoposide.
   c. Chemotherapy in this setting usually consists of 2 cycles of bleomycin, etoposide, and cisplatin (BEP).
   d. Relapses usually occur in the retroperitoneum. Retroperitoneal relapses usually contain teratoma and should be treated with RPLND.
   e. Treatment of relapse—may include RPLND or salvage chemotherapy.

Stage I Nonseminoma	Surveillance	RPLND	Chemotherapy (BEP x 2)
Morbidity	Low	Low	Low
Overall long-term survival	$\geq 98\%$	$\geq 98\%$	$\geq 98\%$
Relapse rate	25-30%	10%*	$\leq 5\%$
Usual location of relapse	Retroperitoneal Nodes	Outside Retroperitoneum	Retroperitoneal Nodes
Treatment of relapse	Chemo	Chemo	RPLND† or chemo

* Relapse rate is 10% when the patient is pathologic stage N0.

† Relapses in the retroperitoneum usually contain teratoma; therefore, they require surgical excision (RPLND).

Nonseminoma Stage I—Risk of Teratoma in Retroperitoneum

1. For nonseminoma tumors, *teratoma may be present in the retroperitoneal lymph nodes despite its absence in the orchiectomy specimen.*

Stage I Nonseminoma Orchiectomy Pathology	Chance of Teratoma in the Retroperitoneal Lymph Nodes
Teratoma absent	6% - 7%
Teratoma present	10% - 19%

2. After primary chemotherapy for stage I nonseminoma, retroperitoneal recurrences usually contain teratoma.
3. Teratoma requires surgical excision because it is unresponsive to chemotherapy and radiation.

Abdominal External Beam Radiation Therapy (XRT) for Seminoma

1. For stage I, 20 Gy appears to be as effective as 30 Gy and seems to reduce acute toxicity, but it is unknown if it reduces late toxicity. Many centers prefer to deliver 25-30 Gy until more data is available.

Stage	XRT Dose	XRT Field
IA or IB	20-30 Gy	Abdominal retroperitoneal nodes below diaphragm* (including the ipsilateral iliac nodes is optional)
IIA or IIB	35-40 Gy	Abdominal retroperitoneal nodes below diaphragm* and ipsilateral iliac nodes

    * Include para-aortic nodes. Shield contralateral testis if it is not involved.

2. When scrotal violation is present, see page 64.
3. Toxicity from abdominal XRT
   a. Acute toxicity—the most common side effect is nausea. Uncommon side effects include vomiting, fatigue, and bone marrow suppression.
   b. Late toxicity—rare instances of peptic ulcer, gastritis, and secondary non-germ cell cancers (e.g. leukemia). The risk of secondary cancer increases with time and may be as high as 18% at 25 years after XRT. Recent data suggests that XRT increases the risk of death (by 2-fold) from cardiac disease and secondary cancer starting 15 years after XRT.
4. The kidney is radiosensitive and can be damaged when radiated.
5. In patients with prior abdominal radiation, inflammatory bowel disease, or a kidney in the expected radiation field (e.g. adenopathy near the kidney, horseshoe kidney, ectopic kidney), consider surveillance for stage IA or IB and chemotherapy for stage IIA or IIB.

Retroperitoneal Lymph Node Dissection (RPLND)

1. Impaired ejaculation after RPLND is caused by injury to post ganglionic sympathetic nerves (T2-L4) and to the hypogastric plexus (sympathetic nerve plexus near the origin of the inferior mesenteric artery [IMA]).
2. Injury to the nerves and the resulting ejaculatory dysfunction can be reduced by two techniques. These two techniques can be used together.
   a. Modified template RPLND—avoids retroperitoneal dissection on the contralateral side (especially below the IMA); therefore, it prevents injury to contralateral nerves (i.e. by reducing the size of the template, it preserves more nerves *outside* the template). The modified template maintains ejaculation in 70-90% of cases.
   b. Nerve sparing—preserves nerves *within* the template.
      i. Nerve sparing is indicated to preserve ejaculatory function or fertility.
      ii. Nerve sparing can be performed in any setting if it does not compromise tumor resection (i.e. post-chemotherapy RPLND, bilateral template RPLND, or modified template RPLND).
      iii. Nerve sparing RPLND maintains ejaculatory function in 99% of appropriately selected men (without compromising tumor removal).

3. RPLND Templates
   a. Margins of resection should never be compromised to maintain the
      template or to preserve ejaculatory function. The template should be
      extended to include nodes suspected of harboring cancer.
   b. Modified templates decrease the morbidity from RPLND (especially
      ejaculatory dysfunction) by limiting dissection on the contralateral side,
      especially below the IMA. A right template is performed for a right
      testis cancer and a left template is performed for a left testis cancer.
      *If palpable nodal metastases are discovered during a modified template,
      a full bilateral template should be performed.*
   c. Full bilateral template—indicated for post-chemotherapy RPLND.
      Limits of resection:
      i.   Superior limit—renal vessels.
      ii. Lateral limit—ureters bilaterally.
      iii. Inferior limit—where ureters cross the iliac arteries.
   d. Bilateral modified template—indicated for clinical stage IIA or IIB
      nonseminoma. Limits of resection:
      i.   Superior limit—renal vessels.
      ii. Ipsilateral limit—ipsilateral ureter.
      iii. Contralateral limit superior to IMA—contralateral ureter.
      iv. Contralateral limit inferior to IMA—aorta and ipsilateral iliac artery.
      v.   Inferior limit—where the ipsilateral ureter crosses the iliac artery.
   e. Unilateral modified template—indicated for clinical stage I
      nonseminoma.
      i.   Limits of resection are the same as for modified bilateral template
           except the contralateral limit superior to IMA is the vena cava for left
           templates and the aorta for right templates.

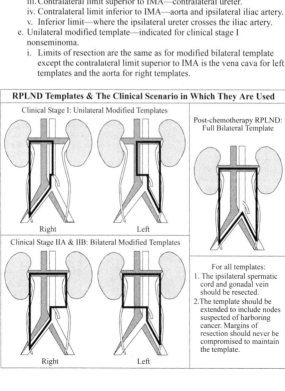

RPLND Templates & The Clinical Scenario in Which They Are Used

Clinical Stage I: Unilateral Modified Templates

Right   Left

Post-chemotherapy RPLND:
Full Bilateral Template

Clinical Stage IIA & IIB: Bilateral Modified Templates

Right   Left

For all templates:
1. The ipsilateral spermatic
   cord and gonadal vein
   should be resected.
2. The template should be
   extended to include nodes
   suspected of harboring
   cancer. Margins of
   resection should never be
   compromised to maintain
   the template.

4. Surgical technique
   a. For nerve sparing, the nerves are *identified prospectively* and preserved.
   b. "*Split and roll*" technique—lymphatic tissue is split on the anterior surface of the great vessel and then rolled off. Ligate the lumbar vessels and remove the lymphatic tissue en bloc.
   c. If necessary, the inferior mesenteric artery can be ligated when the marginal colonic artery is intact.
   d. *The ipsilateral spermatic cord should always be removed.*
5. *Postoperative tachycardia is common and is caused by sympathetic discharge.* Complications include ejaculatory dysfunction, chylous ascites (2%), renal vascular injury (3%), and bowel obstruction (1-3%). The mortality rate of RPLND is approximately 0.3%.
6. The morbidity of post-chemotherapy RPLND is higher than for primary RPLND. The morbidity of post-chemotherapy RPLND is higher for seminoma than for nonseminoma because chemotherapy for seminoma induces a desmoplastic reaction that makes dissection difficult.

Primary Chemotherapy

1. *Platinum (cisplatin) is the most effective agent against germ cell tumors.*
2. The standard chemotherapy regimen is bleomycin, etoposide, and cisplatin (BEP) or etoposide and cisplatin (EP).
3. For clinical stage IIC or III germ cell tumors
   a. *In good risk patients, BEP x 3 cycles is as effective as EP x 4 cycles.* Carboplatin should not be substituted for cisplatin in good risk patients because it results in a lower complete remission rate.
   b. *Intermediate and poor risk patients should receive BEP x 4 cycles.*
4. Bleomycin
   a. Antitumor antibiotic that binds to and breaks DNA.
   b. Side effects—pneumonitis, pulmonary fibrosis, nail and skin changes.
   c. Bleomycin pulmonary toxicity increases the risk of respiratory complications from surgery (e.g. post-chemotherapy RPLND). The risk of complications can be reduced by aggressive monitoring, avoiding over-hydration, preferential use of colloids, judicious use of crystalloids, and keeping fraction of inspired oxygen less than 25% ($FIO_2 < 0.25$).
5. Etoposide (VP-16)
   a. Alkylating agent (covalently binds to DNA).
   b. Dose limiting toxicity = myelosuppression, mucositis. Other side effects include vomiting, alopecia, and *dose related risk of leukemia (rare).*
6. Cisplatin
   a. Cross links DNA.
   b. Dose limiting toxicity = nephrotoxicity. Other side effects include neurotoxicity, ototoxicity, nausea, and vomiting.
   c. *Carboplatin should not be substituted for cisplatin in good risk patients because it results in a lower complete remission rate.* In cases when renal function must be preserved, carboplatin (dose limiting toxicity = myelosuppression) may be substituted for cisplatin (dose limiting toxicity = nephrotoxicity).
7. Carboplatin
   a. Carboplatin is currently being investigated for use in stage I seminoma.
   b. *Carboplatin should not be substituted for cisplatin in good risk patients because it results in a lower complete remission rate.*
   c. Dose limiting toxicity = myelosuppression. Other side effects of carboplatin include nausea, vomiting, and neuropathy.

Salvage Chemotherapy
1. Indicated for men who progress on primary chemotherapy or who relapse after primary chemotherapy.
2. A common salvage chemotherapy regimen is vinblastine, ifosfamide, and cisplatin (VIP) for four cycles.
3. 50% achieve a complete response, but only 25% sustain durable remission.

High Dose Chemotherapy and Autologous Bone Marrow Transplant
1. High dose chemotherapy kills bone marrow; therefore, an autologous bone marrow transplant is given after chemotherapy to reconstitute the marrow.
2. Indicated in patients who had a poor response to standard chemotherapy.
3. Durable remissions are achieved in 10-20% of patients.
4. Treatment related mortality is as high as 10-20%.

Post-Chemotherapy Residual Mass
1. *Residual retroperitoneal masses rarely contain teratoma after primary chemotherapy for seminoma, but 40-50% contain teratoma after primary chemotherapy for nonseminoma.*
2. A residual mass is more likely to contain malignancy after salvage chemotherapy than after primary chemotherapy.

Primary Tumor	Chemotherapy Type	Composition of Post-Chemotherapy Residual Retroperitoneal Mass		
		Malignancy	Teratoma	Necrosis/Fibrosis
Seminoma	Primary	10-20%*	Rare	80-90%
Nonseminoma	Primary	10-20%	40-50%	40%
Any	Salvage	50%	40%	10%

* Malignancy occurs in 10-20% of masses > 3 cm, but is rare in masses < 3 cm.

Survival

Stage	Risk Status	5-Year Overall Survival	
		Seminoma	Nonseminoma
I	—	≥ 98%	≥ 98%
IIA or IIB	—	≥ 95%	≥ 95%
IIC or III	Good	86%	92%
	Intermediate	72%	80%
	Poor	—	48%

REFERENCES

General

Brandes SB: Surgical management of recurrent genitourinary malignancies. AUA Update Series, Vol. 15, Lesson 31, 1996.

Bukowski RM: Management of advanced and extragonadal germ-cell tumors. Urol Clin North Am, 20(1): 153, 1993.

Capelouto CC, Clark PE, et al: A review of scrotal violation in testicular cancer: is adjuvant local therapy necessary? J Urol, 153: 981, 1995.

Dalbagni G, Reuter VE, Fair WR: Testicular carcinoma: in situ. AUA Update Series, Vol. 13, Lesson 38, 1994.

Donohue JP, Foster RS: Management of retroperitoneal recurrences, seminoma and nonseminoma. Urol Clin North Am, 21(4), 1994.

Einhorn LH: Salvage therapy for germ cell tumors. Semin Oncol, 21(4) suppl. 7: 47, 1994.

Greene FL, Page DL, Fleming ID, et al. AJCC Cancer Staging Manual, Sixth Edition. New York: Springer, 2002. (effective January 1, 2003)

International Germ Cell Cancer Collaborative Group. International germ
   cell consensus classification: a prognostic factor-based staging system
   for metastatic germ cell cancers. J Clin Oncol, 15(2): 594, 1997.
National Comprehensive Cancer Network (NCCN) clinical practice
   guidelines in oncology: Testicular cancer. 2007. (http://www.nccn.org).
Richie JP, Steele GS: Neoplasms of the testis. Campbell's Urology. 8th Ed., Ed.
   PC Walsh, et al. Philadelphia: W. B. Sanders Company, 2002, pp 2876-2919.
Roth BJ, Nichols CR: Chemotherapy for testicular cancer: 1994. AUA Update
   Series, Vol. 13, Lesson 22, 1994.
Sagalowsky AI: Current considerations in the diagnosis and initial treatment of
   testicular cancer. Compr Ther, 20(12): 688-694, 1994.
Sheinfeld J, et al: Surgery for testicular cancer. Campbell's Urology. 8th Ed., Ed.
   PC Walsh, et al. Philadelphia: W. B. Sanders Company, 2002, pp 2920-2944.

Nonseminoma & RPLND

Foster RS, Donohue JP: Nerve-sparing RPLND. AUA Update Series, Vol. 12,
   Lesson 15, 1993.
Heidenreich A, Moul JW, et al: The role of retroperitoneal lymphadenectomy in
   mature teratoma of the testis. J Urol, 157(1): 160, 1997.
Herr HW, et al: Management of teratoma. Urol Clin North Am, 20(1): 145, 1993.
Lowe B: Surveillance vs. nerve-sparing retroperitoneal lymphadenectomy in
   stage I nonseminomatous germ-cell tumors. Urol Clin North Am, 20(1): 75,
   1993.
Pohar KS, et al: Results of retroperitoneal lymph node dissection for clinical
   stage I & II pure embryonal carcinoma of the testis. J Urol, 170: 1155, 2003.
Porter J, Obek C, Lange P: The management of stage I nonseminomatous germ
   cell cancer. Campbell's Urology Updates, volume 2, number 3, 2004.
Richie JP: Complications of retroperitoneal lymph node dissection. AUA Update
   Series, Vol. 12, Lesson 16, 1993.
Saxman SB, Nichols CR, Foster RS, et al: The management of patients with
   clinical stage I nonseminomatous testicular tumors and persistently elevated
   serologic markers. J Urol, 155: 587, 1996.
Sheinfeld J, Motzer RJ, et al: Incidence and clinical outcome of patients with
   teratoma in the retroperitoneum following primary retroperitoneal lymph
   node dissection for clinical stages I and IIA nonseminomatous germ cell
   tumors. J Urol, 170: 1159, 2003.

Seminoma & XRT

Aparicio J, et al: Multicenter study evaluating a dual policy of post-orchiectomy
   surveillance and selective adjuvant single agent carboplatin for patients with
   clinical stage I seminoma. Ann Oncol, 14: 867, 2003.
Dieckmann KP, et al: Adjuvant treatment of clinical stage I seminoma: is a single
   course of carboplatin sufficient? J Urol, 55(1): 102, 2000.
Jones WG, et al: Randomized trial of 30 versus 20 Gy in the adjuvant treatment
   of stage I testicular seminoma. J Clin Oncol, 23(6): 1200, 2005.
Oliver RT, et al: Radiotherapy versus single dose carboplatin in adjuvant
   treatment of stage I seminoma. Lancet, 366(9482): 293, 2005.
Wettlaufer JN: The management of advanced seminoma. AUA Update Series,
   Vol. 9, Lesson 11, 1990.
Zagars GK, et al: Mortality after cure of testicular seminoma. J Clin Oncol,
   22(4): 6540, 2004.

Postchemotherapy Residual Mass

Sheinfeld J, Bajorin D: Management of the postchemotherapy residual mass.
   Urol Clin North Am, 20(1): 133, 1993
Sheinfeld J, et al: Management of postchemotherapy residual masses in
   advanced germ cell tumors. AUA Update Series, Vol. 17, Lesson 3, 1997.

PROSTATE CANCER

General Information
1. Prostate cancer is the most common internal tumor in U.S. males and the second leading cause of cancer death in U.S. men.
2. Most prostate cancers do not cause death (< 10% of those with prostate cancer will die from prostate cancer).
3. Only 25% of prostate cancers are thought to be clinically significant.
4. The most common type of prostate cancer is adenocarcinoma.

Presentation
1. Age—usually presents at age ≥ 65 (30-40% of men > 50 years of age have prostate cancer).
2. Most patients are asymptomatic.
3. With advanced cancer, symptoms may include hematuria, urinary obstruction, and bone pain from bone metastases.

Etiology
These populations are at increased risk for prostate cancer:
1. Family history of prostate cancer—the risk is higher when prostate cancer is present in a first degree relative (brother or father) than in a second degree relative (grandfather or uncle). The risk of prostate cancer increases by over 2 fold when a first degree relative has prostate cancer.
2. African American race
3. Higher age (especially age > 65)

Incidental Prostate Cancer
1. 28-61% of patients undergoing radical cystectomy are found to have incidental prostate adenocarcinoma.
2. Up to 10% of patients undergoing TURP are found to have incidental prostate cancer.

Metastasis from the Prostate
Common metastatic locations (listed most common to least common): pelvic lymph nodes, bone, lung, liver.

Prevention
1. Prostate Cancer Prevention Trial (PCPT)—examined finasteride for prevention of prostate cancer. Over 18,000 men with age ≥ 55, normal prostate exam, and PSA ≤ 3.0 were randomized to finasteride 5 mg po q day or to placebo and followed for 7 years. [N Engl J Med, 349: 213, 2003]
   a. Finasteride decreased the risk of developing prostate cancer by 25%, but men taking finasteride were more likely to have high grade cancers and sexual side effects (e.g. erectile dysfunction and loss of libido).
   b. The reduced risk of developing prostate cancer must be balanced against the higher risk of developing sexual side effects and high grade cancer.
   c. Using finasteride for prostate cancer prevention is controversial.
2. The REDUCE trial is evaluating dutasteride for the prevention of prostate cancer. Results are pending.
3. The SELECT trial is currently examining the use of vitamin E and selenium for the prevention of prostate cancer. Men with age ≥ 55, normal prostate exam, and PSA ≤ 4.0 are randomized to one of four treatment arms: placebo, selenium, vitamin E, selenium and vitamin E.
4. Dietary changes may help prevent prostate cancer (see page 84).

Pathology

Types of Prostate Cancer
1. Adenocarcinoma (> 95%)—arises from the prostate gland epithelial cells.
2. Non-adenocarcinomas (< 5%)—transitional cell carcinoma is the most common non-adenocarcinoma. Others: small cell carcinoma, sarcoma, etc.

Diagnostic Criteria
1. Prostate adenocarcinoma originates from prostate *epithelial cells*. These cells stain positive for prostatic acid phosphatase (PAP) and for PSA.
2. Normal prostate glands always have a basal cell layer. *Prostate adenocarcinoma never has a basal cell layer* (not even an incomplete layer). Basal cells stain positive for high molecular weight keratin (HMWK) but negative for PSA and PAP. Therefore, when it is difficult to determine if the cells are malignant, stain the slide with HMWK. If glandular structures lack basal cells (negative HMWK), cancer is present.
3. For grading of prostate adenocarcinoma, see Gleason Score, page 81.

Location of Prostate Cancer
1. *The most common location of prostate cancer is the peripheral zone* (see table).
2. Prostate cancer tends to be multifocal.
3. 60% of cancers are within 5 mm of the urethra, 35% are within 1 mm of the urethra.

Location of Prostate Cancer	
Peripheral Zone	70%
Transition Zone	20%
Central Zone	5-10%
Anterior Prostate	Rare

Local Cancer Spread
1. *Capsular penetration is most common near the neurovascular bundle.*
2. The border between the peripheral and the transition zone may prevent peripheral zone cancers from spreading toward the urethra.
3. Capsular penetration is twice as common in peripheral zone cancers as in transition zone cancers.
4. Capsular penetration is more common in patients with higher clinical stage, higher Gleason score, and higher preoperative PSA.

Prostatic Intraepithelial Neoplasia (PIN)
1. PIN is thought to be a pre-malignant dysplasia of prostatic epithelial cells.
2. These dysplastic cells are located in glands that *have a basal cell layer.*
3. PIN is categorized as low grade or high grade.
4. PIN is seen in 80% of men with prostate cancer.
5. *After a 10-12 core biopsy, 10-20% of men with high grade PIN develop prostate cancer.* After a 6 core biopsy, 20-40% of men with high grade PIN will develop prostate cancer. Low grade PIN does not seem to increase the risk of developing cancer.
6. In patients with high grade PIN, The National Comprehensive Cancer Network (NCCN) guidelines recommend re-biopsy in 1-3 years. See Management of Biopsy Results, page 80.
7. If the patient has low grade PIN without cancer, do an annual digital rectal exam (DRE) and PSA. Biopsy again if indicated based on PSA and DRE.
8. The presence of PIN does not seem to alter the PSA.

Atypia and Atypical Glands
1. These terms are synonymous: atypia, atypical glands, atypical hyperplasia, atypical adenomatous hyperplasia, and atypical small acinar proliferation.
2. *40-60% of men with atypia will develop prostate cancer.* The chance of developing cancer is higher with atypical glands than with high grade PIN.
3. If atypia is present without cancer, the NCCN recommends re-biopsy within 3 months with increased sampling from the atypical region and from adjacent regions. See Management of Biopsy Results, page 80.
4. The presence of atypia does not seem to alter PSA.

Work Up and Diagnosis

Screening for Prostate Cancer

1. Current evidence suggests that screening with PSA may improve survival.
   a. Several trials suggest that screening reduces mortality from prostate cancer. However, there has been methodological problems with these studies. Results from definitive trials (PLCO and ERSPC) are pending.
   b. Prospective randomized trials designed to determine if screening for prostate cancer improves survival. Results are expected soon.
      - PLCO (Prostate, Lung, Colorectal, Ovarian cancer screening trial)
        Men age 55 to 74 are randomized to receive either no screening or an annual PSA and digital rectal exam (DRE). The enrollment was more than 74,000 men (37,000 in each arm). This trial was closed in 2001.
      - ERSPC (European Randomized Study for screening of Prostate Cancer)
        This trial is similar to the PLCO, but is being conducted in Europe. With 10 years of follow up, PLCO has shown that screening reduces the risk of being diagnosed with metastatic prostate cancer by 50%.
2. Current screening recommendations (based on the American Cancer Society, NCCN, and American Urologic Association Guidelines)
   a. Prior to testing, men should have an opportunity to learn about the benefits and limitations of prostate cancer detection and treatment so that they can make an informed decision with a clinician's assistance.
   b. Screening generally consists of an *annual PSA and DRE*.
   c. In men with > 10 years life expectancy, start screening when
      - Age 40-45 in men at high risk for prostate cancer (e.g. African-American men or men with a family history of prostate cancer).
      - Age 40-50 in all other men (NCCN recommends starting at age 40; AUA and ACS recommend starting at age 50).
3. Screening may be continued in men > 70 years of age, especially if they are healthy and have at least 10 years of life expectancy.
4. Prostate imaging is *not* recommended for screening because it does not improve cancer detection compared to DRE.
5. *Over 90% of prostate cancers detected by screening are clinically localized.*

Prostate Biopsy

1. Indications for prostate biopsy
   a. Abnormal digital rectal exam (DRE).
   b. Abnormal PSA (see page 120).
   c. A rising PSA—a significant rise in PSA from test to test or an elevated PSA velocity (PSAV).
2. The chart below recommends when to biopsy

PSA	DRE	Diagnostic Action
PSA ≤ Age specific reference range†, *and* PSA Velocity normal*, *and* No significant PSA rise from test to test	Normal	Annual DRE and PSA
PSA > Age specific reference range†, *or* PSA Velocity worrisome*, *or* Significant PSA rise from test to test	Normal	Prostate Biopsy
Any value	Abnormal	Prostate Biopsy

† % Free PSA may be helpful in determining need for biopsy (see page 120).
* For total PSA < 4 ng/ml, PSA velocity > 0.35 ng/ml/year is worrisome for prostate cancer. For total PSA > 4 ng/ml, PSA velocity > 0.75 ng/ml/year is worrisome for prostate cancer.

3. Biopsy technique
   a. At least 10 systematic cores improve cancer detection over 6 cores ("sextant biopsy"). One biopsy technique includes 12 cores: standard sextant biopsy (bilateral para-sagittal peripheral zone cores at the base, mid, and apical prostate), 2 laterally directed peripheral zone cores on each side, and an apical-anterior core on each side.
   b. Biopsy all hypoechoic regions and palpable nodules. Prostate cancer is found in 30% of hypoechoic lesions and in 30-50% of palpable nodules.
   c. Pain during prostate biopsy can be alleviated by transrectal injection of local anesthetic (prostate block) before the biopsy.
   d. Transrectal ultrasound is usually used to guide the biopsies.
4. Most prostate cancers appear isoechoic on ultrasound because they are too small to be visualized. *When prostate cancers are large enough to be visualized on ultrasound, they are usually hypoechoic.* Rarely, prostate cancers are hyperechoic.
5. Side effects of biopsy—see table.
6. Antibiotic prophylaxis—the optimal prophylactic regimen is unknown.
7. For patients without an anus (e.g. status post abdominoperineal resection), a transperineal or transgluteal CT or MRI guided prostate biopsy may be performed.

Prostate Biopsy Side Effect	% of Patients
Gross hematuria	$\leq 58\%$
Hematospermia	$< 46\%$
Rectal bleeding	$\leq 37\%$
Fever	$\leq 6.2\%$
Vasovagal episode	5.3%
Urinary retention	$\leq 1.2\%$
Sepsis	$< 0.6\%$

Management of Biopsy Results (based of NCCN 2007 Guidelines)

Abnormal PSA or DRE

Prostate Biopsy

Negative or Low Grade PIN	High Grade PIN	Atypia	Prostate Cancer
Continue to follow PSA & DRE	Re-biopsy* in 1-3 Years	Extended† Re-biopsy* within 3 Months	Work up, Stage & Treat

* Re-biopsy should include sampling from the lateral peripheral zone and apical anterior prostate. Transition zone biopsies are optional.

† Extended re-biopsy should also include increased sampling of the atypical region and its adjacent regions.

Increasing PSA after Negative Prostate Biopsy
1. Options for evaluation include
   a. PCA3—after prostate message, the patient voids. Prostate cells in the urine are analyzed for overexpression of the PCA3 gene. The PCA3 score is the ratio of PCA3 mRNA to PSA mRNA multiplied by 1,000. A PCA3 score ≥ 35 suggests a high risk of prostate cancer.
   b. Re-biopsy—at least 12 cores including cores from the lateral prostate and apical anterior prostate ($\pm$ transition zone).

PCA3 Score	Risk of Cancer
< 5	12%
5-19	17%
20-34	23%
35-49	32%
50-100	45%
>100	50%

   c. Saturation biopsy—more than 16 cores including cores from the lateral prostate, apical anterior prostate, and transition zone. This may be most useful in men with multiple negative 10-12 core biopsies.
   d. Transurethral biopsy (TURP biopsy)—may be useful in men with a negative saturation biopsy.

Work Up

1. PSA $\pm$ % free PSA (see Prostate Specific Antigen, page 119).
2. Prostate exam
3. Prostate biopsy (For biopsy indications, see Prostate Biopsy, page 79).
4. If cancer is present on the biopsy, work up for metastasis may be indicated.
   a. Chest x-ray
   b. Bone scan is recommended in patients with PSA > 20, clinical stage T3-T4, Gleason score $\geq$ 8, bone pain, elevated alkaline phosphatase, or elevated serum calcium (these men have a higher risk of bone metastasis).

Pre-treatment Total PSA (ng/ml)	Probability of Positive Bone Scan
< 10	$\leq 0.8\%$
10-20	< 5%
20-50	11%
> 50	> 40%

   c. Pelvic CT or MRI is indicated in patients with clinical stage T3-T4 or a when a nomogram indicates > 20% risk of lymph node metastasis.
   d. If bone scan and pelvic CT/MRI are negative, Prostascint® scan (see page 158) and/or endorectal MRI may be helpful in patients with a high risk of extra-prostatic cancer.
   e. Work up of a suspected bone metastasis—the initial test is a bone scan. If abnormalities are present but the diagnosis is inconclusive, perform this sequence of tests until metastasis are confirmed or ruled out.

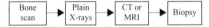

Bone scan → Plain X-rays → CT or MRI → Biopsy

Stage and Grade

Gleason Score

The Gleason grading system is based on the *architectural pattern* of the prostate glands. Cellular characteristics (such as mitoses, nucleoli, etc.) are not used to determine Gleason grade. The two most representative areas of the tumor are graded from 1 to 5. These two grades are added to obtain the Gleason score or Gleason sum. The Gleason score is reported as the most prevalent grade plus the second most prevalent grade, followed by the sum (e.g. 4+3=7). The higher the grade and the sum, the worse the prognosis.

Gleason Grade	Tumor Confined to Well-circumscribed Nodules	Stroma Present Between Each Gland	Variability in Gland Size and Morphology
1	Yes	Yes	None (large uniform glands)
2	Yes	Yes	Minimal
3	No	Yes	Moderate
4	No	No (Fused glands)	Fused ("back to back") glands or cribriform glands
5	No	No glands evident (i.e. tumor cells don't form a lumen). Single tumor cells in the stroma or solid sheets, nests, or cords of tumor.	

TNM Stage (AJCC 2002)

The side on which the lymph nodes are involved does not affect the N stage. This classification applies only to adenocarcinoma. Surgical margin status should be specified with pathologic stage.

Primary Tumor (T) - Clinical Stage
Tx	Primary tumor cannot be assessed
T0	No evidence of primary tumor
T1	Clinically inapparent tumor neither palpable nor visible by imaging
T1a	Tumor incidental histologic finding in $\leq$ 5% of tissue resected
T1b	Tumor incidental histologic finding > 5% of tissue resected
T1c	Tumor identified by needle biopsy (e.g. because of elevated PSA)*
T2	Tumor confined to prostate*
T2a	Tumor involves one-half of 1 lobe or less.
T2b	Tumor involves more than one-half of 1 lobe but not both lobes
T2c	Tumor involves both lobes
T3	Tumor extends through the prostate capsule
T3a	Extracapsular extension (unilateral or bilateral)
T3b	Tumor invades the seminal vesicle(s)
T4	Tumor is fixed or invades adjacent structures other than seminal vesicles: bladder neck, external sphincter, rectum, levator muscles, and/or pelvic wall

* Tumor found in one or both lobes by needle biopsy, but not palpable or reliably visible by imaging, is classified as T1c.

Primary Tumor (T) - Pathologic Stage
pT2†	Organ confined (i.e. no capsular penetration)
	pT2a Unilateral, involving one-half of 1 lobe or less
	pT2b Unilateral, involving more than one-half of 1 lobe, but not both lobes
	pT2c Bilateral disease
pT3	Extraprostatic extension
	pT3a Extraprostatic extension**
	pT3b Seminal vesicle invasion
pT4	Invasion of the bladder, rectum

† There is no pathologic T1 classification

**Positive surgical margin should be indicated by an R1 descriptor (residual microscopic disease).

Regional Lymph Nodes (N) - Clinical Stage
Nx	Regional lymph nodes cannot be assessed or were not sampled
N0	No regional lymph node metastasis
N1	Metastasis in regional lymph node(s)

Regional Lymph Nodes (N) - Pathologic Stage
pNx	Regional nodes not sampled
pN0	No positive regional lymph nodes
pN1	Metastasis in regional node(s)

M Stage
Mx	Distant metastasis cannot be assessed
M0	No distant metastasis
M1	Distant metastasis
	M1a Non-regional lymph node(s)
	M1b Bone(s)
	M1c Other site(s) with or without bone disease

Used with the permission of the American Joint Committee on Cancer (AJCC), Chicago, Illinois. The original source for this material is the *AJCC Cancer Staging Manual, Sixth Edition* (2002) published by Springer Science and Business Media LLC, www.springerlink.com.

Risk Categories

1. *A pretreatment PSA velocity > 2.0 ng/ml per year, high PSA at diagnosis, biopsy Gleason score 8-10, and a palpable nodule all increase the risk of death from prostate cancer.*
2. PSA, biopsy Gleason score, and clinical T stage can be used to stratify the risk for biochemical failure and cancer specific mortality after treatment.

Risk Level†	Criteria		
Low	PSA < 10 &	Gleason score ≤ 6 &	Clinical stage T1 or T2a
Intermediate*	PSA = 10-20 or	Gleason score = 7 or	Clinical stage T2b or T2c
High	PSA > 20 or	Gleason score ≥ 8 or	Clinical stage T3

* Patients with multiple risk factors may be upgraded to high risk.
† Some urologists increase the risk to the next higher level when the prostate biopsy reveals abundant cancer (e.g. prostate cancer in > 50% of cores).

Treatment

General Concepts of Treatment

1. For low risk prostate cancer, radical prostatectomy (RP), external beam radiation (XRT), and permanent brachytherapy have similar cure rates.
2. For high risk prostate cancer, RP, XRT alone, and XRT with brachytherapy have higher cure rates than permanent brachytherapy alone. Therefore, *brachytherapy alone is not recommended for high risk patients.*
3. Prospective randomized trials comparing curative treatments
   a. XRT vs. cryotherapy—men with T1-3, NxM0, and PSA < 20 were treated with neoadjuvant androgen deprivation and randomized to XRT (68-73 Gy) or cryotherapy. At a median follow up of 73 months, overall survival and PSA recurrence are similar [J Urol, 177(4): 376, 2007].
   b. SPIRIT—RP vs. brachytherapy. Cancelled because of poor accrual.
   c. SWOG 8890—RP vs. XRT. Cancelled because of poor accrual.
4. Primary treatment options for localized prostate cancer
   a. Radical prostatectomy (see page 85)
   b. External beam radiation (see page 87)
   c. Brachytherapy (interstitial radiation)
      i. Permanent brachytherapy ± XRT (see page 89)
      ii. Temporary (high dose rate) brachytherapy ± XRT (see page 90)
   d. Cryotherapy (see page 84)
   e. Particle beam therapy (see page 90)
   f. Surveillance (see page 83)
5. Treatment options for local control of advanced progressive cancer—see Treatment Options for Advanced/Metastatic Disease, page 95
6. Treatment options for metastatic cancer—see page 93.

Surveillance ("Watchful Waiting")

1. The best candidates for surveillance have low risk prostate cancer and a life expectancy < 10 years.
2. The optimal surveillance protocol is unknown. Surveillance may include periodic PSA, prostate exam, and prostate biopsy (check for an increase in Gleason score and tumor volume).
3. During surveillance, dietary modification may be helpful (see page 84). Some dietary substances may lower the PSA. It is possible that these substances reduce PSA without altering the cancer itself. Thus, a lower PSA from dietary modification may provide a false sense of security.
4. 50% of men undergoing surveillance elect to undergo treatment within 2 to 5 years. The cure rate of men who opt for treatment after surveillance appears to be similar to men who undergo therapy at the time of diagnosis.

5. Most cancers have an indolent course for 10-15 years. However, the risk of metastasis and death from prostate cancer increases after 15 years of observation. Mortality is greatest for tumors with a higher Gleason score.

Gleason Score	Approximate Percent of Conservatively Treated Men that Die of Prostate Cancer Within 15 years of Diagnosis*	
	Diagnosed at Age 55-64	Diagnosed at Age 65-74
2-4	4-5%	6-7%
5	6-8%	10-11%
6	18-23%	27-30%
7	62-70%	42-53%
8-10	81-87%	60-72%

* Based on data collected prior to the PSA era and most cancers diagnosed by TURP.

6. Surveillance versus treatment
   a. *A prospective randomized trial compared surveillance versus radical prostatectomy* in men with mean age of 65, PSA < 50, and clinical stage T1 or T2. Distribution of cancers in this study showed 76% were clinical stage T2, 48% were Gleason score 5-6, 23% were Gleason score 7, 37% had PSA 4-10, and 47% had PSA 20-50. At 10 years follow up, *men undergoing surveillance had a significantly higher rate of local progression (44% vs. 19%), a higher rate of distant metastasis (25% vs. 15%), and were more likely to die from prostate cancer (death rate 15% vs. 10%).* Radical prostatectomy reduced disease-specific mortality mainly in men age < 65 years. [N Engl J Med, 352: 1977, 2005]
   b. PIVOT trial (Prostate cancer Intervention Vs. Observation Trial)—Men age ≤ 75 with T1 or T2 prostate cancer and PSA ≤ 50 were randomized to surveillance or radical prostatectomy. Results are pending.

Diet Modification

1. Laboratory and epidemiologic data suggest that certain dietary elements may inhibit the growth of prostate cancer. Some diet modifications have been shown to prolong PSA doubling time. It is unknown if these modifications prevent prostate cancer or if they improve survival.
2. The risk, optimal dose, and efficacy of these substances are unknown.
3. Diet supplements and modifications that may be helpful
   a. Low fat diet
   b. Soy protein—the beneficial effects are thought to arise from *isoflavones* (primarily genistein and daidzein).
   c. Vitamin E
   d. Vitamin D
   e. Selenium
   f. Green Tea—the beneficial effects are thought to arise from *polyphenols*.
   g. Lycopene—present in tomatoes, tomato paste, and tomato juice.
   h. High fiber diet and whole grains

Cryotherapy

1. Using transrectal ultrasound guidance, percutaneous cryoprobes are inserted through the perineum and into the prostate. The tips of these probes freeze the prostate. This can be performed in a minor surgical procedure in which the patient goes home within 24 hours.
2. The advancing edge of the ice ball is monitored by transrectal ultrasound. Thermocouples can be used to monitor critical areas such as the sphincter.
3. A urethral warming device helps prevent freezing injury to the urethra.
4. Adequate cell kill requires 2 freeze-thaw cycles. The optimum freezing temperature is unknown, but recent data suggests that reaching at least -40° C during each freeze will induce adequate prostate necrosis.

Radical Prostatectomy (RP)

General Information

1. Predicting recurrence free survival after radical prostatectomy
   a. Kattan preoperative nomogram [J Natl Cancer Inst, 98(10): 715, 2006].
   b. Kattan postoperative nomogram [J Clin Oncol, 23(28): 7005, 2005].
   c. Hopkins pre- and post-operative nomogram [J Urol, 169: 517, 2003].
2. Predicting surgical pathology based on preoperative (clinical) factors—see the Partin Nomogram [Urology, 69(6): 1095, 2007].
3. *A preoperative PSA velocity > 2.0 ng/ml per year, high PSA at diagnosis, Gleason score 8-10, and a palpable nodule all increase the risk of death from prostate cancer.*
4. Pelvic lymph node dissection (PLND)
   a. Some urologists recommend omitting PLND if the PSA < 20, Gleason score < 7, *and* clinical stage is T1-T2 (pelvic imaging and seminal vesical biopsy should also be negative if they were performed).
   b. Complications of PLND—these complications are rare.
      i. Iliac vessel injury
      ii. Lymphocele—if the lymphocele is symptomatic or infected, place a percutaneous drain. Send the fluid for spot creatinine and culture. Spot creatinine will be 25-450 mg/dl for a urine leak (urinoma), but it will be similar to serum creatinine for a lymphocele (0.5-1.5 mg/dl for normal kidney function). Remove the drain when output is minimal and infection has resolved. If lymph output persists, consider infusing a sclerosing agent (e.g. doxycycline) into the lymphocele or performing a peritoneal window (laparoscopic or open). Consider a follow up pelvic ultrasound to rule out recurrence.
      iii. Leg lymphedema—if leg swelling occurs postoperatively, obtain a lower extremity doppler to check for deep venous thrombosis. If this is negative, obtain a pelvic CT to check for lymphocele.
      iv. Obturator nerve injury—if the nerve is severed, the nerve ends can be re-approximated. Obturator nerve injury may impair leg adduction. If this symptom persists, consider obtaining a pelvic CT (a lymphocele may be compressing the nerve) and referral to neurologist.
5. Bladder neck preservation
   a. Does not improve the final degree of urinary continence, but it may permit continence to return sooner after surgery.
   b. Results in a lower rate of bladder neck contracture.
   c. Cancer control is probably not compromised. Intraoperative bladder neck biopsies can be performed to exclude residual tumor.
6. Surgical margins during prostatectomy
   a. The most common site of a positive margin is the *apex* for retropubic prostatectomy and *anterior* for perineal prostatectomy.
   b. Positive margins are more likely to occur with
      • Higher preoperative PSA (especially PSA > 10 ng/ml)
      • High Gleason score (especially Gleason > 7)
      • High clinical tumor stage (especially T2b-T4)
      • High number of positive prostate biopsies
   c. Men with positive margins are more likely to recur. Approximately 50% of men with positive margins recur.
   d. In men with positive margins, adjuvant XRT decreases biochemical and local recurrence, but has not been shown to improve survival.
   e. *The size of a negative margin does not impact prognosis. In other words, a close margin achieves the same cure rate as an ample margin; therefore a close margin should be considered as truly negative.*

7. Radical prostatectomy reduces local progression, metastasis, and death from prostate cancer compared to surveillance, especially in age < 65.
8. Complications and side effects of RP include
   a. Erectile dysfunction—see below and see page 245.
   b. Stress urinary incontinence (SUI)–often occurs, but usually improves during the year after surgery. Younger men recover continence more completely than older men. Chronic severe SUI probably occurs in <5%. See Post-prostatectomy Incontinence, page 200.
   c. Infertility and aspermia—always occurs.
   d. Bladder neck contracture—uncommon.
   e. Other risks include infection, bleeding, inguinal hernia (uncommon), shortening of penile length, and rectal injury (rare). Also see Complications of PLND, page 85.

Erectile Dysfunction After Radical Prostatectomy

1. After RP, approximately 70% of men will have a decrease in penile length (mean loss of length = 1 cm, range = 0 to 5 cm).
2. Potency after radical prostatectomy is better when
   a. Preoperative erectile function is good.
   b. Age is less than 60.
   c. Nerve sparing is performed—bilateral nerve sparing results in a higher chance of potency than unilateral nerve sparing.
3. Nerve Sparing
   a. The *neurovascular bundles (NVB) course posterior-lateral to the prostate* and are composed of cavernous blood vessels and nerves (which induce erections). During nerve sparing, the NVB are preserved by dissecting them away from the prostate.
   b. In appropriately selected patients, cancer control is probably not compromised by nerve sparing. Intraoperative frozen sections of the prostate may help exclude cancer near the neurovascular bundle.
   c. The ideal candidate for nerve sparing would have clinical stage T1 or T2, PSA < 10, Gleason score < 7, small volume of cancer on prostate biopsies, and good preoperative potency. These patients tend to have organ confined cancer that has not invaded the neurovascular bundle.
4. For further details, see ED After Radical Prostatectomy, page 245.

Treatment of Positive Lymph Nodes Found During RP

1. The "Messing" trial (ECOG 3886) included men who underwent radical prostatectomy and pelvic lymph node dissection for clinical stage T1-T2 prostate cancer and who had *microscopic* pelvic lymph node metastasis. Men were prospectively randomized immediately after surgery to surveillance or long-term hormone therapy (LHRH agonist or orchiectomy). At a median follow up of 12 years, disease-specific survival and overall survival were significantly better for immediate hormone therapy than for surveillance. *Thus, immediate hormone therapy after prostatectomy in men with stage N1 improves survival.*
2. In EORTC 30846, men with *microscopic or gross* pelvic lymph node metastasis who did *not* undergo prostatectomy were randomized to surveillance or immediate hormone therapy (LHRH agonist or orchiectomy). With a median follow up of 9.6 years, there was no difference in disease-specific survival.
3. Postoperative pelvic radiation in patients with positive lymph nodes does not appear to be beneficial.
4. When grossly positive lymph nodes are found during surgery, many urologists do not proceed with prostatectomy because there is no convincing evidence that prostatectomy improves survival in this setting.

Neoadjuvant Androgen Deprivation (NAD) before RP

1. *Neoadjuvant androgen deprivation (NAD) has not improved disease-free or overall survival. Thus, NAD is not recommended before RP.*
2. NAD decreases the incidence of positive surgical margins and capsular penetration (and thus increases incidence of organ confined disease).
3. NAD does not appear to alter tumor grade, seminal vesicle invasion, or incidence of lymph node metastasis.
4. NAD does not affect operative time, operative blood loss, or hospital stay.

Radiation Therapy After RP

1. Adjuvant XRT—administered shortly after RP for adverse pathologic findings. It is usually administered after the patient regains urinary continence (e.g. within 4-9 months of RP).
   a. In men with a positive surgical margin, extracapsular extension, or seminal vesicle invasion, adjuvant XRT reduces biochemical and local recurrence, but has not been shown to improve survival. Adjuvant XRT may reduce distant metastasis (evidence is conflicting).
   b Adjuvant XRT increases the risk of urinary incontinence, proctitis, erectile dysfunction, and urethral stricture.
   c. Some patients receiving adjuvant XRT will be treated unnecessarily because they would be cured by RP alone.
2. Salvage XRT—administered when biochemical or local relapse occurs. Waiting until the patient recurs avoids unnecessary XRT in patients who are cured by RP alone. See Salvage XRT, page 92.
3. Retrospective data suggests that the biochemical relapse is similar when comparing patients who do not undergo adjuvant XRT (RP with or without salvage XRT) and patients who undergo adjuvant XRT. In other words, *when the postoperative PSA is undetectable in men with adverse pathologic findings, it is unknown whether it is better to administer adjuvant XRT or to delay XRT until the PSA becomes detectable.*
4. In men undergoing salvage or adjuvant XRT who had lymph node metastasis, seminal vesicle invasion, capsular penetration, preoperative PSA > 20, or Gleason score $\geq$ 8, whole pelvic XRT with concurrent androgen deprivation results in higher relapse free survival than XRT only to the prostate bed. *For salvage or adjuvant XRT after RP in men whose cancer has adverse prognostic factors, consider XRT to the whole pelvis with concurrent androgen deprivation.*

Radiation Therapy

External Beam Radiation (XRT)

1. Predicting biochemical disease-free survival after XRT—see pretreatment nomogram for 3D C-XRT and IMRT [Urology, 70(2): 283, 2007].
2. Common XRT Techniques
   a. Four field box technique—superseded by 3D C-XRT and IMRT.
   b. Three dimensional conformal radiation therapy (3D C-XRT)—permits higher prostate doses compared to 4 field box XRT, but delivers less radiation to surrounding tissue. 3D C-XRT causes less acute and long-term side effects than 4 field box XRT.
   c. Intensity modulated radiation therapy (IMRT)—achieves higher prostate doses compared to 4 field box XRT, but delivers less radiation to surrounding tissues than 4 field box or 3D C-XRT because of exquisite control over the radiation field. IMRT causes less acute and long-term side effects than 4 field box XRT.
   d. Radiation is usually fractionated over approximately 6 weeks.

3. Low risk prostate cancer—the NCCN recommends 70-75 Gy to the prostate ($\pm$ seminal vesicles). Androgen deprivation is not recommended.
4. Intermediate risk prostate cancer—the NCCN recommends 75-80 Gy to the prostate and seminal vesicles. Radiation to the pelvic lymph nodes and 4-6 months of androgen deprivation are optional. Six months of androgen deprivation (2 months before, 2 months during, and 2 months after XRT) improves cancer specific and overall survival in men with intermediate risk prostate cancer.
5. High risk prostate cancer
   a. Without androgen deprivation, XRT to the entire pelvis does not improve local cancer control, the rate of distant metastases, or overall survival compared to prostate radiation alone. However, RTOG 93-13 showed that whole pelvic radiation with neoadjuvant and concurrent androgen deprivation (2 months before and 2 months during XRT) may decrease progression in men with at least 15% risk of pelvic lymph node metastasis (this risk can be assessed with the Partin tables). *XRT to the pelvic lymph nodes with neoadjuvant and concurrent androgen deprivation should be considered in men with a relatively high risk of pelvic lymph node metastasis.*
   b. *Long-term adjuvant androgen deprivation (started shortly before XRT and continued for 2-3 years) improves disease-free survival and overall survival in men with high grade cancer (Gleason score 8-10) or high clinical stage (T3 or T4) or regional lymph node metastasis (N1).*
      i. The "Bolla" trial randomized men with N0M0 cancer and either Gleason score 8-10 or clinical stage T3-T4 to XRT alone or XRT with hormone therapy (LHRH agonist started the first day of XRT and continued for 3 years). 5-year clinical disease-free survival (75% versus 40%) and overall survival (78% versus 62%) were significantly better with XRT and hormones than with XRT alone.
      ii. RTOG 85-31, 86-10, and 92-02 randomized men with advanced clinical T stage and N0-N1 to XRT alone or XRT with hormone therapy. Hormone therapy was long-term (LHRH agonist started near time of XRT and continued $\geq$ 2 years) or short-term (LHRH agonist and flutamide started 2 months before XRT and continued until XRT completed). Men with Gleason score 8-10 had a significantly higher disease-free survival, a higher overall survival, a lower rate of local progression, and a lower rate of distant metastasis when treated with long-term compared to short-term hormone therapy.

Prostate Cancer Risk Level	Common XRT Regimens		
	XRT Field	Prostate Dose	Androgen Deprivation Therapy (ADT)
Low	Prostate $\pm$ SV	70-75 Gy	None
Intermediate	Prostate $\pm$ SV $\pm$ Pelvic LN	75-80 Gy	Consider 4-6 months ADT*
High	Prostate + SV + Pelvic LN	75-80 Gy	2-3 years ADT*

XRT = external beam radiation; SV = seminal vesicles; LN = lymph nodes
   * Started 2 months before XRT

6. After XRT without androgen deprivation, a lower PSA nadir and a longer time to achieve the PSA nadir are associated with higher disease free survival. When PSA nadir < 0.5 (without androgen deprivation), relapse is unlikely.
7. For combination of XRT and brachytherapy, see Permanent Brachytherapy, page 89 and Temporary Brachytherapy, page 90.

Permanent Brachytherapy (Low Dose Rate Brachytherapy; "Seeds")

1. Permanent seed implants only (monotherapy)—radioactive pellets of Iodine 125 (I-125), Palladium 103 (Pd-103), or Cesium 131 (Cs-131) are placed through the perineum into the prostate using transrectal ultrasound guidance. This can be accomplished during a minor surgical procedure.

Seed Type	Half Life (days)	Time it Takes to Deliver 90% of its Radiation	Recommended Prescription Dose* for Seeds	
			Seeds Only	Seeds + XRT
I-125	60	204 days (~ 7 months)	145 Gy	100-110 Gy
Pd-103	17	58 days (~ 2 months)	125 Gy	100 Gy
Cs-131	9.7	33 days (~ 1 month)	**	**

* Based on American Brachytherapy Society (ABS) recommendations.
[Int J Radiat Oncol Biol Phys, 44(4): 789, 1999 and 47(2): 273, 2000]
** Cs-131 was marketed after the ABS guidelines were released.

2. Seed monotherapy has a higher failure rate in patients with Gleason score ≥ 7, PSA ≥ 10 or clinical stage $\geq$ T2b. Therefore, patients with intermediate or high risk should receive and seeds with XRT.

Prostate Cancer Risk Level	Common Brachytherapy Regimens		
	Radiation	XRT Dose	Androgen Deprivation
Low	Seeds	—	None
Intermediate	Seeds ± XRT	40-50 Gy	Optional‡
High	Seeds + XRT	40-50 Gy	Yes‡

‡ The optimal duration of androgen deprivation is unclear, but many physicians use the same regimens that are used for XRT alone.

3. After seed placement, post-implant dosimetry should be performed.
4. Predicting biochemical disease-free survival after brachytherapy—see pretreatment nomogram [Urology, 58(3): 393, 2001].
5. *Brachytherapy is usually avoided in men with prostate size > 60 g, previous TURP, or significant voiding symptoms because they have a higher risk of urinary side effects.*
6. The pubic arch may interfere with seed placement in large prostates. Large prostates may be down-sized with androgen deprivation to reduce pubic arch interference, but it is unknown if downsizing the prostate decreases the risk of urinary retention.
7. Complications
   a. Urinary incontinence—occurs in 0-7%. It is more common when TURP is performed before or after brachytherapy (1% without TURP; 10-30% with TURP). Peripheral loading of seeds (away from the urethra) in men who had a TURP can reduce the incidence of incontinence to < 5%; however, it is unknown if peripheral loading of seeds compromises cure.
   b. Urinary retention—occurs in 2-15%. The risk of retention is higher for men with prostate size > 60 g or with significant pre-brachytherapy voiding symptoms (higher AUA symptom score). Retention is managed by indwelling catheter or by clean intermittent catheterization. Up to 8% of men require TURP/TUIP for persistent retention after brachytherapy. Non-invasive treatment that may help the patient void:
      i. Antibiotics for symptomatic urinary tract infection.
      ii. Alpha-blockers
      iii. Nonsteroidal anti-inflammatory drugs (NSAIDs)
      iv. Course of steroids (taper dose when course is complete)
      v. 5α-reductase inhibitors or other forms of androgen deprivation
   c. Other side effects—see Side Effects from Radiation Therapy, page 90.

Temporary Brachytherapy (High Dose Rate Brachytherapy)
1. High dose rate brachytherapy (HDR) is usually combined with 4-5 weeks of XRT.
2. HDR is delivered using Iridium 192 (Ir-192).
3. Using transrectal ultrasound guidance, percutaneous cannulas are inserted through the perineum and into the prostate. Over 1-2 days, several HDR sessions are conducted. During these sessions, iridium is placed into each cannula for a specific duration. This permits fine control over radiation delivery (which can be adjusted during therapy to improve radiation to "cold spots"). After each session, the iridium is removed. When the HDR is complete, the cannulas are removed.
4. Side effects—see below.

Particle Beam Therapy (Proton or Neutron Therapy)
1. This is conceptually similar to XRT but uses a different form of energy.
2. Proton therapy delivers minimal energy to surrounding tissues because radiation scatter is less than with XRT. However, it is often combined with XRT. Most data on proton therapy has less than 10 years of follow up.
3. Toxicity from neutron therapy is high; therefore it is seldom used.

Side Effects from Radiation Therapy
1. Erectile dysfunction—with radiation, erections are preserved initially but worsen over several years, whereas with nerve sparing RP, erections are worse initially and tend to improve over 1-2 years.
2. Bladder irritation (urgency, dysuria, etc.)—common during radiation, but severe and chronic in < 5%.
3. Rectal irritation (diarrhea, rectal bleeding)—common during radiation, but severe and chronic in < 5%.
4. Urine retention—up to 15% after brachytherapy. Uncommon with XRT.
5. Infertility and decreased ejaculate volume—common.
6. Hemorrhagic cystitis*—up to 8% with long-term follow up.
7. Urethral stricture*—approximately 3% with long-term follow up.
8. Urinary incontinence*—approximately 3% with long-term follow up.
9. Bowel incontinence or rectal stricture*—rare.
10. Small risk of secondary malignancy (e.g. bladder cancer)*—rare.
    * These side effects can develop even up to 15 years after radiation.

PSA Bounce after Radiation Therapy
1. PSA bounce is a temporary increase in PSA after radiation.
2. PSA bounce usually occurs 18-24 months after radiation, but may occur up to 5 years after therapy. PSA bounces up to 16 ng/ml have been observed. Several bounces may occur.
3. 20-30% of patients have a PSA bounce after radiation.
4. PSA bounce is probably caused by radiation induced prostate injury and inflammation, but may be caused by cancer recurrence in some patients.
5. After external beam radiation—PSA bounce (especially > 1.4 ng/ml) is associated with a higher risk of biochemical recurrence. It may also be associated with a higher risk of metastasis and death from prostate cancer.
6. After brachytherapy—PSA bounce may actually be associated with a lower risk of biochemical recurrence.

Recurrence

General Concepts

1. Follow up after treatment for cure
   a. Prostate exam and PSA every 3-6 months for one year, then every 6 months for 4 years, then every year thereafter.
   b. Bone scan when PSA > 10 ng/ml, rapid PSA doubling time (e.g. PSA doubling time < 6 months), bone pain, or pathologic fracture.

2. Post treatment elevation in PSA (biochemical recurrence) is an accurate marker for recurrence and is usually the earliest sign of recurrence.

3. Risks of recurrence
   a. High grade tumors (especially Gleason $\geq$ 7)
   b. High stage tumors (especially T3 or higher)
   c. High pre-treatment PSA levels (especially PSA $\geq$ 10 ng/ml)
   d. Positive surgical margins
   e. Seminal vesicle invasion
   f. Capsular penetration
   g. Positive lymph nodes

Identifying the Location of Recurrence

1. Biopsy of the prostatic fossa
   a. After radiation—*the ASTRO consensus in 1999 concluded that prostate re-biopsy is not necessary for recurrence after radiation unless the patient is a candidate for local salvage therapy* (e.g. RP or cryotherapy). Prostate cancer dissipates slowly after radiation; therefore, biopsy should probably not be done within 18-24 months of radiation. Post-radiation biopsies are difficult to interpret because the prostate may meet the pathologic criteria for cancer, but it may be biologically inactive.
   b. After radical prostatectomy—transrectal biopsy of the prostatic fossa reveals prostate cancer in up to 50% of men with biochemical recurrence. A positive biopsy is more likely in patients with a palpable lesion or a PSA > 2.0. *Biopsy of the prostatic fossa is usually unnecessary after RP,* even when salvage therapy is planned, because the biopsy results do not predict the outcome of salvage therapy.

2. PSA doubling time (PSADT)—local recurrence is more likely when the PSADT is long (e.g. > 1 year), whereas systemic recurrence is more likely when PSADT is short (e.g. < 6 months).

3. CT scan and bone scan—rarely helpful when PSA < 10 and PSADT > 6 months. In men recurring after RP (not treated with hormone therapy), bone scan and pelvic CT were always negative when PSADT > 6 months and PSA < 10 (Okotie et al, J Urol, 2004). In hormone refractory men on androgen deprivation (initially treated with RP $\pm$ postoperative XRT), bone scan was always negative when PSA < 15 (Cher et al, J Urol, 1998).

4. Prostascint® scan (Indium 111 capromab pendetide)
   a. For details, see Prostascint® scan, page 158.
   b. Prostascint® may be indicated in men with biochemical recurrence, negative bone scan, and negative or equivocal pelvic CT/MRI who are candidates for curative salvage therapy. Prostascint® may identify men with local recurrence and improve patient selection for salvage therapy.

5. After radical prostatectomy, local recurrence is more likely in patients with
   a. Biochemical recurrence > 1-2 years after prostatectomy.
   b. Long PSA doubling time (especially doubling time > 1 year).
   c. The following pathologic characteristics in the prostatectomy specimen:
      • No lymph node metastasis
      • No seminal vesicle invasion
      • Gleason score $\leq$ 7

Post Radiation Recurrence

1. Recurrence is present when any of the following criteria are found.
   a. A rising or elevated PSA—*the RTOG-ASTRO consensus defines biochemical failure after radiation (with or without hormone therapy) as a rise of 2 ng/ml or more above the nadir PSA.* The old 1997 ASTRO definition (three consecutive increases in PSA) should no longer be used. PSA can increase during radiation, but this is generally not caused by cancer progression. PSA can "bounce" up and down after radiation. Thus, a single increase in PSA should not be interpreted as recurrence.
   b. A positive prostate biopsy $\geq$ 18-24 months after radiotherapy.
   c. A distant metastasis is detected.
2. Treatment options for local recurrence without metastasis
   a. Salvage radical prostatectomy—high risk of surgical complications (e.g. rectal injury, impotence, and urinary incontinence). The ideal candidate:
      i. Clinical stage T1-T2, N0M0, Gleason score $\leq$ 7, and PSA < 10 at the time of radiation *and* at the time of recurrence (i.e. clinically organ confined cancer before initial therapy and before salvage therapy).
      ii. Positive prostate biopsy after radiation.
      iii. Life expectancy > 10 years.
   b. Cryotherapy—higher complication rate than primary cryotherapy.
   c. Re-irradiation—high complication rate, persistence of radio-resistant tumors, and most patients still develop distant metastasis.
   d. Other options: androgen deprivation, surveillance, and research trials.

Post Prostatectomy Recurrence

1. Recurrence is present when any of the following criteria are found.
   a. Failure of the PSA to fall to an undetectable level after prostatectomy.
   b. Rising PSA—*the 2007 NCCN guideline defines biochemical recurrence as a detectable PSA that increases on 2 subsequent measurements.*
   c. A positive biopsy of the urethral anastomosis or a local lesion.
   d. A distant metastasis is detected.
2. The best PSA threshold for defining recurrence is unknown, but it is probably from 0.2-0.4 (see table).
3. 45% of recurrences occur within 2 years of RP, 77% within 5 years of RP, and 96% within 9 years of RP.
4. From the time of PSA recurrence, the median time to detectable metastasis is 8 years and the median time to death from prostate cancer is 13 years.

PSA Threshold	% of patients whose PSA continues to rise within 3 years
0.2	49%
0.3	62%
0.4	72%

From Amling et al: J Urol 165: 1146, 2001.

5. Treatment options for biochemical or local recurrence without metastases
   a. Salvage XRT—best when a local recurrence is likely (see Identifying the Location of the Recurrence, page 91).
      i. A higher disease-free survival is achieved when the PSA is low (especially PSA $\leq$ 1.5) at the time of salvage XRT.
      ii. The ideal candidate has PSA $\leq$ 1.5, long PSA doubling time, PSA recurrence > 1-2 years after prostatectomy, uninvolved seminal vesicles and lymph nodes, Gleason score $\leq$ 7, and no metastasis.
      iii. *XRT dose to the prostatic fossa should be at least 64 Gy* (ASTRO consensus, J Clin Oncol, 17: 1155, 1999). If possible, XRT should be administered when continence and erections have recovered after RP.
      iv. Salvage radiation reduces potency. However, it usually does not have a significant impact on urinary continence (when administered after maximal recovery of continence).
      v. In appropriately selected men, 6-year disease-free survival = 50%.
   b. Other options: androgen deprivation, surveillance, and research trials.

Advanced/Metastatic Prostate Cancer

Androgen Deprivation (Based on the ASCO Clinical Guidelines 2006)

1. Definitions
   a. Androgen deprivation therapy (ADT)—any therapy that prevents androgens from activating the androgen receptor, including castration, antiandrogen therapy, and combinations thereof.
   b. Castration—bilateral orchiectomy (surgical castration) or LHRH suppressor (medical castration).
   c. Combined androgen blockade—castration and an antiandrogen.
   d. Monotherapy—using one of the following regimens: an LHRH suppressor, bilateral orchiectomy, or an antiandrogen.

2. *"Bilateral orchiectomy or medical castration with...LHRH agonists are the recommended initial treatments for metastatic prostate cancer." —ASCO guidelines 2006.*

3. Asymptomatic men—the optimal time to start ADT in asymptomatic men is unclear. When ADT is started at the time of recurrence, mortality from prostate cancer is slightly decreased, but mortality from other causes is slightly increased. Overall survival is similar regardless of when ADT is started. The ASCO guideline 2006 "cannot make a strong recommendation for the early use of androgen deprivation therapy." Thus, asymptomatic men are candidates for surveillance.

4. Symptomatic men—*men with symptoms of locally advanced or metastatic cancer should be started on androgen deprivation therapy.*

5. Monotherapy with non-steroidal antiandrogens
   a. Monotherapy with non-steroidal antiandrogens may be discussed as an alternative to castration.
   b. *Monotherapy with a nonsteroidal antiandrogen appears to be less effective at controlling prostate cancer than castration.* Compared to castration, nonsteroidal antiandrogen monotherapy:
      i.   Results in a lower overall survival.
      ii. Has a higher rate of withdrawal from therapy.
      iii. Has a higher rate of gynecomastia and breast pain.
      iv. Causes less hot flashes and fatigue.
      v.   Achieves significantly better quality of life in the domains of sexual interest and physical capacity.
      vi. Does not impair libido.
      vii. Does not cause osteoporosis.
   c. *High dose bicalutamide monotherapy (150 mg per day) should not be used to treat localized prostate cancer.* In men with localized prostate cancer who would have undergone watchful waiting, early results show more deaths with high dose bicalutamide than with placebo.
   d. Dose—bicalutamide 50-150 mg po q day, flutamide 250 mg po TID (These antiandrogens are FDA approved for prostate cancer when used with castration, but they are *not* FDA approved for monotherapy).

6. Steroidal anti-androgens should not be offered as monotherapy because they have a more rapid time to progression than LHRH agonists.

7. *Combined androgen blockade should be considered in men on androgen deprivation.* A 1-5% benefit in overall survival after 5 years of combined androgen blockade must be balanced against the greater side effects and cost. The ASCO guidelines state "Combined androgen blockade confers a statistically significant but questionable clinical improvement in survival over orchiectomy or LHRH monotherapy."

8. There is insufficient information on intermittent ADT; therefore, it is still considered experimental.

Hormone Refractory Prostate Cancer

1. Prostate cancer responds to LHRH agonists for an *average of 2 years*, then PSA begins to rise (i.e. it is "hormone refractory"). However, the duration of response can range from a few months to 10-15 years.
2. The androgen receptor remains active in hormone refractory prostate cancer, thus androgen deprivation should be continued.
3. Work up and initial therapy of hormone refractory prostate cancer

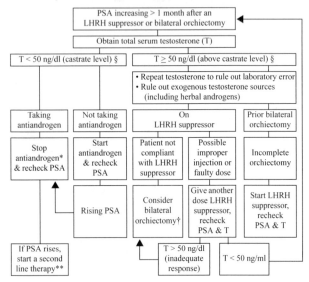

§ Some use a cut off of T < 20 ng/ml instead of T < 50 ng/ml.
* see Antiandrogen Withdrawal, page 106.
† If the patient refuses orchiectomy, add an antiandrogen.
** See Second Line Therapies, below.

Second Line Therapies

1. Most second line therapies have not been shown to improve survival.
2. If the patient was on flutamide, high dose bicalutamide (150-200 mg po q day) may decrease PSA in 22-38% of patients.
3. Ketoconazole and steroids (see Ketoconazole, page 104)
   a. PSA decreases by $\geq$ 50% in 63-78% of patients.
   b. Usually sustains PSA reduction for 3-8 months.
4. Aminoglutethimide and steroids (see Aminoglutethimide, page 104).
5. Diethylstilbestrol 1 mg po q day—up to 43% have a PSA reduction. Other estrogenic compounds, may have similar effects (see Estrogens, page 103).
6. Chemotherapy—*the NCCN 2007 guideline recommends a docetaxel based regimen as first line chemotherapy because it has been shown to improve survival compared to mitoxantrone and prednisone*; median survival was 2-3 months longer with docetaxel (SWOG 9916 and TAX327).
7. Investigational treatments

Treatment of Locally Advanced/Metastatic Prostate Cancer

1. *Men with symptoms of locally advanced or metastatic cancer should be started on androgen deprivation therapy* (ASCO Guidelines).
2. Bladder outlet obstruction—treated with TURP, suprapubic tube, urethral catheter, or urethral stent.
3. Ureteral obstruction—treated with ureteral stents or nephrostomy tubes.
4. Bone metastasis
   a. Bisphosphonates
      i. Guidelines from 3rd International Consultation on Prostate Cancer
         • An IV bisphosphonate should be initiated *in all men with hormone refractory prostate cancer and bone metastasis*.
         • An IV bisphosphonate should be *strongly considered in men with hormone sensitive prostate cancer and bone metastasis*.
         • Intravenous bisphosphonate therapy should be continued while other indicated treatments are administered.
      ii. In hormone refractory men with bone metastasis, zoledronic acid (Zometa®) 4 mg IV (over 15 minutes) every 3 weeks for 20 cycles reduced skeletal related events (SREs) such as pathologic fracture and delayed the onset of SREs by nearly 6 months. It may reduce pain from bone metastasis. Zoledronic acid can cause renal insufficiency, pancytopenia, and electrolyte abnormalities. Check creatinine before each dose. Potassium, calcium, phosphate, magnesium, hemoglobin, and hematocrit should be monitored regularly. During therapy, 500 mg calcium and 400 IU vitamin D should be taken orally each day.
   b. Symptomatic bone metastasis—focal lesions can be treated with external beam radiation. Diffuse lesions may be treated with bone seeking radionucleotides (e.g. strontium or samarium) or chemotherapy.
   c. Significant threat of fracture in a weight bearing bone—usually requires orthopedic surgery.
   d. Pathologic fracture—usually requires orthopedic surgery.

Acute Spinal Cord Compression from Metastasis

1. Symptoms from acute spinal cord compression depend on the level and degree of compression. Metastases from prostate cancer often occur in the lumbar spine, which corresponds to the sacral spinal cord and cauda equina. Therefore, neurologic symptoms tend to involve the lower extremities, bowel, and bladder. Symptoms may include weakness or paresis below the level of injury, sensation loss below the level of injury, urinary/fecal incontinence or retention, and back pain.
2. Start intravenous steroids—the usual recommended dose is dexamethasone 100 mg IV bolus, followed by dexamethasone 25 mg po QID x 3 days. Thereafter, the dose is tapered.
3. Start immediate androgen deprivation by one of the following methods:
   a. Bilateral orchiectomy—testosterone reaches castrate level in 2-12 hours.
   b. Start ketoconazole 400 mg po q 8 hours—castrate testosterone levels are often reached 8 hours after a 400 mg oral dose (See page 104).
   c. LHRH antagonists—these agents do not cause flare. *Do not give LHRH agonists* because the flare can make spinal compression acutely worse.
   d. Start diethylstilbestrol 1 g IV q 24 hours (dissolve 1 g in 250 cc normal saline. Infusion rate is 20-30 drops/minute for the first 15 minutes. The remaining solution is infused over at least one hour). Intravenous diethylstilbestrol decreases testosterone by 50% in 24 hours.
4. Spine x-rays assess for fracture and localize the involved spinal region. Obtain an MRI of the entire spine (this will identify not only symptomatic lesions, but also lesions that may cause impending problems).

5. Surgical decompression may be indicated in any of the following cases:
   • Failure of androgen deprivation and radiation.
   • Spinal instability from vertebral body collapse.
   • Bone protrusion into the spinal cord.
   • Recurrent spinal compression in an area of previous radiation therapy.
6. External beam radiation therapy to the spinal metastases should be instituted immediately if surgical therapy is not indicated.
7. Neurosurgery, radiation oncology, and medical oncology consults may be helpful in managing patients with cord compression.

REFERENCES

General

Abbas F, Hochberg D, Civantos F, Soloway M: Incidental prostatic adenocarcinoma in patients undergoing radical cystoprostatectomy for bladder cancer. Eur Urol, 30: 322, 1996.

Bruner DW, et al: Relative risk of prostate cancer for men with affected relatives: systematic review and meta-analysis. Int J Cancer, 107: 797, 2003.

Carter HB, Partin AW: Diagnosis and staging of prostate cancer. Campbell's Urology. 8th Edition. Ed. PC Walsh, et al. Philadelphia: W. B. Sanders Company, 2002, pp 3055-3079.

D'Amico AV, et al: Preoperative PSA velocity and the risk of death from prostate cancer after radical prostatectomy. N Engl J Med, 351: 125, 2004.

Freedland SJ, Wieder JA, et al: Improved risk stratification for biochemical recurrence after radical prostatectomy using a novel risk group system based on prostate specific antigen density and biopsy Gleason score. J Urol, 168: 110, 2002.

Greene FL, Page DL, Fleming ID, et al. AJCC Cancer Staging Manual, Sixth Edition. New York: Springer, 2002. (effective January 1, 2003)

Gleave ME, Coupland D, Drachenberg D, et al: Ability of serum prostate-specific antigen levels to predict normal bone scan in patients with newly diagnosed prostate cancer. Urology, 47: 708, 1996.

Thompson I, et al: Guideline for the management of clinically localized prostate cancer: 2007 update. AUA Education and Research, Inc., 2007. (www.auanet.org).

National Comprehensive Cancer Network (NCCN) clinical practice guidelines in oncology: Prostate cancer. 2007. (http:\\www.nccn.org)

Reiter RE, deKernion JB: Epidemiology, etiology, and prevention of prostate cancer. Campbell's Urology. 8th Edition. Ed. PC Walsh, et al. Philadelphia: W. B. Sanders Company, 2002, pp 3003-3024.

Prevention

SELECT trial—http://cancer.gov

Thompson IM, et al: The influence of finasteride on the development of prostate cancer. N Engl J Med, 349: 213, 2003.

Scardino, PT: The prevention of prostate cancer - the dilemma continues. N Engl J Med, 349: 295, 2003.

Pathology

Bostwick DG: Progression of prostatic intraepithelial neoplasia to early invasive adenocarcinoma. Eur Urol, 30:145, 1996.

Epstein JI: Pathology of prostatic neoplasia. Campbell's Urology. 8th Edition. Ed. PC Walsh, et al. Philadelphia: W. B. Sanders Co., 2002, pp 3025-3037.

Epstein JI, Potter SR: The pathologic interpretation and significance of prostate needle biopsy findings: implications and current controversies. J Urol, 166: 402, 2001.

Goldknopf JL, et al: Relationship of prostate cancer to the prostatic urethra: implications for cryoablation. J Urol, 165(5 suppl): 323 (abstract 1326), 2001.

Prostate Biopsy

Marks, LS, et al: PCA3 molecular urine assay for prostate cancer in men undergoing repeat biopsy. Urology, 69: 532, 2007.

Matlaga BR, Eskew LA, McCullough DL: Prostate biopsy: indications and technique. J Urol, 169: 12, 2003.

Rodriguez LV, Terris MK: Risks and complications of transrectal ultrasound guided prostate needle biopsy: a prospective study and review of the literature. J Urol, 160: 2115, 1998.

Screening

ERSPC trial—Aus G, et al: Prostate cancer screening decreases the absolute risk of being diagnosed with advance prostate cancer - results from a prospective, population based randomized controlled trial. Eur Urol, 51(3): 659, 2007.

ERSPC trial—http://www.erspc.org

Hankey BF, et al: Cancer surveillance series: interpreting trends in prostate cancer part I: evidence of the effects of screening in recent prostate cancer incidence, mortality, and survival rates. J Natl Cancer Inst, 91: 1017, 1999.

Labrie F, et al: Screening decreases prostate cancer mortality: 11-year follow-up of the 1988 Quebec prospective randomized controlled trial. Prostate, 59: 311, 2004. [This is an update of Labrie F, et al: Prostate, 38: 83, 1999].

NCCN guidelines: Prostate cancer early detection, 2007. (http:\\www.nccn.org)

Paquette EL, et al: Improved prostate cancer-specific survival and other disease parameters: impact of prostate-specific antigen. Urology, 60: 756, 2002.

PLCO trial—http://cancer.gov/clinicaltrials

PLCO trial—http://www3.cancer.gov/prevention/plco/participation.html

Smith RA, Cokkinides V, Eyre HJ: American Cancer Society Guidelines for the Early Detection of Cancer, 2003. CA Cancer J Clin, 53: 27, 2003.

Thompson I, Carroll P, Coley D, et al: Prostate specific antigen (PSA) best practice policy. Oncology, 14(2): 267, 2000.

Surveillance (also see Survival & Comparison of Treatments)

Albertsen PC, et al: 20-year outcomes following conservative management of clinically localized prostate cancer. JAMA, 293(17): 2095, 2005. [update of Albertsen PC, et al. JAMA, 280(11): 975, 1998.]

Carter CA, et al: Temporarily deferred therapy for men younger than 70 years and with low-risk localized prostate cancer in the prostate specific antigen era. J Clin Oncol, 21: 4001, 2003.

Johansson JE, et al: Natural history of early, localized prostate cancer. JAMA, 291(22): 2713, 2004.

Patel MI, et al: An analysis of men with clinically localized prostate cancer who deferred definitive therapy. J Urol, 171: 1520, 2004.

Diet Modifications

Aronson W, Yip J, deKernion J: Prostate cancer. Nutritional Oncology. Ed. D Heber, et al. San Diego: Academic Press, 1999, pp 453-461.

Kamat AM, et al: Chemoprevention of urologic cancer. J Urol: 161, 1748, 1999.

Moyad MA, Pienta KJ: Complementary medicine for prostatic diseases: a primer for clinicians. Urology, 59 (suppl 4a), 2002.

Cryotherapy

Shinohara K, et al: Cryotherapy for prostate cancer. Campbell's Urology. 8th Ed. Ed. PC Walsh, et al. Philadelphia: W. B. Sanders Co., 2002, pp 3171-3181.

Wieder J, et al: Transrectal ultrasound guided transperineal cryoablation in the treatment of prostate carcinoma: preliminary results. J Urol, 154: 435, 1995.

External Beam Radiation

D'Amico AV, et al: Radiation therapy for prostate cancer. Campbell's Urology. 8th Edition. Ed. PC Walsh, et al. Philadelphia: W. B. Sanders Co., 2002, pp 3147-3170.

Gardner BG, et al: Late normal tissue sequela in the second decade after high dose radiation therapy with combined photons and conformal protons for locally advanced prostate cancer. J Urol, 167: 123, 2002.

Garzotto M, Fair WR: Outcome of external beam radiation therapy of clinically localized prostate cancer. AUA Update Series, Vol. 19, Lesson 27, 2000.

Ray M, et al: PSA nadir predicts biochemical and distant failures after external beam radiotherapy for prostate cancer. Int J Radiat Oncol Biol Phys, 64(4): 1140, 2006.

Brachytherapy

Beyer D, et al: American Brachytherapy Society recommendations for clinical implementation of NIST-99 standards for [103]Palladium brachytherapy. Int J Radiat Oncol Biol Phys, 47(2): 273, 2000.

Blasko JC, Mate TP: Brachytherapy. Genitourinary Oncology. 2nd Edition, Ed. NJ Vogelzang, et al. Philadelphia: Lippincott Williams & Wilkins, 2000, pp 754-761.

D'Amico AV, et al: Radiation therapy for prostate cancer. Campbell's Urology. 8th Edition. Ed. PC Walsh, et al. Philadelphia: W. B. Sanders Company, 2002, pp 3147-3170.

Nag S, Beyer D, Friedland J, et al: American Brachytherapy Society (ABS) recommendations for transperineal permanent brachytherapy of prostate cancer. Int J Radiat Oncol Biol Phys, 44(4): 789, 1999.

Terek MD, et al: Identification of patients at increased risk for prolonged urinary retention following radioactive seed implantation. J Urol, 160: 1379, 1998.

Wang H, Wallner K, Sutlief S, et al: Transperineal brachytherapy in patients with large prostate glands. Int J Cancer (Radiat Oncol Invest): 90, 199, 2000.

Hormone Therapy with Radiation

Bolla M, et al: Long-term results with immediate androgen suppression and external irradiation in patients with locally advanced prostate cancer (an EORTC study): a phase III randomized trial. Lancet, 360 (9327): 103, 2002. [update of Bolla M, et al: N Engl J Med, 337: 295, 1997].

D'Amico AV, et al: 6-month androgen suppression plus radiation therapy vs. radiation therapy alone for patients with clinically localized prostate cancer. JAMA, 292: 821, 2004.

Horwitz EM, Winter K, et al: Subset analysis of RTOG 85-31 and 86-10 indicates an advantage for long term vs. short term adjuvant hormones for patients with locally advanced non-metastatic prostate cancer treated with radiation therapy. Int J Radiat Oncol Biol Phys, 49: 947, 2001.

RTOG 85-31—Pilepich MV et al: Androgen suppression adjuvant to definitive radiotherapy in prostate adenocarcinoma - long term results of phase III RTOG 85-31. Int J Radiat Oncol Biol Phys, 61: 1285, 2005. [update of Int J Radiat Oncol Biol Phys, 49: 937, 2001].

RTOG 86-10—Pilepich MV, et al: Phase III RTOG trial 86-10 of androgen deprivation adjuvant to definitive radiotherapy in locally advanced carcinoma of the prostate. Int J Radiat Oncol Biol Phys, 50: 1243, 2001.

RTOG 92-02—Hanks, et al: Phase III trial of long term adjuvant androgen deprivation after neoadjuvant hormonal cytoreduction and radiotherapy in locally advanced carcinoma of the prostate: RTOG 92-02. J Clin Oncol, 21: 3972, 2003. [update of Int J Radiat Oncol Biol Phys, 48(suppl 3): 112, 2000].

RTOG 94-13—Lawton CA, et al: An update of the phase III trial comparing whole pelvic to prostate only radiotherapy and neoadjuvant to adjuvant total androgen suppression. Int J Radiat Oncol Biol Phys, 2007. E-published ahead of print [update of J Clin Oncol, 21 (10): 1904, 2003].

PSA Bounce after Radiation

Ciezki JP, et al: PSA kinetics after prostate brachytherapy: PSA bounce phenomenon and its implications for PSA doubling time. Int J Radiat Oncol Biol Phys, 62(2): 512, 2006.

Critz FA, Williams WH, et al: Prostate specific antigen bounce after radioactive seed implantation followed by external beam radiation for prostate cancer. J Urol, 163: 1085, 2000.

Feigenberg SJ, et al: A prostate specific antigen bounce greater than 1.4 ng/ml is clinically significant after external beam radiotherapy for prostate cancer. Am J Clin Oncol, 29: 458, 2006.

Hanlon AL, Pinover WH, et al: Patterns and fate of PSA bouncing following 3D-CRT. Int J Radiat Oncol Biol Phys, 50: 845, 2001.

Horwitz EM, et al: Biochemical and clinical significance of the post-treatment prostate specific antigen bounce for prostate cancer patients treated with external beam radiation therapy alone: a multi-institutional pooled analysis. Cancer, 107: 1496, 2006.

Patel AR: PSA bounce predicts early success in patients with permanent iodine-125 prostate implant. Urology 63(1): 110, 2004.

Rosser CJ, et al: Prostate specific antigen bounce phenomenon after external beam radiation for clinically localized prostate cancer. J Urol, 168: 2001, 2002.

Radical Prostatectomy

Walsh PC: Anatomic radical retropubic prostatectomy. Campbell's Urology. 8th Edition. Ed. PC Walsh, et al. Philadelphia: W. B. Sanders Co., 2002, pp 3107-3029.

Wieder JA, Soloway M: Incidence, etiology, location, prevention, and treatment of positive surgical margins after prostatectomy for prostate cancer. J Urol, 160: 299, 1998.

Neoadjuvant Androgen Deprivation with Radical Prostatectomy

Scolieri MJ, Altman A, et al: Neoadjuvant hormonal ablative therapy before radical prostatectomy: a review. Is it indicated? J Urol, 164: 1465, 2000.

Soloway MS, et al: Neoadjuvant androgen ablation before radical prostatectomy in cT2bNxM0 prostate cancer: 5 year results. J Urol: 167: 112, 2002.

Wieder JA, Soloway M: Neoadjuvant androgen deprivation before radical prostatectomy for prostate adenocarcinoma. Prostate Cancer: Principles and Practice. Ed. PW Kantoff, P Carroll, A D'Amico. Philadelphia. Lippincott Williams and Wilkins, 2002, pp 425-437.

XRT after Radical Prostatectomy

Bolla M, et al: Postoperative radiotherapy after radical prostatectomy: a randomized controlled trial (EORTC 22911). Lancet, 366(9485): 572, 2005.

Swanson GP, et al: Predominant treatment failure in postprostatectomy patients is local: analysis of patterns of treatment failure in SWOG 8794. J Clin Oncol, 25(16): 2225, 2007.

Spiotto MT, et al: Radiotherapy after prostatectomy: improved biochemical relapse free survival with whole pelvic compared with prostate bed only for high risk patients. Int J Radiat Oncol Biol Phys, 69(1): 54, 2007.

Thompson IM, et al: Adjuvant radiotherapy for pathologically advanced prostate cancer. JAMA, 296: 2329, 2006.

Vargas C, et al: Improved biochemical outcome with adjuvant radiotherapy after radical prostatectomy for prostate cancer with poor pathologic features. Int J Radiat Oncol Biol Phys, 61(3): 714, 2005.

Treatment of Positive Pelvic Lymph Nodes after Radical Prostatectomy

ECOG 3886—Messing EM, et al: Immediate versus deferred androgen deprivation treatment in patients with node-positive prostate cancer after radical prostatectomy and pelvic lymphadenectomy. Lancet Oncol, 7(6): 472, 2006 [update of Messing E, et al: N Engl J Med, 341:1781, 1999].

EORTC 30846—Schroder FH, et al: Early versus late endocrine treatment of pN1-3 M0 prostate cancer without local treatment of the primary tumor: results of the EORTC 30846. J Urol 172: 923, 2004.

Recurrence and Salvage Therapy

ASTRO Consensus Panel: Consensus statements on radiation therapy of prostate cancer: guidelines for prostate re-biopsy after radiation and for radiation therapy with rising prostate-specific antigen levels after radical prostatectomy. J Clin Oncol, 17: 1155, 1999.

Amling CL, et al: Defining prostate specific antigen progression after radical prostatectomy: What is the most appropriate cut point? J Urol, 165:1146, 2001.

Cher ML, Bianco Jr FJ, Lam JS, et al: Limited role of radionuclide bone scintigraphy in patients with prostate specific antigen elevations after radical prostatectomy. J Urol, 160: 1387, 1998.

Han M, Partin AW, Zahurak M, et al: Biochemical (prostate specific antigen) recurrence probability following radical prostatectomy for clinically localized prostate cancer. J Urol, 169: 517, 2003.

Jhaveri FM, Klein EA: How to explore the patient with a rising PSA after radical prostatectomy: defining local versus systemic failure. Sem Urol Oncol, 17(3): 130, 1999.

Zelefsky MJ, et al: Pretreatment nomogram predicting ten year biochemical outcome of three dimensional conformation radiotherapy and intensity modulated radiotherapy for prostate cancer. Urology, 70(2): 283, 2007. [update of J Clin Oncol, 18(19): 3352, 2000].

Kattan MW, et al: Pretreatment nomogram for predicting freedom from recurrence after permanent prostate brachytherapy in prostate cancer. Urology, 58(3): 393, 2001.

Neulander EZ, Soloway MS: Failure after radical prostatectomy. Urology, 61: 30, 2003.

Okotie OT, Aronson WJ, Wieder JA, et al: Predictors of metastatic disease among men with biochemical failure following radical prostatectomy. J Urol, 171: 2260, 2004.

Pound CR, Partin AW, et al: Natural history of progression after PSA elevation following radical prostatectomy. JAMA, 281: 1591, 1999.

Roach M, et al: Defining biochemical failure following radiotherapy with or without hormonal therapy in men with clinically localized prostate cancer: recommendations of the RTOG-ASTRO Phoenix consensus conference. Int J Radiat Oncol Biol Phys, 65(4): 965, 2006 [update of Int J Radiat Oncol Biol Phys, 37(5): 1035, 1997].

Stephenson AJ, et al: Preoperative nomogram predicting the 10-year probability of prostate cancer recurrence after radical prostatectomy. J Natl Cancer Inst, 98(10), 715, 2006 [update of J Natl Cancer Inst, 90: 766, 1998].

Stephenson AJ, et al: Postoperative nomogram predicting the 10-year probability of prostate cancer recurrence after radical prostatectomy. J Clin Oncol, 23(28): 7005, 2005 [update of J Clin Oncol, 17(5): 1499, 1999].

Wieder JA, Belldegrun A: The utility of PSA doubling time for prostate cancer recurrence. Mayo Clin Proc, 76(6): 571, 2001.

Zietman AL: Salvage and adjuvant radiation after radical prostatectomy. Genitourinary Oncology. 2nd Edition. Ed. NJ Vogelzang, PT Scardino, et al. Philadelphia: Lippincott Williams and Wilkins, 2000, pp 804-813.

Survival and Comparison of Treatments

Bill-Axelson A, et al: Radical prostatectomy versus watchful waiting in early prostate cancer. N Engl J Med, 352: 1977, 2005. [update of Holmberg L, et al. N Engl J Med, 347: 781, 2002].

D'Amico AV, et al: Biochemical outcome after radical prostatectomy, external beam radiation therapy, or interstitial radiation therapy for clinically localized prostate cancer. JAMA, 280: 969, 1998.

Donnelly BJ, et al: A randomized controlled trial comparing external beam radiation and cryoablation in localized prostate cancer. J Urol, 177(4): 376 (abstract #1141), 2007.

Kupelian PA, Potters L, et al: Radical prostatectomy, external beam radiotherapy < 72 Gy, external beam radiotherapy ≥ 72 Gy, permanent seed implantation, or combined seeds/external beam radiotherapy for stage T1-T2 prostate cancer. Int J Radiat Oncol Biol Phys, 58(1): 25, 2004.

Martinez AA, et al: A comparison of external beam radiation therapy versus radical prostatectomy for patients with low risk prostate carcinoma diagnosed, staged, and treated at a single institution. Cancer, 88: 425, 2000.

PIVOT trial—http://cancer.gov/clinicaltrials

Advanced/Metastatic Prostate Cancer (see also Androgen Deprivation)

Abraham JL, ACP-ASIM End-of-Life Care Consensus Panel: Management of pain and spinal cord compression in patients with advanced cancer. Ann Intern Med, 131: 37, 1999.

AstraZeneca Canada Inc.: Health Canada important drug safety information - Casodex® 150 mg, 2003.

Carroll PR, Altwein J, et al: Management of disseminated prostate cancer. Prostate Cancer: 3rd International Consultation on Prostate Cancer - Paris. Ed. L Denis, et al. Paris: Health Publications, 2003, pp 249-284.

Hahn SM, et al. Oncologic emergencies. Cecil Textbook of Medicine. 19th ed, Ed. Wyngaarden, et al. Philadelphia: W. B. Sanders, 1992, pp 1067-1071.

Iversen P, et al: Bicalutamide monotherapy compared with castration in patients with non-metastatic locally advanced prostate cancer: 6.3 years of follow up. J Urol, 164: 1579, 2000.

Iversen P, et al: Bicalutamide 150 mg for early non-metastatic prostate cancer in patients who would otherwise undergo watchful waiting: latest results at a median 5.4 years follow-up. J Urol, 171(4 suppl): 280 (abstract 1061), 2004.

Loblaw DA, et al: Initial hormone management of androgen sensitive metastatic, recurrent, or progressive prostate cancer: 2006 update of an American Society of Clinical Oncology practice guideline. J Clin Oncol, 25(12) 1596, 2007. [Update of J Clin Oncol, 22(14): 1, 2004.]

Saad F, Gleason DM, et al: A randomized, placebo controlled trial of zoledronic acid in patients with hormone refractory metastatic prostate cancer. J Natl Cancer Inst, 94(19): 1458, 2002.

Seidenfeld J, et al: Single-therapy androgen suppression in men with advanced prostate cancer: a systematic review and meta-analysis: Ann Intern Med, 132: 566, 2000.

Smith MR, et al: Bicalutamide monotherapy versus leuprolide monotherapy for prostate cancer: effects on bone mineral density and body composition. J Clin Oncol, 22(13): 2546, 2004.

Studer UE, et al: Immediate versus deferred hormonal treatment for patients with prostate cancer who are not suitable for curative local treatment: results of the randomized trial SAKK 08/88. J Clin Oncol, 22(20): 4109, 2004.

SWOG 9916—Petrylak DP, et al: Docetaxel and estramustine compared with mitoxantrone and prednisone for advanced refractory prostate cancer. N Engl J Med, 351: 1513, 2004.

TAX327—Tannock IF, et al: Docetaxel plus prednisone or mitoxantrone plus prednisone for advanced prostate cancer. N Engl J Med, 351: 1502, 2004.

ANDROGEN DEPRIVATION

Androgens
1. Sources of androgens in men
   a. Testes—produce 90-95% of circulating androgens in the form of testosterone. Luteinizing hormone (LH) stimulates testosterone production in the testicular Leydig cells.
   b. Adrenal glands—produce $\leq 10\%$ of circulating androgens in the form of androstenedione and dehydroepiandrosterone (DHEA).
2. In most reproductive tissues, testosterone is converted by 5α-reductase to dihydrotestosterone (DHT), which has a higher affinity for androgen receptors than testosterone.

Prolactin
1. Prolactin, which is secreted by the anterior pituitary, decreases testosterone by inhibiting GnRH release from the hypothalamus.
2. Conditions that increase prolactin—prolactinoma, hypothyroidism, stress, estrogen exposure, chronic renal failure, and antipsychotic drugs (especially phenothiazines).
3. Prolactin may directly stimulate prostate growth.

Definitions
1. Androgen deprivation therapy (ADT)—any therapy that prevents androgens from activating the androgen receptor.
2. Castration—bilateral orchiectomy (surgical castration) or LHRH suppressor (medical castration).
3. Combined androgen blockade—castration and an antiandrogen.
4. Monotherapy—using either castration or an antiandrogen.
5. Neoadjuvant—before curative therapy
6. Adjuvant—after curative therapy.

General Treatment Principles
1. LHRH agonist and bilateral orchiectomy are equally effective.
2. Combined androgen blockade provides limited benefit over an LHRH suppressor or bilateral orchiectomy alone.
3. The long-term efficacy of intermittent androgen deprivation is unknown.
4. The optimal type of androgen deprivation, the optimal time to initiate it, and the optimal duration of therapy are not known.
5. See also Advanced/Metastatic Prostate Cancer, page 93.

Summary of Androgen Deprivation
1. Surgical
   a. Bilateral orchiectomy {T}
   b. Hypophysectomy {A+T}
   c. Bilateral adrenalectomy {A}
2. Pharmacological
   a. Estrogens {T}
   b. Progestins {T}
   c. Prolactin antagonists
   d. LHRH agonists {T}
   e. LHRH antagonists {T}
   f. Inhibitors of androgen synthesis {A+T}
   g. Anti-androgens {R}—non-steroidal or steroidal
   h. 5α-reductase inhibitors

> Special notations used in this chapter.
> {T} = inhibits testicular androgen production
> {A} = inhibits adrenal androgen production
> {A+T} = inhibits adrenal & testicular androgen production
> {R} = blocks androgen receptors in the target tissue.

Surgical Androgen Deprivation

Bilateral Orchiectomy {T}

1. Orchiectomy is the gold standard for androgen deprivation. Castrate testosterone levels occur 2-12 hours postoperatively.
2. Mechanism of action—removes the testis as a source of testosterone.
3. Eliminates ≥ 90% of androgens (the remaining androgens arise from the adrenal gland).
4. Advantages—low cost, compliance not required after castration.
5. *Orchiectomy does not cause a testosterone flare.*
6. Side effects—see Morbidity From Medical or Surgical Castration, page 107.

Hypophysectomy (Ablation of the Pituitary) {A+T}

1. Mechanism of action—the source of LH and ACTH is removed; therefore, testicular *and* adrenal androgen production is inhibited.
2. Not used anymore—pharmaceuticals are now used instead.

Bilateral Adrenalectomy {A}

1. Mechanism of action—removes the adrenals as a source of testosterone.
2. Not used anymore—pharmaceuticals are now used instead.

Pharmacological Androgen Deprivation

Estrogens {T}

1. Mechanism of action—inhibits the hypothalamic-pituitary axis, which decreases luteinizing hormone (LH) secretion and, therefore, decreases testosterone production. Estrogens *increase serum prolactin*. Testosterone reaches castrate levels in approximately 10-14 days (range =10-60 days).
2. Examples—diethylstilbestrol (DES), Premarin®, estradiol, PC-SPES (PC-SPES was taken off the market. It is an herbal mixture that has estrogenic activity; therefore, it has side effects that are similar to estrogen. There is no evidence that PC-SPES has an advantage over prescription estrogen. It was expensive and not covered by insurance. Dose varied from 1-9 capsules po daily).
3. Side effects—embolic (pulmonary embolism, deep venous thrombosis, stroke), cardiac (myocardial infarction), peripheral edema, painful gynecomastia, impotence, weight gain, and altered fat distribution. *Estrogens do not cause hot flashes or osteoporosis.*
4. When using estrogens, consider prescribing an anticoagulant (such as aspirin or coumadin) to reduce the potential for embolic complications.
5. DES 3-5 mg/day has significant cardiovascular risk. DES 1 mg/day delays the progression of advanced prostate cancer, but has a much lower cardiovascular risk. However, castrate testosterone levels are not reliably reached with 1 mg per day. DES may also be given IV (see page 95).

Progestins {T}

1. Mechanism of action—inhibits the hypothalamic-pituitary axis, which decreases LH secretion and, therefore, decreases testosterone production. Progestins do *not* increase serum prolactin.
2. Progestins cause a transient reduction in plasma testosterone is followed by a gradual rise in testosterone (i.e. there is an *escape phenomenon*). Thus, they are usually not used alone to treat prostate cancer.
3. These agents do not cause hot flashes.
4. Examples—megestrol acetate (Megace®), cyproterone acetate (cyproterone is not available in the United States).

Prolactin Antagonists
1. Mechanism of action—blocks prolactin secretion by the pituitary.
2. In those who are no longer responsive to standard hormone therapy, these agents can relieve symptoms, especially bone pain.
3. Examples—bromocriptine, levodopa.

Luteinizing Hormone Releasing Hormone (LHRH) agonists {T}
1. Mechanism of action—stimulation of LHRH receptors in the pituitary produces an initial increase in LH and FSH, which causes an initial increase in testosterone ("flare phenomenon", see page 106). Further LHRH agonism suppresses LH and FSH secretion, resulting in a decrease in testosterone. Testosterone reaches castrate levels within 30 days.
2. Examples–leuprolide (Lupron®, Eligard™, Viadur™), histrelin (Vantas™) goserelin (Zoladex®), triptorelin (Trelstar®). For doses, see page 418.
3. *"Flare phenomenon"* can make tumor associated symptoms worse. See Flare Phenomenon, page 106.
4. Side effects–see Morbidity From Medical or Surgical Castration, page 107

LHRH antagonists {T}
1. Mechanism of action—antagonizing LHRH receptors in the pituitary decreases LH and testosterone. *LHRH antagonists do not cause a flare.*
2. Examples—abarelix (Plenaxis™). Abarelix is no longer available in the United States. Only physicians enrolled in a special program may prescribe abarelix. Abarelix has a cumulative risk of systemic allergic reaction, and this risk increases as the duration of treatment increases. Patients must be monitored for at least 30 minutes after each injection. 20% of patients stop responding to abarelix within the first year of treatment.
3. Side effects—see Morbidity From Medical or Surgical Castration, page 107.

Inhibitors of Androgen Synthesis
1. Ketoconazole {A+T}
   a. Mechanism of action—reduces gonadal and adrenal androgen synthesis by inhibiting cytochrome P-450.
   b. Castrate levels of testosterone may occur by 8 hours after a 400 mg oral dose. The effects are dose dependent (testosterone is diminished with 800 mg/day, and eliminated with 1600 mg/day). High doses decrease corticosteroid levels; thus, steroid supplementation may be necessary (e.g. hydrocortisone 10 mg po TID or prednisone 5 mg po BID).
   c. Side effects—*hepatotoxicity*, weakness, lethargy, nausea, vomiting, decreased libido. The dose limiting side effect is nausea/vomiting.
   d. Adult dose = ketoconazole 400 mg po TID [Tabs: 200 mg]. Side effects may be reduced by starting at 200 mg po TID and increasing the dose to 400 mg po TID as tolerated.
   e. Requires stomach acid for dissolution and absorption. Therefore, give all anti-ulcer medications 2 hours after the ketoconazole dose.
   f. Decreases warfarin metabolism (and increases PT).
   g. Avoid use with hypoglycemic agents (causes severe hypoglycemia).
2. Aminoglutethimide {A+T}
   a. Mechanism of action—blocks the transformation of cholesterol to pregnenolone by inhibiting cytochrome P-450, and thus blocks the formation of glucocorticoids, mineralocorticoids, and sex steroids. Therefore, glucocorticoid and mineralocorticoid supplements are necessary to prevent adrenal insufficiency (Addison's) crisis.
   b. Side effects—hypotension, nausea, vomiting, fatigue, anorexia, depression, edema, skin rashes.
   c. Adult dose = aminoglutethimide 250 mg po q 6 hours.

5α-reductase Inhibitors—see page 114.

Nonsteroidal Antiandrogens {R}

1. Mechanism of action—antiandrogens block the binding of DHT and testosterone to the androgen receptor. Adrenal and gonad androgen increases because androgen receptors in the pituitary and hypothalamus are also blocked, which prevents negative feedback and increases LH.
2. Libido and potency are preserved because testosterone is not reduced.
3. Excess testosterone may be converted to estrogen by aromatase (which is in adipose tissue), resulting in gynecomastia.
4. Examples
   a. Flutamide (Eulexin®)
      • Flutamide half life = 6-8 hours.
      • Adult dose = flutamide 250 mg po TID [Caps: 125 mg].
      • Side effects—hepatotoxicity, gynecomastia, diarrhea, nausea, and vomiting. Gastrointestinal side effects are the dose limiting factor.
   b. Bicalutamide (Casodex®)
      • Bicalutamide half life = approximately 5.8 days.
      • Adult dose = bicalutamide 50 mg po q day [Tabs: 50 mg].
      • Side effects–similar to flutamide but less gastrointestinal effects.
   c. Nilutamide (Nilandron™)
      • Nilutamide half life = approximately 45 hours.
      • Adult dose = nilutamide 300 mg po q day for 30 days, then 150 mg po q day thereafter [Tabs: 50 mg].
      • Side effects—visual disturbances, alcohol intolerance, rarely interstitial pneumonitis, nausea, vomiting.

Steroidal Antiandrogens

1. Mechanism of action—inhibits binding of DHT and testosterone to the nuclear androgen receptors, inhibits 5α-reductase, and has negative feedback on the hypothalamic-pituitary axis.
2. Side effects—include weight gain.
3. Examples—megestrol acetate (Megace®), cyproterone acetate (cyproterone is not available in the United States).

Effects of Androgen Deprivation

Pathologic Changes in Prostate From Androgen Deprivation

1. The most common pathological changes
   a. Atrophy of the glands—this compresses the basal cells closer so they look multi-layer (i.e. basal cell prominence).
   b. Decreased gland density.
   c. Increased fibromuscular stroma.
2. Other changes that can also be seen—apoptosis (cell death), nuclear pyknosis (dense nuclei), intracytoplasmic vacuolization, inflammation.
3. *Necrosis is rarely seen.*

Testosterone Levels After Androgen Deprivation

Therapy	Mean Time to Castrate Testosterone (range)
Orchiectomy	3 hours (2-12 hours)
Ketoconazole†	8 hours (8-72 hours)
LHRH agonists	30 days
LHRH antagonist	8-15 days
DES 1 g IV q 24 hours	*
Oral DES	(10-60 days)

† At dose of 400 mg po q 8 hours.

* Approximately 50% decrease in testosterone levels within 24 hours.

Flare Phenomenon

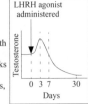

1. When an LHRH agonist is initiated, testosterone increases transiently and can exacerbate cancer related symptoms (e.g. spinal cord compression, bone pain, urinary obstruction) and can cause death from life-threatening metastases. The increase in testosterone over baseline levels (the "flare") peaks in 3-4 days and lasts for approximately 7 days.
2. Flare *is not* caused by orchiectomy, antiandrogens, LHRH antagonists, or estrogens.
3. Preventing flare
   a. Use an LHRH antagonist or orchiectomy instead of an LHRH agonist.
   b. Antiandrogens—these block the testosterone receptor and prevent flare related side effects, but do not prevent the rise in testosterone with flare. Start an antiandrogen *before* giving the LHRH agonist. Theoretically, it may be beneficial to achieve steady state antiandrogen levels before starting the LHRH agonist. To achieve steady state levels, the antiandrogen should be started 4 half lives before the LHRH agonist (see below). Continue the antiandrogen for at least one week after the LHRH agonist because the flare in testosterone (above baseline) lasts one week.
      • Start flutamide $\geq$ *32 hours* before the LHRH agonist ($T_{1/2}$ = 6-8 hours)
      • Start nilutamide $\geq$ *8 days* before the LHRH agonist ($T_{1/2}$ = 45 hours)
      • Start bicalutamide $\geq$ *24 days* before the LHRH agonist ($T_{1/2}$ = 6 days)
   c. Use ketoconazole before the LHRH agonist.

Antiandrogen Withdrawal (AAW)

1. AAW is a decline in PSA (and possible clinical response) that occurs after stopping the antiandrogen component of combined androgen blockade.
2. On average, AAW occurs in approximately 25% of patients (although up to 50% has been reported).
3. The range of PSA reduction varies considerably.
4. The reduction in PSA usually lasts 3-6 months.
5. When flutamide is stopped, PSA decline begins within a few days.
6. When bicalutamide is stopped, PSA decline begins in 4-8 weeks.

Hot Flashes

1. Hot flashes can be caused by LHRH agonists, LHRH antagonists, bilateral orchiectomy and nonsteroidal antiandrogens.
2. Estrogens and progesterones do not cause hot flashes.
3. Preventing hot flashes
   a. Endocrine treatments—estrogenic [E] and progestational [P]. Estrogens may cause painful gynecomastia, thrombosis, and cardiac side effects.
      i. Megestrol acetate 20 mg po BID [P]—most effective with the least side effects. Titrate the dose as necessary. Weight gain is common.
      ii. Transdermal estradiol 0.05-0.10 mg patch applied twice a week [E]
      iii. Diethylstilbestrol 0.5 mg po q day [E].
   b. Non-endocrine treatments
      i. Clonidine 0.1 mg po q day—venlafaxine is more effective.
      ii. Venlafaxine—starting dose is often 37.5 mg/day. If necessary, it can be titrated up to 75 mg/day.
      iii. Vitamin E 800 IU po q day—recent evidence suggests that long-term use (> 1 year) of more than 400 IU per day may increase the risk of heart failure and mortality.
      iv. Gabapentin—reports suggest that it is effective, including in patients refractory to venlafaxine.
      v. Acupuncture

Morbidity From Medical or Surgical Castration

1. Long-term androgen deprivation with medical or surgical castration increases the risk of
   a. Adverse lipid profile—elevated cholesterol and LDL.
   b. Diabetes
   c. Cardiovascular disease—LHRH agonists increase the risk of coronary artery disease, heart attack, and sudden cardiac death. However, orchiectomy does not appear to increase the risk of these cardiac events.
   d. Osteoporosis
   e. Anemia—normocytic anemia (normal MCV). Hemoglobin may decline within the first month of therapy and often reaches its nadir by 6 months of therapy. This anemia can be corrected by either stopping hormone therapy or by administering erythropoietin.
   f. Periodontal disease—no increase in cavities, but a higher risk of plaque, gingival recession, and other indicators of periodontal disease.
   g. Sexual dysfunction—decreased libido and erectile dysfunction.
   h. Changes in body habitus—gynecomastia (sometimes painful), testicular atrophy, weight gain, loss of muscle mass, increased subcutaneous fat.
   i. Fatigue—may be caused by anemia or low testosterone.
   j. Hot flashes—hot flashes can be frequent and bothersome.
2. Recent data suggests that depression and cognitive deficits (such as impaired memory) occur with equal frequency in men undergoing and not undergoing androgen deprivation. Thus, it appears that androgen deprivation may not cause depression or cognitive deficits.

Osteoporosis from Androgen Deprivation

1. LHRH agonists/antagonists and orchiectomy can cause osteoporosis. Antiandrogen monotherapy and estrogens to do not cause osteoporosis.
2. *A longer duration of androgen deprivation is associated with a greater decline in bone mineral density (BMD) and a higher risk of skeletal fractures.* Bone density may decline as much as 10% during the first year of therapy and by 1-3% per year thereafter.
3. Men on long-term androgen deprivation appear to have at least a 5 fold higher risk of osteoporosis related fractures than healthy age matched controls. Some fractures occur during the first year of treatment. *Pathologic fractures in men receiving androgen deprivation have been correlated with decreased overall survival.*
4. Men about to undergo androgen deprivation for prostate cancer have a lower BMD than healthy age matched controls. Thus, men with prostate cancer are at risk for osteoporosis before androgen deprivation is started.
5. Other risk factors for osteoporosis—smoking, alcohol intake, steroid use, physical inactivity, thin body habitus, and advancing age.
6. Methods to prevent osteoporosis caused by androgen deprivation include
   a. Reduce risk factors for osteoporosis—stop smoking, avoid alcohol intake, avoid steroid use, and engage in physical activity.
   b. Vitamin D 400-800 IU po q day and calcium 500-1000 mg po q day.
   c. Bisphosphonate therapy—see below.
7. Treatment guidelines (Based on the 3rd International Consultation on Prostate Cancer and the NCCN 2007 Guidelines)
   a. Patients on long-term androgen deprivation should have baseline and periodic bone densitometry scans to assess BMD.
   b. In patients with a substantial decrease in BMD from androgen deprivation, consider using a bisphosphonate.
   c. Vitamin D and calcium supplements are recommended in men receiving androgen deprivation.

Gynecomastia from Androgen Deprivation

1. Gynecomastia (GM) is enlargement of the breasts. In some cases, GM can be painful.
2. GM can be caused by medical castration, surgical castration, antiandrogens, 5α-reductase inhibitors, and estrogens.
3. GM is more common with estrogens and antiandrogens than with medical or surgical castration. 5α-reductase inhibitors rarely cause GM (< 1%).
4. GM may resolve after stopping androgen deprivation. However, it is more likely to resolve when the duration of therapy was short (e.g. < 6 months).
5. Evaluation includes a breast and lymph node exam. Classify the breast size by Tanner stage or by measuring the breast. A mammogram and biopsy may be indicated in men with a family history of breast cancer, focal breast enlargement/pain, or a suspicious breast exam (lump, dimple, etc.).
6. Treatment
   a. If possible, stop the causative agent.
   c. External beam radiation (XRT)—a single fraction of 12-15 Gy to the breasts *before* administering an antiandrogen or an estrogen has been shown to decrease the risk of GM. The long-term risks of breast XRT are unknown and some patients still develop GM.
   c. Tamoxifen—10 to 20 mg per day can reduce breast size and pain. It is most effective when it is started before or soon after GM develops.
   d. Breast reduction surgery—reduces breast size and can reduce breast pain. Surgery is often necessary when GM is severe (Tanner stage ≥ III) or long standing (> 1 year). Surgery may include liposuction or excision of breast tissue.

REFERENCES

General

Daneshgari F, Crawford ED: Endocrine therapy of advanced carcinoma of the prostate. Cancer of the prostate. Ed. S Das, ED Crawford. New York: Marcel Dekker, Inc., 1993, pp. 333-354.

Maatman TJ, Gupta MK, Montie JE: Effectiveness of castration versus intravenous estrogen therapy in producing rapid endocrine control of metastatic cancer of the prostate. J Urol, 133: 620, 1985.

Schellhammer PF, Venner P, Haas GP, et al: Prostate specific antigen decreases after withdrawal of antiandrogen therapy with bicalutamide or flutamide in patients receiving combined androgen blockade. J Urol, 157: 1731, 1997.

Smith Jr. JA, et al: Clinical effects of gonadotropin-releasing hormone analog in metastatic carcinoma of the prostate. Urology, 25(2): 106, 1985.

Hot Flashes

Barton DL, Loprinzi CL, Quella SK, et al: Prospective evaluation of vitamin E for hot flashes in breast cancer survivors. J Clin Oncol, 16(2): 495, 1998.

Hammar M, Frisk J, et al: Acupuncture treatment of vasomotor symptoms in men with prostatic carcinoma: a pilot study. J Urol, 161(3): 853, 1999.

Loprinzi CL, Michalak JC, Quella SK, et al: Megestrol acetate for the prevention of hot flashes. N Engl J Med, 331(6): 347, 1994.

Gerber GS, Zagaja GP, Ray PS, et al: Transdermal estrogen in the treatment of hot flushes in men with prostate cancer. Urology, 55: 97, 2000.

Quella SK, Loprinzi CL, Sloan J, et al: Pilot evaluation of venlafaxine for the treatment of hot flashes in men undergoing androgen ablation therapy for prostate cancer. J Urol, 162(1): 98, 1999.

Quella SK, Loprinzi CL, Sloan JA, et al: Long term use of megestrol acetate by cancer survivors for the treatment of hot flashes. Cancer, 82(9): 1784, 1998.

Smith Jr. JA: Management of hot flushes due to endocrine therapy for prostate carcinoma. Oncology, 10(9): 1319, 1996.

Ketoconazole

Pont A: Long-term experience with high dose ketoconazole therapy in patients with D2 prostate carcinoma. J Urol, 137: 902, 1987.

Trachtenberg J: Ketoconazole therapy in advanced prostate cancer. J Urol, 132: 61, 1984.

Flare and Flare Prevention

Labrie F, Dupont A, Belanger A, et al: Flutamide eliminates the risk of disease flare in prostatic cancer patients treated with a luteinizing hormone-releasing hormone agonist. J Urol, 138: 804, 1987.

Noguchi K, et al: Inhibition of PSA flare in prostate cancer patients by administration of flutamide for 2 weeks before initiation of treatment with slow-releasing LH-RH agonist. Int J Clin Oncol, 6(1): 29, 2001.

Tsushima T, et al: Optimal starting time for flutamide to prevent disease flare in prostate cancer patients treated with a gonadotropin-releasing hormone agonist. Urol Int, 66(3): 135, 2001.

Osteoporosis

Carroll PR, Altwein J, et al: Management of disseminated prostate cancer. Prostate Cancer: 3rd International Consultation on Prostate Cancer - Paris. Ed. L Denis, et al. Paris: Health Publications, 2003, pp 249-284.

Daniell HW: Osteoporosis due to androgen deprivation therapy in men with prostate cancer. Urology, 58 (suppl 2A): 101, 2001.

Moyad MA, Pienta KJ: Complementary medicine for prostatic diseases: a primer for clinicians. Urology, 59 (suppl 4a), 2002.

Kiratli BJ, et al: Progressive decrease in bone density over 10 years or androgen deprivation therapy in patients with prostate cancer. Urology, 57:127, 2001.

Oefelein MG, et al: Skeletal fracture associated with androgen suppression induced osteoporosis: the clinical incidence and risk factors for patients with prostate cancer. J Urol, 166: 1724, 2001.

Smith MR, et al: Bicalutamide monotherapy versus leuprolide monotherapy for prostate cancer: effects on bone mineral density and body composition. J Clin Oncol, 22(13): 2546, 2004.

Stoch SA, et al: Bone loss in men with prostate cancer treated with gonadotropin-releasing hormone agonists. J Clin Endocrinol Metab 86: 2787, 2001.

Townsend MF, et al: Bone fractures associated with luteinizing hormone-releasing hormone agonists used in the treatment of prostate carcinoma. Cancer, 79: 545, 1997.

Other Side Effects of Androgen Deprivation

Dobs A, Darkes MJM: Incidence and management of gynecomastia in men treated for prostate cancer. J Urol, 174(5): 1737, 2005.

Famili P, et al: The effect of androgen deprivation therapy on periodontal disease in men with prostate cancer. J Urol, 177(3): 921, 2007.

Joly F, et al: Impact of androgen deprivation therapy on physical and cognitive function, as well as quality of life of patients with non-metastatic prostate cancer. J Urol, 166(6, part1): 2443, 2006.

Keating NL, et al: Diabetes and cardiovascular disease during androgen deprivation therapy for prostate cancer. J Clin Oncol, 24(27): 4448, 2006.

Kumar RJ, et al: Adverse events associated with hormonal therapy for prostate cancer. Rev Urol, 7(suppl 5): S37, 2005.

Shahinian VB, et al: Risk of the "androgen deprivation syndrome" in men receiving androgen deprivation for prostate cancer. Arch Intern Med, 166(4): 465, 2006.

BENIGN PROSTATIC HYPERPLASIA (BPH)

General Information
   1. *BPH occurs in the transition zone*. Prostate cancer may also occur in the transition zone (see Location of Prostate Cancer, page 78).
   2. Most of the α-adrenergic receptors in the prostate are α-1A receptors. These α-1A receptors mediate contraction of prostatic smooth muscle and are located predominantly in the prostate stroma.
   3. 5α-reductase converts testosterone to dihydrotestosterone. Most of the 5α-reductase in the prostate is type II 5α-reductase. Type II 5α-reductase is present in stromal and basal prostate cells (but not epithelial cells).
   4. As men age, the following changes occur in the prostate. These changes may lead to clinical BPH.
      a. *Increase in the amount of prostate stroma*—prostate stroma growth into the lumen of the prostatic urethra can obstruct the flow of urine. 5α-reductase inhibitors treat BPH by shrinking the prostate stoma.
      b. *Increase in the number of α-1 receptors in the prostate stroma*—this augments smooth muscle contraction in the bladder neck and prostate stroma, which can obstruct the flow of urine. *This is the most important factor contributing to lower urinary tract symptoms (LUTS) from BPH.* α-1 blockers block these receptors and relax the smooth muscle.

Bladder Outlet Obstruction (BOO) From BPH
   1. Increased bladder outlet resistance in BPH may occur from
      a. Increased tone of the prostate stroma and bladder neck.
      b. Prostate growth into the lumen of the urethra.
   2. *Degree of BOO does not correlate with severity of BPH symptoms*. Men with severe obstruction may have few LUTS and men with minimal obstruction may have severe LUTS.
   3. The best test to determine the presence of BOO is video urodynamics. Prostate size and radiographic imaging are of little use in evaluating BOO.

Presentation and Symptoms
   1. Lower urinary tract symptoms (LUTS) from BPH include decreased force of stream, hesitancy, intermittent stream, post void dribbling, and nocturia. These symptoms usually occur in men over the age of 60 years and are often called *"LUTS suggestive of BPH."*
   2. With progressive BOO, the bladder may become overworked, leading to symptoms of "overactive bladder" such as urgency and frequency.
   3. If BPH is severe and prolonged, the bladder may decompensate, resulting in absent or ineffective contractions that do not empty the bladder. Inability to empty the bladder can cause elevated post void residual, urine retention, sensation of incomplete emptying of the bladder, and overflow incontinence. Hydronephrosis from bladder outlet obstruction is rare, but it can lead to renal insufficiency.
   4. *The severity of urinary symptoms do not correlate with prostate size*. Small prostates can cause severe symptoms. Large prostates can be asymptomatic.
   5. *The severity of urinary symptoms do not correlate with degree of bladder outlet obstruction*. Men with severe obstruction may have few symptoms and men with minimal obstruction may have severe symptoms.
   6. BPH can cause hematuria—see page 123.

Work up of BPH (Based on 2003 AUA Guideline)

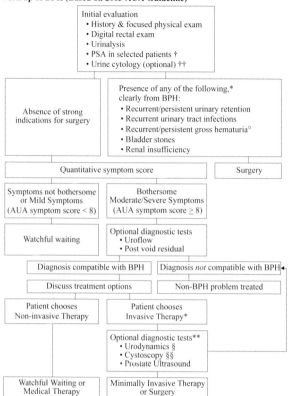

* See Indications for Surgical Management, page 115.
** Some diagnostic tests are used in predicting response to therapy.
† PSA may be offered to men in whom PSA would change management or to men
   with at least 10-year life expectancy in whom the diagnosis of prostate
   cancer would change management.
†† Especially useful in men with irritative symptoms or at risk for bladder cancer.
§ Urodynamic testing should be considered in patients with
   • Known or suspected neurologic dysfunction
   • Lifelong symptoms
   • Persistent symptoms after prior surgical treatment of BPH
   • Young men
§§ Cystoscopy is recommended in men with
   • Hematuria
   • History of bladder tumors or at risk for bladder tumors
   • At risk for urethral stricture or bladder neck contracture
° Some patients may benefit from a 5α-reductase inhibitor.

Test Results That Suggest Bladder Outlet Obstruction
1. Low flow rate on uroflowometry.
2. Elevated post void residual—stasis of urine can increase the risk of urinary tract infection and bladder stones.
3. Trabeculation of the bladder and enlarged prostate on cystoscopy.
4. Low flow rate and high detrusor pressure on urodynamics—advanced stages may also reveal detrusor overactivity or acontractile bladder.

Natural History and Progression of BPH
1. BPH does not progress in all patients. In men with mild LUTS, 57% progress to worse LUTS in 4 years; however, only 10% require surgical intervention. In men with severe LUTS, one third undergo prostate surgery within 4 years.

Symptoms at Initial Diagnosis	Symptoms 4 Years after Diagnosis			
	Better	Unchanged	Worse	Undergo Surgery
Mild	-	33%	57%	10%
Moderate	13%	46%	17%	24%
Severe	23%	38%	-	39%

2. In men with BPH, higher PSA values increase the risk of prostate growth, worsening LUTS, decline in urine flow rates, acute urinary retention, need for surgical intervention, and progression of BPH.
3. The risk of BPH progression (to worse symptoms, acute urinary retention, or surgical intervention) is higher in men with larger prostate size, higher PSA, older age, lower urine flow rates, and more severe LUTS.
4. The MTOPS trial showed that α-blockers and 5α-reductase inhibitors can prevent BPH progression (see Combination Therapy, page 114).

Non-invasive Therapy

General Recommendations
1. Avoid substances that can exacerbate symptoms or cause urinary retention.
   a. α-agonists—examples include decongestants that contain pseudoephedrine and the diet supplement ephedra.
   b. Anticholinergics—including those prescribed for "overactive bladder." In some cases, anticholinergic medications can cause urinary retention; however, they usually help voiding symptoms in patients with BPH.
   c. Caffeine and alcohol—lower intake of these may reduce LUTS.
   d. Spicy and acidic foods—reducing these substances in the diet may help minimize voiding symptoms.
2. Nocturia can be reduced by
   a. Decreasing fluid intake in the evening.
   b. Avoiding diuretics in the evening.
   c. When men have lower extremity edema, they can elevate their legs for one hour before bedtime (this mobilizes lower extremity fluid into the circulation and helps eliminate it before going to sleep).

Surveillance ("Watchful Waiting")
1. Watchful waiting is the preferred management for men whose urinary symptoms are mild and not bothersome (i.e. AUA symptom score < 8).
2. Surveillance consists of repeating the initial evaluation described on page 111 at least once a year.

Phytotherapy

1. The AUA guideline did not recommend phytotherapy as a standard therapy; however, it may have a therapeutic benefit.

2. Saw palmetto is the most widely used phytotherapy for BPH. It does not appear to change PSA.

3. The mechanism of action for these agents is largely unknown.

Common Name	Species
Saw Palmetto, American dwarf palm	*Serenoa repens, Sabal serrulata*
African plum tree	*Pygeum africanum*
Stinging nettle	*Urtica dioica, Urtica urens*
Pumpkin Seed	*Cucurbita pepo*
African star grass	*Hypoxis rooperi*
Rye pollen	*Secale cereale*

α-Blockers

1. Examples: Terazosin (Hytrin®), immediate release doxazosin (Cardura®), extended release doxazosin (Cardura® XL), tamsulosin (Flomax®), alfuzosin (Uroxatral®).

2. *α-1A adrenergic receptors are the primary subtype of α-1 receptor in the prostate.* Tamsulosin is the only α-blocker that is α-1A selective.

3. α-blockers relax smooth muscle in the prostate fibromuscular stroma. They may also act in the central nervous system to improve symptoms.

4. These drugs achieve a *dose dependant* improvement in maximum urinary flow rate and symptom score and *appear to have equal clinical efficacy.*

5. α-blockers can prevent BPH progression (see page 114).

6. Maximal response is usually observed in approximately 1-2 weeks.

7. Side effects—dizziness, fatigue (asthenia), nasal congestion, syncope, orthostatic hypotension, and retrograde ejaculation.

   a. Tamsulosin, alfuzosin, and extended release (ER) doxazosin are less likely to cause orthostatic hypotension compared to terazosin and immediate release (IR) doxazosin.

   b. Tamsulosin has the highest rate of retrograde ejaculation.

   c. Intraoperative floppy iris syndrome (IFIS)—patients who have taken α-blockers are at risk for IFIS during cataract surgery. Permanent visual problems can arise when cataract surgery is not modified to account for IFIS. It is unknown if stopping α-blockers before cataract surgery reduces the risk of IFIS. *IFIS has been reported mainly with tamsulosin.* IFIS appears to be less likely with other α-blockers, presumably because they are not α-1A selective.

8. IR doxazosin and terazosin can be used to treat hypertension (HTN). Tamsulosin, alfuzosin, and ER doxazosin are *not* used to treat HTN.

9. The ALLHAT study randomized men with HTN and at least one other risk factor for heart disease to treatment with various antihypertensive drugs. Hypertensive men treated with IR doxazosin (the only α-blocker in the study) had a significantly higher incidence of congestive heart failure, stroke, angina, and coronary revascularization. Thus, care should be taken when prescribing α-blockers to men with HTN.

10. Tamsulosin, alfuzosin, and ER doxazosin may be started at a therapeutic dose. IR doxazosin and terazosin should be titrated to a therapeutic dose to avoid hypotension. Adult dose:

Generic Name	Brand Name	Initial Dose	Max Dose for BPH	Max Dose for HTN
Terazosin	Hytrin®	1 mg po q HS	10 mg po q HS	20 mg po q HS
Doxazosin IR	Cardura®	1 mg po q day	8 mg po q day	16 mg po q day
Doxazosin ER	Cardura XL®	4 mg po q day	8 mg po q day	—
Tamsulosin	Flomax®	0.4 mg po q day	0.8 mg po q day	—
Alfuzosin	Uroxatral®	10 mg po q day	10 mg po q day	—

IR = immediate release; ER = extended release; Max = maximum

5α-Reductase Inhibitors
1. Finasteride (Proscar®) inhibits type II 5α-reductase.
   Dutasteride (Avodart™) inhibits type I and II 5α-reductase.
2. By blocking the enzyme that converts testosterone to dihydrotestosterone (DHT), these drugs lower DHT and promote the following effects.
   a. Reduces prostate volume by 20% to 25%.
   b. Increases maximum urinary flow rate by approximately 10%.
   c. Improves symptom scores by approximately 20 to 30%.
   d. Reduces the risk of urinary retention by approximately 50%.
   e. Reduces the need for surgical BPH therapy by approximately 50%.
   f. Reduces the risk of BPH progression (see page 114).
   g. Decreases total PSA by 50% after 6 months of treatment. In men taking a 5α-reductase inhibitor for ≥ 6 months, the PSA during treatment should be doubled in order to compare it to PSA levels before treatment.
   h. Increases testosterone by 10-20% (usually clinically insignificant).
   i. May help stop chronic hematuria from the prostate.
3. Symptom improvement and the effects listed above may begin within several weeks; however, it takes 6-9 months to achieve maximum benefit.
4. Clinical effects are observed mainly in men with a large prostate; therefore, these medications are indicated in men with a large prostate (e.g. > 40 cc).
5. Adult dose—finasteride 5 mg po q day, dutasteride 0.5 mg po q day.
6. Adverse effects include—impotence (< 5%), decreased libido (< 4%), decrease volume of ejaculate (< 3%), gynecomastia (<1%).

Combination Therapy (α-Blocker and 5α-Reductase Inhibitor)
1. The Medical Therapy of Prostate Symptoms (MTOPS) trial randomized 3047 men age ≥ 50 years to doxazosin, finasteride, or both. At trial entry, men had PSA ≤ 10, maximum urine flow rate of 4-15 ml/sec, and AUA symptom score of 8-30. Progression was defined as AUA symptom score increase ≥ 4, urinary incontinence, recurrent urinary tract infection (UTI), acute urine retention, or renal insufficiency. Mean follow up was 4.5 years.
2. The MTOPS trial showed that both α-blockers and 5α-reductase inhibitors prevent progression of BPH; however, *the combination of an α-blocker and a 5α-reductase inhibitor prevents progression of BPH better then either agent alone*. The benefit of combination therapy was greatest in men with PSA > 4.0 ng/ml and prostate volume > 40 cc. Therapy did not reduce renal insufficiency, UTI, or urine incontinence, but it did reduce progression of voiding symptoms, acute urinary retention, and subsequent need for BPH surgery.

	Reduction in Given Endpoint Compared to Placebo		
	Any Progression	Acute Urinary Retention	Need For Surgery
Doxazosin	39%	No change	No change
Finasteride	34%	68%	64%
Combination	66%	81%	67%

3. The AUA guideline did not specify a PSA or prostate volume beyond which prevention should be initiated. All risk factors for BPH progression (large prostate, high PSA, older age, low urine flow rate, severe LUTS) should be considered.
4. Although the MTOPS study examined doxazosin and finasteride, the AUA guideline "assumes...the combination of any effective α-blocker and 5α-reductase inhibitor probably produces a comparable benefit."

Minimally Invasive Therapy

TUNA (Transurethral Needle Ablation)
1. *Radiofrequency (RF) waves* heat the prostate and create thermal necrosis.
2. Under direct vision, 2 curved needles (which extend from the tip of a special cystoscope sheath) deliver RF energy into the prostate.
3. Examples—Prostiva™
4. The ideal patient for TUNA is a man with obstructive voiding symptoms, prostate size ≤ 60 grams, and mainly lateral lobe prostate enlargement.
5. Irritative symptoms can persist for several weeks after the procedure.
6. TUNA seems to require more sedation and analgesia than TUMT.
7. See page 117 for efficacy and side effects.

TUMT (Transurethral Microwave Thermotherapy)
1. *Microwaves* heat the prostate and create thermal necrosis.
2. The microwaves are delivered using a catheter type device.
3. Examples—Prostatron®, TherMatrx™, CoreTherm™, Targis®
4. Irritative symptoms can persist for several weeks after the procedure.
5. See page 117 for efficacy and side effects.

Emerging Minimally Invasive Therapies
Examples include interstitial laser coagulation, absolute ethanol injection, water induced thermal therapy, high intensity focused ultrasound (HIFU).

Surgical Therapy

Indications for Surgical Management
1. Strong indications
   a. Refractory urinary retention
   b. Recurrent urinary tract infections
   c. Refractory gross hematuria
   d. Bladder stones
   e. Renal insufficiency from BPH
2. Moderate indication—AUA symptom score ≥ 8 *and* any of the following:
   a. Substantial bother from symptoms.
   b. Increasing postvoid residual on serial exams.
   c. Low maximum flow rate (esp. < 15 ml/sec).

TUIP (Transurethral Incision of Prostate)
1. Using cutting current, 1 or 2 endoscopic incisions in the prostatic urethra (at 5 and/or 7 o'clock) are extended from the bladder neck to a location immediately cephalad to the verumontanum. The depth of the incision should be down to the fibrous prostate capsule.
2. Compared to TURP, TUIP has similar efficacy, but a *lower rate of retrograde ejaculation* and other complications (see page 117).
3. TUIP is best suited for men with smaller prostates (< 30 g resectable weight) and for men who wish to reduce the risk of retrograde ejaculation.

TURP (Transurethral Resection of Prostate)
1. A resection loop is used to remove "chips" of prostate tissue. Resection is accomplished circumferentially from the bladder neck to a location immediately cephalad to the verumontanum
2. The success rate of TURP is higher when the following are present:
   a. Preoperative maximum flow rate < 15 ml/sec.
   b. Men are substantially bothered by their urinary symptoms.
3. TURP has a higher risk of bleeding requiring transfusion than TUIP or minimally invasive therapies.

4. Complications—see also page 117.
   a. Postoperative bleeding is the most common complication.
   b. TUR syndrome—excessive absorption of hypotonic irrigation fluid from the prostatic vascular bed results in hyponatremia, hypervolemia, hypertension, mental confusion, nausea, vomiting, and visual disturbances. Treatment includes diuresis and fluid restriction. TUR syndrome occurs in 2% of cases.
5. Up to 10% of men undergoing TURP have foci of prostate cancer in the resected prostate chips.

Open Prostatectomy

1. Open prostatectomy is usually reserved for men with *large prostates* (e.g. > 80 cc) or men who cannot tolerate a transurethral procedure.
2. Surgical approaches include suprapubic, retropubic, and perineal.
3. The suprapubic approach is ideal for patients who also require removal of bladder stones or excision of a bladder diverticulum.
4. See page 117 for efficacy and side effects.

Other Surgical BPH Therapies

1. Holmium laser resection/enucleation of the prostate
2. Transurethral laser coagulation (VLAP, visual laser ablation of prostate)— laser energy coagulates prostate tissue (but does not vaporize it).
3. Transurethral laser vaporization—laser energy vaporizes prostate tissue.
4. Transurethral electrovaporization—electric (cutting) current vaporizes prostate tissue. Efficacy is similar to TURP, but post-operative irritative voiding symptoms and urine retention occur more often than with TURP.

Persistent Symptoms After Surgical Treatment

1. Symptoms persist in 15-20% of men after invasive treatment for BPH.
2. When voiding symptoms persist after invasive treatment of BPH, obtain urodynamics. Urodynamic testing reveals the following results:
   • 38% remain obstructed
   • 25% have poor detrusor contraction
   • 50% have detrusor overactivity when a neurologic disorder is *absent*. Detrusor overactivity may persist up to one year after invasive therapy.
   • 70% have detrusor overactivity when a neurologic disorder is *present*.
3. The most common causes of urinary incontinence after invasive treatment for BPH are *detrusor overactivity and sphincter damage*.

Comparison of Therapies for BPH

1. Minimally invasive therapy improves urinary flow rate and symptom score more than medical therapy, but less than surgery.
2. Surgery improves urinary flow rate and symptom score more than other therapies.
3. See page 117.

Comparison of Treatments for BPH

BPH Therapy	Invasiveness	Symptom Score Improvement*	Flow Rate Improvement*	Urinary Retention	BNC	Urinary Incontinence	Retro Ejac	ED	Blood Transfusion	Secondary Procedure Rate
Watchful Waiting	Non-invasive	0.5	—	3%	—	2%	—	21%	0%	55%
α-Blockers	Non-invasive	6	2-3	0-4%	—	—	≤10%	—	—	—
5α-Reductase Inhibitors	Non-invasive	3.4	1.7	2%	—	—	†	3%†	—	†
TUMT	Minimal	9-11	3	6-15%	3%	2%	5-16%	3%	≤2%	10-16%
TUNA	Minimal	9	4	20%	3%	1%	4%	3%	3%	23%
Holmium Resection Enucleation	Surgical	18	11	8%	5%	1%	59%	3%	2%	1%
Transurethral Laser Coagulation	Surgical	20	11	21%	5%	1%	17%	6%	2%	7%
Transurethral Laser Vaporization	Surgical	14	11	13%	3%	3%	42%	7%	3%	8%
Transurethral Electro Vaporization	Surgical	16	13	12%	5%	3%	65%	8%	1%	8%
TUIP	Surgical	15	7	6%	6%	2%	18%	13%	3%	14%
TURP	Surgical	15	11	5%	7%	3%	65%	10%	8%	5%
Open Prostatectomy	Surgical	10	14	1%	8%	6%	61%	?	27%	1%

* At 10-16 months after beginning treatment. AUA Symptom score improvement is in points. Flow rate improvement is in ml/second.
† 5α-reductase inhibitors have a low risk of reversible ED, low libido, and low volume ejaculate. They reduce the need for surgery by 50%.
BNC = bladder neck contracture; Retro Ejac = retrograde ejaculation; ED = erectile dysfunction; TUMT = transurethral microwave thermotherapy
TUNA = transurethral needle ablation; TUIP = transurethral incision of prostate; TURP = transurethral resection of prostate

REFERENCES

General

ALLHAT Collaborative Research Group: Major cardiovascular events in hypertensive patients randomized to doxazosin vs. chlorthalidone: The Antihypertensive and Lipid Lowering treatment to prevent Heart Attack Trial (ALLHAT). JAMA, 283(15): 1967, 2003.

Barry MJ, et al: The natural history of patients with benign prostatic hyperplasia as diagnosed by North American Urologists. J Urol, 157: 10, 1997.

Chadha V, et al: Floppy iris behavior during cataract surgery: associations and variations. Br J Opthalmol, 91(1): 40, 2007.

Jacobsen SJ, Jacobsen DJ, et al: Natural history of prostatism: risk factors for acute urinary retention. J Urol, 158: 481, 1997.

McConnell JD, Barry MJ, Bruskewitz RC, et al: Benign prostatic hyperplasia: diagnosis and treatment. Clinical practice guideline, Number 8. AHCPR publication No. 94-0582. Rockville, Maryland: Agency for Health Care Policy and Research, Public Health Service, U.S. Department of Health and Human Services, February 1994.

Oshika T, et al: Incidence of intraoperative floppy iris syndrome in patients on either systemic or topical alpha(1)-adrenoreceptor antagonist. Am J Opthalmol, 143(1): 150, 2007.

AUA Practice Guidelines Committee: AUA guideline on the management of benign prostatic hyperplasia. J Urol, 170: 530, 2003.

Medical Therapy

Lepor H, Vaughan ED Jr.: Medical management of BPH part I. AUA Update Series, Vol. 15, Lesson 3, 1996.

Lepor H, Vaughan ED Jr.: Medical management of BPH part II. AUA Update Series, Vol. 15, Lesson 4, 1996.

Lepor H, Williford WO, Barry MJ, et al: The efficacy of terazosin, finasteride, or both in benign prostatic hyperplasia. N Engl J Med, 335(8): 533, 1996.

Lowe FC, Ku JC: Phytotherapy in the treatment of benign prostatic hyperplasia: a critical review. Urology, 48(1): 12, 1996.

McConnell JD, et al for the MTOPS research group: The long term effect of doxazosin, finasteride, and combination therapy on the clinical progression of benign prostatic hyperplasia. N Engl J Med, 349: 285, 2003.

McConnell JD, et al: The effect of finasteride on the risk of acute urinary retention and the need for surgical treatment among men with benign prostatic hyperplasia. N Engl J Med, 338(9):557, 1998.

Roehrborn CG, et al: Efficacy and safety of a dual inhibitor of 5-alpha-reductase types 1 and 2 (dutasteride) in men with benign prostatic hyperplasia. Urology, 60: 434, 2002.

Tempany CMC, et al: The influence of finasteride on the volume of the peripheral and periurethral zones of the prostate in men with benign prostatic hyperplasia. Prostate, 22: 39, 1993.

Invasive Therapy

Blute ML: Transurethral microwave thermotherapy: minimally invasive therapy for benign prostatic hyperplasia. Urology, 50: 163, 1997.

Madsen FA, Bruskewitz RC: Role of prostatectomy in the management of benign prostatic hyperplasia. AUA Update Series, Vol. 15, Lesson 5, 1996.

Mebust WK, Holtgrewe HL, Cockett ATK, et al: Transurethral prostatectomy: immediate and postoperative complications. Cooperative study of 13 participating institutions evaluating 3,885 patients. J Urol 141: 243, 1989.

Naslund MJ: Transurethral needle ablation of prostate. Urology, 50: 167, 1997.

Nudell DM, Cattolica EV: Transurethral prostatectomy: an update. AUA Update Series, Vol. 19, Lesson 5, 2000.

Perlmutter AP: New uses of energy for the treatment of BPH. AUA Update Series, Vol. 16, Lesson 32, 1997.

PROSTATE SPECIFIC ANTIGEN (PSA)

General Information
1. PSA is a serine protease of the kallikrein family produced by the prostate.
   - Seminogelin, a protein in seminal fluid, is cleaved by PSA. This cleavage is an important step in semen liquefaction.
   - PSA half life is approximately 2.2-3.2 days.
   - PSA does *not* vary during the day (no variance with circadian rhythms).
   - PSA is androgen dependent (i.e. its production is stimulated by androgens).
2. The use of PSA in screening for prostate cancer has resulted in
   - Detecting more prostate cancers—PSA detects more organ confined cancers than digital rectal exam. Therefore, PSA and DRE detect more cancers than DRE alone.
   - Detecting prostate cancers earlier.
   - No proven increase in survival in those with PSA detected cancers.
3. Conditions that can elevate PSA
   - Prostate cancer
   - Benign conditions (e.g. BPH, prostatitis). PSA is not elevated in nonbacterial prostatitis, but may be elevated in bacterial prostatitis.
   - Manipulation or trauma (e.g. cystoscopy, prostatic massage, prostate biopsy, extensive ambulation or cycling). Prostate exam (without excessive prostate pressure) does not appear to alter PSA appreciably.
   - Ejaculation may increase PSA levels.
   - PSA increases with age.
   - In rare instances, PSA can be falsely elevated after Prostascint® scan because of human anti-murine antibody (HAMA) formation.
4. Conditions that can reduce PSA
   - 5α-reductase inhibitors (finasteride, dutasteride)—these drugs reduce total PSA by approximately 50% after 6 months of treatment, but do not appear to change the % Free PSA (free PSA/total PSA ratio).
   - Androgen deprivation or castration.
   - Prostatic surgery—removes or destroys a significant portion of the prostate (PSA may increase immediately after prostate surgery because of prostatic manipulation or infarction; however, with longer follow up, PSA will usually decline).
   - Radiation therapy often elevates PSA during and immediately after radiation; however, with longer follow up, PSA will usually decline.

Prostate Cancer and PSA

Using PSA to Screen for Prostate Cancer
See Screening for Prostate Cancer, page 79.
See Prostate Biopsy, page 79.

Methods to Improve Prostate Cancer Detection
1. Age specific serum PSA reference ranges (based on Caucasian men)

Age (years)	"Normal" PSA Range (ng/ml)
40-49	0-2.5
50-59	0-3.5
60-69	0-4.5
70-79	0-6.5

2. Race specific serum PSA reference ranges—still under investigation.
3. PSA velocity (PSAV)
   a. For total PSA < 4 ng/ml, PSA velocity > 0.35 ng/ml/year is worrisome for prostate cancer.
   b. For total PSA = 4-10 ng/ml, PSA velocity > 0.75 ng/ml/year is worrisome for prostate cancer.
   c. PSAV requires at least 3 PSA levels taken at least 6 months apart.
   d. Calculation

$$PSAV = 0.5 \times \left(\frac{PSA_2 - PSA_1}{Time_1} + \frac{PSA_3 - PSA_2}{Time_2} \right)$$

PSA_1 = 1st PSA (ng/ml); PSA_2 = 2nd PSA (ng/ml); PSA_3 = 3rd PSA (ng/ml).
$Time_1$ = time from PSA_1 to PSA_2 (years); $Time_2$ = time from PSA_2 to PSA_3 (years).

4. PSA density (PSAD)
   a. PSAD should not be used as the primary determinant for biopsy because it has many factors affecting its accuracy.
   b. PSAD $\geq$ 0.15 suggests prostate cancer.
   c. PSAD requires transrectal ultrasound measurement of prostate volume.
   d. Calculation

$$PSAD = \frac{PSA \ (ng/ml)}{Prostate \ Volume \ (cc)}$$

5. Free PSA and Percent Free PSA (% Free PSA)
   a. Total PSA = free PSA + complexed PSA. Standard PSA tests measure total serum PSA. Free PSA is not complexed with other proteins.
   b. Both total serum PSA and free PSA increase with age. The ratio of free PSA/total PSA (% Free PSA) may increase with age as well.
   c. The FDA approved % free PSA for prostate cancer screening when total PSA is 4 to 10 ng/ml.
   d. When PSA is from 4 to 10 ng/ml in patients with a *normal* prostate exam, % free PSA can help further define the risk of prostate cancer.

% Free PSA	Probability of Cancer
< 10%	56%
10-15%	28%
15-20%	20%
20-25%	16%
> 25%	8%

6. Complexed PSA
   a. PSA is complexed mostly with α1-antichymotrypsin. A smaller amount is complexed with α2-macroglobulin.
   b. The higher the complexed PSA, the higher the risk for cancer.
   c. The clinical use of complexed has not been well-defined.

Detecting Prostate Cancer with PSA
1. At least 15% of men with PSA < 4.0 ng/ml have prostate cancer.
2. Cancer detection rates are higher in men with an abnormal prostate exam.

Prostate Exam	Total PSA (ng/ml)	Probability of Cancer
Normal	≤ 0.5	6.6%
Normal	0.6-1.0	10%
Normal	1.1-2.0	17%
Normal	2.1-3.0	24%
Normal	3.1-4.0	27%
Normal	4.1-10.0	at least 25%
Normal or Abnormal	4.1-10.0	45%
Normal or Abnormal	10.1-20.0	49%
Normal or Abnormal	> 20.0	68%

Prostate Cancer and Pre-treatment PSA
1. Higher pre-treatment PSA increases the risk for capsular penetration, seminal vesicle invasion, lymph node metastasis, and distant metastasis.
2. An annual PSA velocity of > 2 ng/ml before treatment is associated with a significantly higher death rate from prostate cancer.
3. PSA and pretreatment bone scan—see Prostate Cancer, Work Up, page 81.

Prostate Cancer and Post-treatment PSA
See Prostate Cancer, Recurrence, page 91.

BPH and PSA

PSA and Progression of BPH
1. In men with BPH, higher PSA values increase the risk of prostate growth, deterioration of urinary symptoms, decline in urine flow rate, acute urinary retention, surgery for BPH, and BPH progression.
2. In men with BPH, PSA is directly proportional to prostate volume. Thus, men with higher PSA tend to have larger prostates.
3. For prevention of progression, see Combination Therapy, page 114.

REFERENCES

Catalona WJ, Partin A, Slawin KM, et al: Use of the percentage of free prostate-specific antigen to enhance differentiation of prostate cancer from benign prostatic disease. JAMA, 279 (19): 1542, 1998.

D'Amico AV, et al: Preoperative PSA velocity and the risk of death from prostate cancer after radical prostatectomy. N Engl J Med, 351: 125, 2004.

Partin AW, et al: Complexed prostate specific antigen improves specificity for prostate cancer detection: results of a prospective multicenter clinical trial. J Urol, 170, 1787, 2003.

Partin AW, Oesterling JE: Prostate-specific antigen in clinical urologic practice. AUA Update Series, Vol. 14, Lesson 1, 1995.

Presti JC, et al: Extended peripheral zone biopsy schemes increase cancer detection rates and minimize variance in prostate specific antigen and age related cancer rates. J Urol, 169: 125, 2003.

Slawin KM, Ohori M, Dillioglugil O, et al: Screening for prostate cancer: an analysis of the early experience. CA Cancer J Clin, 45(3): 134, 1995.

Thompson I, Carroll P, Coley D, et al: Prostate specific antigen (PSA) best practice policy. Oncology, 14(2): 267, 2000.

Thompson IM, Pauler DK, et al: Prevalence of prostate cancer among men with a prostate specific antigen level ≤ 4.0 ng/ml. N Engl J Med, 350: 2239,2004.

HEMATURIA

General Information
1. Significant hematuria—see Work Up, page 123.
2. Hemorrhagic cystitis is persistent or recurrent hematuria caused by bladder inflammation. Bleeding is often severe. Causes of this syndrome include radiation cystitis and chemotherapy induced cystitis (e.g. from cyclophosphamide).

Differential Diagnosis (mnemonic: "Pee Pee ON THIS—with 4 T's")

P   Period (i.e. menses)—results in cyclic pseudohematuria*
P   Prostate (prostatitis, prostate cancer, BPH)
O   Obstructive uropathy
N   Nephritis (glomerulonephritis, Alport's syndrome, Berger's IgA nephropathy, interstitial nephritis, etc.)
T   Trauma
T   Tumor (renal, urothelial, prostate, urethral, etc.)
T   Tuberculosis
T   Thrombosis (renal vein thrombosis)
H   Hematologic (anticoagulation, bleeding disorders, sickle cell disease)
I   Infection/inflammation†
S   Stones

* Cyclic pseudohematuria is contamination of the urine by vaginal menstrual blood. True cyclic hematuria (i.e. not caused by vaginal blood) should raise the suspicion of endometriosis of the urinary tract or utero-urinary fistula.
† Cystitis causes include radiation, infection, cyclophosphamide (from acrolein), interstitial cystitis, etc.

Drugs That May Cause Red Urine

Pyridium®	Ibuprofen	Quinine
Sulfamethoxazole	Phenytoin (Dilantin®)	Chloroquine
Nitrofurantoin	Levodopa	Phenacetin
Rifampin	Methyldopa	

Findings During Hematuria Work Up
1. Urologic malignancy is more common in patients with gross hematuria (23%) than in patients with microscopic hematuria (5%).
2. In adults with microscopic hematuria, the initial evaluation fails to identify an etiology in 43% of patients. Approximately 1-3% of these patients eventually develop urologic malignancy.
3. In adults with gross hematuria, the initial evaluation fails to identify an etiology in 8% of patients. Approximately, 18% of these patients eventually develop urologic malignancy.

Severity of Hematuria	Findings on Initial Hematuria Evaluation		Chance of Developing Urologic Cancer after Negative Initial Hematuria Work Up
	Urologic Cancer	No Etiology	
Microscopic	5%	43%	1-3%
Gross	23%	8%	18%

Urinary Tests for Red Blood Cells (RBCs)
1. Urine should be a freshly voided, clean catch, midstream specimen or a freshly catheterized specimen. A first morning void is best because the urine is less likely to be hypotonic; thus, it is less likely to lyse RBCs.
2. Dipstick for heme
   a. Confirm a heme positive dipstick by performing a microscopic analysis. RBCs may lyse when the urine specific gravity is less than 1.007, causing a heme positive dipstick without RBCs on microscopic analysis.
   b. Causes of a false positive test—myoglobinuria, hemoglobinuria, and povidone/iodine contamination.
   c. Causes of a false negative test—high vitamin C intake.
   d. Urine dipsticks detect as few as 2-5 RBCs per high power field (HPF).
   e. Gross hematuria can cause a false positive for protein on a dipstick.
3. Microscopic urine analysis for RBCs
   a. Centrifuge 10 ml of urine at 2000 rpm for 5 minutes. 9.0-9.5 ml of the supernatant is poured out and the sediment is resuspended in the remaining 0.5-1.0 ml of urine. A drop of this resuspended sediment is examined microscopically under the high power field (x 400).
   b. Many squamous epithelial cells suggest skin or vaginal contamination.
   c. The presence of RBC casts (often found at the edges of the cover glass) and dysmorphic RBCs suggest *glomerular bleeding*.

Work Up
1. For evaluation of pregnant patients, see Hematuria During Pregnancy, page 220. For evaluation of traumatic hematuria, see page 301.
2. Non-traumatic hematuria in adults warrants work up if *any* of the following criteria are present.
   a. Low grade microscopic hematuria—2 of 3 properly collected urine specimens that show ≥ 3 RBCs per HPF when centrifuged.
   b. High grade microscopic hematuria—any episode of properly collected urine that shows >100 RBCs/HPF when centrifuged.
   c. Gross hematuria—any episode of grossly visible blood in the urine.
3. Evaluation in the adult may consist of the following elements:
   a. History and physical, including blood pressure measurement.
   b. Urinalysis—confirm a positive dipstick with a microscopic examination.
   c. Urine culture
   d. Urine cytology and/or other urothelial tumor markers.
   e. Blood tests—BUN and creatinine. Check PSA in older men. Consider CBC with differential, platelets, PT, PTT, and bleeding time if indicated.
   f. Upper tract imaging—may be accomplished by CT urogram (CTU) or a combination of intravenous pyelogram (IVP) and renal ultrasound. When it is available, *CTU is preferred because it has a higher sensitivity for detecting upper tract pathology than IVP.* When CTU is not available, a combination of IVP and renal ultrasound is suggested (renal imaging is usually insufficient on IVP, so ultrasound is added). If the patient is allergic to iodine or at risk for contrast induced toxicity (see page 153), then consider retrograde pyelograms and renal ultrasound.
   g. Cystoscopy—if blood arises from the ureter, consider ureteroscopy.
4. If the hematuria work up is normal, consider checking urinalysis, urine tumor marker, and blood pressure at 6, 12, 24, and 36 months later, especially in "high risk patients" (i.e. age > 40, voiding symptoms, smoker, chemical exposure, gross hematuria, other urologic diseases). If the work up is still negative after 36 months, some advocate no further evaluation.
5. If the patient has renal insufficiency, hypertension, significant proteinuria, RBC casts, or predominately dysmorphic RBCs in the urine, refer the patient to a nephrologist for the work up of renal parenchymal disease.

Treatment of Gross Hematuria
1. Treat the underlying cause of the hematuria (e.g. correct coagulopathy).
2. Consider stopping NSAIDs, heparin, warfarin, and other anticoagulants.
3. If the patient is anemic, consider a blood transfusion.
4. Place a 3-way hematuria catheter.
   a. Hand irrigate and evacuate all the blood clots from the bladder.
   b. If bleeding may be coming from the prostate or urethra, placing the catheter on light traction may tamponade the bleeding and may minimize back bleeding into the bladder (thus decreasing hematuria).
   c. Consider starting continuous bladder irrigation with normal saline.
5. If bleeding persists, perform a cystoscopy under anesthesia.

Options for Treating Refractory Bleeding
1. Renal bleeding
   a. Embolization
   b. Partial or total nephrectomy
2. Prostate bleeding
   a. Aminocaproic acid (Amicar®)
   b. Androgen deprivation
   c. 5α-reductase inhibitors—see page 114.
   d. Prostate surgery—electrocautery, TURP, or open prostatectomy.
   e. Prostate radiation
3. Bladder bleeding
   a. Aminocaproic acid (Amicar®)
   b. Transurethral electrocautery
   c. Intravesical agents—when the bladder has a diffuse abnormality (e.g. radiation cystitis), intravesical therapy (which contacts the entire bladder surface) may be used. Examples: alum, formalin, silver nitrate, phenol.
   d. Hyperbaric oxygen—used primarily for hemorrhagic cystitis caused by radiation or chemotherapy.
   e. Diverting urine with nephrostomy tubes—bleeding often resolves within 1 week.
   f. Embolization or ligation of the internal iliac arteries.
   g. Cystectomy

Aminocaproic Acid (Amicar®)
1. Aminocaproic acid is an *inhibitor of plasmin*; therefore, it prevents clot lysis. It may counteract urokinase and help stop refractory hematuria.
2. Contraindications
   a. Disseminated intravascular coagulation (DIC)
   b. Upper urinary tract bleeding—it can induce glomerular capillary thrombosis and clots can obstruct the ureters.
   c. Patients with thrombosis or at risk for thrombosis.
3. Complications of therapy
   a. Rhabdomyolysis (including cardiac necrosis) especially when therapy lasts > 24 hours. Monitor CPK levels if therapy continues > 24 hours.
   b. Hypotension
   c. Nausea, diarrhea, dizziness, nasal congestion, headache, rash, fatigue.
4. For bladder bleeding, intravesical use may be safer because intravascular exposure to aminocaproic acid may be minimized.
5. Dose
   • IV: aminocaproic acid 5 g IV over one hour followed by 1 g/hour continuous infusion.
   • PO: aminocaproic acid 5 g po the first hour followed by 1 g po q 1 hour.
   • Intravesical: continuous bladder irrigation with 0.1% aminocaproic acid (mix 1 g aminocaproic acid per liter normal saline).

Hyperbaric Oxygen (HBO)

1. The patient is placed in a chamber, which is pressurized from 1.4-3.0 atm. While in the chamber, the patient breaths 100% oxygen. Each session in the chamber (called a "dive") lasts approximately 90 minutes.
2. HBO increases the amount of dissolved oxygen in the blood and tissues.
3. Effects of HBO
   a. Enhanced healing of damaged or inflamed tissue—HBO improves angiogenesis and formation of granulation tissue.
   b. Vasoconstriction—may decrease bleeding during HBO treatment.
   c. Enhances the efficacy of many of antibiotics.
   d. Enhances immune function—enhances the ability of neutrophils to kill bacteria through oxygen dependant reactions.
4. *Hematuria caused by malignancy must be ruled out prior to HBO.*
5. Absolute contraindications—concurrent cisplatin or doxorubicin treatment, untreated pneumothorax, and active viral infections.
6. Relative contraindications—at risk for seizures (e.g. alcohol withdrawal, history of seizures), poorly controlled diabetes mellitus, emphysema with carbon dioxide retention, optic neuritis, glaucoma, pregnancy, high fever, active malignancy, history of sinus/ear surgery or infection, history of spontaneous pneumothorax, congenital spherocytosis, and claustrophobia.
7. Hemorrhagic cystitis from radiation
   a. 14-60 HBO sessions are administered.
   b. Severe bleeding resolves in 70% of cases after 1-2 years of follow up. Long-term success rates appear to be lower because radiation continues to cause progressive damage after HBO.
   c. *Recurrent bleeding after HBO is often caused by malignancy; therefore, complete evaluation of hematuria is recommended in this setting.*

Formalin

1. Formalin hydrolyzes proteins and coagulates tissues.
2. Up to 10% formalin has been used, but a maximum concentration of 4% formalin has been advocated to minimize complications. Formalin is prepared by mixing formalin in distilled water. Formalin is a volume dilution of formaldehyde. [1% formalin = 0.37% formaldehyde].
3. Before instillation
   a. Evacuate all clots out of the bladder before instilling formalin.
   b. Cystogram—a cystogram is required before each instillation. Intravesical formalin is contraindicated in the presence of extravasation or vesicoureteral reflux (severe complications have been reported when these findings are present). If reflux is present, the ureters may be occluded with Fogarty catheters. If a cystogram reveals no reflux while the Fogarty catheters are in place, formalin may be instilled.
   c. Formalin is painful and requires general or spinal anesthesia.
4. Instillation—the initial dose is intravesical 1% formalin instilled passively by gravity through a Foley catheter. This catheter is placed on light traction during instillation to prevent urethral exposure to formalin. The bladder is usually filled to capacity, but a smaller volume may be used. The catheter is clamped and kept on light traction and the formalin is left in the bladder for approximately 10 minutes. After draining the formalin, the bladder is irrigated with a liter of distilled water or normal saline. A hematuria catheter is usually left in place until the hematuria resolves.
5. Resolution of hematuria usually occurs within 48 hours, but may take up to 5 days. If bleeding persists, the concentration of formalin and the duration of instillation can be increased, but this increases the risk of complications.
6. Intravesical formalin can severely scar the bladder.

1% Alum
1. Alum is an astringent that causes protein precipitation over the bleeding surface, which induces clotting.
2. 1% alum is prepared by mixing 10 grams of aluminum potassium sulfate (or aluminum ammonium sulfate) per liter of distilled water.
3. Before instillation
   a. Evacuate all clots out of the bladder before starting alum.
   b. Alum can be given even when there is vesicoureteral reflux; thus a cystogram is unnecessary.
   c. Alum is not painful, and thus can be given without anesthesia.
4. Instillation
   a. The maximum dose is continuous intravesical irrigation with 1% alum at 300 cc per hour (i.e. 3 grams per hour).
   b. Alum can be absorbed systemically; therefore, use it cautiously in patients with renal failure. Consider monitoring aluminum levels and either potassium or ammonia levels (depending on which solution is used). If symptoms develop (e.g. mental status changes, arrhythmia, etc.), stop the irrigation and check serum levels of these substances.
   c. A hematuria catheter is usually left in place until the hematuria resolves.
5. Once therapy is started, hematuria usually resolves in 3-4 days.
6. Alum does not cause major bladder changes or scaring.

Silver Nitrate (0.5% to 1% in water)
1. Silver nitrate causes protein precipitation, which induces clotting.
2. Mix silver nitrate in water—if saline is used, the silver will precipitate out of solution.
3. Before instillation
   a. Evacuate all clots out of the bladder before instilling silver nitrate.
   b. Cystogram—a cystogram is required before each instillation. Intravesical silver nitrate is contraindicated in the presence of extravasation or vesicoureteral reflux (severe complications have been reported when these findings are present). If reflux is present, the ureters may be occluded with Fogarty catheters. If a cystogram reveals no reflux while the Fogarty catheters are in place, silver nitrate may be instilled.
   c. Silver nitrate is painful, and requires general or spinal anesthesia when high concentrations (> 0.5%) are used.
4. Instillation—silver nitrate is instilled passively by gravity through a Foley catheter. This catheter is placed on light traction during instillation to prevent urethral exposure to silver nitrate. The catheter is clamped and kept on light traction and the silver nitrate is left in the bladder for approximately 15 minutes. After draining the silver nitrate, the bladder is irrigated with a liter of normal saline. A hematuria catheter is usually left in place until the hematuria resolves.
5. Resolution of hematuria usually occurs within 48 hours.
6. Intravesical silver nitrate can severely scar the bladder.

Intravesical Agent	Causes Pain	Anesthesia Required	Can be given with VUR	Causes Bladder Scaring
Amicar®	No	No	Yes	No
Alum	No	No	Yes	No
Silver nitrate	Yes	Yes*	No	Yes
Formalin	Yes	Yes	No	Yes

VUR = vesicoureteral reflux
* Anesthesia may not be required when using a low concentration (0.5%).

REFERENCES

General

Garber BB, Wein AJ: Common urologic bleeding problems part I. AUA Update Series, Vol. 8, Lesson 33, 1989.

Garber BB, Wein AJ: Common urologic bleeding problems part II. AUA Update Series, Vol. 8, Lesson 34, 1989.

Grossfield GD, Litwin MS, Wolf Jr JS, et al: Evaluation of asymptomatic microscopic hematuria in adults: the American Urological Association best practice policy-part I & II. Urology, 57(4): 599, 2001.

Restrepo NC, Carey PO: Evaluating hematuria in adults. Am Fam Physician, 40(2): 149, 1989.

Sutton JM: Evaluation of hematuria in adults. JAMA, 263(18): 2475, 1990.

CT Urogram

Albani JM, et al: The role of computerized tomography urography in the initial evaluation of hematuria. J Urol, 177: 644, 2007.

Gray Sears CL, et al: Prospective comparison of computerized tomography and excretory urography in the initial evaluation of asymptomatic microhematuria. J Urol, 168: 2457, 2002.

Finasteride

Carlin BI, Bodner DR, Spirnak JP, et al: Role of finasteride in the treatment of recurrent hematuria secondary to benign prostatic hyperplasia. Prostate, 31: 180, 1997.

Foley SJ, Soloman LZ, Wedderburn AW, et al: A prospective study of the natural history of hematuria associated with benign prostatic hyperplasia and the effect of finasteride. J Urol, 163: 496, 2000.

Miller MI, Puchner PJ: Effects of finasteride on hematuria associated with benign prostatic hyperplasia: long-term follow-up. Urology, 51: 237, 1998.

Sieber PR, Rommel FM, Huffnagle HW, et al: The treatment of gross hematuria secondary to prostatic bleeding with finasteride. J Urol, 159:1232, 1998.

Formalin

Donahue LA, Frank IN: Intravesical formalin for hemorrhagic cystitis: analysis of therapy. J Urol, 141: 809, 1989.

Fair WR: Formalin in the treatment of massive bladder hemorrhage, techniques, results and complications. Urology, 3(5): 573, 1974.

Kumar S, Rosen P, Grabstald H: Intravesical formalin for the control of intractable bladder hemorrhage secondary to cystitis or cancer. J Urol, 114: 540, 1975.

Alum

Goel AK, Rao MS, Bhagwat AG, et al: Intravesical irrigation with alum for the control of massive bladder hemorrhage. J Urol, 133: 956, 1985.

Kennedy C, Snell ME, Witherow RO: Use of alum to control intractable vesical haemorrhage. Br J Urol, 56: 673, 1984.

Ostroff EB, Chenault Jr. OW: Alum irrigation for the control of massive bladder hemorrhage. J Urol, 128: 929, 1982.

Nephrostomy Tubes

Sneiders A, Pryor JL: Percutaneous nephrostomy drainage in the treatment of severe hemorrhagic cystitis. J Urol, 150(3): 966, 1993.

Zagoria RJ, et al: Percutaneous nephrostomy for the treatment of intractable hemorrhagic cystitis. J Urol, 149(6): 1449, 1993.

Hyperbaric Oxygen

Capelli-Schellpfeffer M, Gerber GS: The use of hyperbaric oxygen in urology. J Urol, 162: 647, 1999.

O'Reilly KJ, et al: Hyperbaric oxygen in urology. AUA Update Series, Vol. 21, Lesson 4, 2002.

UROLITHIASIS

General Information
1. 90% of kidney stones are radio-opaque.
2. A metabolic etiology can be found in ≥ 97% of patients with stone disease.
3. The most common stone in industrialized countries is *calcium oxalate*.
4. The most common metabolic cause of stones is *hypercalciuria*.

Stone Composition
1. Calcium oxalate stones
   a. Most common cause—*dehydration*. The most common metabolic cause of calcium oxalate stones is absorptive hypercalciuria type II.
   b. Forms in urine with a *wide range of pH*.
   c. Radio-opaque
   d. Extremely difficult to dissolve.
   e. Calcium oxalate is the most common type of stone in American adults and children, hyperuricosuria, intestinal bypass, inflammatory bowel disease, and renal failure (on dialysis).
   f. Calcium oxalate is the most common type of bladder stone.
2. Uric acid (urate) stones
   a. Most common cause—*dehydration*. See also Hyperuricosuria, page 135.
   b. Forms in *acidic urine* (usually pH < 6.0)
   c. Radiolucent
   d. Dissolves with urinary alkalization (see Dissolution of Stones, page 144)
   e. *Patients with uric acid stones usually have normal serum and urine uric acid levels.*
3. Magnesium ammonium phosphate (struvite, triple phosphate)
   a. Usually *associated with urinary tract infection (UTI)*.
   b. Forms in *alkaline urine*.
   c. Radio-opaque
   d. Can be dissolved (see Dissolution of Stones, page 144).
   e. Most staghorn calculi are composed of struvite.
4. Matrix stones
   a. Often associated with *Proteus UTI*.
   b. Forms in *alkaline urine*.
   c. Radiolucent
5. Ammonium acid urate
   a. Associated with UTI, urinary phosphate deficiency, and *laxative abuse*.
   b. Radiolucent
6. Indinavir (Crixivan®)
   a. Indinavir is an antiviral protease inhibitor used to treat HIV.
   b. Stones are composed of precipitated indinavir.
   c. Radiolucent and not visible on non-contrast CT scan.
   d. Forms in urine with pH ≥ 5.0. Indinavir is soluble in acid; however, acidifying the urine to prevent or dissolve these stones is not practical.
7. Cystine
   a. Caused by Cystinuria (usually homozygotes), see page 139.
   b. Forms in acid urine.
   c. Radio-opaque
   d. Dissolves with urinary alkalization.
   e. Resistant to ESWL and to the pulsed (coumarin) dye laser.
   f. May form staghorns.

Stone Composition and Crystal Shape

Stone Composition	Mineral	Crystal Shape
Calcium oxalate monohydrate*	Whewellite	Oval, Dumbbells
Calcium oxalate dihydrate	Weddellite	Octahedral, Envelopes
Magnesium ammonium phosphate	Struvite	Coffin lids
Calcium hydrogen phosphate	Brushite	Needles
Calcium phosphate	Apatite	Amorphous
Cystine	-	Hexagonal
Uric acid*	-	Rhomboids, Rosettes
Tyrosine	-	Needles
Leucine	-	Spheres

* Crystals demonstrate birefringence.

Radiolucent Stones

1. Urate stones—uric acid, sodium urate, ammonium urate.
2. Xanthine
3. Matrix
4. 2,8 - dihydroxyadenine
5. Triamterene
6. Protease inhibitor stones—Indinavir (Crixivan®) and nelfinavir stones are *not* visualized on x-ray or non-contrast CT scan.
7. Silica

Etiology of Urolithiasis

Summary of Etiologies

1. Anatomic—urinary obstruction or stasis.
2. Urine composition—pH, crystal inhibitors, stone forming substances.
3. Urine volume/hydration status—low urine volume and dehydration can lead to crystal formation in the urine.
4. Diet—consumption of stone forming or stone inhibiting substances.
5. Metabolic
   a. The four most common metabolic causes of stone formation are hypercalciuria, hypocitraturia, hyperoxaluria, hyperuricosuria.
   b. Other metabolic causes include hypomagnesiuria and xanthinuria.
   c. Hypokalemia—causes an intracellular acidosis.
6. Disease states
   a. Metabolic acidosis
   b. Type I renal tubular acidosis (RTA)—see page 134.
   c. Sarcoidosis—granulomas convert 25-hydroxyvitamin D to 1,25-dihydroxyvitamin D, resulting in hypercalciuria. Steroids often correct the hypercalciuria.
   d. Chronic diarrhea
   e. Cystinuria—see Cystinuria, page 139.
   f. Inflammatory bowel disease—see Hyperoxaluria, page 138.
   g. Hyperparathyroidism—see Resorptive Hypercalciuria, page 136.
   h. Medullary sponge kidney—up to 20% have calcium urolithiasis.
   i. Adult polycystic kidney disease—up to 20% have urolithiasis.
7. Urinary tract infection—see page 130.
8. Sedentary lifestyle/immobilization—increases bone resorption; therefore, it increases urine calcium.
9. Medications—see page 131.

Inhibitors of Crystallization
1. Organic
   a. Citrate—decreases calcium stone formation by
      • Complexing with calcium and lowering calcium saturation.
      • Directly inhibiting calcium crystallization.
   b. Urea—decreases uric acid stone formation by
      • Increasing the solubility of uric acid.
      • No effect on calcium stones.
   c. Nephrocalcin
   d. Tamm-Horsfall protein
   e. Glycosaminoglycans
2. Inorganic
   a. Pyrophosphate—no way to increase this in the urine.
   b. Magnesium—increases solubility of calcium, phosphate, and oxalate.
   c. Trace elements, especially zinc.

How Acidosis Increases Stone Risk
1. The following types of acidosis may exist.
   a. Systemic acidosis—extracellular with or without intracellular acidosis.
   b. Intracellular acidosis—caused by hypokalemia. When serum potassium decreases, intracellular potassium diffuses out of cells. To balance electrical potential, the potassium that exits the cell is exchanged for hydrogen that enters the cell. This leads to an intracellular acidosis.
2. Acidosis causes the following changes in urinary composition.
   a. Increased urine calcium
   b. Increased urine phosphate
   c. Decreased urine citrate
3. Prolonged acidosis causes bone demineralization, which increases calcium delivery to the kidney and results in hypercalciuria.
4. If acidosis is from volume depletion/dehydration (such as in chronic diarrhea), the low urine volumes contribute to stone formation. In addition, hypomagnesiuria is associated with low urine volumes 33% of the time.

How Urine pH Affects Stone Risk
1. Stones that form in acid urine
   a. Amino acid stones (e.g. cystine, leucine, and tyrosine)
   b. Uric acid (usually pH < 6.0)
   c. Cholesterol
2. Stones that form in alkaline urine
   a. Matrix
   b. All stones that include phosphate, carbonate, or ammonia
      • Magnesium ammonium phosphate (struvite)
      • Calcium phosphate
      • Calcium carbonate
3. Stones that form over a wide range of urine pH
   a. Calcium oxalate
   b. Hippuric acid

How Urinary Tract Infection (UTI) Increases Stone Risk
1. UTI causes hypocitraturia (low urine citrate increases stone risk).
2. Urease producing organisms (Proteus, Klebsiella, Pseudomonas, Serratia, and Staphylococcus) split urea into ammonia and bicarbonate, which causes alkalization of the urine and increases the risk of stones formed in alkaline urine, especially struvite. Matrix stones are often associated with Proteus UTI. Note that *E. Coli does not produce urease*.
3. UTI may decrease ureteral peristalsis.
4. Stones often associated with UTI—struvite, matrix, carbonate apatite.

Medications That May Induce Urolithiasis
1. Vitamin C—metabolized to oxalate. A dose of 1000 mg daily increases urinary oxalate by 20-60%.
2. Vitamin D (high doses)—increases calcium absorption, which increases the calcium delivered to the kidney.
3. Triamterene—precipitates in the urine and forms radiolucent stones.
4. Protease inhibitors—Indinavir (Crixivan®) and nelfinavir precipitate in the urine and form stones composed of the protease inhibitor itself. These stones are radiolucent and are *not* seen on x-rays or non-contrast CT scan.
5. Furosemide—increases calcium excretion in the urine.
6. Acetazolamide—a carbonic anhydrase inhibitor (CAI) that causes the physiologic equivalent of distal RTA through bicarbonate diuresis. CAIs also alkalize the urine; however, they are not used for stone prevention because they tend to increase the risk of stones by causing distal RTA.
7. Uricosuric agents—e.g. salicylates, probenecid.

Metabolic Evaluation

Metabolic Work Up
1. All patients with urolithiasis should have an initial metabolic work up.
2. Perform the metabolic work up at least one month after obstruction has resolved, stents have been removed, and infection has been treated.
3. Patients with any of the following characteristics are at "high risk" for developing recurrent stones or complications from stones.
   a. Pediatric stone formers
   b. Solitary kidney
   c. Staghorns or multiple stones
   d. Stones composed of cystine, uric acid, or struvite
   e. Nephrocalcinosis
   f. Gout
   g. Chronic urinary tract infection
   h. Family history of stones
   i. Gastrointestinal diseases associated with urolithiasis (e.g. Crohn's)
   j. Bone diseases (e.g. pathologic fractures, osteoporosis)
   k. Professions such as pilots, bus drivers, truck drivers, etc. (stone pain in these people while they are working can cause danger to others).
4. Metabolic work up—initial evaluation
   a. History and physical—including diet, fluid consumption, medications, urinary tract infections, prior urolithiasis, family history of urolithiasis.
   b. Analyze the composition of any recovered stones.
   c. Urinalysis and urine culture.
   d. Serum chemistry panel (sodium, potassium, chloride, bicarbonate, uric acid, calcium, phosphate, alkaline phosphatase, and creatinine). If the serum calcium is elevated, obtain a parathyroid hormone (PTH) level.
5. If the initial evaluation is normal and the patient is not "high risk", suggest dietary modifications (see General Dietary Recommendations, page 133).
6. In patients with abnormal serum chemistry panel or at "high risk" obtain
   a. 24-hour urine on a *random diet*. 24-urine should include urinary pH, volume, sodium, potassium, calcium, magnesium, phosphate, uric acid, oxalate, citrate, protein, creatinine, and qualitative cystine. If the qualitative cystine is normal on the first 24-hour urine, further cystine testing is not necessary. Some recommend obtaining two 24-hour urines on a random diet, with the tests one week apart.
   b. After one week on a *restricted diet* (see Dietary Recommendations, page 133), obtain a 24-hour urine, serum chemistry panel, and PTH.

7. See also Metabolic Work Up and Initial Preventative Management of Urolithiasis, page 140.

24 Hour Urine Test	Normal Values	
	Adult	Pediatric
Total Volume	> 2 liters	> 20 ml/kg/day
Creatinine	≤ 2.0 g/day*	
Protein	< 150 mg/day	< 100 mg/m²/day
Sodium	< 200 meq/day	
Potassium	≤ 80 meq/day	
Calcium	≤ 200 mg/day	< 4 mg/kg/day
Magnesium	≥ 50 mg/day	
Phosphate	< 1100 mg/day	
Uric acid	≤ 600 mg/day	< 10 mg/kg/day
Oxalate	≤ 45 mg/day	< 0.57 mg/kg/day
Citrate	≥ 300 mg/day	> 6 mg/kg/day
Cystine	≤ 30 mg/day	≤ 30 mg/day

* females have ≤ 1.8 g/day urinary creatinine

Findings on Metabolic Work Up and Initial Management

1. If the serum calcium is elevated, obtain a PTH level. Work up and treat hyperparathyroidism appropriately.
2. If the serum potassium and bicarbonate are low and the urine pH >6.0, the patient probably has type I renal tubular acidosis (RTA)—see page 134.
3. 24-hour urine volume < 2 liters—increase oral fluid intake (keep urine volume 2-3 liters per day).
4. High urine sodium—low sodium diet.
5. Low urine magnesium—magnesium supplementation (see Hypomagnesiuria, page 135.
6. Proteinuria—consider referral to nephrologist.
7. Elevated creatinine—rule out urinary obstruction. Refer to nephrologist as indicated.
8. High urine uric acid—see Hyperuricosuria, page 135.
9. High urine calcium—see Hypercalciuria, page 136.
10. Low urine citrate—see Hypocitraturia, page 138.
11. High urine oxalate—see Hyperoxaluria, page 138.
12. High urine cystine—see Cystinuria, page 139.
13. See also Metabolic Work Up and Initial Preventative Management of Urolithiasis, page 140.

Prevention & Treatment of Metabolic Disorders

General Dietary Recommendations

1. Oral fluid intake (keep urine volume 2-3 liters per day).
2. Low sodium diet
3. Low animal protein diet (0.8-1.0 grams of protein/kg/day)—the amino acids in protein increase the circulating acid. This "chronic acidosis" causes increased bone resorption and reduced tubular reabsorption of calcium, resulting in a higher risk of calcium stones.
4. Low oxalate diet
5. Moderate calcium intake (800-1000 mg/day).
6. Avoid high doses of vitamin C (>500 mg) and vitamin D.

Drugs Used in Medical Management of Urolithiasis

1. Potassium citrate
   a. Corrects hypokalemia—hypokalemia causes intracellular acidosis.
   b. Corrects acidosis—citrate is converted to bicarbonate by the liver.
   c. Increases urinary citrate—correction of acidosis increases urinary citrate. There may also be direct delivery of citrate to the kidney.
   d. Alkalizes the urine
   e. Side effects include hyperkalemia and peptic ulcers. Use carefully in patients with renal failure, uncontrolled diabetes mellitus, peptic ulcers, delayed gastric emptying, and those taking potassium sparing diuretics.
   f. Adult dose = potassium citrate 20 meq po TID
2. Thiazide
   a. Inhibits active sodium reabsorption in the distal convoluted tubule, leading to sodium diuresis (and therefore water diuresis). It can cause hypokalemia, metabolic alkalosis, increased reabsorption of calcium and uric acid, and increased serum glucose and lipids.
   b. Prevents stone formation by decreasing urinary excretion of calcium. *A low sodium diet enhances this action by augmenting the relative volume depletion.* Thiazides may also prevent stones by correcting acidosis.
   c. Contributes to stone formation by causing hypokalemia (and thus it is usually given with potassium citrate or potassium chloride).
   d. Thiazides have a *declining* therapeutic effect on absorptive hypercalciuria, but a *sustained* effect on renal leak hypercalciuria.
   e. Adult dose = hydrochlorothiazide 50 mg po q day or BID [Tabs: 25, 50, 100 mg]. Pediatric dose = hydrochlorothiazide 1 mg/kg/day divided BID [solution: 5 mg/5 ml].
   f. Thiazides can cause weakness and fatigue. By starting at a lower dose and titrating the dose up, these side effects can be minimized.
3. Allopurinol
   a. Allopurinol inhibits the enzyme xanthine oxidase. Xanthine oxidase converts hypoxanthine to xanthine and xanthine to uric acid.
   b. Since hypoxanthine is eventually converted to uric acid, allopurinol decreases serum uric acid levels, and thus decreases urine uric acid.
   c. Allopurinol prevents calcium oxalate stone formation in those with hyperuricosuria and normal urine calcium.
   d. Allopurinol prevents uric acid stones *only* in hyperuricosuria.
   e. It may cause xanthinuria and xanthine stones (which are radiolucent).
   f. Allergic reactions to allopurinol occur more often if used with thiazides.
   g. Adult dose = allopurinol 300 mg po q day [Tabs: 100, 300 mg]
4. Water
   a. Oral water intake prevents concentrated urine; therefore, it prevents the saturation of urine with stone forming substances.
   b. Encourage fluid intake to keep urine volume at 2-3 liters per day.

5. Magnesium
   a. Be cautious when giving magnesium to patients with renal failure.
   b. May be useful in patients with hypomagnesiuria and calcium stones.
   c. The main side effect is diarrhea. Titrate the dose to prevent diarrhea.
   d. Magnesium is used with cellulose sodium phosphate, see page 137.
   e. Dose—see Hypomagnesiuria, page 135.
6. Pyridoxine (vitamin B6)
   a. Used to treat primary hyperoxaluria (see Hyperoxaluria, page 138).
   b. Given with D-penicillamine to prevent neurologic side effects.
   c. Adult dose = pyridoxine 25-50 mg po q day [Tabs: 25, 50, 100 mg],
      Pediatric dose = pyridoxine 1-2 mg/kg/day po q day.
7. Acetohydroxamic acid (Lithostat®)
   a. Acetohydroxamic acid inhibits urease; therefore, it prevents the
      formation and growth of struvite stones. Treat UTI concurrently.
   b. Side effects—nausea/vomiting, anorexia, tremor, anxiety, headache
      (30%), hemolytic anemia (15%), alopecia (rare), deep venous
      thrombosis (rare), rash after drinking alcohol.
   c. Do not use with creatinine > 2.5 (it will not be excreted in the urine).
   d. Check CBC, reticulocyte count, and liver function tests after two weeks
      of treatment and at least every 3 months during treatment.
   e. Adult dose = acetohydroxamic acid 250 mg po TID or QID [Tabs: 250 mg]
8. Cellulose sodium phosphate and orthophosphate—see Absorptive
   Hypercalciuria, page 137.
9. Cholestyramine—see Hyperoxaluria, page 138.
10. Thiola™ and D-Penicillamine—see Cystinuria, page 139.

Real Tubular Acidosis (RTA) Type 1

1. Type 1 RTA is the only RTA associated with urolithiasis and is the most
   common form of RTA.
2. It is caused by impaired secretion of hydrogen ions in the *distal nephron*.
3. Clinical Manifestations
   a. Hyperchloremic metabolic acidosis—acidosis can cause osteomalacia
      (see Osteomalacia/Bone Demineralization page 415).
   b. Hypokalemia—may cause muscle weakness or paralysis.
   c. Urine pH > 6.0 (non-infected urine).
   d. Urolithiasis—occurs in approximately 75% of patients with type 1 RTA.
      Stones are composed primarily of *calcium phosphate*, although calcium
      oxalate stones form as well. Stones are usually multiple and bilateral.
   e. Nephrocalcinosis
   f. Renal cysts—usually multiple and bilateral.
4. Complete RTA—presents with pH > 6.0, metabolic acidosis, and
   hypokalemia.
5. Incomplete RTA—presents with urine pH > 6.0, but metabolic acidosis
   and/or hypokalemia are absent. An oral ammonium chloride loading test is
   often necessary to diagnose incomplete RTA.
6. Patients with calcium phosphate stones, nephrocalcinosis, bilateral stones,
   or multiple/recurrent stones should be evaluated for RTA.
7. Acidosis and hypokalemia increase the risk of stone formation by causing
   hypocitraturia, hypercalciuria, and hyperphosphaturia (see How Acidosis
   Increases Stone Risk, page 130). *Hypocitraturia is probably the most
   important factor that leads to stone formation in type 1 RTA.*
8. Treatment—oral citrate or bicarbonate (1-3 meq/kg/day in adults, children
   may require higher doses). This therapy often resolves the acidosis,
   hypokalemia, and urolithiasis. Consider referral to nephrologist.
9. Follow patients with periodic KUB and serum bicarbonate and potassium.

Hyperuricosuria (Urinary Uric Acid > 600 mg/day)
1. Characteristics of stone disease associated with hyperuricosuria
   a. High urine uric acid level.
   b. Stones may be composed of calcium oxalate or uric acid (i.e. hyperuricosuria increases your risk for both of these stone types).
   c. Urine pH < 5.5 in absence of other causes of acidosis.
2. Causes
   a. Gout
   b. Lesch-Nyhan Disease—defect in HGPRT enzyme.
   c. Myeloproliferative disorders
   d. Chemotherapy—results in massive cellular destruction.
   e. Glycogen storage diseases
   f. Chronic diarrhea—results in acid urine and low urine output.
   g. Excessive oral intake of purine rich foods.
   h. Uricosuric medications—salicylates, probenecid.
3. Mechanism of stone formation
   a. Urate crystals can form a nidus for the formation of calcium or urate stones (a process called nucleation).
   b. Uric acid antagonizes naturally occurring macromolecular inhibitors of calcium stone formation.
4. Treatment
   a. Treat obstructing stones accordingly.
   b. Eliminate possible causes (e.g. treat diarrhea, etc.).
   c. Because those on chemotherapy cannot afford to lose any kidney function from an obstructing stone, allopurinol is often started before chemotherapy to prevent formation of uric acid stones.
   d. You should start allopurinol (adult dose = allopurinol 300 mg po q day) and alkalize the urine to pH $\geq$ 6.5 (which may be accomplished with potassium citrate). When the patient is stone free, adjust the medications as follows:
      • If the patient had an elevated serum uric acid, continue the allopurinol and stop the urine alkalization.
      • If the patient did not have an elevated serum uric acid, stop the allopurinol and continue the urine alkalization.
   e. Moderate sodium restriction
   f. Low purine diet—decrease red meat, poultry, and fish.
   g. Hydration
   h. With the above treatments, urate stones dissolve in less than 3 months.

Hypomagnesiuria (Urinary Magnesium < 50 mg/day)
1. Magnesium increases the solubility of calcium, phosphate and possibly oxalate. Therefore, it inhibits calcium stone formation.
2. Hypomagnesiuria is associated with hypocitraturia 66% of the time.
3. Treatment—increase dietary magnesium or use magnesium supplement (adult dose = magnesium oxide 140 mg po QID or 400-500 mg po BID [Caps: 140, 250, 400, 420, 500 mg], magnesium gluconate 500 mg po BID [Tabs: 500 mg]). Titrate the dose to prevent diarrhea. Use cautiously in patients with renal insufficiency.

Xanthinuria
1. May cause xanthine stones, which are radiolucent.
2. Causes
   a. Inherited deficiency in xanthine oxidase.
   b. Allopurinol (xanthine oxidase inhibitor).
3. Treatment—low purine diet, stop allopurinol. Alkalization is *not* effective.

Hypercalciuria (Urinary Calcium > 200 mg/day)

Type of Hypercalciuria	Serum Calcium	PTH	Fasting Urinary Calcium	Intestinal Calcium Absorption	Treatment
Absorptive	N	N or ↓	N	↑ (1)	See page 137
Renal	N	↑ (2)	↑	↑ (2)	Low Na Diet, Thiazide, K-Citrate
Resorptive	↑	↑ (1)	↑	↑ (2)	Parathyroid-ectomy
Unclassified	N	N	↑	↑	?

    ↑ = increased from normal   N = no change from normal
    ↓ = decreased from normal   K = potassium; Na = sodium
    (1) = primary change (i.e. a primary effect of the disease)
    (2) = secondary change (i.e. a response to the primary problem)

Renal Hypercalciuria

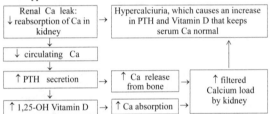

1. Primary defect—*impaired renal tubular reabsorption of calcium.*
2. Treatment
   a. Thiazide—corrects renal calcium leak (effect begins in 2-3 days and is a *sustained* effect).
   b. Low sodium diet—maximizes thiazide effect by contributing to volume depletion.
   c. Potassium—prevents hypokalemia caused by thiazide.
   d. Low calcium diet is *not warranted* because it may exacerbate the hyperparathyroid state.

Resorptive Hypercalciuria (Primary Hyperparathyroidism)

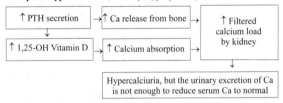

1. Primary defect—*hypersecretion of PTH.*
2. Treatment—parathyroidectomy

Unclassified Hypercalciuria
   One cause is excess dietary carbohydrate intake, which results in a brief hypercalciuria after a high carbohydrate meal.

Absorptive Hypercalciuria

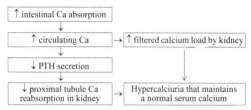

1. Primary defect—*excess intestinal absorption of calcium.*
2. Types and treatment

Type	Hypercalciuria occurs if dietary calcium intake is			Serum levels			Treatment
	None	Low	High	Ca	PO4	PTH	
I	−	+	+	N	N	N/↓	① or ②
II	−	−	+	N	N	N/↓	③
III*	−	+	+	N	↓	N/↓	④

↑ = Increased from normal   N = No change from normal
↓ = Decreased from normal   + = Yes; − = No; PO4 = phosphate
* Renal leak of phosphate stimulates overproduction of 1,25-OH vitamin D.

① Cellulose sodium phosphate (CSP)—a non-absorbable oral resin that binds calcium in the gut and prevents calcium absorption. CSP is used only in type I absorptive hypercalciuria.
  a. CSP may cause a negative calcium balance, so it is contraindicated in patients with bone loss (e.g. osteoporosis) and in patients at risk for bone loss (postmenopausal women, growing children, steroid use).
  b. CSP is contraindicated in patients with poor renal function because it provides a large phosphate load.
  c. CSP binds magnesium in the gut, so check serum magnesium levels or give a magnesium supplement.
  d. CSP increases oxalate absorption, which can increase the risk of calcium oxalate stones. Therefore, administer CSP with a low oxalate diet.
  e. CSP causes gastrointestinal upset if not taken with meals and can cause diarrhea. If diarrhea occurs, reduce the dose.
  f. Adult dose = cellulose sodium phosphate 5 gm po BID or TID
② Thiazide (with potassium and a low sodium diet)—a diuretic that decreases urine calcium. This is the *first line therapy* because it is effective, cheap, and you can use it in those with or at risk for bone loss. In fact, thiazides induce an increase in bone density. The therapeutic effect of thiazides in absorptive hypercalciuria is *not sustained*. They lose their effectiveness in approximately 6 months. If you stop thiazides for a while and then restart them, they will be effective for another 6 months. In absorptive hypercalciuria, you can alternate 6 months of thiazide followed by 6 months of CSP to avoid risks of prolonged CSP treatment (including bone loss).
③ Low calcium diet, low sodium diet, high fluid intake to keep urine output > 2 liters per day.
④ Orthophosphate—inhibits 1,25-OH vitamin D synthesis and therefore decreases intestinal absorption of calcium. This leads to decreased urine calcium. Contraindicated in patients with poor renal function (because of its high phosphate content) and with struvite stones (increases the risk of struvite stones). Its main side effect is diarrhea. Adult dose = phosphate 500 mg (e.g. K-Phos™ Neutral two tablets) po TID or QID.

Hypocitraturia (Urinary Citrate < 300 mg/day)
1. Causes
   a. Acidosis
   b. Hypokalemia—causes an intracellular acidosis.
   c. Urinary tract infection (UTI)
2. Mechanism of stone formation
   a. Citrate complexes with calcium and inhibits calcium crystallization. If urinary citrate is low, calcium stones are more likely to form.
   b. Acidosis decreases citrate in the urine and increases calcium and phosphate in the urine. These all contribute to stone formation.
   c. Hypomagnesiuria is associated with hypocitraturia in 66% of cases.
3. Treatment—potassium citrate (corrects both acidosis and hypokalemia, and alkalizes the urine).

Hyperoxaluria (Urine Oxalate > 45 mg/day)
1. Urinary oxalate has two sources
   • Liver—80% of serum oxalate is synthesized by the liver.
   • Dietary—20% arises from intake of oxalate or vitamin C.
2. Causes
   a. High dietary intake of oxalate (e.g. beets, spinach, chocolate/cocoa, liver, tea, peanuts, rhubarb, strawberries, potatoes) or its precursors (e.g. vitamin C).
   b. Pyridoxine (vitamin B6) deficiency—pyridoxine is a cofactor for alanine-glyoxalate aminotransferase (AGT), a liver enzyme that metabolizes oxalate.
   c. Primary hyperoxaluria—defect of the AGT enzyme, causing excess oxalate release by the liver. Oxalate deposition in the kidneys causes renal failure by age 20 in 90% of these patients. Many patients also develop urolithiasis and/or nephrocalcinosis. A young patient with renal failure and either urolithiasis or nephrocalcinosis should be evaluated for primary hyperoxaluria with a 24 hour urinary oxalate. When primary hyperoxaluria is suspected, a liver biopsy will confirm the diagnosis.
   d. Enteric hyperoxaluria—Crohn's disease, ileal resection, and jejuno-ileal bypass can cause fat malabsorption. The unabsorbed fat in the intestinal lumen causes increased oxalate absorption by
      • Chelating calcium—less calcium is available to bind to oxalate; therefore, oxalate is more freely absorbed.
      • Increasing colonic permeability to oxalate—colonic exposure to fat and bile acids causes increased oxalate absorption.
      Chronic diarrhea from the states listed above can cause dehydration and hypokalemic metabolic acidosis, reducing urinary citrate levels. Low urine citrate, low urine volumes from dehydration, and high urine oxalate increase the risk of urolithiasis.
3. Treatment
   a. Primary hyperoxaluria is treated with pyridoxine 25-50 mg po q day to QID, low oxalate diet, and fluid intake. Liver transplant (corrects the enzyme defect) and renal transplant (for renal failure) may be required.
   b. Treat the underlying cause (e.g. dietary excess, Crohn's, etc.).
   c. If the patient has diarrhea, give an anti-diarrhea drug.
   d. Hydrate well, increase fluid intake.
   e. Low oxalate, low fat diet—low fat prevents increased oxalate uptake.
   f. Oral calcium supplements to saturate oxalate and prevent oxalate uptake. Aluminum antacids have the same effect.
   g. Cholestyramine 12 gm po daily divided TID or QID (adult dose)— chelates bile acids, preventing them from increasing colonic oxalate permeability. It does not cause a sustained reduction in urinary oxalate.

Cystinuria (Urinary Cystine > 30 mg/day)
1. Cystinuria is an inherited autosomal recessive disorder. *Urolithiasis is the only known pathology of cystinuria.*
2. A defect in the transport of the dibasic amino acids cystine, ornithine, lysine, and arginine (COLA) is present in the
   a. Kidney—impaired tubular reabsorption of COLA.
   b. Gastrointestinal tract—impaired absorption of COLA.
3. Diagnosis is made by a positive *cyanide nitroprusside test*.
4. Family members should be screened with the cyanide nitroprusside test.
5. Heterozygotes usually have urinary cystine < 400 mg/day and usually do *not* form cystine stones. Homozygotes usually have urinary cystine > 400 mg/day and usually *do* form cystine stones.
6. Methionine is the major dietary precursor of cystine.
7. Cystine stones form in *acid urine* and may form staghorns. They are resistant to ESWL and pulsed (coumarin) dye laser, but may be dissolved with urine alkalization. *Cystine crystals are hexagon shaped.*
8. Treatment
   a. Treat large or obstructing stones accordingly.
   b. General recommendations for cystine stones
      i.   Oral hydration
      ii. Low sodium diet—decreases COLA excretion.
      iii. Low methionine diet—minimize meats, milk, eggs, wheat, etc.
   c. Dissolution—alkalize the urine to pH > 7.5 with oral potassium citrate or bicarbonate, oral hydration, low sodium diet, low methionine diet.
   d. Prevention—in patients who form stones, *alkalize the urine to pH > 7.5,* hydrate, and start low sodium, low methionine diet. In patients who do not form stones, offer the same therapy if urinary cystine > 300 mg/day. If this fails to prevent stones, try Thiola™, D-penicillamine, or captopril (adjust the medications to *keep urinary cystine < 200 mg/day*).
9. Thiol therapy for cystinuria
   a. Thiola™ (α-mercaptopropionylglycine, tiopronin)
      i.   Binds to cystine and increases its solubility.
      ii. Less toxic than D-penicillamine, but may have similar side effects.
      iii. Adult dose = Thiola™ 1-2 g per day divided QID
           Pediatric dose = Thiola™ 15 mg/kg/day divided QID
   b. D-penicillamine
      i.   Binds to cystine and increases its solubility.
      ii. Side effects
           • Hematologic—leukopenia, thrombocytopenia, anemia.
           • Renal—proteinuria/nephrotic syndrome, hematuria.
           • Gastrointestinal—nausea, vomiting, diarrhea, loss of taste.
           • Pulmonary—dyspnea, hemoptysis, pulmonary infiltrates.
           • Drug fever—usually occurs 2-3 weeks after starting therapy.
           • Skin—rash, wrinkling of skin.
           • Neurologic—can occur if not given with vitamin B6 (pyridoxine).
      iii. Adult dose = D-penicillamine 250-1000 mg po QID with pyridoxine 25-50 mg po q day; Pediatric dose = D-penicillamine 30 mg/kg/day divided QID with pyridoxine 1-2 mg/kg day po.
      iv. Side effects may be reduced by starting D-penicillamine at a low dose once a day and gradually increasing the dose.
   c. At least every 3-6 months during thiol therapy, check: urinary cystine level, urinalysis, urine pH, 24 hour urinary protein, CBC, serum albumin, and liver function tests. Consider KUB every 6-12 months.
10. Captopril has been shown to reduce urinary cystine.

Metabolic Work Up and Initial Preventative Management of Urolithiasis

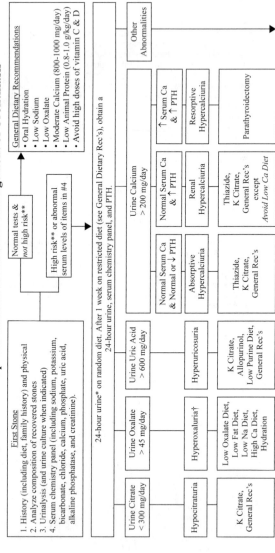

First Stone

1. History (including diet, family history) and physical
2. Analyze composition of recovered stones
3. Urinalysis (and urine culture when indicated)
4. Serum chemistry panel (including sodium, potassium, bicarbonate, chloride, calcium, phosphate, uric acid, alkaline phosphatase, and creatinine).

Normal tests & *not high risk***

High risk** or abnormal serum levels of items in #4

General Dietary Recommendations
- Oral Hydration
- Low Sodium
- Low Oxalate
- Moderate Calcium (800-1000 mg/day)
- Low Animal Protein (0.8-1.0 g/kg/day)
- Avoid high doses of vitamin C & D

Other Abnormalities

24-hour urine* on random diet. After 1 week on restricted diet (see General Dietary Rec's), obtain a 24-hour urine, serum chemistry panel, and PTH.

Urine Citrate < 300 mg/day	Urine Oxalate > 45 mg/day	Urine Uric Acid > 600 mg/day	Urine Calcium > 200 mg/day		
Hypocitraturia	Hyperoxaluria†	Hyperuricosuria	Normal Serum Ca & Normal or ↓ PTH	Normal Serum Ca & ↑ PTH	↑ Serum Ca & ↑ PTH
			Absorptive Hypercalciuria	Renal Hypercalciuria	Resorptive Hypercalciuria
K Citrate, General Rec's	Low Oxalate Diet, Low Fat Diet, Low Na Diet, High Ca Diet, Hydration	K Citrate, Allopurinol, Low Purine Diet, General Rec's	Thiazide, K Citrate, General Rec's	Thiazide, K Citrate, General Rec's except *Avoid Low Ca Diet*	Parathyroidectomy

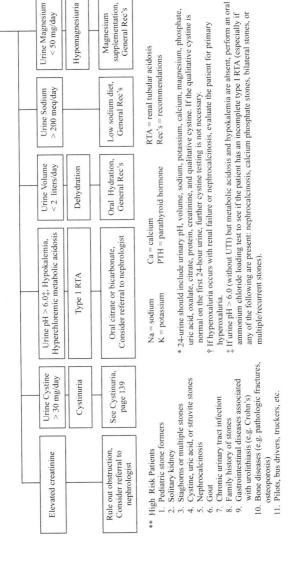

Elevated creatinine	Urine Cystine > 30 mg/day	Urine pH > 6.0‡, Hypokalemia, Hyperchloremic metabolic acidosis	Urine Volume < 2 liters/day	Urine Sodium > 200 meq/day	Urine Magnesium < 50 mg/day
	Cystinuria	Type 1 RTA	Dehydration		Hypomagnesiuria
Rule out obstruction, Consider referral to nephrologist	See Cystinuria, page 139	Oral citrate or bicarbonate, Consider referral to nephrologist	Oral Hydration, General Rec's	Low sodium diet, General Rec's	Magnesium supplementation, General Rec's

Na = sodium   Ca = calcium
K = potassium   PTH = parathyroid hormone
RTA = renal tubular acidosis
Rec's = recommendations

* 24-urine should include urinary pH, volume, sodium, potassium, calcium, magnesium, phosphate, uric acid, oxalate, citrate, protein, creatinine, and qualitative cystine. If the qualitative cystine is normal on the first 24-hour urine, further cystine testing is not necessary.

† If hyperoxaluria occurs with renal failure or nephrocalcinosis, evaluate the patient for primary hyperoxaluria.

‡ If urine pH > 6.0 (without UTI) but metabolic acidosis and hypokalemia are absent, perform an oral ammonium chloride loading test to see if the patient has an incomplete type I RTA (especially if any of the following are present: nephrocalcinosis, calcium phosphate stones, bilateral stones, or multiple/recurrent stones).

** High Risk Patients
1. Pediatric stone formers
2. Solitary kidney
3. Staghorns or multiple stones
4. Cystine, uric acid, or struvite stones
5. Nephrocalcinosis
6. Gout
7. Chronic urinary tract infection
8. Family history of stones
9. Gastrointestinal diseases associated with urolithiasis (e.g. Crohn's)
10. Bone diseases (e.g. pathologic fractures, osteoporosis)
11. Pilots, bus drivers, truckers, etc.

Acute Stone Episode

Work Up

1. History and physical exam
2. WBC with differential, urinalysis, BUN, creatinine, and electrolytes. If the patient is febrile, obtain a urine culture and sensitivity.
3. Imaging—see also Imaging of Urolithiasis, page 165.
   a. KUB—a simple, rapid screening test, but it misses many stones.
   b. Non-contrast abdominal/pelvic CT scan—detects most stones (including radiolucent stones). Non-contrast CT is often the first study obtained because it detects most stones and screens for other causes of pain.
   c. Renal and bladder ultrasound—may identify hydronephrosis; however, it will completely miss most ureteral stones.
   d. Non-contrast CT scan and renal ultrasound *cannot* rule out obstruction (these are *anatomic* studies and *not* functional studies).
   e. Contrast studies—these functional studies can identify the stone and determine the presence of obstruction.
      i. IVP—obtain delayed films until the level of obstruction is seen. Oblique films help differentiate urologic from non-urologic calcifications (e.g. phleboliths).
      ii. CT urogram—provides more detail than IVP.
      iii. If IV iodine is contraindicated, nuclear renal scan may be used to determine the presence of obstruction.

Indications for Admission and Surgical Intervention

1. Complete or high grade unilateral urinary obstruction.
2. Any degree of bilateral urinary obstruction.
3. Any degree of urinary obstruction in a solitary kidney.
4. Any degree of urinary obstruction with fever or leukocytosis.
5. Any degree of urinary obstruction with azotemia.
6. Obstruction in patients who are immunocompromised or diabetics.
7. Inability to tolerate food because of severe nausea or vomiting.
8. Severe pain not controlled by oral analgesics.
9. A stone that is unlikely to pass spontaneously.
10. If admission is not indicated, the patient is given a "trial of stone passage" (see Treatment of Urolithiasis, Surveillance, page 144).

Acute Ureteral Obstruction

1. Changes in the kidney and ureter
   a. Hypertrophy of ureteral musculature—may begin within 3 days.
   b. Scarring and fibrosis of ureter—may begin within 2 weeks.
   c. If a stone is causing complete obstruction, permanent renal damage is thought to occur after approximately one month.

Hours After Obstruction	Ureteral Pressure	Ipsilateral RBF	Contralateral RBF
0-1.5	Increased	Increased	-
1.5-5.0	Increased	Decreased	Increased
5-18	Decreased	Decreased	Increased

RBF = renal blood flow

2. If obstruction exists without infection, you can place a ureteral stent cystoscopically, place a nephrostomy tube, or remove the stone.
3. If infection and obstruction exist, give IV antibiotics and place a stent cystoscopically or place a nephrostomy tube. *Nephrostomy is the best option for those with high fevers or sepsis.* Wait until infection has cleared before treating the stone and obstruction definitively.

Treatment of Urolithiasis

Interventions for the Treatment of Stones
1. Surveillance ("trial of passage")
2. Ureteral stent placement and trial of passage (for small obstructing stones)
3. Extracorporeal shock wave lithotripsy (ESWL) ± ureteral stent
4. Ureteroscopy $\pm$ endoscopic lithotripsy
5. Percutaneous nephrolithotomy (PCNL)—used for calyceal, renal, and proximal ureteral stones.
6. Dissolution (chemolysis)
7. Open surgery

First Line Treatment Recommendations
(Based on AUA Clinical Guidelines Panel, J Urol, 158: 1915, 1997)
1. Ureteral stones
   a. High probability of spontaneous passage (especially stone size < 5 mm): trial of spontaneous passage
   b. Low probability of spontaneous passage
      i. Proximal ureter
         • Stone size $\leq$ 10 mm: ESWL
         • Stone size > 10 mm: ESWL, PCNL, or ureteroscopy
      ii. Distal ureter
         • Any stone size: ESWL or ureteroscopy
2. Renal pelvis or calyceal stones
   a. High probability of spontaneous passage (especially stone size < 5 mm): trial of spontaneous passage
   b. Low probability of spontaneous passage
      • Stone size $\leq$ 2.5 cm: ESWL
      • Stone size > 2.5 cm: PCNL alone or PCNL + ESWL
3. The gold standard for determining the stone free status after treatment is non-contrast CT scan.

Staghorn Stones
1. Most staghorn calculi are struvite and, therefore, they tend to be associated with UTI and alkaline urine. Staghorns may also be composed of uric acid and cystine. Calcium oxalate and calcium phosphate rarely form staghorns.
2. The majority of staghorns are symptomatic.
3. Staghorns should be treated even when asymptomatic because they cause progressive renal damage and persistent infection. Furthermore, the mortality rate of 11-30% when staghorns are observed is much higher compared to when they are treated.
4. Treatment (based on the AUA Staghorn Clinical Guidelines, 2005)
   a. The goal of treatment is complete stone removal.
   b. For most patients, PCNL alone is the preferred treatment.
   c. If combination therapy is planned (ESWL and PCNL), ESWL should be performed first and PCNL should be performed last.
   d. ESWL should not be used as monotherapy for most patients. It is a reasonable option in patients with small volume staghorn calculi and normal collecting system anatomy. If ESWL is used, a ureteral stent or nephrostomy tube should be placed.
   e. Open stone surgery should not be used in most patients, but may be a reasonable option for staghorns in a kidney with negligible function (nephrectomy may be the treatment of choice) or when removal of the stone will take an unreasonable amount of endoscopic procedures (see Indications for Open Stone Surgery, page 149).
5. Treatment of staghorn calculi usually requires multiple procedures.

Surveillance ("Trial of Passage")
1. A stone is more likely to pass when
   a. It is located more distal in the ureter.
   b. It is small in size (stone width is more important than stone length).
2. *95% of stones ≤ 5 mm in width will pass within 40 days.*
3. If admission is not indicated and the stone has a high probability of passing, consider surveillance, which includes
   a. Oral hydration
   b. Oral pain medications (opioids usually control pain best).

Stone Width (mm)	Approx. % of Stones Passed*	Mean Time to Stone Passage†
1	90 %	8 days
2	85 %	
3	83 %	11 days
4	77 %	
5	56 %	22 days
6	41 %	
7	30 %	
8	21 %	?
9	3 %	

* Urology 10(6): 544, 1977 & Am J Roentgenol 178: 101, 2002.
† J Urol, 162: 688, 1999.

   c. α–blockers—tamsulosin (0.4 mg po q day) has been most studied, but other α–blockers are probably equivalent. *The ureter smooth muscle contains α_1 receptors.* α–blockers relax the ureter smooth muscle, and they
      i. Increase the stone passage rate by approximately 44%.
      ii. Decrease the time to stone passage by 2-4 days.
      iii. Decrease pain during stone passage.
   d. Calcium channel blockers (e.g. nifedipine 10 mg po QID) and steroids (e.g. methylprednisolone 4 mg po QID) have also been used to help stone passage, but they do not appear to be as effective as α–blockers.
   e. A urine strainer to capture any passed stones.
   f. Follow-up radiographs—to monitor the stone and/or obstruction.
   g. The patient should return for fever, pain unresponsive to analgesics, impaired oral intake from nausea or vomiting, or significant hematuria.

Dissolution of Stones
1. Uric acid stones can be dissolved by alkalizing the urine to pH ≥ 6.5. Uric acid stones usually dissolve within 3 months.
2. Cystine stones can be dissolved by alkalizing the urine to pH ≥ 7.5.
3. Struvite stones can be dissolved by acidifying the urine, which is most commonly done for persistent stones after PCNL, ESWL, or ureteroscopy.
   a. Acidic solutions for dissolution: Suby's G solution, Renacidin®.
   b. Struvite stones may be dissolved if the following criteria are met:
      • A nephrostogram shows no extravasation and no ureteral obstruction.
      • Urine culture shows no growth.
   c. 1-2 days postoperatively, start irrigating with normal saline at 60 cc/hour through the nephrostomy tube. If the patient does not have pain or fever, change the normal saline to Suby's G solution or Renacidin®. The infusion rate is slowly increased to a maximum of 120 ml/hour as tolerated. Keep the infusion pressure ≤ 25 cm of water.
   d. Continue antibiotics during the irrigation.
   e. Monitor serum magnesium, especially in patients with renal failure (Suby's G solution and Renacidin® contain large amounts magnesium). Symptoms of hypermagnesemia include confusion, drowsiness, coma, paralysis, nausea, vomiting, hypotension, and prolonged QT interval. Treatment of hypermagnesemia includes stopping the irrigation and
      • Asymptomatic—treat with hydration and furosemide.
      • Symptomatic—treat with calcium gluconate, hydration, and furosemide. Severely symptomatic patients may require dialysis.
   f. Monitor dissolution with serial KUBs.
   g. If pain, fever, or magnesium toxicity develop, stop the irrigation. Otherwise, the irrigation is stopped when the stones have dissolved.

Extracorporeal Shock Wave Lithotripsy (ESWL)
1. Advantages—noninvasive, only sedation is required, outpatient surgery.
2. Disadvantages—stone fragments are not removed (they must pass).
3. Contraindications to ESWL
   a. Absolute contraindications
      • Pregnancy
      • Coagulopathy
      • Urinary tract infection
      • Urinary obstruction distal to the stone
      • Intrarenal vascular calcifications near the shock wave focus
      • Abdominal aortic aneurysm (esp. if > 4 cm in diameter)
   b. Relative contraindications
      • Cystine, matrix, or calcium oxalate stones (usually resistant to ESWL)
      • Radiolucent stones (however, these may be localized with ultrasound, IVP, or retrograde pyelogram during ESWL).
      • Chronic pancreatitis with pancreatic calcification
4. Performing ESWL on both kidneys at the same time should be done with caution. ESWL compromises renal function, therefore, you will be compromising both kidneys if you ESWL them at the same time.
5. Possible reasons for ESWL failure
   a. Stone burden (# of stones and stone size)—a greater stone burden correlates with greater ESWL morbidity and lower stone free rates. Stones > 2.5 cm frequently result in obstruction and are most often treated with PCNL ± ESWL.
   b. Stone composition—calcium oxalate monohydrate, cystine, and matrix stones are difficult to fragment with ESWL.
   c. Obesity—adipose absorbs the shock wave prior to its arrival at the stone.
   d. Impacted stone—the stone may fragment, but it certainly will not pass.
   e. Stone location—for renal stones, the stone free rate is less for lower pole stones (60%) than for upper and middle pole stones (70-90%).
   f. Renal anatomy—for lower pole stones, a decreased stone free rate is associated with infundibular length > 3 cm, infundibular width < 5 mm, and infundibulopelvic angle < 90°.
6. Stone free rates—see Efficacy of Stone Treatment, page 148.
7. Ureteral stent placement before ESWL does not alter stone free rates, but it prevents obstruction from passing fragments (especially for stones > 1-2 cm). A stent should probably be placed before ESWL on a solitary kidney.
8. Temporary effects of ESWL on the kidney
   a. The predominant injury when shock waves impact the kidney is *venous rupture*, especially of the arcuate veins.
   b. ESWL causes decreased renal blood flow and decreased renal function for up to 3 weeks. During this time, renal scan shows decreased uptake (reduced blood flow) and increased transit time (decreased function).
9. Complications of ESWL
   a. Renal hematoma or retroperitoneal hematoma occurs in ≤ 0.5% of cases. *Patients with hypertension have a higher risk of hematoma. Suspect a hematoma when the patient complains of an unusual amount of pain.* If a hematoma is suspected, obtain an abdominal/pelvic CT, draw a type and cross, check serial hematocrits, and place the patient on bed rest.
   b. Petechiae/ecchymosis—may occur at the shock wave entry site or at the exit site and are more likely to occur in thin patients.
   c. Pain—associated with passing of stone fragments.
   d. Sepsis—more likely to occur in presence of UTI or struvite stones. UTI is a contraindication to ESWL. Treat a UTI adequately prior to ESWL. Preoperative antibiotics reduce the risk of sepsis.

e. Steinstrasse—stone fragments line up in the ureter, resulting in pain or obstruction. Many advocate operative intervention for steinstrasse. Often, an obstructing lead fragment can be removed ureteroscopically.

f. *Retrospective data suggests that with long-term follow up (19 years), ESWL for renal and proximal ureter stones may increase the risk of diabetes mellitus and hypertension.* The risk of diabetes was higher in patients receiving a greater number and greater intensity of shocks. The risk of hypertension was higher in patients undergoing bilateral ESWL.

Percutaneous Nephrolithotomy (PCNL)

1. PCNL removes calculi through a percutaneous access that traverses through the back and into the kidney.

2. Stone free rate is 95% for renal calculi and 75% for ureteral calculi (see Efficacy of Stone Treatment, page 148). *The success rate of PCNL is independent of stone size, whereas the success rate of ESWL is dependent on stone size.*

3. Indications for PCNL may include failure of other less invasive therapies, renal stone burden > 2.5 cm, proximal ureteral stone burden > 1.0 cm, stone in calyceal diverticulum, and ureteropelvic junction obstruction with renal stones when an endopyelotomy is planned at the same time.

4. Contraindications of PCNL
   a. Urinary tract infection
   b. Coagulopathy
   c. Safe renal access is not possible

5. Access to the kidney
   a. Renal access is usually performed antegrade (access achieved from the skin to the collecting system). However, retrograde access can be accomplished by guiding a wire from the collecting system to the skin using endoscopy or fluoroscopy.
   b. To avoid intraperitoneal injury and colonic injury, access should be posterior to the posterior axillary line because the peritoneum rarely reflects posterior to this landmark.
   c. To avoid vascular injury
      i. Avoid direct access to the renal pelvis because there is no parenchyma covering this area to tamponade bleeding. Direct posterior access into the renal pelvis can injure the posterior segmental artery.
      ii. Direct access into the infundibulum should be avoided because the peri-infundibular area is highly vascular.
      iii. If possible, access the kidney through a posterior-lateral approach because Brodel's avascular plane is located in this area of the kidney.
   d. Supracostal—supracostal access almost always traverses the diaphragm. *Access should be performed during end expiration to reduce the risk of lung injury.* Risks of supracostal access include hydrothorax, pneumothorax, and lung injury. When a supracostal puncture is performed, fluoroscopy of the chest should be done at the end of the procedure and a post-operative upright chest x-ray should be performed.
   e. The preferred point of entry into the collecting system for PCNL is along the axis of the calyx through the papilla.
   f. For stones in a calyceal diverticulum, the preferred access is directly into the diverticulum.
   g. When instrumentation of the ureter or ureteropelvic junction is required, middle or upper pole renal access is preferred.

6. Irrigate with sterile normal saline to decrease the risk of hyponatremia and hemolysis. Ideally, irrigation should be warmed to body temperature to prevent hypothermia.

7. Complications of PCNL
   a. Bleeding—the risk of transfusion is approximately 3%.
      i. Hemodynamically unstable—the patient should undergo open surgery to control bleeding (partial or total nephrectomy).
      ii. Hemodynamically stable—if intraoperative bleeding is substantial, stop the PCNL and ensure that blood is available for transfusion. Place a large diameter nephrostomy tube and clamp it for 30-45 minutes to tamponade the bleeding. If bleeding persists, a nephrostomy tamponade balloon catheter (nephrostomy tube encased in a low pressure balloon) may be used. If bleeding still persists, perform arteriography and selective embolization. If embolization fails, the patient should undergo open surgery (partial or total nephrectomy).
   b. Sepsis—occurs in ≤ 1.5%.
   c. Renal pelvis perforation—extravasation of fluid can be detected by intra-operative monitoring of fluid input and output. Stop the PCNL when significant perforation or extravasation occurs. Electrolytes and fluid status should be monitored postoperatively. The nephrostomy tube should be maintained until a nephrostogram shows no extravasation.
   d. Pneumothorax/hydrothorax—occurs in 10% of supracostal punctures. When significant pneumothorax or hydrothorax exists, insert a chest tube and place it to suction. When drainage is minimal and air leak is absent, the chest tube may be removed.
   e. Intraperitoneal injury (rare)—usually requires laparotomy.
      i. Splenic injury—occurs during left renal access and is more common with splenomegaly. It usually requires surgical repair or splenectomy.
      ii. Liver injury—occurs during right renal access. Minor injuries have been managed conservatively. Some injuries require surgical repair.
      iii. Bowel injury—usually requires open surgical repair.
   f. Extraperitoneal injury (rare)
      i. Colon injury—this injury occurs by trans-colonic access into the renal pelvis. It can occur on the right or left. Colonic injury is more common with left renal access, females, enlarged colon, and lean patients (minimal retroperitoneal fat increases the risk of a retro-renal colon). The injury may be noticed intraoperatively or postoperatively. Postoperative findings may include blood per rectum, fecaluria, pneumaturia, ileus, fever, leukocytosis, and contrast in the colon during nephrostogram. Treatment includes all of the following steps:
         • Withdraw the trans-colonic nephrostomy tube from the renal pelvis into the colon (it will serve as a colostomy tube).
         • Place a nephrostomy tube through a new tract or insert a ureteral stent. If a ureteral stent is placed (or if vesicoureteral reflux is present), maintain bladder drainage with a Foley catheter.
         • Broad spectrum antibiotics.
         • After 7 days, image the urinary tract (a retrograde pyelogram if a stent was placed or nephrostogram if a nephrostomy tube was placed) and image the gastrointestinal tract (colostogram through the colostomy tube). If there is no extravasation, remove the colostomy tube, stent, and nephrostomy tube.
      ii. Duodenum injury—this injury occurs when an instrument is advanced through the *right* renal pelvis into the duodenum. Treatment includes placing a nephrostomy tube into the renal pelvis, broad spectrum antibiotics, NPO status, total parenteral nutrition, and a nasogastric tube to suction. In 2 weeks, perform a nephrostogram and upper gastrointestinal study. If no fistula is observed, remove the nasogastric tube, feed the patient, and remove the nephrostomy tube.

Ureteroscopy

1. Ureteroscopy is usually combined with endoscopic lithotripsy and stone extraction (with a basket or grasper).
2. For stone free rates, see Efficacy of Stone Treatment below.
3. Complications
   a. Ureteral avulsion—occurs in 0.5%. It usually occurs in the *proximal ureter* because greater fibroconnective tissue and less prominent muscular layers engender less ureteral resilience in this location. Avulsion usually occurs when trying to extract a stone that is too large to be removed in one piece. If a stent cannot be placed, immediate open surgical repair is required. If a stent can be placed, a trial of stent drainage may be attempted; however, a stricture often results and an open repair is often required.
   b. Ureteral perforation—it usually occurs in the *proximal ureter* because the proximal ureter is not as thick as the distal ureter. Perforation occurs in $\leq 4\%$ of cases. Treatment consists of placing a stent for 6 weeks. If a stent cannot be placed, a nephrostomy tube should be placed.
   c. Submucosal tunnelling—it usually occurs in the *distal ureter* because the transitional layer is more bulky and redundant in this location.
   d. Ureteral stricture—usually occurs in $\leq 3\%$ of cases. It is not clear whether the strictures are caused by the stone, the ureteroscopy, or both.
   e. Extrusion of a ureteral stone into the peri-ureteral tissue—if this occurs, do not "chase" the stone; leave it outside the ureter and place a ureteral stent.
   f. Other complications include bleeding, infection, and pain.

Efficacy of Stone Treatment

	Renal		Proximal Ureter		Distal Ureter	
	Non-Staghorn	Staghorn	Stone size ≤ 1.0 cm	Stone size > 1.0 cm	Stone size ≤ 1.0 cm	Stone size > 1.0 cm
ESWL	65-75%	54%	84%	72%	85%	74%
Ureteroscopy	85%	—	56%	44%	89%	73%
PCNL	95%	78%	76%	74%	—	—
Open Surgery	—	71%	99%	71%	90%	84%

Endoscopic Lithotripsy Devices

1. Pneumatic impactor (PI)—uses a pneumatically driven rigid solid probe to fragment calculi (it works like a jackhammer).
2. Ultrasonic lithotripsy (US)—uses ultrasonic vibrations transmitted through a rigid probe to fragment stones. Some of the larger probes permit simultaneous aspiration of stone fragments.
3. Electrohydraulic lithotripsy (EHL)—an electrical discharge causes vaporization of the surrounding fluid creating a cavitation bubble. The bubble rapidly expands and contracts, producing a hydraulic shock wave that impacts the stone and fragments it.
4. Laser lithotripsy
   a. Holmium-YAG laser (Ho:YAG)—the mechanism of stone fragmentation is unclear. Ho:YAG will destroy a stone basket.
   b. Pulsed (coumarin) dye—the laser induces a plasma cloud on the surface on the stone that rapidly expands and collapses, producing an acoustic shock wave that impacts the stone and fragments it. Stone baskets can be used to immobilize the stone.

5. Comparison of endoscopic lithotripsy devices

Device	Scope it can be used with	Stone Contact Required	Capable of Thermal Injury	Resistant Stones
P I	Rigid	Yes	No	None
US	Rigid	Yes	Yes	CaOx Mono, Cystine, Matrix
E H L	Rigid, Flexible	No*	Yes	None
Ho:YAG	Rigid, Flexible	Yes	Yes	None
Pulsed Dye	Rigid, Flexible	Yes	Rare	CaOx Mono, Cystine

CaOx Mono = calcium oxalate monohydrate
* Probe tip should be less than 1 mm away from the stone, but not in contact with it.

Indications for Open Stone Surgery
1. Failed endoscopic procedure.
2. Contraindication to endoscopic procedure.
3. Stone in a nonfunctioning or poorly functioning kidney (nephrectomy may be the treatment of choice).
4. Stone removal will take an unreasonable amount of endoscopic procedures (e.g. > 3 percutaneous tracts or a prolonged procedure).

Open Stone Surgery
1. Cystolithotomy—usually performed for a large stone burden or if suprapubic prostatectomy is performed at the same time.
2. Pyelolithotomy—performed using a *transverse incision* in the renal pelvis.
3. Ureterolithotomy—performed using a *vertical incision* in the ureter.
4. Anatrophic nephrolithotomy—indicated mainly for a highly branched staghorn calculus, especially one with branches into narrow infundibula. A vertical renal incision is made into Brodel's avascular plane.

REFERENCES

General

Gentle DL, Stoller ML, Jarrett TW, et al: Protease inhibitor-induced urolithiasis. Urology, 50: 508, 1997.

Shekarriz B, Stoller ML: Uric acid nephrolithiasis: current concepts and controversies. J Urol, 168: 1307, 2002.

Spontaneous Stone Passage

Coll DM, et al: Relationship of spontaneous passage of ureteral calculi to stone size and location as revealed by unenhanced helical CT. Am J Roentgenol, 178: 101, 2002.

Miller OF, Kane CJ: Time to stone passage for observed ureteral calculi: a guide for patient education. J Urol, 162: 688, 1999.

Ueno A, Kawamura T, Ogawa A, et al: Relation of spontaneous passage of ureteral calculi to size. Urology, 10(6): 544, 1977.

Pediatric Stones

Battino BS, et al: Metabolic evaluation of children with urolithiasis: are adult references for supersaturation appropriate? J Urol, 168: 2568, 2002.

Cohen TD, Ehreth J, King LR, et al: Pediatric urolithiasis: medical and surgical management. Urology, 47(3): 292, 1996.

Stapleton FB: Current approaches to pediatric stone disease. AUA Update Series, Vol. 19, Lesson 40, 2000.

Alpha-blockers

Lipkin M, Shah O: The use of alpha-blockers for the treatment of nephrolithiasis. Reviews in Urology, 8(4): S35, 2006.

Parsons JK, et al: Efficacy of α-blockers for the treatment of ureteral stones. J Urol, 177: 983, 2007.

Medical Management/Prevention

Drach GW: Urinary lithiasis: etiology, diagnosis, and medical management. Campbell's Urology. 6th Edition. Ed. PC Walsh, AB Retik, TA Stamey, et al. Philadelphia: W. B. Sanders Company, 1992, pp 2085-2156.

Kinkead TM, Menon M: Renal tubular acidosis. AUA Update Series, Vol. 14, Lesson 7, 1995.

Leveillee RJ, Wong C: Metabolic evaluation of renal calculus disease. Mediguide® to Urology, 13(6): 1, 2000.

Preminger GM: Medical management of urinary calculus disease part I. AUA Update Series, Vol. 14, Lesson 5, 1995.

Preminger GM: Medical management of urinary calculus disease part II. AUA Update Series, Vol. 14, Lesson 6, 1995.

Rodman JS, Vaughan Jr ED: Chemolysis of urinary calculi. AUA Update Series, Vol. 11, Lesson 1, 1992.

Shetty SD, et al: A practical approach to the evaluation and treatment of nephrolithiasis. AUA Update Series, Vol. 19, Lesson 30, 2000.

Surgical Management

Dretler SP: Management of the lower ureteral stone. AUA Update Series, Vol. 14, Lesson 8, 1995.

Elbahnasy AM, Shalhav AL, Hoenig DM, et al: Lower calyceal stone clearance after shock wave lithotripsy or ureteroscopy: the impact of lower pole radiographic anatomy. J Urol, 159: 676, 1998.

Krambeck AE, et al: Diabetes mellitus and hypertension associated with shock wave lithotripsy of renal and proximal ureteral stones at 19 years follow up. J Urol, 175(5): 1742, 2006.

Lingeman JE, Lifshitz DA, Evan AP: Surgical management of urinary lithiasis. Campbell's Urology. 8th Edition. Ed. PC Walsh, et al. Philadelphia: W. B. Sanders Company, 2002, pp 3361-3451.

Mcdougall EM, et al: Percutaneous approaches to the upper urinary tract. Campbell's Urology. 8th Edition. Ed. PC Walsh, et al. Philadelphia: W. B. Sanders Company, 2002, pp 3320-3360.

Pearle MS, Roehrborn CG: Antimicrobial prophylaxis prior to shock wave lithotripsy in patients with sterile urine before treatment: a meta-analysis and cost effectiveness analysis. Urology, 49: 679, 1997.

Razvi H, Denstedt JD, Sosa RE, et al: Endoscopic lithotripsy devices. AUA Update Series, Vol. 14, Lesson 36, 1995.

Segura JW, et al: Ureteral stones clinical guidelines panel summary report on the management of ureteral calculi. J Urol, 158: 1915, 1997.

Segura JW: Complications of shock wave lithotripsy. Urologic Complications, 2nd Ed. Ed. F. Marshall. St. Louis: Mosby Year Book, 1990, pp. 215-219.

Staghorns

Assimos DG, Martin JH: Treatment options for staghorn calculi. AUA Update Series, Vol. 21, Lesson 1, 2002.

Blandy JP, Singh M: The case for a more aggressive approach to staghorn stones. J Urol, 115: 505, 1976.

Koga S, Arakaki Y, Matsuoka M, et al: Staghorn calculi—long-term results of management. Br J Urol, 68: 122, 1991.

Meretyk S, et al: Complete staghorn calculi: random prospective comparison between extracorporeal shock wave lithotripsy monotherapy and combined with percutaneous nephrolithotomy. J Urol, 157: 780, 1997.

Rous SN, Turner WR: Retrospective study of 95 patients with staghorn calculus disease. J Urol, 118: 902, 1977.

Preminger GM, et al: Report on the management of staghorn calculi. AUA Education and Research, Inc., 2005 (http://www.auanet.org).

Singh M, Chapman R, Tresidder GC, et al: The fate of the unoperated staghorn calculus. Br J Urol, 45: 581, 1973.

IMAGING & RADIOLOGY

General Information

Types of Radiation and Units of Measurement

1. Non-ionizing radiation—studies that emit non-ionizing radiation include ultrasound and magnetic resonance imaging (MRI).
2. Ionizing radiation—studies that emit ionizing radiation include x-rays, fluoroscopy, CT scans, and nuclear scans.
   a. Absorbed dose—the amount of radiation deposited in tissue. It is measured in rads or Gray (Gy): 1 Gy = 100 rads
   b. Relative effective dose—the potential for biologic damage caused by a given absorbed dose of radiation. It is calculated by
      Relative effective dose = absorbed dose x quality factor
      The quality factor (QF) includes the potential for tissue damage caused by a given type of radiation. For example, α-particles cause more tissue damage than x-rays when delivered in the same dose. Relative effective dose is measured in rem or Sievert (Sv): 1 Sv = 100 rem
   c. *For radiation used in diagnostic imaging, QF = 1; therefore, absorbed dose and relative effective dose are equivalent (1 rem = 1 rad).*

Measure	Definition	Unit
Exposure	# of ions produced by X-rays per kilogram of air	Roentgen (R)
Absorbed Dose	Amount of energy deposited per unit of tissue mass	rad or Gray (Gy)
Relative Effective Dose	Absorbed dose adjusted to include the potential for tissue damage	rem or Sievert (Sv)

Radiation Safety

1. The most important rule of radiation safety is to keep the radiation exposure "as low as reasonably achievable" (acronym = ALARA).
   a. Maximize distance of medical personnel from the patient—the dose from scattered radiation declines as the distance from the patient increases.

   $$\text{Scattered radiation dose} \propto \frac{1}{\text{Distance}^2}$$

   b. Limit the time of exposure—use "spot" (single images) or pulsed (intermittent images) fluoroscopy rather than continuous fluoroscopy.
   c. Use shielding—use a full length lead apron and thyroid shield. Consider using lead lined glasses when you are close to the patient.
   d. Keep your hands and other body parts out of the x-ray beam.
   e. When the image is underpenetrated, the kVp should be increased rather than the mA (increasing mA will increase the radiation exposure).
   f. Use a fluoroscopy system with the x-ray tube below the table and the image intensifier above the table.
2. Risks of radiation exposure include cataracts from eye radiation, thyroid cancer from neck radiation, and leukemia.

Radiation Dose Received by the Patient for Common Imaging Studies
For fetal doses during pregnancy, see page 217.

Study	Typical Radiation Dose
KUB	0.1 - 0.2 rad
CT abdomen/pelvis	1-2 rad
CT urogram	4 rads
Fluoroscopy	5 rad/minute
Renal scan	≤ 0.5 rad
Bone scan	0.4-0.5 rad

Proper Terminology
1. *Hydronephrosis is a descriptive term and it does not imply cause.*
   Hydronephrosis may have an obstructive cause (such as an obstructing stone) or a non-obstructive cause (such as excessive hydration or prominent extrarenal pelvis).
2. Appropriate terminology should be used when describing the visual appearance of something on the image.

Imaging Modality	Proper Descriptive Terms	
	General Term	Example Terms
Plain x-ray	Radiodensity	Radiodense, radiolucent
Ultrasound	Echogenicity	Echogenic, hyperechoic, isoechoic, hypoechoic, anechoic
CT	Attenuation	High, intermediate, or low attenuation
MRI	Signal Intensity	High, intermediate, or low intensity

Definition of Enhancement
1. *To determine whether a lesion enhances, you must compare images obtained with and without intravenous contrast.*
2. CT scan
   a. For a specific lesion, measure the difference in Housfield units (HU) between the contrast and non-contrast images.

$$\frac{\text{Increase in HU}}{\text{with IV contrast}} = \frac{\text{HU of lesion on}}{\text{contrast images}} - \frac{\text{HU of lesion on}}{\text{non-contrast images}}$$

   b. There is no universally accepted Hounsfield boundary that distinguishes an enhancing lesion from a non-enhancing lesion. The following definitions have been suggested.

Increase in HU with IV contrast	Lesion Characteristic
< 10	Non-enhancing
10-20	Indeterminate*
> 20	Enhancing

   * These lesions should be better defined by obtaining a MRI or a more optimized CT. Renal ultrasound may also be helpful.
3. MRI—there is no standard method to determine enhancement on MRI; however, relative signal intensity (expressed as relative value units or RVU) can be compared between contrast and non-contrast images.
4. *Enhancement is proportional to the vascularity of the lesion.* Highly vascular lesions will enhance prominently (large increase in HU), while hypovascular lesions will enhance minimally (small increase in HU).
5. The presence of enhancement is one of the most important criteria for determining whether a renal mass should be managed surgically or non-surgically. Enhancing renal masses are often malignant.

Iodine Intravenous Contrast

Risks of Intravenous Iodine Contrast

1. Contraindications to intravenous (IV) iodine contrast
   a. Risk factors for contrast induced nephrotoxicity.
   b. Taking metformin or exposure to interleukin-2.
   c. At risk for exacerbation of underlying medical conditions.
   d. At risk for iodine allergy.
2. Risk factors for contrast induced nephrotoxicity
   a. Creatinine > 1.5 (patients with diabetes and chronic renal insufficiency are at especially high risk).
   b. Dehydration
   c. Currently receiving other nephrotoxic agents (such as NSAIDs).
   d. Recent IV iodine contrast load (especially within 24 hours).
   e. Congestive heart failure (New York Heart Association classes III & IV).
   f. Multiple myeloma (especially without adequate hydration).
   g. Older age
3. Medications that cause complications when given with IV iodine
   a. Metformin (Glucophage®)—acute renal failure in patients taking metformin can precipitate lactic acidosis. Discontinue metformin prior to or at the time of IV iodine injection and withhold it until 48 hours later. Resume metformin when renal function is found to be normal.
   b. Interleukin-2—patients who are currently receiving IL-2 or who have received IL-2 in the past are at risk for fevers, chills, flushing, dizziness, and occasionally hypotension when exposed to IV iodine.
4. Examples of medical conditions that may be exacerbated by IV iodine
   a. Pheochromocytoma—can develop hypertensive crisis.
   b. Cardiac disease—can develop angina, heart failure, or arrhythmia.
   c. Hyperthyroidism—can develop thyroid storm.
   d. Sickle cell anemia—can develop sickle cell crisis.
   e. Myasthenia gravis—acute worsening of symptoms including respiratory distress (from dysfunction of the respiratory muscles).

Allergic Reactions to Iodine Contrast

1. Risk factors for allergic reaction to IV iodine
   a. Prior IV iodine contrast reaction—associated with a 3-7 fold higher risk.
   b. History of asthma—associated with a 1-3 fold higher risk.
   c. Allergies—associated with a 1-3 fold higher risk. Patients with an allergy to shellfish or seafood do *not* have a higher risk of contrast allergy than people with allergies to other substances.
2. Low osmolality contrast causes fewer allergic reactions than high osmolality contrast. Low osmolality contrast agents are usually non-ionic.
3. Adverse reactions can occur when contrast contacts only the urothelium. Intravascular exposure may occur even without an intravascular injection (contrast can be absorbed into the blood stream after extravasation, leak around a percutaneous tube, pyelovenous backflow, etc.)
4. *Patients that have had an anaphylactic reaction should not be exposed to iodine contrast again.* For patients with a history of non-anaphylactic reaction, see Prophylaxis for Allergy to Iodine Contrast, page 154.
5. Testing for iodine allergy (skin test or a small IV test dose) is usually of no clinical value. In fact, a test dose can cause an anaphylactic reaction.
6. The majority of contrast reactions occur shortly after the contrast injection. *Almost all life-threatening reactions occur within 15 minutes after injection.* Mild reactions (e.g. pruritus, rash) may occur up to 48 hours after injection.
7. The risk of death after ionic IV iodine contrast is 1 in 40,000.

Prophylaxis for Allergy to Iodine Contrast

1. *Patients that have had an anaphylactic reaction to IV iodine should not be exposed to iodinated contrast again.*
2. Current evidence suggests that H1 blockers (such as diphenhydramine) and corticosteroids prevent allergic reactions to iodine contrast media.
3. *Severe allergic reactions can occur despite prophylaxis.*
4. Prophylaxis for adults undergoing an outpatient study
   - Low osmolality contrast.
   - Oral steroids—use *one* of the following agents:
     - Prednisone 50 mg po 13 hrs, 7 hrs, and 1 hr before contrast infusion, or
     - Methylprednisolone 32 mg po 12 hrs and 2 hrs before contrast infusion
   - Histamine blockers—consider adding both of the following agents:
     - Diphenhydramine 50 mg po 1 hour before contrast infusion
     - H2 blocker 1 hour before contrast infusion (e.g. cimetidine 300 mg po, ranitidine 150 mg po, or famotidine 20 mg po).
5. Prophylaxis for adults undergoing an intra-operative study
   - General anesthesia—the patient is intubated; therefore, the airway is protected if an anaphylactic reaction develops.
   - Low osmolality contrast.
   - Methylprednisolone 125 mg IV preoperatively.
   - H2 blocker preoperatively (e.g. cimetidine 300 mg IV, ranitidine 50 mg IV, or famotidine 20 mg IV)
   - Diphenhydramine 50 mg IV preoperatively.

Preventing Nephrotoxicity Caused by Iodine Contrast

1. Stop nephrotoxic agents (e.g. NSAIDs) 48-72 hours before the procedure.
2. Stop ACE inhibitors and diuretics 24 hours before the procedure.
3. Use low osmolality contrast.
4. Minimize the volume of contrast used for the procedure.
5. Hydration—for patients at high risk for nephrotoxicity, consider administering half normal saline IV at 1.0-1.5 ml/kg/hr starting 8-12 hours before the procedure and continuing 8-24 hours after the procedure.
6. Acetylcysteine 600 mg po BID the day before and the day of the procedure [Solution: 10%, 20%]. It may be mixed in water. It is not clear whether this substance truly protects against nephrotoxicity.
7. Theophylline 200 mg po 30 minutes before contrast administration. Theophylline appears to be more effective than acetylcysteine. Combining theophylline with acetylcysteine does not improve outcome.

Alternatives to IV Iodine Contrast

1. Alternatives to IVP
   a. KUB
   b. Nuclear renal scan
   c. Renal and bladder ultrasound (check for ureteral jets)
   d. Retrograde pyelograms (RPG)—RPGs with iodine contrast can still cause an allergic reaction, especially if injection results in pyelovenous backflow. RPGs should be performed with caution in patients with significant iodine allergy. Consider using the regimen for surgical procedures listed under Prophylaxis for Allergy to Iodine Contrast.
2. Alternatives to abdominal/pelvic CT scan with IV contrast
   a. Abdominal and pelvic ultrasound
   b. CT scan without IV contrast
   c. MRI with gadolinium—gadolinium can be used safely in patients with iodine allergy. Consider avoiding gadolinium in patients with advanced renal insufficiency (see page 158).
3. Alternatives to cystogram with iodine contrast—nuclear cystogram.

Imaging Studies

Imaging During Pregnancy—see page 216.

Contraindications to IV Iodine—see page 153.

Intravenous Pyelogram (IVP)/Intravenous Urogram (IVU)
1. Important things to observe when reading an IVP
    a. Bones—note presence of spinal dysraphism or metastasis.
    b. Soft tissues—note bowel gas pattern, psoas margin, and visible portions of the lung fields. The psoas margins should be symmetric. An obliterated psoas margin suggests an abnormal retroperitoneal process.
    c. Kidney
        i. Size—normal kidney length = 3-4 x height of the L2 vertebra.
        ii. Location—usually located between T11 and L3 vertebral level. The left kidney is usually 2 cm higher than the right. Look for abnormalities such as renal ptosis and ectopic kidney.
        iii. Axis—the longitudinal axis drawn through each kidney should intersect at T10 and should be parallel to the psoas shadow. If the axis is abnormal, the kidney may be malrotated or distorted by a mass.
        iv. Contour—should be smooth. Some normal variations are pseudotumors (see Pseudotumors, page 3).
        v. Nephrograms—are they prompt, delayed, or absent? Normally, symmetric nephrograms appear within *one* minute of IV contrast injection. Delayed or absent nephrograms may be caused by
            • Decreased blood entering kidney (renal artery compromise)*
            • Decreased blood exiting kidney (renal vein compromise)*
            • Obstruction of the collecting system
            • Non-functioning or poorly functioning kidney
            • Absent kidney (congenital absence or prior nephrectomy)
            • Ectopic kidney out of x-ray field (e.g. pelvic or thoracic kidney)
                * e.g. thrombosis, spasm, avulsion, stenosis.
    d. Collecting system
        i. Is excretion prompt, delayed, or absent? Calyces are usually visualized within 2 minutes.
        ii. Ureter position—the ureters usually course lateral to the vertebral bodies and overlie the transverse processes.
            • J-hooking of ureters often implies prostatic enlargement.
            • Medial deviation of the ureters or extremely straight ureters implies a retroperitoneal process such as retroperitoneal fibrosis.
        iii. Presence of filling defects or extravasation.
        iv. Presence of hydronephrosis.
    e. Bladder—identify filling defects, extravasation, post void residual.
    f. Presence of calcifications
2. Potential causes of filling defects in upper urinary tract
    a. Vascular impression (crossing vessel)—the most common filling defect.
    b. Intrinsic defect—urothelial tumor, radiolucent stones, sloughed papilla, blood clot, air bubble injected during a radiographic study, etc.
    c. Extrinsic compression—vascular impression, mass compressing collecting system, etc.
    d. Artifact—overlying bowel gas, stool.

On The O.R. Table IVP
1. An "on the table IVP" is performed by giving 1 ml/lb or 2.2ml/kg (maximum = 150 ml) contrast IV bolus followed by KUB in 2-10 minutes.
2. Are there two kidneys? Do the kidneys function? Is there extravasation?

Fluoroscopy

1. A fluoroscopy unit consists of the following elements:
   a. X-ray tube—generates the x-rays.
   b. Collimator—restricts the x-ray beam to the area of interest (which reduces radiation exposure).
   c. Image intensifier—receives the x-rays and processes them into a digital signal that can be displayed on a monitor.
2. X-rays generated by the x-ray tube pass through the collimator and into the patient, and then have one of the following fates.
   a. Absorbed by the patient
   b. Scattered by the patient—radiation scattered from the patient is the largest source of radiation exposure to medical personnel.
   c. Pass through the patient and transmitted to the image intensifier—this radiation generates the image.
3. There is less radiation exposure to medical personnel when the x-ray tube is below the table (compared to when the x-ray tube is above the table).
4. The image can be adjusted by manipulating these variables.
   a. X-ray tube current (milliamperes; mA)—proportional to the number of x-rays generated (reflects the radiation dose delivered to the patient).
   b. X-ray tube voltage (kilovolts; kVp)—proportional to the penetration achieved by a given number of x-rays.
5. When the image is underpenetrated, the kVp should be increased rather than the mA (increasing mA will increase the patient's radiation exposure).

Ultrasound (Sonography)

1. Tissue penetration increases as the ultrasound frequency is reduced.
2. Spacial resolution increases as the ultrasound wavelength is increased.
3. Frequency and wavelength are inversely proportional (as frequency increases, the wavelength decreases). Therefore, *low frequency probes achieve deeper penetration and lower resolution, whereas high frequency probes achieve less penetration and higher resolution.*
4. When imaging tissue far away from the probe, greater ultrasound penetration is required and a low frequency probe is used (e.g. 3 to 5 MHz probe for renal or abdominal ultrasound).
5. When imaging tissue close to the probe, less penetration is required and a high frequency probe is used (e.g. 6 to 7.5 MHz probe for transrectal ultrasound, 7.5 or 10 MHz probe for scrotal ultrasound). Using a higher frequency probe improves the resolution.
6. Highly echogenic substances usually have an acoustic shadow (lack of echoes beyond the echogenic focus).

Substance	Echogenicity
Water	Anechoic
Soft Tissue or Dense fluid	Low to moderate
Fat	Moderate to high
Calculi or Calcification	High
Bone	High
Air	High

7. Doppler ultrasound
   a. Pulse Doppler measures the direction and velocity of flow at a designated point and displays this information as a continuous waveform on a time-velocity graph. Real time ultrasound imaging allows you to designate the point at which pulse Doppler is measured. When real time ultrasound imaging and pulse Doppler are used together, it is called duplex Doppler ultrasound.

b. *Color Doppler shows the velocity and direction of flow* using a scale of colors that are superimposed on the real time ultrasound image.

c. Power Doppler detects slower flow than color Doppler; therefore, *it can evaluate flow in much smaller vessels. However, power Doppler does not provide information on the velocity or direction of flow.* Flow is depicted as a color superimposed on the real time ultrasound image.

d. Doppler ultrasound is usually used to evaluate blood flow.

8. Renal ultrasound

a. *Renal ultrasound CANNOT diagnose ureteral obstruction.* Neither hydronephrosis nor resistive index are reliable indictors of obstruction. See Imaging of Upper Urinary Tract Obstruction, page 163.

b. Lack of hydronephrosis usually indicates the absence of obstruction; however, obstruction without hydronephrosis may occur in early obstruction, poor renal function, and after forniceal rupture.

c. *Ultrasound cannot diagnose the pathology of a solid renal mass.* Many radiologists incorrectly interpret a highly echogenic solid renal mass as angiomyolipoma; however, malignancy may also be highly echogenic.

d. *Renal ultrasound should not be used to classify complex renal cysts* (i.e. it is not used to determine Bosniak classification for complex cysts). Ultrasound may be used to confirm that a cystic lesion is simple.

e. *Ultrasound cannot assess the entire ureter*; therefore, ureteral stones and ureteral lesions are usually missed by ultrasound. Ultrasound may identify stones in the proximal ureter or intramural distal ureter.

9. Bladder ultrasound

a. Assess for the presence of ureteral jets (caused by urine efflux from the ureteral orifice into the bladder). The absence of a ureteral jet may be caused by high grade obstruction, poor hydration, renal insufficiency, or an absent kidney. The presence of a ureteral jet does not rule out obstruction (partial obstruction may be present).

b. Ureteral jets are best seen using Doppler ultrasound.

10. Prostate ultrasound

a. Most prostate cancers are detected when they are too small to be visible on ultrasound; therefore, they appear isoechoic.

b. *Prostate cancers that are large enough to be seen on ultrasound are usually hypoechoic.* Rarely, prostate cancers are hyperechoic.

Computerized Tomography (CT)

1. Hounsfield units (HU) are a measure of x-ray attenuation (amount of absorbed radiation) at a designated point. HU range from -1000 (lowest attenuation) to +1000 (highest attenuation).

Substance	Approximate Hounsfield Units on Non-contrast Images	Attenuation
Air	-1000	Lowest
Fat	-100 to -20	
Water	0 to 20	
Soft Tissue or Dense Fluid	10 to 50	
Calculi or Calcification	> 160	
Bone	1000	Highest

2. Enhancement is important in assessing urologic lesions (see page 152).

3. CT Urogram (CTU) is a combination of IVP and abdominal CT that provides excellent imaging of the collecting system and kidneys.

4. *Calcifications are well-visualized with CT.* Non-contrast CT is an excellent way to screen for urolithiasis. IV contrast and urolithiasis have a similar appearance on CT; therefore, IV contrast may obscure a stone.

Magnetic Resonance Imaging (MRI)

1. MRI images the body using a strong magnetic field. MRI parameters that may be manipulated to generate an image include
   a. Time to repetition (TR) and time to echo (TE)—T1 images have a short TR and TE, whereas T2 images have a long TR and TE.
   b. Gradient Echo (GE)—a technique to make blood flow appear bright. Gradient echo is use for MR angiography (MRA).
   c. Fat suppression—a technique that suppresses the fat signal to help improve the contrast between tissues.
   d. Gadolinium (Gd)—a non-iodine contrast agent that is *used only with T1 imaging*. Gd is excreted by glomerular filtration, improves renal visualization, can be used safely in patients with iodine allergy, and is cleared by dialysis. In patients with advanced renal insufficiency, Gd rarely causes nephrogenic systemic fibrosis (fibrosis of body tissue that can lead to death). FDA advisory: "Gadolinium...especially at high doses, should be used only if clearly necessary in patients...requiring dialysis or with glomerular filtration rate = 15 cc/min or less." If these patients must receive gadolinium, consider prompt dialysis after the MRI (although it is unclear if dialysis prevents the syndrome).
2. Calcification is not well-visualized on MRI.
3. MRI is the best study for determining the presence of tumor thrombus in the renal vein and vena cava.
4. Pheochromocytoma appears bright on T2.
5. To determine the type of MRI you are reading, look at the subcutaneous fat, the kidneys, and the cerebrospinal fluid (CSF) in the spinal canal.
   a. T1—fat is bright (T*1* bright *l*ipid), CSF dark.
   b. T1+Gd—kidneys bright (*g*adolinium bright *g*lomerular), CSF dark.
   c. T2—CSF bright (T*2* bright H*2*0).

	TR (msec)	TE (msec)	Fat	Fluid	Kidney	Blood Flow
T1	Short (<600)	Short (< 20)	*Bright*	Dark	Dark	Dark
T1 + Gd	Short (<600)	Short (< 20)	Intermediate	Dark	*Bright*	Dark
T2	Long (>1000)	Long (≥ 60)	Intermediate	*Bright*	Bright	Dark
GE	—	—	Dark	Dark	Dark	*Bright*

Dark = low signal intensity; Bright = high signal intensity

Prostascint® Scan

1. Indium 111 capromab pendetide (Prostascint®) scan uses radiolabeled monoclonal IgG murine antibodies against prostate specific membrane antigen (PSMA) to detect prostate cancer.
2. The sensitivity is 70% and the specificity is 80%.
3. Prostascint® may be indicated in the following patients.
   • Men with newly diagnosed prostate cancer who are at high risk for metastasis but have negative bone scan and negative pelvic CT/MRI.
   • Men with recurrent prostate cancer who are candidates for curative local salvage therapy and who have a negative bone scan and negative or equivocal pelvic CT/MRI.
4. Prostascint® may induce human anti-murine antibodies (HAMA) in ≤ 8% of patients. When HAMA are present, they can interfere with subsequent Prostascint® scans and with antibody based immunoassays for PSA and digoxin. When HAMA alters PSA, it typically causes *falsely elevated PSA levels*. Hybritech Tandem-R and Abbott IMX PSA assays may be resistant to HAMA interference. The laboratory may need to modify testing to accurately measure PSA when HAMA are present.

Bone Scan (Bone Scintigraphy)
1. Bone scan shows the metabolic activity in bones using a radioactive tracer.
2. Metastases to bone often appear as areas of increased activity. Other causes of increased activity include arthritis, infection, and fracture.
3. Symmetric activity in the joints often represents arthritis.
4. A prostate cancer metastasis seen on bone scan may take up to one year to go away after hormone therapy is started.

Renal Scan (Renal Scintigraphy)
1. Renal scan quantifies renal function, assesses renal excretion, and determines the presence of renal obstruction. Renal scan can identify the presence of obstruction, but not the cause of obstruction.
2. After intravenous injection of a radioactive tracer (radiotracer), continuous imaging is performed while the kidneys excrete the radiotracer.
3. Common radiopharmaceuticals (radiotracers)
   a. DTPA (Technetium-99m diethylenetriamine pentaacetic acid)—*DTPA is eliminated mainly by glomerular filtration (and is therefore called a glomerular agent)*. DTPA may be used to quantitate glomerular filtration rate (GFR). DTPA is not useful in patients with renal insufficiency because low GFR leads to inadequate excretion of DTPA.
   b. MAG3 (Technetium-99m mercaptoacetyltrigylcine)—*MAG3 is eliminated mainly by secretion from the proximal renal tubules (tubular agent)*. MAG3 is the radiotracer of choice for most urologic indications.
   c. DMSA (Technetium-99m dimercaptosuccinic acid)—*DMSA binds to the proximal renal tubules in the renal cortex for a prolonged period of time (cortical binding agent, tubular fixation agent)*. Retention of DMSA in the renal cortex allows relatively high resolution renal images. Thus, DMSA is often used to differentiate a true solid renal mass from a pseudotumor (see page 1 and page 3) and to demonstrate renal scarring.
4. When renal function is normal, DTPA and MAG3 can be used interchangeably. With mild to moderate renal dysfunction, DTPA elimination (which is dependant on GFR) is insufficient while MAG3 elimination (which is dependant on tubular function) is maintained. Therefore, MAG3 is superior when renal function is impaired.
5. Diuretic renal scan—used to differentiate obstructive hydronephrosis from non-obstructive hydronephrosis. Intravenous diuretic (usually furosemide) is administered 15 minutes before radiotracer injection or at the time of peak radiotracer activity in the kidneys.
   a. Hydronephrosis without obstruction—prolonged retention of radiotracer is caused by a reservoir effect. Diuresis with furosemide produces a rapid elimination of the radiotracer from the reservoir ("wash out").
   b. Hydronephrosis with obstruction—prolonged retention of radiotracer is caused by obstruction. Diuresis with furosemide does not produce washout because obstruction restricts elimination of the radiotracer.
   c. Poor renal function—diuretic renal scan becomes less reliable as renal function worsens. There is no standard for determining when renal dysfunction is severe enough to render the renal scan unreliable. With impaired renal function, the kidney may not respond to diuresis, creating a delay in radiotracer washout that may be misinterpreted as obstruction.
   d. Poor hydration—can also cause poor response to the diuretic.
6. Vesicoureteral reflux (VUR) and ureteral stents during renal scan—with VUR or an indwelling ureteral stent, radiotracer can flow back toward the kidney as the bladder fills. This leads to persistent radiotracer in the renal pelvis that may give the false impression of obstruction. To obtain an accurate study, patients with VUR or a ureteral stent should have a catheter draining the bladder during the renal scan.

7. Phases of the renal scan

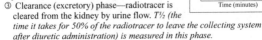

① Flow (vascular) phase—radiotracer is delivered to the kidney by arterial blood flow (this phase normally lasts 60 seconds). *Flow curves are generated during this phase.*

② Extraction (parenchymal) phase—radiotracer is taken up into the renal parenchyma (this phase normally lasts 1 to 3 minutes). *Differential renal function is measured in this phase.*

③ Clearance (excretory) phase—radiotracer is cleared from the kidney by urine flow. *T½ (the time it takes for 50% of the radiotracer to leave the collecting system after diuretic administration) is measured in this phase.*

8. Renal scans typically consist of the following elements.

   a. Images

      i. Flow (perfusion) series—images taken every few seconds during the flow phase. For normal kidneys, the renal outlines (nephrograms) are symmetric and appear within 4 to 6 seconds. Asymmetry of the nephrograms suggests decreased renal perfusion to the side with the delayed nephrogram.

      ii. Excretion (function) series—images taken every few minutes during the parenchymal and clearance phases. For a normal kidney, radiotracer appears within the collecting system within 5 minutes after radiotracer injection. The ureters are not always visualized. Bladder activity is often seen 10-15 minutes after radiotracer injection. A photopenic region ("cold spot") in the nephrogram is a poorly functioning or non-functioning area that may be caused by a mass (cyst, tumor), scar, infarct, focal pyelonephritis, or dilated intrarenal collecting system. Delayed filling of the photopenic area with radiotracer suggests that the cold spot is a calyceal diverticulum, a prominent intrarenal calyx, or a prominent intra-renal pelvis.

   b. Graphs

      i. Flow (perfusion) curve—time-activity curves from the flow phase.

      ii. Renogram—time-activity curves from all phases.

9. Interpretation of flow curves

   a. When blood flow to the kidney is normal, the aorta and kidney flow curves have a similar steep initial rise in slope. When blood flow to the kidney is impaired, the slope of the aorta flow curve remains steep, but the slope of the kidney flow curve is less steep. When the bolus of the radiotracer is inadequate (e.g. infiltrated IV), then both the aorta and renal flow curves are less steep.

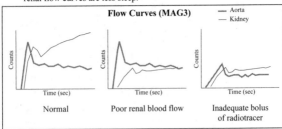

b. *In patients with a renal transplant, flow curves are useful for differentiating acute rejection from other causes of acute renal failure* (such as acute tubular necrosis and cyclosporine toxicity). Flow curves are usually normal with acute tubular necrosis and acute cyclosporine toxicity, whereas the flow curves show poor renal perfusion with acute rejection. Renogram is not helpful in distinguishing these situations because all causes of acute renal failure have a similar renogram.

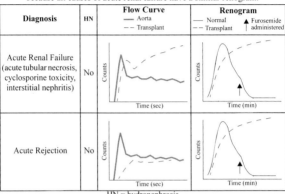

Diagnosis	HN	Flow Curve — Aorta -- Transplant	Renogram — Normal ▲ Furosemide -- Transplant ↑ administered
Acute Renal Failure (acute tubular necrosis, cyclosporine toxicity, interstitial nephritis)	No		
Acute Rejection	No		

HN = hydronephrosis

10. Interpretation of renograms
    a. In a normal kidney, peak activity usually occurs 2-4 minutes after radiotracer injection. Without furosemide, radiotracer is completely cleared from the kidneys by 45-50 minutes. When furosemide is administered, clearance is usually complete in less than 45 minutes.
    b. $T\frac{1}{2}$ is the time it takes for 50% of the radiotracer to leave the collecting system after diuretic administration and is measured during the clearance phase. *$T\frac{1}{2}$ after furosemide administration is helpful*

$T\frac{1}{2}$ (minutes) after Furosemide	Interpretation
<10	Not obstructed
10-20	Indeterminate
>20	Obstructed

   for assessing the presence of obstruction. $T\frac{1}{2} > 20$ minutes suggests the presence of obstruction. Determining obstruction should not be based on $T\frac{1}{2}$ alone; it should be based on all aspects of the renal scan.
    c. Hydronephrosis without obstruction—MAG3 renal scan demonstrates accumulation of activity in the hydronephrotic kidney, but this activity washes out rapidly after furosemide injection ($T\frac{1}{2} < 10$ minutes). Examples include spacious renal pelvis and extrarenal pelvis.
    d. Hydronephrosis with obstruction—MAG3 renal scan demonstrates accumulation of activity in the hydronephrotic kidney, but this activity does not wash out sufficiently after furosemide injection.
       i. High grade or complete obstruction—none of the activity washes out. Since activity continues to accumulate, $T\frac{1}{2}$ cannot be calculated.
       ii. Low or moderate grade obstruction—some activity washes out, but the $T\frac{1}{2} > 20$ minutes.
    e. Acute renal failure—MAG3 renal scan demonstrates accumulation of activity in the affected kidney, but this activity does not wash out or partially washes out after furosemide injection (impaired response to furosemide). Examples include acute tubular necrosis (ATN), interstitial nephritis, and cyclosporine toxicity.

f. When the renal scan is indeterminate, a more definitive test may be required to determine if renal obstruction exists (e.g. Whitaker test). See Imaging of Upper Urinary Tract Obstruction, page 163.

Clinical Scenario †	Hydronephrosis	Renogram — Normal ▲ Furosemide -- Abnormal ↑ administered	T½ (minutes)
Hydronephrosis without obstruction	Yes		< 10
Hydronephrosis with obstruction (moderate or low grade)	Yes		>20
Hydronephrosis with obstruction (complete or high grade)	Yes		—
Acute Renal Failure (acute tubular necrosis, cyclosporine toxicity, interstitial nephritis) or Acute Rejection or Very early obstruction*	No		—
Acute Renal Failure with partial recovery or Acute Rejection with partial recovery or Very early obstruction*	No		—
Poor renal function	Maybe		—

* Obstruction duration less than 24 hours may show no hydronephrosis. Follow up studies may be helpful to determine if obstruction is present.

† Poor response to diuretic (from significant renal insufficiency, dehydration, etc.) can also cause abnormal findings.

Imaging of Upper Urinary Tract Obstruction

1. Hydronephrosis is a descriptive term and does not imply the cause of hydronephrosis. Hydronephrosis may have an obstructive cause (e.g. obstructing stone) or a non-obstructive cause (e.g. excessive hydration or prominent extra-renal pelvis).
2. Anatomic studies (such as KUB, renal ultrasound, CT without IV contrast, and MRI without gadolinium) cannot diagnose ureteral obstruction.
3. Diagnosing ureteral obstruction requires one of the following study types.
   a. Functional study—images are obtained as contrast is excreted into the collecting system. *Functional tests depend on sufficient renal function.*
      i. Examples—diuretic renal scan, IVU, CT with IV contrast, and MRI with gadolinium. Delayed images are often helpful.
      ii. *Findings that suggest obstruction include delayed nephrogram, delayed excretion, and hydronephrosis.*
   b. Infusion study—images are obtained as contrast is infused into the collecting system. *Infusion tests are not dependant on renal function.*
      i. Examples—pyelogram (antegrade or retrograde) and Whitaker test.
      ii. *Findings that suggest obstruction include delayed drainage and hydronephrosis.*
4. The optimal non-invasive test for evaluating ureteral obstruction is diuretic renal scan because it provides images and objective measurements of urine flow (such as $T\frac{1}{2}$).
5. When other imaging studies are inconclusive (e.g. hydronephrosis with poor renal function), a Whitaker test may be required.
6. Whitaker test
   a. Ureteral resistance is determined by measuring the pressure gradient across the suspected obstruction.
   b. A cannula in the renal pelvis and a catheter in the bladder are each connected to a pressure transducer. With the *patient in the prone position*, a mixture of saline and contrast is infused through the renal cannula at a constant infusion rate (usually 10 ml/minute).
   c. During infusion, the pressure gradient between the renal pelvis and bladder is monitored and fluoroscopic imaging is performed to define the site of obstruction.

Pressure Gradient (mm H_2O)	Interpretation
< 15	Not obstructed
15-22	Indeterminate
> 22	Obstructed

   d. The presence of obstruction is based on fluoroscopic imaging and the pressure gradient (see chart).
   e. False negative, false positive, and indeterminate results may occur.

Imaging of Renal Cysts

General Information
1. Simple renal cyst—a fluid filled lesion that meets the certain criteria (see page 164). Simple cysts are the most common renal lesion.
2. Complex renal cyst—a fluid filled lesion that does not meet the criteria for a simple cyst.
   a. *Imaging with and without IV contrast is required to evaluate complex renal cysts.*
   b. Complex cysts have at least one of the following characteristics: high density fluid, calcification, septation, solid elements, or enhancement.
   c. High attenuation complex cysts (also called high density cysts) are characterized by Hounsfield units (HU) > 20 on non-contrast CT.
   d. The Bosniak classification is used to characterize complex renal cysts.

Imaging Criteria for Simple Renal Cysts

Criteria 1 through 5 must always be met. Criteria 6 is required in certain cases.
1. Round or ovoid shape.
2. Sharply marginated demarcation from surrounding renal parenchyma.
3. Smooth and thin cyst wall.
4. Homogeneous—no calcifications or septation.
5. Content is consistent with water density (no solid components)
   a. On ultrasound, a simple cyst appears anechoic (no internal echoes) and has good through transmission (acoustic enhancement behind the cyst).
   b. On CT scan, a simple cyst has Hounsfield units (HU) from 0 to 20. When HU > 20, ultrasound is required. If ultrasound shows a simple cyst, further work up is unnecessary. If ultrasound does not show simple cyst and the initial CT was without IV contrast, then obtain a CT with and without IV contrast to satisfy criteria "6" below.
   c. On MRI, the cyst is dark on T1 and bright on T2.
6. The cyst does not enhance with IV contrast.
   a. IV contrast is not required to diagnose a simple cyst when criteria 1-5 are met.
   b. On CT, IV contrast is not necessary to diagnose a simple cyst when HU = 0-20. On CT with IV contrast, a simple cyst does not enhance.
   c. On MRI with gadolinium, a simple cyst does not enhance.

Bosniak Classification of Renal Cysts

1. *The Bosniak classification is based on imaging and is used to guide the clinical management of renal cysts. It is not a pathologic classification and it does not take into account symptoms or other clinical factors.*
2. *Bosniak classification can be applied to CT or MRI and requires imaging with and without IV contrast.* Ultrasound is reserved for confirming that a cyst is simple, and should not be used to determine Bosniak category.
3. Bosniak Classification
   a. Category I—simple cysts. These cysts have water density, a thin wall, do not enhance, and do not contain septa, solid elements, or calcifications. This is the most common type of renal cyst.
   b. Category II—these cysts do not enhance, are sharply marginated, have a smooth and thin wall, and have any of the following characteristics:
      i. A few thin "hairline" septa—these septa may have perceived enhancement (enhancement is not measurable because the septa are too thin to accurately determine Hounsfield units, but the septa may appear to enhance when contrast and non-contrast images are compared side by side).
      ii. Fine calcification or a short segment of slightly thickened calcification in the cyst wall or septa.
      iii. Cysts < 3 cm in size with uniformly high attenuation (HU > 20).
   c. Category IIF—these cysts do not enhance, are usually sharply marginated, and have any of the following characteristics:
      i. Multiple thin "hairline" septa or minimal smooth septa thickening—these septa may have perceived enhancement.
      ii. Thick or nodular calcification in the cyst wall or septa.
      iii. Cysts > 3 cm in size with uniformly high attenuation (HU > 20)
      iv. Minimal smooth thickening of the cyst wall—the cyst wall may have perceived enhancement.
   d. Category III—these cysts have any of the following characteristics:
      i. Thickened or irregular septa with measurable enhancement.
      ii. Thickened or irregular cyst wall with measurable enhancement.
   e. Category IV—these cysts contain enhancing soft tissue components adjacent to, but independent of, the cyst wall or septa.

4. Management of complex renal cysts
   a. Bosniak I and II cysts are considered benign and generally require no treatment or follow up.
   b. Bosniak III and IV cysts are usually malignant and surgical management is recommended.
   c. 5-20% of Bosniak IIF cysts are malignant. Serial imaging will usually reveal which lesions are malignant; thus, surveillance is recommended.

Bosniak Category	Approximate Chance of Malignancy	Usual Management
I	Extraordinarily rare	None
II	Very rare	None
IIF	5%-20%	Surveillance*
III	> 50%	Surgery**
IV	> 90%	Surgery**

* Repeat imaging is performed 6 months after the initial imaging study. If the lesion is stable, imaging may be performed every year. If the lesion changes, surgical intervention may be indicated.

**Surgical treatment usually consists of excision.

Imaging of Urolithiasis

1. 90% of ureteral stones are radio-opaque (i.e. they are visible on plain x-rays). Radiolucent stones are not visible on plain x-rays (see page 129).
2. All stones except protease inhibitor stones (see page 131) are visible on CT.
3. Stones are not well-visualized on MRI.
4. A bladder stone can be differentiated from a ureterovesical junction stone by placing the patient lateral or prone and re-imaging. A bladder stone will move to the most dependant portion of the bladder.
5. A phlebolith is a focal calcification in a vein. They are usually located in the pelvis near the distal ureter.
6. Differentiating a ureter stone from a phlebolith
   a. Phleboliths often have a central lucency (a grey center that is most conspicuous on plain films).
   b. On non-contrast CT, a phlebolith is often completely surrounded by fat (encircled by black) or is partially surrounded by fat with a vein emanating from it (comet sign: a grey, often tapering, streamer).
   c. On non-contrast CT, a ureter stone is usually surrounded by edematous ureteral tissue (rim sign: a grey rim encircles the stone). The rim may be indistinct for large stones because they stretch the ureteral wall, which thins the rim. This sign may also be indistinct when edema is minimal.
   d. Tests that can definitively differentiate a phlebolith from a ureter stone include: pyelogram with oblique films, CT urogram, and ureteroscopy. When the diagnosis is in question, obtain one of these tests.
7. Iodine and stones look similar on CT; thus, IV iodine can obscure a stone.

Appearance on Non-contrast CT (transverse)

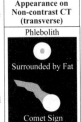

Phlebolith

Surrounded by Fat

Comet Sign

Ureteral Stone

Rim Sign

REFERENCES

Radiation Safety

Health Physics Society: Radiation exposure from medical diagnostic imaging procedures. 8/1/06. (http://hps.org/documents/meddiagimaging.pdf)

Ramakumar S, Jarrett TW: Radiation safety for the urologist. AUA Update Series, Vol. 19, Lesson 26, 2000.

General

Haas CA, Resnick MI: Office based ultrasound for urologists. AUA Update Series, Vol. 26, Lesson 31, 1997.

King Jr BF, Schnall MD, Levy J: Magnetic resonance imaging (MRI) in urology part I. AUA Update Series, Vol. 26, Lesson 38, 1997.

Food and Drug Administration (FDA): Gadolinium containing contrast agents for magnetic resonance imaging. http://www.fda.gov/cder/drug/advisory/gadolinium_agents.htm (accessed March12, 2006).

Schulam PG, et al: Urinary tract imaging - basic principles. Campbell's Urology. 8th Edition. Ed. PC Walsh, et al. Philadelphia: W. B. Sanders Company, 2002, pp 122-168.

Thrall JH, Ziessman HA: Genitourinary system. Nuclear Medicine. St. Louis: Mosby, 1995, 283-320.

Upper Urinary Tract Obstruction

Ames CD, Older RA: Imaging in urinary tract obstruction. Braz J Urol, 27: 316, 2001.

Tchetgen MB, Bloom DA: Robert H. Whitaker and the Whitaker test: a pressure-flow study of the upper urinary tract. Urology, 61: 253, 2003.

Whitaker RH, et al: A comparison of pressure flow studies and renography in equivocal upper urinary tract obstruction. J Urol, 131: 446, 1984.

Adverse Reactions to Iodine Contrast

Cohan RH, Ellis JH: Iodinated contrast material in uroradiology, choice of agent and management of complications. Urol Clin North Am, 24(3): 471, 1997.

Delaney A, et al: The prevention of anaphylactoid reactions to iodinated radiological contrast media. BMC Med Imaging, 6: 2, 2006.

Huber W, et al: Prophylaxis of contrast material induced nephropathy in patients in intensive care: acetylcysteine, theophylline, or both? A randomized study. Radiology, 239: 793, 2006.

Keizer JJ, Das S: Intravascular contrast media in urologic imaging. AUA Update Series, Vol. 15, Lesson 13, 1996.

Pannu N, et al: Prophylaxis strategies for contrast induced nephropathy. JAMA, 295: 2765, 2006.

Tramer MR, et al: Pharmacological prevention of serious anaphylactic reactions due to iodinated contrast media: a systematic review. BMJ, 333(7570): 675, 2006. (BMJ, doi:10.1136/bmj.38905.634132.AE)

Waybill M, Waybill P: Contrast media induced nephrotoxicity: identification of patients at risk & algorithms for prevention. J Vasc Interv Radiol 12: 3, 2001.

Bosniak Classification and Renal Cysts

Harsinghani MG, et al: Incidence of malignancy in complex cystic renal masses (Bosniak category III): should imaging-guided biopsy precede surgery? Am J Roentgenol, 180: 755, 2003.

Israel GM, Bosniak MA: An update of the Bosniak renal cyst classification system. Urology, 66 (3): 484, 2005. [update of Radiology, 158(1): 1, 1986.]

Israel GM, Bosniak MA: How I do it: evaluating renal masses. Radiology, 236: 441, 2005.

Israel GM, Bosniak MA: Follow-up CT of moderately complex cystic lesions of the kidney (Bosniak category IIF). Am J Roentgenol, 181: 627, 2003.

Kausik S, et al: Classification and management of simple and complex renal cysts. AUA Update Series, Vol. 21, Lesson 11, 2002.

Koga S, et al: An evaluation of Bosniak's radiological classification of cystic renal masses. BJU Int, 86 (6): 607, 2000.

Limb J et al: Laparoscopic evaluation of indeterminate renal cysts: long term follow-up. J Endourol, 16(2): 79, 2002.

VOIDING & URODYNAMICS

Bladder Function—Filling (Storage) and Emptying (Voiding)
1. The 2 phases of bladder function are filling and emptying.
2. Normal filling requires
    a. Accommodation with sensation—accommodation refers to physiologic properties of the bladder that permit filling. These properties include
        • Compliance ($C = \Delta V / \Delta P$)—a compliant bladder permits *low pressure filling*. Compliance may be reduced by cystitis, radiation, etc.
        • Sympathetic stimulation—reduces detrusor tone.
        • Parasympathetic inhibition—reduces detrusor tone.
    b. Closed bladder outlet—this is achieved by
        • Sympathetic stimulation–increases smooth (involuntary) sphincter tone
        • Somatic pelvic nerve stimulation—increases striated (voluntary) sphincter tone.
    c. Absence of involuntary bladder contractions.
3. Normal emptying requires
    a. Lowering of smooth and striated sphincter resistance—*relaxation of these pelvic muscles is the first event in micturition* and occurs by
        • Sympathetic inhibition—decreases smooth sphincter tone.
        • Somatic pelvic nerve inhibition—decreases striated sphincter tone.
    b. Coordinated detrusor contraction of adequate magnitude and duration.
        • Parasympathetic stimulation—increases detrusor tone.
        • Sympathetic inhibition—decreases detrusor inhibition.
    c. Absence of obstruction.

Determinants of Urine Flow
1. Urine flow is determined by detrusor function and outlet resistance.
2. Detrusor function is determined by
    a. Bladder muscle fiber function.
    b. Function of nerves that innervate the bladder.
3. Outlet resistance is determined by
    a. Functional factors—voluntary and involuntary urethral sphincters.
    b. Mechanical factors—extrinsic compression of the urethra (e.g. BPH) and intrinsic obstruction of the urethra (e.g. strictures).

Terminology (Based on 2002 ICS Report)
1. Urinary continence—the ability to store urine in the bladder without leakage. *Continence depends mainly on smooth urinary sphincter function.*
2. Urinary incontinence—involuntary leakage of urine.
3. Detrusor sphincter dyssynergia (DSD)—involuntary contraction of the urethral sphincter during a detrusor contraction (causes bladder outlet obstruction). DSD is usually caused by a neurologic condition.
4. Pseudo DSD—*voluntary* sphincter contraction during a detrusor contraction (causes bladder outlet obstruction). Pseudo DSD occurs when the patient actively attempts to inhibit voiding during a bladder contraction. This is usually not caused by a neurologic condition. The term Pseudo-DSD was not defined in the 2002 ICS Report.
5. See page 169.

Neural Control of Voiding

1. The spinal cord ends between T10-L2 *vertebral* level by 5 years of age. Therefore, injury to this vertebral level can injure S2-S4 in the spinal cord.
2. Parasympathetic pathway: S2-S4 spinal cord → pelvic splanchnic nerve (nervus erigentes) → inferior pelvic (hypogastric) plexus → nerves to bladder and penis. Bladder nerves cause detrusor contraction (muscarinic cholinergic receptors). Penile nerves control erection.
3. Sympathetic pathway: T10-L2 spinal cord → hypogastric nerve → inferior pelvic (hypogastric) plexus → nerves to bladder, smooth urinary sphincter, penis, and reproductive glands. Smooth sphincter nerves cause sphincter contraction (α-adrenergic receptors). Detrusor nerves cause detrusor relaxation (β-adrenergic receptors). Other nerve branches control emission and detumescence.

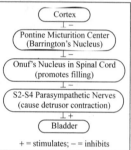

4. Somatic pathway: S2-S4 spinal cord (sacral plexus) → pudendal nerve → nerves to striated sphincter and penile muscles. Striated sphincter nerves cause sphincter contraction (nicotinic cholinergic receptors). Other branches control ejaculation.
5. Control of voiding (see figure).

Location of the Neurologic Lesion and Its Impact on Voiding

1. Cortex—detrusor overactivity with synergy of bladder and sphincter, normal bladder sensation, and usually adequate emptying.
2. Pons and spinal cord above S2 (upper motor neuron damage)—detrusor sphincter dyssynergia (DSD) and spastic paresis of the lower limbs.
3. S2-S4 (lower motor neuron damage)—acontractile (flaccid) detrusor, flaccid striated sphincter, and flaccid paralysis of the lower limbs.
4. Peripheral pelvic nerves—acontractile detrusor and absent bladder sensation.

Lesion Location	Urologic Syndrome	Bladder	Sphincter	Synergy*	Lower Limbs	BCR
Sacral Cord	Acontractile Bladder	Flaccid	Flaccid	–	Flaccid	Absent
Suprasacral Cord	DSD	Spastic	Spastic	No	Spastic	Present
Cerebral Cortex	NDO	Spastic	Normal	Yes	Normal	Present

* Synergistic (synchronized) function of the bladder and urinary sphincter.
BCR = bulbocavernosus reflex; DSD = detrusor sphincter dyssynergia;
NDO = Neurogenic detrusor overactivity (detrusor hyperreflexia)

Disease States and Typical Urodynamic Findings

1. Multiple sclerosis—detrusor overactivity.
2. Stroke—detrusor overactivity without DSD.
3. Parkinson's disease—detrusor overactivity. DSD is usually absent, but "cog wheeling" of the sphincter may result in intermittent DSD.
4. Cauda equina syndrome—acontractile detrusor.
5. Tethered cord—detrusor underactivity.
6. Spinal shock (suprasacral)–acontractile detrusor (the sphincter is often functional resulting in urinary retention). Spinal shock lasts 6-12 weeks.

Terminology For Voiding Abnormalities

	ICS Term	Previous Term	Description
Symptoms (Diagnosis Based on)	Stress Urinary Incontinence (SUI)	Stress Urinary Incontinence	Involuntary leakage of urine on effort, exertion, sneezing, or coughing.
	Urge Urinary Incontinence (UUI)	Urge Urinary Incontinence	Involuntary leakage of urine accompanied by or immediately preceded by urgency.
	Mixed Urinary Incontinence	Mixed Urinary Incontinence	A combination of SUI and UUI.
	Nocturnal Enuresis	Nocturnal Enuresis	Leakage of urine during sleep.
	Continuous Urinary Incontinence	Continuous Urinary Incontinence	Continuous leakage of urine.
Urodynamics (Diagnosis Based on)	Detrusor Overactivity (DO)	Uninhibited Bladder Contractions	Involuntary detrusor contractions (spontaneous or provoked) during the filling phase.
	Idiopathic DO	Detrusor Instability	Detrusor overactivity when the cause is unknown.
	Neurogenic DO	Detrusor Hyperreflexia	Detrusor overactivity with a relevant neurologic condition.
	Acontractile Detrusor	Atonic Bladder	Absent detrusor contraction when the cause is unknown.
		Detrusor Areflexia	Absent detrusor contraction with a relevant neurologic condition.
	Detrusor Sphincter Dyssynergia (DSD)	Detrusor Sphincter Dyssynergia	Involuntary contraction of the urethral sphincter during a detrusor contraction (DSD causes bladder outlet obstruction).
	Incompetent Urethral Closure Mechanism	Intrinsic Sphincter Deficiency	Leakage of urine in the absence of a detrusor contraction.
	Urodynamic SUI	Genuine SUI	SUI in the absence of a detrusor contraction (i.e. SUI confirmed by urodynamics).

ICS = International Continence Society

Useful Ways to Assess Voiding Function
1. Voiding log—record the following information:
   a. Time and date of void, voided volume, and symptoms with each void.
   b. Volume of liquid consumed per day.
   c. Urinary incontinence and the activity when the incontinence occurred.
   d. Number of pads/diapers used and degree of wetness (e.g. soaked, moist).
   e. Recording stools, constipation, and stool incontinence may be helpful.
2. Symptom scores
3. Urodynamic studies, uroflow, and post void residual.
4. Radiography (e.g. retrograde urethrogram, voiding cystourethrogram)
5. Cystoscopy

Urodynamics
Urodynamics is the study of micturition and may include
   1. Uroflowometry—evaluates urine flow.
   2. Cystometry—evaluates of bladder filling (storage).
   3. Pressure flow studies—evaluates of bladder emptying (voiding).
   4. Electromyography—evaluates the voluntary urinary sphincter activity.
   5. Cystogram—images of the bladder during filling and emptying.
   6. Urethral pressure profilometry–evaluates the voluntary urinary sphincter.
   7. Residual urine (post-void residual)

Uroflowometry
1. Uroflowometry evaluates bladder emptying.
2. Technique—the patient voids into a flowometer while in a normal voiding position. Bladder volume should be > 150 ml, but not over distended.
3. Information that can be obtained with uroflowometry
   a. Total voided volume
   b. Total voiding time (voiding duration)
   c. Peak urine flow rate
   d. Mean urine flow rate = total voided volume ÷ total voiding time
      i. This is less clinically useful than peak urine flow rate.
      ii. This calculated value will not be accurate if the patient does not maintain a continuous flow.
4. Normal peak flow rates
   a. Male: 20-25 ml/sec
   b. Female: 25-30 ml/sec
   c. Nomograms exist for age adjustment of flow rates.
   d. Normal flow can occur with abnormal physiology. For example,
      i. Poor detrusor function, compensated by elevated abdominal pressure.
      ii. Weak detrusor, but minimal outlet resistance.
      iii. Increased outlet resistance, but stronger detrusor contraction.
5. Normal flow profile (flow versus time)—looks like bell shaped curve.
6. Abnormal peak flow rates
   a. Suspected obstruction = 10-15 ml/sec.
   b. Probable obstruction < 10 ml/sec.
   c. "Supervoiders" achieve high flow, but are not of clinical concern.
7. Obstruction results in
   a. Low average urine flow rate
   b. Low maximum urine flow rate (especially < 10 ml/sec)
   c. Long flow time
   d. Interrupted flow with subsequent increases in intra-abdominal pressures to restore urine flow.

Residual Urine (Post-void Residual)
  1. Post-void residual (PVR) evaluates bladder emptying.
  2. PVR is influenced by detrusor function and outlet resistance.
  3. PVR is measured by catheterization after voiding, post-void film on cystogram, or post-void ultrasound.
  4. High PVR (> 50-100cc) indicates that one of the following is present: increased bladder outlet resistance, decreased detrusor function, or both.

Filling Cystometry (Cystometrogram, CMG)
  1. Filling cystometry evaluates bladder filling.
  2. Technique—subjective and objective recordings during bladder filling.
     a. Urethral catheter
        i.   Used to fill bladder with sterile water.
        ii. Measures intravesical pressure.
     b. Rectal probe measures intra-abdominal pressure.
     c. EMG measures voluntary sphincter activity.
  3. Information that can be obtained from CMG
     a. Detrusor pressure = intravesical pressure – intra-abdominal pressure
     b. Bladder capacity
     c. Bladder compliance ($C=\Delta V/\Delta P$)—normal compliance is a rise ≤ 6 cm water in detrusor pressure with filling.
     d. Presence of bladder sensation.
     e. Presence of involuntary detrusor contractions.
     f. Voluntary sphincter function and control (based on EMG activity).
     g. Leak point pressure (see Leak Point Pressure, page 172).
  4. These should be noted during CMG
     a. Volume at first sensation of filling (usually at 100-200 ml).
     b. Volume at sensation of fullness (usually at 350-450 ml).
     c. Volume at desire to void (usually at 350-450 ml).
     d. Volume of imminent void (unable to inhibit voiding any more).
     e. Occurrence of a voluntary detrusor contraction when asked to void.
     f. The ability to inhibit a voluntary detrusor contraction.
     g. Leak of urine during a cough and a valsalva.
  5. This study is often combined with pressure flow studies (see next section) to obtain both filling and emptying phases during urodynamics.

Pressure-Flow Studies
  1. Pressure-Flow studies evaluate bladder emptying.
  2. Technique—uses same equipment as filling cystometry.
  3. Information that can be obtained
     a. Maximum urinary flow rate
     b. Average urinary flow rate
     c. Detrusor pressure = intravesical pressure – intra-abdominal pressure
     d. Intravesical Pressure vs. Time
     e. Intravesical Pressure vs. Urinary Flow

Leak Point Pressure
1. Valsalva leak point pressure (VLPP)
   a. The intravesical pressure at which the urine leaks around the filling catheter during an increase in abdominal pressure, but in the absence of a detrusor contraction. If a cystocele is present, this test is invalid. VLPP is usually started with the bladder half full and then repeated at several higher bladder volumes.
   b. VLPP < 60 cm water implies that stress urinary incontinence is caused by intrinsic sphincter dysfunction. VLPP > 100 cm water implies that stress urinary incontinence is not from intrinsic sphincter dysfunction. VLPP from 60 to 100 is indeterminate.
2. Detrusor leak point pressure (DLPP)
   a. The lowest intravesical pressure at which the urine leaks around the filling catheter in the *absence* of a detrusor contraction and in the absence of increased abdominal pressure.
   b. DLPP > 40 cm water means that the upper tracts are at risk for deterioration (hydronephrosis and renal dysfunction). The high intravesical pressure causes functional ureteral obstruction.

Reading Urodynamics
1. Filling phase
   a. Compliance—normal compliance is ≤ 6 cm water change in detrusor pressure during filling.
   b. Capacity—in adults, normal bladder capacity is 400-500 cc. In kids, estimated normal bladder capacity (cc) = (age in years + 2) x 30.
   c. Sensation—normal adult first sensation at 100-200 cc.
   d. Presence of uninhibited bladder contractions—significant if they are > 15 cm water, sensed, or cause leakage.
   e. Is urine leak present?
2. Voiding phase
   a. Maximum flow (Qmax)
      i. Normal—male = 20-25 ml/sec; female = 25-30 ml/sec.
      ii. Suspected obstruction—Qmax = 10-15 ml/sec.
      iii. Probable obstruction—Qmax < 10 ml/sec.
   b. Voided volume
   c. Maximum detrusor pressure (Pdet max)—male normal = 40-60 cm water; female should be less.
   d. Post void residual (PVR)—normal usually < 50 cc.
   e. EMG—Does activity quiet when voiding? DSD? pseudo DSD?
   f. Is the bladder contraction sustained adequately?
3. Video
   a. Bladder contour—filling defects, trabeculation, or diverticula?
   b. Presence of vesicoureteral reflux
   c. Post void residual—does it correlate with measured PVR?
   d. Bladder neck—does it funnel appropriately? Is the bladder neck open?
   e. Urethra—strictures?
4. Flow
   a. Maximum flow (Qmax)
   b. Average flow (Qave)
   c. Total voiding time (including periods of intermittent voiding)
   d. Voided volume

Deflections on Urodynamic Pressure Tracings

	Pressure Tracing Deflection Based on the Pressure Source			
	Abdomen*	Detrusor	Colon†	Abdomen and Detrusor
Pves	↑	↑	-	↑
Pabd	↑	-	↑/↓	↑
Pdet	-	↑	↓/↑	↑

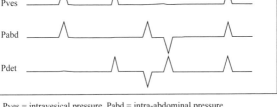

Pves = intravesical pressure, Pabd = intra-abdominal pressure
Pdet = pressure generated by the detrusor (calculated as Pves-Pabd)
* e.g. cough, strain, crede, abdominal tapping, valsalva.
† e.g. peristalsis, flatulence. These pressures are transmitted to the abdominal
  (rectal) transducer but not to the intravesical transducer. When the colon is
  the only source of pressure changes, Pabd and Pdet always deflect in
  opposite directions.

REFERENCES
Abrams P, et al: The standardisation of terminology of lower urinary tract
    function: Report from the Standardisation Sub-committee of the
    International Continence Society. Urology, 61: 37, 2003.
Incontinence: 3rd International Consultation on Incontinence.
    Ed. P Abrams, et al. vols. 1 & 2. Plymouth, United Kingdom: Health
    Publication Ltd., 2005.
Wein AJ: Neuromuscular dysfunction of the lower urinary tract. Campbell's
    Urology. 6th Edition. Ed. PC Walsh, AB Retik, TA Stamey, et al.
    Philadelphia: W. B. Sanders Company, 1992, pp 571-658.

URINARY INCONTINENCE: GENERAL CONCEPTS

Definition and Classification

1. *Urinary incontinence is defined as the involuntary loss of urine.*
2. *Urinary symptoms do not necessarily correlate with the underlying cause of incontinence.* For example, stress incontinence can be caused by sphincter deficiency (urine is pushed through a weak sphincter), urethral hypermobility (urine is pushed through a poorly coapting urethra), overflow (urine is pushed from a full bladder), or detrusor overactivity (stress triggers an involuntary bladder contraction). *Urodynamic testing is required to determine how symptoms correlate with voiding physiology.*
3. Classification based on symptoms (also see page 169)
   a. Stress urinary incontinence (SUI)—episodic involuntary loss of urine that occurs during an increase in abdominal pressure (such as coughing, sneezing, straining, lifting, bending, exercising, and exertion).
   b. Urge urinary incontinence (UUI)—episodic involuntary loss of urine that is accompanied by or immediately preceded by urgency.
   c. Mixed incontinence—a mixture of both SUI and UUI.
   d. Unaware (unconscious) incontinence—involuntary loss of urine without urge, without stress, and without the patient being aware of it.
   e. Nocturnal enuresis—involuntary loss of urine during sleep.
   f. Continuous incontinence—continuous involuntary loss of urine. Continuous incontinence often arises from a fistula.
4. Classification based on the structure from which the urine leaks
   a. Urethral incontinence—urine loss through the urethral meatus.
   b. Extra-urethral incontinence—urine loss through a structure other than the urethral meatus. Examples include vesicovaginal fistula, ureterovaginal fistula, and ectopic ureter.
5. Classification based on underlying pathophysiology (also see page 169)
   a. Intrinsic sphincter deficiency (ISD)—dysfunction of the urinary sphincter. The 2002 International Continence Society (ICS) report prefers the term "incompetent urethral closure mechanism." However, the term ISD is more widely utilized and will be used in this book.
   b. Urethral hypermobility—hypermobility is caused by pelvic floor muscle weakness and is defined as excessive descent of the bladder neck and urethra during increased abdominal pressure. Hypermobility can impair urethral coaptation, and, in some cases, can cause urinary incontinence. Hypermobility and ISD often occur together.
   c. Detrusor overactivity (DO)—involuntary detrusor contractions during the filling phase.
      i. Neurogenic DO (previously called detrusor hyperreflexia)—DO in the presence of a relevant neurologic condition.
      ii. Idiopathic DO (previously called detrusor instability)—DO from an unknown cause.
   d. Low bladder compliance—with low bladder compliance, there is a progressive rise in intravesical pressure during filling. High intravesical pressure may push urine from the bladder and cause incontinence.
   e. Urinary retention—urine leakage may be caused by overfilling of the bladder (overflow incontinence).

6. The optimal way to document the patient's condition is to describe the symptoms and the underlying pathophysiology. Examples: SUI from ISD, UUI from idiopathic DO, SUI from urinary retention (overflow incontinence), continuous incontinence from vesicovaginal fistula.

Classification of Urinary Incontinence	
Based on Symptoms	**Based on Underlying Pathophysiology**
Stress Incontinence Urge Incontinence Mixed Incontinence Unaware Incontinence Nocturnal Enuresis Continuous Incontinence	Urethral Incontinence Intrinsic Sphincter Deficiency (ISD) Urethral Hypermobility Detrusor Overactivity (DO) Low Bladder Compliance Urinary Retention Extra-urethral Incontinence Urinary Fistula Ectopic Ureter

Transient Urinary Incontinence

1. The causes of transient incontinence are summarized using the mnemonic "DIAPPERS" (proposed by Resnick, Urol Clin North Am 23: 55, 1996).
   - D Delirium—cognitive dysfunction can impair voiding.
   - I Infection—bladder irritation may cause incontinence.
   - A Atrophic vaginitis—postmenopausal status may cause nocturia, frequency, urgency, and UUI (but it does not appear to cause SUI).
   - P Pharmaceuticals/polypharmacy
   - P Psychological (especially depression)—severe psychological dysfunction can impair voiding.
   - E Excessive urine production—diuretics, untreated diabetes, and other causes of excessive urine production may overwhelm the bladder and cause urinary incontinence.
   - R Restricted mobility—may cause incontinence because the patient cannot reach the bathroom in time. Causes of restricted mobility include arthritis, Parkinson's disease, and impaired balance.
   - S Stool impaction/constipation—severe constipation may impair bladder function and pelvic floor muscle function.

2. Pharmaceuticals
   a. Diuretics—increased urine output can cause urinary frequency, urgency, polyuria, and incontinence. Examples: furosemide, thiazides.
   b. Anticholinergics—can impair bladder contraction (leading to urinary retention) and can cause constipation. Examples: anti-psychotics, anti-depressants, and anti-histamines.
   c. Sedatives—can cause delirium. Examples: benzodiazepines.
   d. Narcotics—can impair bladder contraction (leading to urinary retention), can cause delirium, and can cause constipation.
   e. α-agonists—can increase urethral sphincter tone (leading to urinary retention). Examples: nasal decongestants, imipramine.
   f. α-antagonists—can decrease urethral sphincter tone (leading to SUI). Examples: terazosin, doxazosin, tamsulosin, and alfuzosin.
   g. Calcium channel blockers—can impair bladder contraction (leading to urinary retention).
   h. Angiotensin converting enzyme (ACE) inhibitors—can cause coughing, which may precipitate SUI.
   i. Alcohol—can increase urine output and cause frequency, urgency, and incontinence. Alcohol can also cause delirium and urinary retention.

Evaluation of Urinary Incontinence

History

1. Precipitating factors—coughing, sneezing, lifting, straining, changes in body position, alcohol, caffeine, constipation, immobility.
2. Severity of incontinence—number of pads used per day, wetness of the pad when it is changed (soaked, few drops).
3. Other voiding symptoms—urgency, frequency, nocturia, intermittent stream, hesitancy, weak stream, etc.
4. Obstetrical history—number of pregnancies (gravida), number of live births (para), number of abortions (gravida, para, and abortions are often abbreviated as GPA). Type of delivery (cesarean section, vaginal delivery, traumatic delivery).
5. History of genitourinary conditions—stricture, diverticulum, sexually transmitted diseases, urinary tract infections, etc.
6. History of pelvic surgery—abdominoperineal resection, incontinence surgery, female genital surgery (hysterectomy, prolapse surgery), prostatectomy, urethral surgery, etc.
7. Neurologic disease (e.g. multiple sclerosis, stroke, Parkinson's disease, lumbar disc disease) and neurologic symptoms (e.g. weakness, numbness, visual changes)
8. Fluid consumption (type and amount of fluid consumed)
9. Medications

Physical Examination

1. Pelvic examination (see below).
2. Neurologic examination may include
   a. Perineal sensation
   b. Anal sphincter tone (at rest and with volitional contraction)
   c. Bulbocavernosus reflex (BCR)—squeezing the glans penis or clitoris causes contraction of the anal sphincter. In males, absence of the BCR reflex is almost always associated with a neurologic abnormality. In females, absence of the BCR reflex may be a normal finding (30% of normal females do not exhibit the BCR) or it may be associated with a neurologic abnormality.
3. Rectal examination—check for stool impaction, sphincter tone, and BCR.
4. Lower extremity—edema of the lower extremity may create excess urine production, leading to incontinence, especially at night.

Pelvic Examination in the Female

1. Pelvic examination is performed with the patient in the lithotomy position during relaxation and during cough or valsalva, and should include inspection of the following regions.
   a. Vaginal epithelium—check for atrophic vaginitis, erythema, lesions.
   b. Anterior vagina—check for urethral hypermobility, cystocele, and urethral diverticulum.
   c. Middle vagina—check for enterocele and uterine prolapse.
   d. Posterior vagina—check for rectocele.
   e. Perineum
2. Cotton swab test—this test assesses the degree of hypermobility. A lubricated cotton swab is placed into the urethra. The axis of the swab is measured at rest and with straining. Urethral hypermobility is present when the swab axis changes by more than 30° from rest to strain.
3. Cough test (stress test)—check for urine leak during cough. When urine leak is not demonstrated during pelvic exam, the cough test may be performed while the patient is standing with a foot on stool.

Laboratory and Imaging Tests
1. Urinalysis $\pm$ urine culture—check for glucosuria and for infection.
2. Post void residual—check for retention.
3. Voiding diary—a record of the patients' voiding pattern. It may include the date and time of each entry, volume and type of fluid consumed, volume of each void, each incontinence episode and the approximate volume of urine lost, urinary symptoms (e.g. urgency), and pad usage (including the degree of wetness when the pad is changed). Documenting bowel movements may also be helpful.
4. Cystoscopy—consider cystoscopy in patients at risk for urethral stricture or bladder cancer. Cystoscopy should be performed when surgery for incontinence is being considered, when empiric therapy is unsuccessful, or when the diagnosis is unclear.
5. Urodynamics—urodynamic testing is usually unnecessary, but it should be performed when surgery for incontinence is being considered, when empiric therapy is unsuccessful, or when the diagnosis is unclear.
6. Imaging studies—imaging may be useful in select cases. Examples include voiding cystourethrogram, pelvic MRI, spinal imaging, and brain imaging.

Treatment: General Concepts

Treatment of Transient Incontinence
1. Delirium—eliminate causes of delirium.
2. Infection—treat urinary tract infection and vaginitis.
3. Atrophic vaginitis—consider administering topical vaginal estrogen.
4. Pharmaceuticals—eliminate unnecessary or offending medications.
5. Psychological—consider referring the patient for treatment of psychological disorders.
6. Excessive urine output—treatment may include restricting fluids, avoiding diuretics when possible, and treating medical disorders that may cause polyuria (e.g. diabetes mellitus, diabetes insipidus, hypercalcemia, congestive heart failure, lower extremity edema). For patients with lower extremity edema, elevating the legs before bed may help eliminate excess fluid before going to sleep.
7. Restricted mobility—this problem can often be overcome by using a hand held urinal or bedside commode. Timed voiding may also help.
8. Stool impaction/constipation—consider laxatives and stool softeners.
9. If incontinence persists after treatment of transient causes, further evaluation is necessary.

Behavioral Therapy
1. Avoid activities that exacerbate incontinence.
2. Voiding diary—provides feedback and helps the patient and physician monitor progress.
3. Timed (scheduled) voiding—voiding by a routine schedule, usually with a constant interval between voids (e.g. voiding every 2-3 hours).
   a. Timed voiding empties the bladder before incontinence occurs.
   b. Incontinence may occur more frequently during certain times of the day. In this case, the voiding interval may be changed throughout the day to match the patients' incontinence pattern (habit training).
   c. Patients with impaired cognition may have difficulty complying with timed voiding. In this case, a care giver may need to prompt the patient when it is time to void (prompted voiding).
   d. A Cochrane review in 2004 found that there is insufficient evidence to determine whether timed voiding is beneficial.

4. Bladder training (also known as bladder retraining or bladder drill)
  a. Bladder training may involve 2 processes: modification of the voiding interval and urge control.
  b. Modification of the voiding interval—voiding by a strict schedule that starts with a short interval between voids and gradually progresses to a longer interval between voids. The initial voiding interval is determined from the pre-treatment voiding diary (initial voiding interval often ranges from 30 to 120 minutes). When continence is achieved at the existing interval (which often takes 1-2 weeks), the voiding interval is increased by 15-60 minutes. This process is continued until an acceptable voiding interval is achieved.
  c. Urge control (bladder inhibition)—suppressing the urge to void using any of following methods: keeping the body still until the urge subsides, taking slow deep breaths, concentrating on eliminating the urge (mental imagery), mental distraction to reduce awareness of the urge (humming a tune, mental calculations), and contracting the pelvic floor muscles (contracting the pelvic floor muscles inhibits detrusor contraction). When the urge subsides, do not urinate until the next scheduled void.
  d. Bladder training requires a motivated patient with sufficient cognitive function to participate in the regimen. In addition, bladder training relies on adequate pelvic floor muscle function.
  e. A Cochrane review in 2004 found that "bladder training may be helpful for the treatment of urinary incontinence, but this conclusion can only be tentative...more research is required." In motivated patients, bladder training may decrease SUI and UUI episodes by up to 50%.
5. Pelvic floor muscle training (see below).
6. Fluid management—avoid excessive fluid intake. Fluid restriction before bed may help reduce nocturnal incontinence.
7. Dietary management—avoiding bladder irritants (caffeine, alcohol, spicy food, acidic food) may improve continence.
8. Weight loss—weight loss in obese patients can reduce SUI.
9. Avoid constipation
10. Stop smoking—smoking may increase the risk of SUI. Although there are no studies showing that smoking cessation improves continence, it may be worth trying.
11. For patients with lower extremity edema, elevating the legs before bed permits elimination of excess fluid before going to sleep.

Treatment: Pelvic Floor Therapy

Pelvic Floor Muscle Training (PFMT)
1. PFMT is a regimen of repeated voluntary pelvic floor muscle contractions taught by a health care professional. Previously used terms include Kegel exercises, pelvic floor exercises, and pelvic floor physiotherapy.
2. *PFMT improves stress, urge, and mixed incontinence.* In motivated patients, PFMT may decrease SUI and UUI episodes by up to 80%. In patients with SUI, PFMT achieves enough improvement that 40% choose to avoid surgery. A 2006 Cochrane review revealed that PFMT is more effective at reducing incontinence than no treatment or placebo.
3. *PFMT should be offered as first line therapy for stress, urge, and mixed incontinence.*
4. The mechanism by which PFMT works is unknown. Theories include pelvic muscle strengthening and suppression of involuntary contractions.

5. To achieve improvement, patients must be motivated, compliant, and properly instructed.
   a. *Inadequate instruction is the most common reason why pelvic floor muscle training fails. Verbal instructions are usually insufficient to teach the patient which muscles to contract.* A physical demonstration of which muscles to contract is often required.
   b. Compliance is often a problem (over 50% stop therapy); therefore, periodic reinforcement is essential.
6. PFMT consists of intermittent maximal isometric contractions of the pelvic floor muscles. Each contraction is held for 6-8 seconds and is followed by brief period of relaxation. A common regimen is a set of 10 contractions three times a day. It may also be helpful to contract the pelvic floor muscles before an activity that causes leakage (e.g. squeeze before a cough, sneeze, or lift).
7. Continence typically improves 6-12 weeks after starting PFMT.

Vaginal Weights
1. A rounded weight is inserted into the vagina. The patient must contract the pelvic floor muscles to prevent the weight from slipping out. The patient begins with a light weight. When she is able to retain the existing weight, she advances to the next heavier weight. Vaginal weights are often used for 10-15 minutes twice a day.
2. A Cochrane review in 2002 indicated that there is "some evidence that weighted vaginal cones are better than no treatment." It appears that combining PFMT with vaginal weights is no better than PFMT alone.

Pelvic Floor Electrical Stimulation (PFES)
1. PFES delivers intermittent electrical pulses to the pelvic floor muscles using an intravaginal probe, an intrarectal probe, or surface (skin) electrodes. Self treatment may be instituted after office based instruction. There is no standard protocol for PFES.
   a. Acute maximal PFES—electrical pulses of high enough intensity to induce maximal contraction of the pelvic floor muscles. Stimulation is often conducted for 15-30 minutes daily to weekly.
   b. Chronic PFES—electrical pulses of low enough intensity to avoid contraction of the pelvic floor muscles. Stimulation is usually conducted 6-12 hours a day for several months.
2. It is unclear if adding PFES to PFMT improves outcomes.

Pelvic Floor Magnetic Stimulation
1. The patient sits in a chair that delivers magnetic pulses to the perineum. These pulses induce contraction of the pelvic floor muscles.
2. There are no invasive probes and the patient can remain fully clothed.

Biofeedback
1. Biofeedback may help "instruct" the patient on which muscles are the proper ones to contract.
2. Sensors are applied to the patient's body (vaginal, rectal, or skin probes). The degree of pelvic floor muscle activity is detected by the sensors and provided to the patient as auditory or visual feedback. This information helps the patient identify when the proper muscles are being utilized.
3. Home and office based systems are available.
4. Based on current data, it is unclear whether outcomes are improved by combining biofeedback with PFMT.

Combination Therapy

1. There is insufficient data to determine whether combining multiple types of pelvic floor therapy is more effective than a single therapy.
2. Combining PFMT with bladder training may be more effective in the short-term than PFMT alone, but the benefit may not be maintained beyond 6 months.
3. Based on current data, it is unclear whether outcomes are improved by combining biofeedback with PFMT.

General

Abrams P, et al: **The standardisation of terminology of lower urinary tract function: Report from the Standardisation Sub-committee of the International Continence Society. Urology, 61: 37, 2003.**

Incontinence: 3rd International Consultation on Incontinence.
    Ed. P Abrams, et al. vols. 1 & 2. Plymouth, United Kingdom: Health Publication Ltd., 2005.

Payne CK: Urinary incontinence: nonsurgical management. Campbell's Urology. 8th Edition. Ed. PC Walsh, AB Retik, TA Vaughan, et al. Philadelphia: W. B. Sanders Company, 2002, pp 1069-1091.

Resnick NM: Geriatric incontinence. Urol Clin North Am 23(1): 55, 1996.

Schwab CW, Rovner ES: Conservative management of urinary incontinence. AUA Update Series, Vol. 24, Lesson 23, 2005.

Ostaszkiewicz J, et al: Timed voiding for the management of urinary incontinence. Cochrane Database Syst Rev, Issue 1: CD002802, 2004.

Wallace SA, et al: Bladder training for urinary incontinence in adults. Cochrane Database Syst Rev, Issue 1: CD001308, 2004.

Pelvic Muscle Training

Berghmans LCM, et al: Conservative treatment of stress urinary incontinence in women: a systematic review of randomized clinical trials. Br J Urol, 82: 181, 1998.

Goode PS, et al: Effect of behavioral training with or without pelvic floor electrical stimulation on stress incontinence in women: a randomized controller trial. JAMA, 290(3): 345, 2003.

Hay-Smith EJ, Dumoulin C: Pelvic floor muscle training versus no treatment, or inactive control treatments, for urinary incontinence in women. Cochrane Database Syst Rev, Issue 1: CD005654, 2006.

Herbison P, et al: Weighted vaginal cones for urinary incontinence. Cochrane Database Syst Rev, Issue 1: CD002114, 2002.

Kegel AH: Physiologic therapy for urinary stress incontinence. JAMA, 146: 915, 1951.

Klarskov P, et al: Pelvic floor exercise versus surgery for female urinary stress incontinence. Urol Int, 41: 129, 1986.

Neumann PB, et al: Pelvic floor muscle training and adjunctive therapies for the treatment of stress urinary incontinence in woman: a systematic review. BMC Women's Health, 6: 11, 2006.

Payne CK: Electrostimulation. Urinary Incontinence. Ed. PD O'Donnell. St. Louis: Mosby Year Book Inc., 2002, pp 287-294.

Shaikh S, et al: Mechanical devices for urinary incontinence in women. Cochrane Database Syst Rev, Issue 2: CD001756, 2006.

Weatherall M: Biofeedback of pelvic floor muscle exercises for female genuine stress incontinence: a meta-analysis of trials identified in a systematic review. BJU Int, 83: 1015, 1999.

Wise BG, et al: A comparative study of vaginal cone therapy, cones and Kegel exercises, and maximal electrical stimulation in the treatment of female genuine stress incontinence. Neurourol Urodyn, 12: 436, 1993 (abstract).

URGE INCONTINENCE & OVERACTIVE BLADDER

General Information
1. *Overactive bladder (OAB) refers to symptoms of urgency with or without urge incontinence.*
2. *Urge urinary incontinence (UUI) is episodic involuntary loss of urine which is accompanied by or immediately preceded by urgency.*
3. Causes and risk factors of OAB
   a. Bladder inflammation—e.g. interstitial cystitis, bacterial cystitis, stones.
   b. Chronic bladder outlet obstruction—chronic strain on the bladder may cause detrusor overactivity and UUI.
   c. Central nervous system disorders—see page 168.
   d. Pregnancy—page 222.
   e. Postmenopausal status
   f. Idiopathic—*the most common cause of UUI and OAB is idiopathic.*

Evaluation
1. Urodynamic testing does not always reveal UUI when it is present.
   a. Leakage may be intermittent and may not occur during urodynamics.
   b. Anxiety or discomfort during urodynamics may alter the normal voiding physiology and mask UUI.
2. See Evaluation of Urinary Incontinence, page 176.

Summary of Treatment Options for OAB and UUI
1. Non-invasive treatment
   a. Behavioral therapy (see page 177)—*first line treatment usually consists of behavioral therapy with or without an anticholinergic medication.*
   b. Estrogen for postmenopausal females
   c. Anticholinergic medications
2. Minimally invasive treatment
   a. Percutaneous tibial nerve stimulation
   b. Sacral neuromodulation
   c. Botulinum
3. Surgical treatment
   a. Augmentation enterocystoplasty
   b. Autoaugmentation
   c. Urinary Diversion

Estrogen in Postmenopausal Women
1. A meta-analysis in 2004 by the Hormones and Urogenital Therapy Committee showed that estrogens were significantly better than placebo for improving UUI, urgency, frequency, and nocturia. Estrogen also improved volume at first sensation and bladder capacity. Topical vaginal administration is superior to oral or systemic administration.
2. Contraindications—history of venous thrombosis or pulmonary embolism, recent stroke or myocardial infarction, estrogen dependant cancer (such as breast cancer), abnormal genital bleeding, and liver dysfunction.
3. Side effects—embolic (pulmonary embolism, deep venous thrombosis, stroke), cardiac (myocardial infarction), increased risk of female cancers (breast, endometrial, and ovarian cancer), slightly increased risk of dementia, gallbladder disease, and visual disturbances.

Anticholinergic Medications

General Information

1. *Anticholinergic drugs competitively inhibit muscarinic cholinergic receptors.*
2. Anticholinergic drugs produce a statistically significant improvement in UUI and overactive bladder symptoms compared to placebo.
3. Anticholinergic drugs improve symptoms to a greater degree than bladder training alone. *Symptom improvement is best when anticholinergic medications are combined with behavioral therapy, such as bladder training and pelvic floor muscle therapy.*
4. Chemical structure
   a. Tertiary amines—more likely to cross the blood brain barrier than quaternary amines and they are usually metabolized by the liver.
   b. Quaternary amines—unlikely to cross the blood brain barrier and are not metabolized by the liver.
5. M3 selectivity—a higher affinity for M3 than for M2 (binding still occurs to other M subtypes). The clinical importance of M3 selectivity is unclear.
   a. Highest selectivity—darifenacin.
   b. Moderate selectivity—solifenacin and oxybutynin.
6. Anticholinergic medications achieve maximal effect after 2-3 months.
7. Contraindications—urinary retention, gastric retention, intestinal obstruction, uncontrolled narrow angle glaucoma, or myasthenia gravis.
8. Side effects—*dry mouth is the most common side effect*. Other side effects include blurry vision, constipation, headache, dizziness, drowsiness, tachycardia (rare), urinary retention (rare), and impaired perspiration.
9. For doses, see page 418.

Tertiary Amines
Oxybutynin
Tolterodine
Darifenacin
Solifenacin
Hyoscyamine
Flavoxate
Dicyclomine

Quaternary Amines
Trospium
Propantheline

Muscarinic Cholinergic Receptors (M receptors)

1. There are 5 subtypes of the muscarinic cholinergic receptor (M1-M5).
2. The bladder contains M1, M2, and M3 receptors. M2 is more numerous, but *M3 is the primary receptor that mediates bladder contraction*. Inhibition of M3 in the bladder reduces detrusor overactivity.
3. Inhibition of M receptors outside the bladder can cause side effects.
   a. Eye—inhibition of M3 causes pupil dilation (blurry vision).
   b. Salivary glands—inhibition of M3 reduces saliva secretion (dry mouth).
   c. Intestines—inhibition of M3 reduces motility (constipation).
   d. Heart—inhibition of M2 causes tachycardia.
   e. Brain—inhibition of M1 probably impairs cognition and memory.

Anticholinergic Agents—Insufficient Evidence to Make Recommendations

1. These agents are categorized as "optional" or "no recommendation possible" by the Third International Consultation on Incontinence 2004 (3rd ICOI) because there is insufficient evidence regarding their efficacy.
2. Hyoscyamine—(tertiary amine, non-selective M receptor inhibitor). FDA approved for OAB.
3. Flavoxate—(tertiary amine, non-selective M receptor inhibitor, smooth muscle relaxant). FDA approved for OAB.
4. Dicyclomine—(tertiary amine, non-selective M receptor inhibitor, smooth muscle relaxant). *Not* FDA approved for OAB.

Agents‡ Recommended by the 3rd International Consultation on Incontinence 2004 for Treatment of Overactive Bladder (OAB) and Urge Urinary Incontinence (UUI)

	Generic Name	Brand Name	Route	M Receptor Selectivity	Metabolism	Active Compound in Urine†	Other Characteristics	FDA Approved for OAB
Tertiary Amines	Tolterodine	Detrol®	Oral	Non-selective	Hepatic	<15%	Bladder selectivity (higher selectivity for the bladder than for the salivary glands, which may reduce dry mouth). May be less effective in poor metabolizers.*	Yes
Tertiary Amines	Oxybutynin	Ditropan®	Oral	M3 Selective	Hepatic	<1%	Highest risk of CNS side effects.	Yes
Tertiary Amines	Oxybutynin	Oxytrol™	Trans-dermal	M3 Selective	Hepatic	<1%	Lowest rate of dry mouth and constipation. May cause skin irritation at patch site.	Yes
Tertiary Amines	Darifenacin	Enablex®	Oral	M3 Selective	Hepatic	3%	Highest rate of constipation. No QT interval prolongation.	Yes
Tertiary Amines	Solifenacin	Vesicare®	Oral	M3 Selective	Hepatic	<15%	Bladder selectivity (higher selectivity for the bladder than for the salivary glands, which may reduce dry mouth).	Yes
Quaternary Amines	Propantheline	Pro-Banthine®	Oral	Non-selective	Not Hepatic	<5%	Requires frequent dosing because of its short half life.	No
Quaternary Amines	Trospium	Sanctura®	Oral	Non-selective	Not Hepatic	60%	Lowest risk of CNS side effects. Highest excretion of active compound in the urine. No QT interval prolongation.	Yes

FDA = Food and Drug Administration; CNS = central nervous system

‡ Agents available in the United States. Propiverine was also recommended, but it is not available in the United States.

† This is the percent of the absorbed dose that is excreted as active compound (drug or active metabolites) in the urine.

* The enzyme that produces active metabolites has reduced activity in 7% of Caucasians and 2% of African Americans (poor metabolizers).

Minimally Invasive Treatment

Botulinum Toxin

1. Botulinum is the toxin that causes botulism. It inhibits muscle contraction by blocking the release of acetylcholine at the neuromuscular junction.
2. When botulinum is injected into the bladder, it reduces urgency and urge incontinence by inhibiting detrusor overactivity.
3. Botulinum is administered by injecting it though a cystoscope and into the detrusor. 10-30 sites are injected throughout the bladder.
4. The effects wear off in 3-12 months; thus, repeat treatments are required.
5. In very rare cases, focal or generalized weakness may occur when botulinum spreads systemically. However, central nervous system effects are unlikely because botulinum does not cross the blood brain barrier.
6. Contraindications—pregnancy, breast feeding, neuromuscular compromise (e.g. myasthenia gravis, amyotrophic lateral sclerosis).
7. Botulinum is not FDA approved.

Percutaneous Tibial Nerve Stimulation (PTNS)

1. A percutaneous needle electrode is inserted slightly cephalad to the medial malleolus of the leg. Electrical pulses delivered through the needle are transmitted along the tibial nerve to the S3 segment of the sacral plexus. Electrical stimulation of the S3 afferent nerve modifies the voiding reflex.
2. PTNS has been shown to improve urgency, frequency, and UUI in 60-80% of patients. The S3 peripheral nerves (including the tibial nerve) must be intact for this therapy to be effective.
3. Treatment duration is 30 minutes each week for a minimum of 12 weeks.
4. The Urgent® PC Neuromodulation System is FDA approved for OAB.

Sacral Neuromodulation (Interstim®)

1. Sacral neuromodulation modifies the voiding reflex using direct electrical stimulation of the S3 afferent nerve. It is ineffective when the S3 nerves are damaged (e.g. from sacral spinal cord injury or pelvic surgery).
2. Sacral neuromodulation is accomplished by a two stage procedure.
   a. First stage—a percutaneous electrode is implanted through the sacral foramen and next to the S3 nerve root. The electrode is connected to a pager like generator that controls the electrical stimulation. The patient undergoes a test period of 2-4 weeks. If the implant does not achieve a satisfactory improvement in urinary symptoms, the percutaneous electrode is removed. If the implant achieves a satisfactory improvement in urinary symptoms (i.e. more than 50% reduction in symptoms), the second stage is performed.
   b. Second stage—the percutaneous lead is connected to a subcutaneous generator and the entire system is internalized.
3. Interstim® is indicated for patients who fail or cannot tolerate conservative treatments and who have one or more of the following conditions: UUI, urinary urgency and frequency, or non-obstructive urinary retention.
4. When used for UUI, up to 50% of patients became dry and 60-90% were dry or improved. The efficacy in men has not been well studied.
5. If the need for postoperative MRI is anticipated, Interstim® should be avoided. The device may be affected by electrical or magnetic exposure such as with MRI, electrocautery, defibrillators, etc.
6. Complications include infection, hematoma, pain at the generator or lead site, lead migration (uncommon), and device malfunction (uncommon). Occasionally, patients may have changes in bowel function, changes in menstrual cycle, and undesirable sensations (shock sensation, numbness).
7. Surgical revision rates (for infection, malfunction, etc.) range from 7-33%.

Surgical Treatment

1. These surgeries may be considered for DO refractory to less invasive treatments and for urinary incontinence caused by reduced bladder capacity.
2. Augmentation enterocystoplasty
   a. A sagittal incision is made in the bladder dome and the bladder is opened up like a clam. A detubularized intestinal segment is sutured to the bladder to "patch" the opening. This intestinal "patch" increases (augments) the bladder capacity. It also lowers the intravesical pressure during a bladder contraction (which minimizes the risk of UUI).
   b. This is the most commonly used surgical option for treating DO.
   c. Approximately 80% of patients become improved or dry; however, 10-40% require intermittent catheterization for urinary retention.
   d. The success rate is lower when augmentation cystoplasty is used in patients with a history of contracted bladder from radiation.
3. Autoaugmentation
   a. The detrusor muscle overlying the bladder dome is either excised from the urothelium (detrusor myectomy) or incised and mobilized away from the urothelium (detrusor myotomy). This permits the exposed urothelial mucosa to balloon out as a wide mouth diverticulum. This diverticulum increases (augments) the bladder capacity. It also lowers the intravesical pressure during bladder contraction (which minimizes the risk of UUI).
   b. *Autoaugmentation achieves a very limited increase in bladder capacity and bladder capacity may decrease with long-term follow up.* It should be used only in patients with good bladder capacity before surgery.
   c. Approximately 75% of patients become improved or dry; however, some patients may require intermittent catheterization for urinary retention.
   d. If autoaugmentation fails, enterocystoplasty can be performed.
4. Urinary diversion
   a. Urinary diversion is usually not used for UUI, but it may be a reasonable option in select cases.
   b. Examples—ileal chimney, conduit, catheterizable diversion, neobladder.

REFERENCES

General

Burgio KL, et al: Combined behavioral and drug therapy for urge incontinence in older women. J Am Geriatr Soc, 48: 370, 2000.

Incontinence: 3rd International Consultation on Incontinence. Ed. P Abrams, et al. vols. 1 & 2. Plymouth, United Kingdom: Health Publication Ltd., 2005.

Payne CK: Urinary incontinence: nonsurgical management. Campbell's Urology. 8th Edition. Ed. PC Walsh, AB Retik, TA Vaughan, et al. Philadelphia: W. B. Sanders Company, 2002, pp 1069-1091.

Staskin DR: Overactive bladder in the elderly. Drugs Aging, 22(12): 1013, 2005.

Estrogens

Cardozo L, et al: A systematic review of estrogens for symptoms suggestive of overactive bladder: fourth report of the Hormones and Urogenital Therapy Committee. Acta Obstet Gynecol Scand, 83(10): 892, 2004.

Moehrer B, et al: Oestrogens for urinary incontinence in women. Cochrane Database Syst Rev, Issue 2: CD001405, 2003.

Robinson D, Cardozo LD: The role of estrogens in female lower urinary tract dysfunction. Urology, 62 (Suppl 4a): 45, 2003.

Anticholinergic Medications

Alhasso AA, et al: Anticholinergic drugs versus non-drug active therapies for overactive bladder syndrome in adults. Cochrane Database Syst Rev, Issue 4: CD003139, 2006.

Chapple CR, et al: A comparison of the efficacy and tolerability of solifenacin succinate and extended release tolterodine at treating overactive bladder syndrome: results of the STAR trial. Eur Urol, 48: 464, 2005.

Diokno AC, et al: Prospective randomized double blind study of the efficacy and tolerability of the extended release formulations of oxybutynin and tolterodine for overactive bladder: results of the OPERA trial. Mayo Clin Proc, 78: 687, 2003.

Dmochowski RR, et al: Comparative efficacy and safety of transdermal oxybutynin and oral tolterodine versus placebo in previously treated patients with urge and mixed urinary incontinence. Urology, 62(2): 237, 2003.

Kim Y, et al: Intravesical instillation of human urine after oral administration of trospium, tolterodine, and oxybutynin in a rat model of detrusor activity. BJU Int, 97(2): 400, 2006.

Nabi G, et al: Anticholinergic drugs versus placebo for overactive bladder syndrome in adults. Cochrane Database Syst Rev, Issue 4: CD003781, 2006.

Ohtake A, et al: In vitro and in vivo selectivity profile of solifenacin succinate (YM905) for urinary bladder over salivary glands. Eur J Pharmacol, 492: 243, 2004.

Sussman D, Garely A: Treatment of overactive bladder with once daily extended release tolterodine or oxybutynin: the antimuscarinic clinical effectiveness trial (ACET). Curr Med Res Opin, 18(4): 177, 2002.

CNS effects of Anticholinergic Medications

Ancelin ML: Non-degenerative mild cognitive impairment in elderly people and use of anticholinergic drugs. BMJ, 332(7539): 455, 2006.

Diefenbach K, et al: Effects on sleep of anticholinergics used for overactive bladder in healthy volunteers aged > or = 50 years. BJU Int, 95: 346, 2005.

Edwards KR: Risk of delirium with concomitant use of tolterodine and acetylcholinesterase inhibitors. J Am Geriatr Soc, 50(6): 1165, 2002.

Kay G, et al: Differential effects of antimuscarinic agents darifenacin and oxybutynin ER on memory in older subjects. Eur Urol, 50(2): 317, 2006.

Pietzko A, et al: Influences of trospium chloride and oxybutynin on quantitative EEG in healthy volunteers. Eur J Clin Pharmacol, 47: 337, 1994.

Staskin DR, et al: Effects of trospium chloride on somnolence and sleepiness in patients with overactive bladder. Curr Sci, 5: 423, 2004.

Sunderland T, et al: Anticholinergic sensitivity in patients with dementia of the Alzheimer's type and age matched controls: a dose response study. Arch Gen Psychiatry, 44: 418, 1987.

Todorova A, et al: Effects of tolterodine, trospium chloride, and oxybutynin on the central nervous system. J Clin Pharmacol, 41(6): 636, 2001.

Invasive Therapy

Kohn IJ, et al: Electrical stimulation and neuromodulation in the treatment of lower urinary tract dysfunction. AUA Update Series, Vol. 22, Lesson 9, 2003.

Latti JM, et al: Efficacy of sacral neuromodulation for symptomatic treatment of refractory urge incontinence. Urology, 67(3): 550, 2006.

Rackley RR, Vasavada SP: Botulinum toxin therapy for pelvic health conditions. AUA Update Series, Vol. 24, Lesson 39, 2005

van Balken MR, et al: Posterior tibial nerve stimulation as neuromodulative treatment of lower urinary tract dysfunction. J Urol, 166: 914, 2001.

STRESS URINARY INCONTINENCE IN THE FEMALE

General Information

1. The 1997 AUA guideline defines stress urinary incontinence (SUI) as "the involuntary loss of urine related to increases in abdominal pressure resulting from activities such as coughing, laughing, lifting, and positional changes."

2. *Stress urinary incontinence refers to the clinical symptoms; it does not imply an underlying cause of incontinence.* SUI can be caused by any of the following underlying conditions.

   a. Urinary retention—when the bladder is full, an increase in abdominal pressure may push urine out of the bladder.

   b. Detrusor overactivity—an increase in abdominal pressure may trigger an involuntary detrusor contraction that pushes urine out of the bladder.

   c. Intrinsic sphincter deficiency (ISD)—when the function of the urinary sphincter is deficient, it may not be able to hold urine in the bladder when there is an increase in abdominal pressure.

   d. Urethral hypermobility—hypermobility can impair urethral coaptation during increased abdominal pressure, which leads to SUI.

3. Urodynamic SUI (previously called genuine SUI) is defined as SUI in the absence of a detrusor contraction and is caused by either intrinsic sphincter deficiency or urethral hypermobility. This condition can only be diagnosed based on urodynamics.

4. The 1997 AUA guideline defines urethral hypermobility (UH) as "the rotational descent of the proximal urethra and bladder neck into the vagina...with increases in abdominal pressure..."

   a. UH is present in most women with SUI; however, UH can be present in absence of SUI.

   b. Hypermobility is caused by pelvic floor weakness.

5. Pelvic organ prolapse in the female pelvis is classified as follows.

   a. Anterior compartment (anterior vagina)
      i. Cystocele
      ii. Urethrocele

   b. Middle compartment (apical vagina)
      i. Enterocele
      ii. Uterine prolapse

   c. Posterior compartment (posterior vagina)
      i. Rectocele
      ii. Perineal defects

Risk Factors for SUI
1. Obesity—obesity increases the risk of SUI, mainly through an increase in intraabdominal pressure. SUI from obesity is reversible with weight loss.
2. Gender—females are more likely to have SUI than males.
3. Pregnancy—SUI is more common during pregnancy. SUI may begin within the first trimester. The chance of incontinence increases as pregnancy progresses. After delivery, SUI usually resolves. However, incontinence during pregnancy increases the risk of persistent incontinence postpartum. See Incontinence and Voiding Symptoms From Pregnancy, page 222.
4. Vaginal delivery—SUI is more likely after a vaginal delivery than after a cesarean section.
5. Hysterectomy—hysterectomy appears to increase the risk of SUI.
6. Postmenopausal status does *not* appear to increase the risk SUI.
7. Prostate surgery—prostate surgery (especially radical prostatectomy) increases the risk of SUI.
8. Medications—α-blockers and diuretics may cause SUI.
9. Family history—women with a family history of SUI are more than 3 times more likely to have SUI than the general population.
10. Race—Caucasian women are more likely to develop SUI than Hispanic and African American women.
11. Participation in strenuous physical activity—women who engage in strenuous activity are more likely to have SUI.
12. Smoking—data are conflicting, but smoking may increase the risk of SUI. However, there are no studies showing that smoking cessation improves continence.

Evaluation
1. Urodynamics does not always reveal SUI when it is present.
   a. Leakage may be intermittent and may not occur during urodynamics.
   b. Anxiety or discomfort during urodynamics may alter the normal voiding physiology and mask SUI.
   c. A cystocele can mask SUI by kinking the urethra (which increases bladder outlet resistance and causes invalid valsalva leak point pressures).
2. See Evaluation of Urinary Incontinence, page 176.

Summary of Treatment Options for Female SUI
1. Non-invasive treatment
   a. Behavioral therapy—see page 177.
   b. Medications
   c. Continence devices (catheter, pessary, stent, plug, etc.)
2. Minimally invasive treatment (no incision required)
   a. Bulking agent injections
   b. Transurethral radiofrequency collagen microremodeling (Renessa™)
3. Surgical treatment (incision required)
   a. Anterior repairs
   b. Retropubic suspensions
   c. Transvaginal suspensions
   d. Sling procedures
   e. Artificial urinary sphincter

<u>Non-invasive Treatment of ISD</u>

Behavioral Therapy - see page 177.

Medication

1. Estrogen in postmenopausal women—*topical and systemic estrogens do not objectively improve SUI*. In fact, some studies show that estrogens increase the risk of SUI. Therefore, *estrogen is not recommended for the treatment of SUI*.

2. α-agonists
   a. α-agonists increase the tone of the urethral sphincter. A Cochrane meta-analysis in 2005 concluded that there was "weak evidence" that α-agonists in women significantly improve continence compared to placebo. However, α-agonists rarely achieve complete dryness.
   b. α-agonists are often avoided because they may cause hypertension and cardiac arrhythmias. They must be used with extreme caution in patients with heart disease.
   c. α-agonists are not FDA approved for the treatment of SUI.
   d. Contraindications include
      i. Cardiac disease (coronary artery disease, angina, congestive heart failure, arrhythmia, recent myocardial infarction)
      ii. Untreated or uncontrolled hypertension
      iii. Narrow angle glaucoma
      iv. Hyperthyroidism or patient on thyroid replacement
      v. Diabetes
      vi. Patients taking a monoamine oxidase inhibitor (MAOI) or who have stopped an MAOI within the past 14 days.
      vii. At risk for seizures
   e. Doses
      i. Pseudoephedrine—60 mg po q day to QID [Tabs: 30, 60 mg]; extended release 120 mg po BID [Tabs: 120 mg]; extended release 240 mg po q day [Tabs: 240 mg].
      ii. Imipramine 25 mg po BID [Tabs: 10, 25, 50 mg]
      iii. Ephedrine sulfate 50 mg po QID [Caps: 25, 50 mg]
      iv. Phenylpropanolamine 75 mg po BID—no longer available in the United States. The FDA removed it from the market because of the risk of hemorrhagic stroke.

3. Duloxetine
   a. Duloxetine is a serotonin and norepinephrine reuptake inhibitor that increases the concentration of these neurotransmitters at the synapse.
   b. Duloxetine reduces SUI by 50% and improves quality of life.
   c. Up 17% of patients discontinue duloxetine because of adverse side effects (mainly nausea). In open-label extensions of controlled trials, there was a higher than expected rate of suicide attempts.
   d. Currently, the use if duloxetine for SUI is not recommended. It has not been approved by the FDA this indication.

Continence Devices

1. Pessary—these devices are inserted into the vagina and are primarily used to treat pelvic prolapse; however, some designs also have a nodular protrusion that can compress the urethra and reduce SUI.
2. Indwelling catheter—an indwelling catheter (urethral or suprapubic) may be a reasonable treatment for some patients with SUI.
3. Urethral occlusive devices—these stents, plugs, and caps occlude the urethra, but must be removed to void. They may cause bladder spasms, which can exacerbate incontinence.

Minimally Invasive Treatment

Bulking Agent Injection Therapy

1. During cystoscopy, a bulking agent is injected into the submucosa of the proximal urethra and/or bladder neck to coapt the urethral mucosa. This increases bladder outlet resistance and reduces the risk of SUI.
2. Routes of administration
   a. Periurethral—used in females. A needle is inserted next to the meatus and advanced parallel to the urethra to the injection site.
   b. Suprapubic—a suprapubic needle is advanced to the injection site.
   c. Transurethral—a needle is placed through the cystoscope and inserted into the injection site. Most agents are injected via this route.
3. Contraindications
   a. Genital or urinary tract infection.
   b. Inflammation of the bladder or urethra.
   c. Weak or fragile urethral tissue.
   d. Untreated urethral stricture or urethral obstruction.
   e. Pregnancy
   f. History of pelvic radiation
   g. For Contigen®, contraindications also include history of collagen allergy and hypersensitivity on the skin test. Caution is advised in patients with beef allergy or who are immunosuppressed.
4. Bulking agents that are FDA approved for the treatment of SUI
   a. Contigen® (gluteraldehyde cross-linked bovine collagen)—4% develop a hypersensitivity reaction. An intradermal skin test must be performed at least 1 month before the planned procedure. If hypersensitivity is identified on the skin test, then Contigen® should not be used.
   b. Durasphere® (carbon coated beads)—these particles are not resorbed, are visible on x-rays, and may migrate into the lymphatic system. Durasphere® seems to be as effective as Contigen®, but Durasphere® may have a higher rate of postoperative urgency and urinary retention.
   c. Tegress™ (dimethyl sulfoxide and ethylene vinyl alcohol copolymer)—Tegress™ is a liquid that changes into a spongy mass after injection.
   d. Coaptite® (calcium hydroxylapatite)—Coaptite® is visible on x-rays.
   e. Macroplastique® (silicone elastomer)—migration is unlikely, but possible (one report of a large size silicone particle migrating in dogs).
5. Bulking agents that are *not* FDA approved for treatment of SUI
   a. Teflon (polytetrafluoroethylene)—particle migration has been reported.
   b. Autologous fat—seldom used. Harvesting fat adds morbidity. Fat is difficult to inject and most of it is resorbed. Fat embolism has been reported. FDA approval is not required to use autologous fat.

Bulking Agent	FDA Approval for SUI from ISD		Migration Reported	Allergic Reactions
	Patient Group	Route†		
Contigen®	Adult Males & Females	Any	No	Yes*
Durasphere®	Adult Females	Any	Yes	No
Tegress™	Adult Females	Transurethral	No	No
Coaptite®	Adult Females	Transurethral	No	No
Macroplastique®	Adult Females	Transurethral	Yes	No
Autologous Fat	Approval not required	Any	No	No
Teflon	Not FDA Approved	Any	Yes	No

SUI = stress urinary incontinence; ISD = intrinsic sphincter deficiency
† Routes of administration include transurethral, periurethral, and suprapubic.
* Preoperative skin test must be performed and must show no hypersensitivity.

6. Complications include pain at the injection site, de novo urgency (up to 13%), urinary retention (2%-10%), worse urinary incontinence (8-10%), hematuria, infection, periurethral abscess (rare), urethral necrosis (rare), urethral erosion (rare), extrusion of bulking agent (rare), and particle migration (rare). Materials that are injected intravascularly or that migrate intravascularly have the potential to cause emboli.

7. Patients often require multiple procedures to achieve maximum continence. Periodic "maintenance" injections may be required to sustain continence.

8. Efficacy
   a. Short-term success—at 1 year of follow up, the average chance of being completely dry is approximately 30-40% and the chance of being dry or improved is approximately 50-60%.
   b. Long-term success—with long-term follow up, success rates generally decrease.
   c. The success rate is lower when bulking agents are used for severe SUI, when there is extensive periurethral scarring, or after pelvic radiation.
   d. Surgical therapies (e.g. slings) have a higher long-term success rate.

Transurethral Radiofrequency Collagen Microremodeling (Renessa™)

1. Renessa™ is FDA approved for the treatment of urodynamic SUI caused by urethral hypermobility in women who have failed conservative therapy.

2. The safety and efficacy of Renessa™ has not been evaluated in women with urge incontinence, mixed incontinence, overactive bladder, absent urethral hypermobility, valsalva leak point pressure < 60 cm water, post void residual > 50 cc, severe pelvic prolapse, or previous urinary incontinence surgery.

3. A 21 French catheter-like probe is placed though the urethra and into the bladder. The probe's balloon is inflated inside the bladder and positioned at the bladder neck. Four needles are deployed from the probe into the bladder neck and proximal urethra. Radiofrequency energy is delivered though the needles for 60 seconds, which generates low temperature heating around the needle tips. The probe is repositioned 9 times, resulting in 36 treatments sites (4 needles deployed for each balloon position).

4. The low temperature heating denatures collagen. Upon healing, the treated tissue becomes firmer, which increases urethral resistance and reduces the risk of SUI.

5. The procedure can be done in the office under local anesthetic and oral sedation. The procedure lasts approximately 20-30 minutes.

6. Contraindications—coagulopathy, pregnancy, immunosuppression, collagen vascular disease, and urinary tract infection.

7. Long-term data are lacking. However, 12 months after treatment, the following outcomes were reported.
   a. 67% of women reported improved quality of life.
   b. There was a significant improvement in valsalva leak point pressure.
   c. 76% of women experienced fewer daily incontinence episodes.
   d. 68% of women used fewer pads each day.
   e. 58% of women stopped using pads.
   f. 35% of women were completely dry.

8. It may take 60-90 days to achieve maximal improvement.

9. Complications—*the most common side effect is dysuria*, which is present in up to 60% during the first month after treatment and up to 9% at one year after therapy. Urgency, frequency, and hematuria are also common in the first month after therapy, but rarely persist. Urine retention and infection are rare.

Surgical Treatment

General Information

1. *Surgical therapy offers the highest long-term cure rates for SUI.*
2. The tendinous arch is a condensation of connective tissue that extends from the pubic bone to the ischial spine. The endopelvic fascia (urethropelvic ligament) passes anterior to the urethra. The periurethral fascia passes posterior to the urethra and extends laterally, where it fuses with the endopelvic fascia.
3. Anterior repair—the periurethral fascia is imbricated under the bladder neck and urethra.
4. Suspension—sutures are placed in the periurethral and/or perivesical tissue and then fixed to pubic or suprapubic structures. These sutures suspend the bladder and urethra from the pubic or suprapubic tissue.
5. Sling—a strip of material is placed under the urethra (like a hammock).
6. Slings and retropubic suspensions are more effective for treating SUI than transvaginal suspensions and anterior repairs. *Transvaginal suspensions and anterior repairs are mainly of historical interest and are no longer used to treat SUI.*

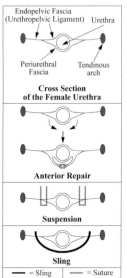

Endopelvic Fascia
(Urethropelvic Ligament)   Urethra

Periurethral Fascia   Tendinous arch

Cross Section of the Female Urethra

Anterior Repair

Suspension

Sling

— = Sling   ---- = Suture

7. Slings and retropubic suspensions have a similar success rate. Mid urethral and distal urethral slings provide the best combination of long-term efficacy and minimal invasiveness.
8. Retropubic suspensions increase the risk of pelvic organ prolapse (including rectocele, uterine prolapse, and enterocele), whereas slings do not increase the risk of pelvic organ prolapse.
9. Hysterectomy is not utilized to treat SUI.
10. Efficacy
    a. The success rate is lower when surgery is performed for failure of a previous procedure for SUI.
    b. In general, the cure rates for retropubic suspensions and slings are relatively durable, whereas the cure rates decline with time for anterior repairs, transvaginal suspensions, and bulking agent injections.

Invasive Treatment for SUI in the Female	Chance of Being Dry*
Artificial Urinary Sphincter	
Sling	80-85%
Retropubic Suspensions	
Transvaginal Suspension	67%
Anterior Repair	61%
Renessa™	35%†
Bulking Agent Injection	35%†

* At 4 years after treatment unless specified otherwise.
† At 1 year after treatment.

Artificial Urinary Sphincter (AUS)

1. AUS is seldom used for female SUI (a sling is usually preferred). However, the AUS may be better than a sling in women with an acontractile bladder because it may be less likely to cause postoperative urinary retention.
2. When an AUS is used for female SUI, the patient should have a well supported urethra and an adequate ability to operate the AUS.
3. AUS in the female can be placed through a vaginal or a retropubic incision.
4. For details, see page 203.

Anterior Repair (Anterior Colporrhaphy)

1. When applied to SUI, anterior repairs have a higher failure rate than slings and retropubic suspensions. Thus, *anterior repairs are not recommended for treatment of SUI.*
2. *Anterior repairs are primarily used to treat a midline cystocele.* They may be combined with a sling when a cystocele and SUI coexist.
3. The pubocervical fascia is imbricated under the cystocele to restore the support for the bladder. The periurethral fascia is often imbricated under the bladder neck and urethra.
4. Examples include the Kelly plication and the Kennedy procedure.

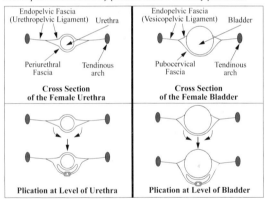

Transvaginal Suspension (Transvaginal Urethropexy, Needle Suspension)

1. Through a vaginal and an abdominal incision, the urethra and bladder neck are suspended by suturing perivesical and periurethral tissue to the rectus fascia. A needle-like instrument is used to pass sutures from the vaginal incision to the abdominal incision (thus the term needle suspension).
2. Examples include the Pereyra procedure, Stamey procedure, Raz procedure, and Gittes procedure.
3. Cochrane reviews show that transvaginal suspensions have a lower success rate and have a higher complication rate than retropubic suspensions.
4. *Transvaginal suspensions are not recommended for treatment of SUI* because they have a relatively high failure rate and complication rate.

Retropubic Suspension
1. Through a lower abdominal (retropubic) incision, the urethra and bladder neck are suspended by suturing the perivesical and/or periurethral tissue to the pubic periosteum or the pubic ligaments.
2. Marshall-Marchetti-Krantz (MMK)—periurethral tissue is sutured to the periosteum or midline cartilage of the symphysis pubis. 2.5% of patients develop osteitis pubis, a painful chronic inflammation of the pubic bone.
3. Burch—perivesical tissue is sutured to Cooper's ligament. The Burch procedure requires enough vaginal mobility to permit vaginal elevation.
4. *A Cochrane review in 2003 stated that the Burch procedure may have a higher long-term success rate that the MMK procedure.* Beyond 4-5 years, success is sustained with the Burch procedure but declines with the MMK.
5. Laparoscopic retropubic suspensions—with long-term follow up, the laparoscopic approach may have a higher failure rate than the open approach. The laparoscopic suspension was developed to make incontinence procedures less invasive; however, it is still more invasive (and may be less effective) than mid urethral and distal urethral slings.
6. Retropubic suspensions increase the risk of pelvic organ prolapse (including rectocele, uterine prolapse, and enterocele), whereas slings do not. After a retropubic suspension, prolapse develops in 12-14% of cases.
7. A retropubic suspension does not adequately repair a midline cystocele. An anterior repair is more appropriate for treating a midline cystocele.

Sling Procedure
1. These procedures place a sling under the urethra or bladder neck. The sling provides urethral support and helps reduce SUI.
2. The term "pubovaginal sling" is a non-specific term that may refer to any sling that is placed through retropubic and vaginal incisions.
3. Sling material
   a. Autologous (the patient's own tissue)—*autologous tissue appears to have the lowest erosion rate*, but harvesting the tissue adds morbidity. Examples: rectus fascia, fascia lata, dura, skeletal muscle.
   b. Allograft (cadaveric human tissue)—allograft tissue has the theoretical risk of disease transmission. Examples: fascia lata, dermis.
   c. Xenograft (non-human animal tissue)—xenograft tissue has the theoretical risk of disease transmission. Examples: porcine dermis, bovine pericardium, porcine small intestinal mucosa.
   d. Synthetic—examples: polypropylene, polyethylene.
4. Sling anchoring
   a. Anchored slings—these slings are anchored using sutures. The sutures are secured by either tying them anterior to the rectus fascia or by fixing them to the pubic bone with bone anchors.
   b. Non-anchored slings—these slings are not sutured to anything.
5. Sling position
   a. Bladder neck/proximal urethra—these slings are placed under the bladder neck or proximal urethra. They are usually anchored. Examples include autologous fascia sling and xenograft bone anchored sling.
   b. Mid urethra/distal urethra—these slings are placed loosely under the mid or distal urethra. Most of these slings are synthetic, non-anchored, and are performed by passing the sling via one of these approaches:
      i. Retropubic—tension free vaginal tape (TVT™), SPARC™, distal urethral polypropylene sling (DUPS), etc.
      ii. Transobturator—Monarc™, ObTape™, etc.
6. Slings and retropubic procedures have a similar success rate, and are the most successful surgical treatments for SUI.

7. Although data are premature for mid urethral slings, it appears that the retropubic and transobturator approaches achieve similar outcomes.
8. *When a sling is performed in women with mixed urinary incontinence, urge incontinence resolves in 50-75% of cases.*
9. Autologous fascia sling—harvesting the fascia adds morbidity; therefore, it is more invasive than slings using non-autologous materials. Autologous fascia slings and the mid urethral slings appear to have similar efficacy.

Complications of Continence Procedures for SUI

1. Bleeding—bleeding requiring transfusion is rare.
2. Pelvic or abdominal organ injury—vascular, bladder, and bowel injuries are rare, but can occur with laparoscopic retropubic suspensions or when passing trocars or needles into the retropubic space. The transobturator sling almost eliminates the risk of pelvic and abdominal organ injury.
3. Pelvic organ prolapse—retropubic suspensions increase the risk of rectocele, uterine prolapse, and enterocele. The risk of pelvic prolapse after a retropubic suspension is approximately 12-14%.
4. Pubic pain—when periosteum or bone is penetrated, there is a small risk of osteomyelitis (bacterial bone infection) and osteitis pubis (painful pubic bone inflammation). These complications are mainly reported with the MMK procedure or when using bone anchors.
5. Infection—recurrent UTI can be caused by retention, erosion, fistula, or suture/sling placement through the bladder or urethra. Sling infection may present with pain, discharge, or voiding symptoms.
6. Vaginal pain and dyspareunia—may be caused by infection or erosion.
7. Sling erosion—*erosion is rare, but is more common with synthetic slings.*
   a. Erosion into vagina—may present with dyspareunia, vaginal pain, vaginal bleeding, or vaginal discharge. Treatment usually requires sling removal, with or without a repeat sling. After TVT, success has been reported with re-closure of the vaginal mucosa over the sling.
   b. Erosion into urethra/bladder—may present with recurrent UTI, recurrent SUI, hematuria, dysuria, urgency, frequency, and vaginal pain. Treatment usually requires sling removal and urethral repair.
8. Worse voiding symptoms—reasons for persistent, recurrent, or worse voiding symptoms include infection, obstruction, and erosion.
   a. If voiding symptoms or retention persist, perform a physical exam, urine culture, post void residual, urodynamics, and cystoscopy.
   b. Urinary retention—retention is usually temporary and is managed by intermittent catheterization or an indwelling catheter. See Urethral Obstruction, page 198.
   c. De novo urgency—new onset urgency or detrusor overactivity after the procedure. De novo urgency is often refractory to anticholinergics and behavioral therapy. Irritative symptoms, such as urgency, may indicate the presence of urethral obstruction, See Urethral Obstruction, page 198.

Invasive Treatment for Female SUI	Urine Retention Longer Than 4 Weeks	De Novo Urgency†
Artificial Urinary Sphincter	Rare	at least 4%
Sling	0-11%	2-11%
Retropubic Suspensions	3-7%	1-16%
Transvaginal Suspension	4-8%	3-10%
Anterior Repair	< 5%	≤ 6%
Renessa™	0%	17%
Bulking Agent Injection	2-10%	0-13%

† For patients with no urgency and no detrusor overactivity preoperatively.

9. Urethral obstruction
   a. Urethral obstruction usually presents within several months after surgery; however, it can present at anytime, even years later.
   b. Urethral obstruction immediately postoperative is often caused by inflammation and swelling and usually resolves within 1-3 months.
   c. Persistent urethral obstruction may be caused by making the suspension or sling too tight, by placing suspension sutures too close to the urethra, or by injecting too much bulking agent.
   d. *After an incontinence procedure, urethral obstruction usually presents with irritative voiding symptoms (urgency, urge incontinence, frequency).* Elevated post void residual is present in approximately 60% of cases. Decreased force of stream is uncommon.
   e. Urodynamic testing shows increased maximum detrusor pressure and decreased flow rate (especially compared to preoperative urodynamics).
   f. When obstruction is present, it is reasonable to wait 1-3 months after surgery to see if the obstruction resolves without invasive intervention.
   g. Treatment options for persistent obstruction after a sling or suspension
      i. Clean intermittent catheterization or indwelling catheter for retention.
      ii. Sling/suspension release—for suspensions and anchored slings, the suspending sutures are cut. For non-anchored slings, the sling is cut. These maneuvers usually relieve obstruction, often without causing recurrent incontinence. This option is usually limited to the early postoperative period (before scarring causes fixation of the urethra).
      iii. Urethrolysis—performed when scaring and fixation of the urethra precludes sling/suspension release. The urethra is mobilized from the surrounding scar, usually via a transvaginal approach. Urethrolysis is often combined with a sling to avoid recurrent SUI.

REFERENCES

General

Incontinence: 3rd International Consultation on Incontinence.
   Ed. P Abrams, et al. vols. 1 & 2. Plymouth, United Kingdom: Health Publication Ltd., 2005.
Klausner AP, Steers WD: Risk factors for stress urinary incontinence in women. AUA Update Series, Vol. 22, Lesson 33, 2003.

Oral Medications for SUI

Alhasso A, et al: Adrenergic drugs for urinary incontinence in adults. Cochrane Database Syst Rev, Issue 3: CD001842, 2005.
Duloxetine—FDA website. www.fda.gov/cder/drug/infopage/duloxetine/ default.htm (accessed June 2007).
Mariappan P, et al: Duloxetine, a serotonin and noradrenaline reuptake inhibitor for the treatment of stress urinary incontinence: a systematic review. Eur Urol, 51(1): 67, 2007.
Mariappan P, et al: Serotonin and noradrenaline reuptake inhibitors (SNRI) for stress urinary incontinence in adults. Cochrane Database Syst Rev, Issue 3: CD004742, 2005.
Phenylpropanolamine—FDA website. www.fda.gov/cder/drug/infopage/ppa/ (accessed June 2007).

Estrogens for SUI

Fantl JA, et al: Estrogen therapy in the management of urinary incontinence in postmenopausal women: a meta-analysis. First report of the Hormones and Urogenital Therapy Committee. Obstet Gynecol, 83(1): 12, 1994.
Grady D, et al: Postmenopausal hormone and incontinence: the Heart and Estrogen/Progesterone Replacement Study. Obstet Gynecol, 97: 116, 2001.
Robinson D, Cardozo LD: The role of estrogens in female lower urinary tract dysfunction. Urology, 62 (Suppl 4a): 45, 2003.

Renessa™

Appell RA, et al: Transurethral radiofrequency energy collagen microremodeling for the treatment of female stress urinary incontinence. Neurourol Urodyn, 25(4): 331, 2006.

Novasys Medical® website. www.novasysmedical.com (accessed May 2007).

Sotomayor M, Bernal GF: Transurethral delivery of radiofrequency energy for tissue microremodeling in the treatment of stress urinary incontinence. Int Urogynecol J Pelvic Floor Dysfunct, 14(6): 373, 2003.

Bulking Agent Injection Therapy

Henly DR, et al: Particulate silicone for use in periurethral injections: local tissue effects and search for migration. J Urol, 153(6): 2039, 1995.

Itano NB, et al: The use of bulking agents for stress incontinence. AUA Update Series, Vol. 21, Lesson 5, 2002.

Lightner D, et al: A new injectable bulking agent for the treatment of stress urinary incontinence: results of a multicenter, randomized, controlled, double blind study of Durasphere. Urology, 58(1): 12, 2001.

Pannek J, et al: Particle migration after transurethral injection of carbon coated beads for stress urinary incontinence. J Urol, 166(4): 1350, 2001.

Picard R, et al: Periurethral injection therapy for urinary incontinence in women. Cochrane Database Syst Rev, Issue 2: CD003881, 2003.

Surgical Treatment for SUI

Amaro JL, et al: A prospective randomized trial of autologous fascial sling versus tension free vaginal tape for treatment of stress urinary incontinence. J Urol, 177(4): 482, 2007 (abstract # 1460).

Amundsen CL, et al: Urethral erosion after synthetic and nonsynthetic pubovaginal slings: differences in management and continence outcome. J Urol, 170(1): 134, 2003.

Blaivas JG, Sandhu J: Urethral reconstruction after erosion of slings in women. Curr Opin Urol, 14(6): 335, 2004.

Dean NM, et al: Laparoscopic colposuspension for urinary incontinence in women. Cochrane Database Syst Rev, Issue 3: CD002239, 2006.

Foster Jr HE, McGuire EJ: Urethrolysis. Ed. PD O'Donnell. St. Louis: Mosby Year Book Inc., 2002, pp 253-257.

Giri SK, et al: Management of vaginal extrusion after tension free vaginal tape procedure for urodynamic stress incontinence. Urology, 69: 1077, 2007.

Glazner CM, Cooper K: Anterior vaginal repair for urinary incontinence in women. Cochrane Database Syst Rev, Issue 1: CD001755, 2001.

Glazner CM, et al: Bladder neck needle suspension for urinary incontinence in women. Cochrane Database Syst Rev, Issue 2: CD003636, 2004.

Kocjancic E, et al: Tension free vaginal tape and trans-obturator suburethral tape: a prospective randomized trial. J Urol, 177(4): 483, 2007 (abstract # 1462).

Lapitan MC, et al: Open retropubic colposuspension for urinary incontinence in women. Cochrane Database Syst Rev, Issue 3: CD002912, 2005.

Leach GE, et al: Report on the surgical management of female stress urinary incontinence. AUA Education and Research, Inc., 1997. (http://www.auanet.org).

Royal College of Obstetricians and Gynecologists: Surgical treatment of urodynamic stress incontinence. Guideline 35, 2003: www.rcog.orh.uk/index.asp?pageID=538 (accessed May 2007).

Ward KL, Hilton P: A prospective randomized trial of tension free vaginal tape and colposuspension for primary urodynamic stress incontinence. Am J Obstet Gynecol, 190: 324, 2004.

STRESS URINARY INCONTINENCE
IN THE MALE

General Information
1. For the definition of SUI, see page 189.
2. Stress urinary incontinence (SUI) in the male may be caused by the following conditions.
   a. Detrusor overactivity (DO)—abdominal pressure can trigger an involuntary detrusor contraction. When DO is present before prostate surgery, it may persist for up to 1 year postoperatively.
   b. Urine retention—abdominal pressure can push urine from a full bladder.
   c. Intrinsic sphincter deficiency (ISD)—causes of ISD include radical prostatectomy, procedures for benign prostate hyperplasia, pelvic fracture with posterior urethral injury, and neurologic disorders.
3. *The most common cause of SUI in the male is ISD from radical prostatectomy (RP) or procedures for BPH (see page 117).*

Post-Prostatectomy Urinary Incontinence

General Information
1. For the purposes of this chapter, post-prostatectomy SUI refers to SUI after any invasive prostate procedure.
2. *Most cases of post-prostatectomy SUI are caused by ISD.*
3. The risk of post-prostatectomy SUI is higher in men who have had pelvic radiation.
4. After radical prostatectomy (RP), SUI often occurs, but usually improves during the year after surgery. Chronic severe SUI occurs in < 5% of men.
   a. Younger men (age < 65) recover continence more quickly and more completely than older men (age > 70).
   b. Preserving adequate urethral length during RP helps maintain urinary continence.
   c. Bladder neck preservation does not improve the final degree of urinary continence, but continence may return sooner after surgery.
   d. Pelvic floor muscle therapy does not improve the final degree of urinary continence, but continence may return sooner after surgery.
5. *Surgical therapy for post-prostatectomy SUI should be delayed until at least 6-12 months after prostatectomy.* In most cases, SUI improves during this time, which may obviate the need for invasive treatment of SUI.
6. *In general, an artificial urinary sphincter (AUS) is the preferred management of persistent problematic post-prostatectomy SUI caused by ISD.*

Evaluation and Treatment
1. The evaluation and treatment of post-prostatectomy incontinence depends on the time since surgery.
   a. Early postoperative period (less than 1 year after surgery)—SUI usually improves during this period. Thus, management consists of identifying exacerbating factors and instituting conservative therapy.
   b. Late postoperative period (more than 1 year after surgery)—SUI does not improve substantially after 1 year postoperatively. Therefore, treatment is aimed at a long-term solution.

Evaluation of Post-prostatectomy Urinary Incontinence

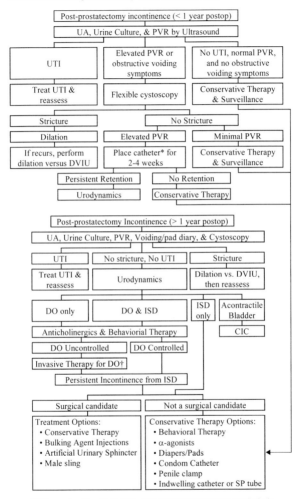

PVR = post void residual; UTI = urinary tract infection; UA = urinalysis
DO = detrusor overactivity; ISD = intrinsic sphincter dysfunction; SP = suprapubic
DVIU = direct vision internal urethrotomy; CIC = clean intermittent catheterization
* A silicone or silicone coated catheter may reduce reactive tissue response.
† Invasive options for refractory DO include tibial or sacral neuromodulation,
  botulinum, and bladder augmentation. See page 186 and page 187.
Adapted from Leach GE: J Urol, 138: 529, 1987.

Conservative Therapy
1. Management of leaking urine
    a. Diapers/pads
    b. Condom catheter
    c. Penile clamp—should not be used at night when the patient is sleeping because the bladder may become overdistended during sleep. Excessive compression can cause skin break down and tissue necrosis.
    d. Indwelling catheter (urethral or suprapubic).
2. Behavioral therapy—the efficacy of these therapies for post-prostatectomy incontinence is unclear. See also page 177.
    a. Pelvic floor muscle training (PFMT)—doing PFMT (e.g. Kegel exercises) too often can fatigue the sphincter and make incontinence worse (the patient should not over do it). PFMT does not improve the final degree of continence, but it may promote earlier return of continence after surgery.
    b. Timed (scheduled) voiding—voiding by a routine schedule (usually every 2-3 hours) and voiding before exercising. If the bladder is kept empty, incontinence may be less likely.
    c. Fluid management—avoid excessive fluid intake. Fluid restriction before bed may help reduce nocturnal incontinence.
    d. Dietary management—avoid bladder irritants (e.g. caffeine, alcohol, spicy food, acidic food).
    e. Avoid activities that exacerbate incontinence.
3. Avoid α-adrenergic blockers—some patients may be taking α-blockers for other medical problems (e.g. hypertension). When possible, change the α-blocker to a different type of medication.
4. Anticholinergic medications—when detrusor overactivity (DO) is present before prostatectomy, it may persist for up to 1 year after surgery. Occasionally, de novo DO may develop after surgery. See page 182.
5. α-agonists—for details see page 191.

Bulking Agent Injection Therapy
1. Contigen® (gluteraldehyde cross-linked bovine collagen) is the only bulking agent that is FDA approved for use in men.
2. Contigen® injections are less successful in men with severe SUI, significant urethral scarring, or previous pelvic radiation.
3. See Bulking Agent Injection Therapy, page 192.

Male Sling
1. These slings are positioned at the bulbar urethra. Sling materials are similar to those used for female slings (see Sling Materials, page 196).
2. Types of slings
    a. Anchored slings—these slings are anchored by suturing the sling to pubic or suprapubic tissue. Examples include the InVance™ system (a synthetic mesh sling anchored to the pubic bone).
    b. Non-anchored slings—these slings are placed loosely and are not sutured to anything. Examples include the AdVance™ system (a transobturator synthetic mesh sling).
3. Ideal candidates are men with mild to moderate SUI from ISD who are not a candidate for the AUS (e.g. cognitive dysfunction or impaired dexterity).
4. Men with poor detrusor function who undergo a sling may have a higher risk of urinary retention than men who undergo an AUS.
5. Approximately 55-80% are dry and up to 25% are improved (but not dry).
6. Complications include scrotal or perineal pain (16%, but often resolves within a few months postoperatively), urinary retention (3%), sling erosion (rare), infection (rare), and de novo urgency (rare).

Artificial Urinary Sphincter (AUS)

General Information

1. The currently available AUS (AMS Sphincter 800™) is made of a solid silicone elastomer and has 3 main components: an inflatable cuff, a reservoir, and a control pump.

   a. Reservoir—an elastic balloon that is manufactured in several predetermined pressure ranges (41-50, 51-60, 61-70, 81-80, and 81-90 cm water). The reservoir is implanted in the retropubic space. A lower pressure reservoir may be used in patients with a high risk of tissue ischemia (e.g. history of pelvic radiation or urethral stricture surgery).

   b. Pump—permits activation and deactivation of the AUS. The pump is placed in the scrotum for males and in the labia majora for females.

   c. Cuff—when inflated, the cuff occludes the urethra and impedes the flow of urine. *After prostatectomy, the cuff is placed around the bulbar urethra. In all other circumstances, the cuff is placed around the bladder neck.* Twelve cuff sizes are available: 4.0, 4.5, 5.0, 5.5, 6.0, 6.5, 7.0, 7.5, 8, 9, 10, and 11 cm.

2. In the default mode, the cuff is inflated with fluid. The inflated cuff compresses the urethra and prevents the flow of urine. When the pump is squeezed several times, fluid is transferred from the cuff to the reservoir and the cuff deflates. Deflating the cuff reduces urethral compression and allows urine to flow. After 3-5 minutes (long enough to void), fluid automatically flows back into the cuff and restores urethral compression.

3. Contraindications

   a. Impaired cognitive function or impaired manual dexterity—patients must be capable of operating the AUS.

   b. Unresolved urethral stricture or bladder outlet obstruction.

   c. Unresolved detrusor overactivity.

   d. Existing infection.

4. AUS placement can be performed after bulking agent injection therapy.

5. The ideal candidate for AUS has the following characteristics: ISD as the only cause of urinary incontinence, normal bladder compliance, normal detrusor function, no prior history of pelvic radiation, and enough manual dexterity and cognitive ability to operate the AUS.

6. Success rate in males—70-80% are dry, 85-95% are dry or improved.

7. AUS in the adult male

   a. Cuff size is 4.5 cm for most adult males. For post-prostatectomy SUI, the cuff is placed around the bulbar urethra (because the bladder neck is scarred). The pump is placed in the scrotum. Reservoir size is usually 61-70 cm water; however, a 51-60 cm water reservoir may be selected to minimize the risk of erosion in patients with a history of pelvic radiation or bulbar urethral stricture surgery.

   b. *AUS for post-prostatectomy SUI should be delayed until at least 6-12 months after prostatectomy.* SUI improves during this time, which may obviate the need for invasive treatment for SUI.

8. AUS in the adult female

   a. The cuff is placed at the bladder neck. The pump is placed in the labia majora.

   b. AUS placement may be accomplished by a transvaginal or transabdominal approach.

   c. For management of the AUS during pregnancy, see page 225.

9. AUS in children—the cuff is placed at the bladder neck in both male and female children.

10. When the AUS is used in patients with neurogenic bladder, they can develop decreased bladder compliance and high intravesical pressure, which may ultimately lead to hydronephrosis and renal insufficiency.

11. A penile prosthesis and AUS can be performed under the same anesthetic. The pumps are placed on opposite sides of the scrotum.

12. AUS implantation and augmentation cystoplasty can be performed under the same anesthetic.

Postoperative Management

1. Oral antibiotics are often continued for at least 1 week postoperatively.

2. When urethral injury was not encountered, the catheter may be removed on postoperative day 1.

3. The cuff is deactivated (cuff open) after AUS implantation (this allows healing occur without compression on the urethra). The patient should not operate the AUS during the postoperative period. 6 to 8 weeks postoperatively, the physician activates the AUS (initial AUS activation) and the patient is instructed on how to use the AUS. Patients should be proficient at using the AUS before leaving the office.

4. Instructions for the patient immediately postoperative
   a. An ice pack is applied to the labia or scrotum for 24-48 hours to reduce swelling.
   b. The patient should gently pull down on the pump once each day for 6-8 weeks postoperatively. This prevents cephalad migration of the pump during healing.
   c. Patients with a bulbar urethral cuff are instructed to permanently avoid activity that produces significant perineal compression (e.g. bicycle riding, motorcycle riding, horseback riding, etc.). Ideally, they should not sit on firm surfaces (a pad may be used when sitting).
   d. Patients should take prophylactic antibiotics during dental procedures or surgical procedures to prevent AUS infection.

5. Instructions for the patient during initial AUS activation
   a. When leakage is absent at night, deactivate the AUS at night to reduce the risk of cuff erosion.
   b. Patients should notify medical personal that the AUS must be deactivated before urethral instrumentation (e.g. urethral catheter placement, cystoscopy). This information may be placed on a Medic Alert bracelet so it is available when the patient is unable to communicate.

Intraoperative Complications

1. Urethral Injury
   a. Small urethral injury—a small urethral injury can be repaired with absorbable suture.
      i. Satisfactory urethral repair—continue with AUS implant and place the cuff around a different segment of urethra (i.e. do not place the cuff around the urethral repair). A urethral catheter is left in place for approximately one week.
      ii. Questionable urethral repair—AUS placement is abandoned and a urethral catheter is left in place postoperatively.
   b. Large urethral injury—AUS placement is abandoned, the urethral injury is closed with absorbable suture, and a urethral catheter is left in place postoperatively.
   c. An unrecognized intraoperative urethral injury may present as an early postoperative cuff erosion.

2. Rectal injury—AUS placement is abandoned. Close the rectal injury in 2 layers, dilate the anus, and place the patient on a low residue diet.

Postoperative Complications
1. Hematoma is the most common complication after AUS implantation.
2. Infection—AUS infection can occur at anytime; however, most infections occur within 2 months postoperatively. Infections usually present with pain, erythema, and swelling near the cuff or pump. Fever and leukocytosis may also be present. The infection rate is approximately 3-5%. Most infections are caused by E. coli or staphylococcus. Treatment requires antibiotics and AUS removal.
3. Urinary retention before initial AUS activation (early postoperative period)
   a. *Urethral edema is the most common cause of urinary retention in the immediate postoperative period.* However, it may also be caused accidently leaving the cuff inflated after surgery; therefore, check to make sure the AUS is deactivated.
   b. If the patient is unable to void after catheter removal, start clean intermittent catheterization (CIC) with a small caliber catheter. Prolonged urethral catheterization should be avoided because it may increase the risk of cuff erosion. When CIC cannot be performed and prolonged bladder drainage is required, place a suprapubic tube.
4. Urinary retention after initial AUS activation (late postoperative period)— causes include the following conditions.
   a. Urethral stricture or bladder neck contracture—*urethral stricture and bladder neck contracture are the most common causes of urinary retention after initial AUS activation.*
   b. Erosion—when a cuff erodes into the urethra, it may rarely obstruct the flow of urine and cause urinary retention.
   c. AUS malfunction—the cuff may be stuck in the inflated position.
   d. "Patient malfunction"—the patient may be operating the AUS incorrectly. This may occur in patients whose cognitive capacity or manual dexterity have deteriorated since placement of the AUS.
   e. "Bladder malfunction"—impaired detrusor contraction may cause urinary retention.
   f. Urinary tract infection
5. Recurrent urinary incontinence—may be caused by any of the following conditions.
   a. Urethral atrophy—*urethral atrophy is the most common cause of recurrent urinary incontinence after initial AUS activation.*
   b. Erosion—when a cuff erodes into the urethra.
   c. Urethral stricture
   d. AUS malfunction
   e. "Patient malfunction"—the patient may be operating the AUS incorrectly. This may occur in patients whose cognitive capacity or manual dexterity have deteriorated since placement of the AUS.
   f. "Bladder malfunction"—new onset detrusor overactivity or impaired detrusor contractility.
   g. Urinary tract infection
6. Urethral atrophy—atrophy of the tissue encircled by the cuff.
   a. Urethral atrophy occurs 10% of patients.
   b. *Urethral atrophy is the most common cause of recurrent urinary incontinence after initial AUS activation.*
   c. Methods to treat urinary incontinence caused by urethral atrophy.
      i. Increase the reservoir pressure.
      ii. Reduce the cuff size.
      iii. Reposition the cuff to a normal urethral segment.
      iv. Place a second cuff in tandem with the first cuff.

7. Erosion of the cuff into the urethra
   a. *In the early postoperative period, cuff erosion is usually related to an unrecognized intraoperative urethral injury.*
   b. Urethral erosion occurs in 5% of patients and often presents with dysuria, hematuria, or recurrent urinary incontinence. In rare cases, it may present with urinary retention.
   c. Urethral erosion can be prevented by the following maneuvers.
      i. Use a lower pressure reservoir in patients with a history of pelvic radiation or bulbar urethral stricture surgery.
      ii. Deactivate the AUS at night when asleep.
      iii. Deactivate the AUS before instrumentation of the urethra.
      iv. In patients with a bulbar urethral cuff, avoid activity that causes significant perineal compression (e.g. bicycle riding, motorcycle riding, horseback riding, etc.) and avoid sitting on firm surfaces (a pad may be used when sitting).
   d. Urethral erosion requires removal of the AUS. The urethra is repaired primarily with absorbable suture and a urethral catheter is left for 14-21 days postoperatively. At least 3 months after AUS removal, a new AUS may be implanted with the cuff positioned away from the erosion site.
8. AUS malfunction (mechanical failure)—mechanical failure usually presents with recurrent urinary incontinence. Mechanical failure occurs in up to 15% of cases at 5 years postoperatively.
9. Pain—new onset of pain may be caused by AUS infection or urethral erosion. Chronic pain after AUS placement has been reported.
10. Re-operation (AUS revision or removal)—with long-term follow up, the average reoperation rate is approximately 17%. Reasons for reoperation include AUS infection, urethral atrophy, urethral erosion, AUS malfunction, chronic pain, and urinary incontinence (recurrent or persistent).
11. Detrusor dysfunction—*in patients with neurogenic bladder, placement of an AUS increases to risk of developing detrusor overactivity and low bladder compliance*. These conditions can increase intravesical pressure when the AUS is closed, resulting in high pressure vesicoureteral reflux and renal deterioration. Patients with neurogenic bladder and an AUS should have close life-long renal and bladder surveillance.

Evaluation of Urinary Retention and Recurrent Incontinence
1. History and physical examination—determine if cognitive capacity or manual dexterity have deteriorated since placement of the AUS.
2. Determine if the patient is operating the AUS correctly.
3. Check the function of the AUS
   a. Does the pump cycle?
   b. Does the cuff inflate and deflate? In some cases, this may require radiographs during activation and deactivation (this is only helpful if contrast was used to fill the AUS). Alternatively, the AUS can be activated and deactivated during urethroscopy.
4. Urinalysis $\pm$ urine culture
5. Post void residual
6. Uroflow
7. Cystoscopy—check for urethral atrophy, urethral erosion, and urethral stricture. The AUS can be activated and deactivated during urethroscopy to determine if it functioning appropriately.
8. Urodynamics—may be necessary when bladder dysfunction is suspected.

REFERENCES

General

Hunter K, et al: Conservative management for postprostatectomy urinary incontinence. Cochrane Database Syst Rev, Issue 2: CD001843, 2007.

Incontinence: 3rd International Consultation on Incontinence. Ed. P Abrams, et al. vols. 1 & 2. Plymouth, United Kingdom: Health Publication Ltd., 2005.

Levy JB, et al: Postprostatectomy incontinence. AUA Update Series, Vol. 15, Lesson 8, 1996.

Mourtzinos A, et al: Treatments for male urinary incontinence: a review. AUA Update Series, Vol. 24, Lesson 15, 2005.

Parekh AR, et al: The role of pelvic floor exercises on post-prostatectomy incontinence. J Urol, 170(1): 130, 2003.

Artificial Urinary Sphincter

Elliott DS, et al: Does nocturnal deactivation of the artificial urinary sphincter lessen the risk of urethral atrophy? Urology, 57: 1051, 2001.

Elliott DS, Barrett DM: The artificial urinary sphincter. Digital Urology Journal, http://www.duj.com/article/elliott/elliott.html (accessed May 2007).

Hussain M, et al: The current role of the artificial urinary sphincter for the treatment of urinary incontinence. J Urol, 174: 418, 2005.

Lai HH, et al: 13 years of experience with artificial urinary sphincter implantation at Baylor College of Medicine. J Urol, 177(3): 1021, 2007.

Petrou SP, et al: Artificial urinary sphincter for incontinence. Urology, 56: 353, 2000.

Roberts SG, Barrett DM: Troubleshooting the artificial genitourinary sphincter device. AUA Update Series, Vol. 18, Lesson 7, 1999.

Stone KT, Diokno AC: Artificial urinary sphincter. Ed. PD O'Donnell. St. Louis: Mosby Year Book Inc., 2002, pp 258-264.

Male Sling

Comiter CV: The male sling for stress urinary incontinence: a prospective study. J Urol, 167(2): 597, 2002.

Fischer MC, et al: The male perineal sling: assessment and prediction of outcome. J Urol, 177(4). 1414, 2007.

Madjar S, et al: Bone anchored sling for the treatment of post-prostatectomy incontinence. J Urol, 165(1): 72, 2001.

Migliari R, et al: Male bulbourethral sling after radical prostatectomy: intermediate outcomes at 2 to 4 year follow up. J Urol, 176(5): 2114, 2006.

Rehder P, Gozzi C: Transobturator sling suspension for male urinary incontinence including post-radical prostatectomy. Eur Urol, 52(3): 860, 2007.

EMBRYOLOGY

Germ Cell Layers
1. The mesoderm gives rise to all genitourinary organs except:
   a. Urogenital sinus structures (endoderm)
   b. Genital swellings (endoderm)
   c. Adrenal medulla (ectoderm)
2. Germ cells layers and the embryological structures they give rise to
   a. Mesoderm
   - Pronephros
   - Pronephric duct
   - Mesonephros
   - Mesonephric (Wolffian) duct
   - Metanephros (metanephric blastema or metanephric cap)
   - Ureteric bud
   - Paramesonephric (Mullerian) duct
   - Genital tubercle
   - Cloacal folds (which give rise to the urethral folds and anal folds)
   - Adrenal cortex
   b. Endoderm
   - Urogenital sinus
   - Genital swellings
   c. Ectoderm
   - Adrenal medulla

Nephric System
1. Three embryological nephric systems
   a. Pronephros—principal excretory unit < 4 weeks of gestation. Degenerates after week 4.
   b. Mesonephros—principal excretory unit 4-8 weeks of gestation. Degenerates after week 8 (except for the gonadal ridge).
   c. Metanephros—principal excretory unit >8 weeks of gestation. *The metanephros eventually develops into the mature kidney.*
2. Critical steps in the metanephric development
   a. Ureteric ingrowth—differentiation of the metanephros into the mature kidney is dependent on the ingrowth of the ureteric bud into the metanephros.
   b. Ascendance—the metanephros begins at the sacral segments and migrates to the lower thoracic segments. Ascendance may be impaired if the kidney is abnormally shaped (e.g. horseshoe kidney), the renal vasculature is abnormal, or if a mass is impeding its progress. Failure of ascendance can cause a pelvic kidney.
   c. Rotation—during ascent, the kidney internally rotates approximately 90°. Initially, the renal pelvis is anterior. After rotation, the renal pelvis is medial and slightly posterior. Failure of rotation causes a malrotated kidney.
   d. Revascularization—during ascent, the kidney is supplied by successive arteries from the iliac vessels and the aorta. If the preceding arteries do not degenerate, multiple renal arteries result. Also, at each segmental level, a vascular plexus exists that degenerates and leaves only a single renal artery. If this plexus does not degenerate completely, multiple renal arteries occur. Venous anatomy develops in a similar fashion.

Collecting System

1. Ureteric bud
   a. Arises from the distal posterior medial mesonephric (Wolffian) duct.
   b. Grows into and induces differentiation of the metanephros.
   c. As the renal unit ascends, the ureteric bud bifurcates repeatedly giving rise to the renal pelvis, calyces, infundibula, and collecting ducts.
2. Anomalies
   a. If two ureteric buds arise from the Wolffian duct, an ipsilateral complete duplication occurs.
   b. If a single bud bifurcates prematurely, an ipsilateral incomplete duplication or bifid renal pelvis occurs.
   c. If the ureteric bud is absent, ipsilateral renal agenesis occurs and the ureteral orifice is absent.
   d. If ureteral atresia occurs after ureteric ingrowth into the metanephros, ipsilateral multicystic dysplastic kidney may occur (see page 27).

Adrenal Gland

1. Cortex—arises from the *mesoderm* on the root of the dorsal mesentery.
2. Medulla—arises from the *ectodermal* sympathetic ganglion cells that migrate to the root of the dorsal mesentery and become encapsulated by the adrenal cortex.
3. If the kidney is ectopic, the adrenal gland is usually orthotopic because they have a different embryological origin.

Lower Urinary Tract

1. Cloaca—a common chamber into which the urinary, genital, and gastrointestinal tracts converge. It arises from the endoderm. At the surface of the fetus, the cloaca is covered by the cloacal membrane.
2. At approximately 30 days gestation, the urorectal septum grows through the cloaca and divides it into the urogenital (UG) sinus and the anorectal canal (see figure). The fusion of the urorectal septum with the cloacal membrane forms the perineal body and divides the cloacal membrane into the urogenital membrane and the anorectal membrane.

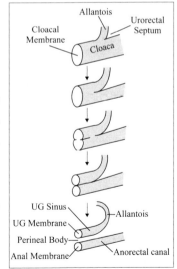

3. Bladder and trigone
   a. As the UG sinus enlarges, it absorbs the portion of the Wolffian duct that is distal to the ureteric bud. This absorbed part becomes the trigone.
   b. The ureteric bud insertion migrates cephalad and lateral and becomes the ureteral orifice.
   c. The insertion of the Wolffian duct migrates caudal and medial and becomes the ejaculatory duct.
   d. The remainder of the bladder forms from the UG sinus. The allantois also forms from the UG sinus.
4. Urachus—as the fetus grows, the bladder descends and the allantois stretches and narrows until it becomes obliterated by month 4 of gestation, forming the urachus (median umbilical ligament).
5. Prostate—the prostate develops from UG sinus near week 10 of gestation. However, the central prostate probably comes from the Wolffian duct.
6. Urethra
   a. Female—the entire urethra forms from the UG sinus.
   b. Male—the prostatic urethra forms from the UG sinus. The penile urethra forms from the urethral folds.

Important Factors For Development
1. SRY (testis determining factor)
   a. SRY is a gene that is located on the short arm of the Y chromosome.
   b. SRY induces the gonadal ridge to become a testis.
2. Mullerian inhibiting factor (MIF)
   a. MIF is produced by sertoli cells in the testis.
   b. MIF causes degeneration of the Mullerian ducts.
3. Testosterone
   a. Testosterone is produced by leydig cells in the testis.
   b. It causes male differentiation of the Wolffian duct.
4. Dihydrotestosterone (DHT)
   a. Testosterone is converted to DHT by 5α-reductase.
   b. DHT causes male differentiation of the UG sinus and external genitalia.
   c. DHT has a much higher affinity for androgen receptors than testosterone.

Summary of Male Differentiation

Weeks of gestation	Event
1-6	Bipotential gonads, Wolffian duct, Mullerian duct
7	Testis begins forming because SRY is present (*the first event is formation of sertoli cells and secretion of MIF*)
8-10	Leydig cells form and begin secreting testosterone, Wolffian ducts & genitals begin male differentiation, Mullerian duct regresses in response to MIF.

Summary of Female Differentiation

Weeks of gestation	Event
1-6	Bipotential gonads, Wolffian duct, Mullerian duct
8-10	Mullerian ducts and external genitalia begin female differentiation, Wolffian duct regresses.
11	Ovary begins developing

Embryological Structures and What They Develop Into

Embryological Structure	Differentiation Regulated By	In the Male, it Develops Into	In the Female, it Develops Into
Pronephros	—	(Degenerates)	(Degenerates)
Pronephric duct	—	(Degenerates)	(Degenerates)
Mesonephros (genital ridge)	SRY*	Testis	Ovary
Mesonephric (Wolffian) duct	Testosterone**	Bladder trigone† Epididymis, Ductus deferens, Seminal vesicles, Ejaculatory ducts	Bladder trigone† (the rest degenerates in the absence of testosterone)
Ureteric bud (arises from Wolffian duct)	—	Ureter, Renal pelvis, Calyces, Distal collecting ducts	Ureter, Renal pelvis, Calyces, Distal collecting ducts
Metanephros	Ureteric Ingrowth	Kidney (nephrons)	Kidney (nephrons)
Paramesonephric (Mullerian) duct	MIF°	(Degenerates in response to MIF)	Fallopian tubes Uterus, Cervix, Upper $1/3$ of vagina
Urogenital sinus	DHT°°	Prostatic urethra, Cowper's glands, Prostate, § Part of bladder, Urachus	Entire urethra, Bartholin's glands, Skene's glands, Part of bladder, Urachus, Hymen, Lower $2/3$ of vagina
Genital tubercle	DHT°°	Penis	Clitoris
Genital swellings	DHT°°	Scrotum	Labia majora
Urethral folds	DHT°°	Penile urethra	Labia minora
Urogenital groove	—	Lumen of penile urethra	Vestibule
Caudal genital ligament	—	Gubernaculum	Round ligament, Ovarian ligament

* SRY (testis determining factor) regulates differentiation of the gonadal ridge (bipotential gonad). When SRY is present, the genital ridge becomes a testis. If SRY is absent, the genital ridge becomes an ovary.

** When testosterone is present, the Wolffian duct differentiates into male structures. If testosterone is absent the Wolffian duct degenerates.

† The trigone of the bladder arises from the portion of the mesonephric duct that is distal to the ureteric bud.

° Mullerian inhibiting factor (MIF) regulates differentiation of the Mullerian duct. When MIF is absent, the Mullerian duct differentiates into female structures. When MIF is present, the Mullerian duct degenerates.

°° Dihydrotestosterone (DHT) mediates the male differentiation of these structures. If DHT is present, these structures differentiate into male structures. If it is absent, these structures differentiate into female structures.

§ The central zone of the prostate may actually derive from the Wolffian duct.

Vestigial Structures

1. Wolffian (mesonephric) remnants in males
   a. Appendix epididymis—persistent cranial end.
   b. Paradidymis (Organ of Giraldes)—tubules between efferent ducts and the vas deferens.
   c. vas aberrans of Haller
2. Wolffian (mesonephric) remnants in females
   a. Appendix vesiculosa—persistent cranial end.
   b. Epoophoron (parovarium, organ of Rosenmuller)—persistent tubules in broad ligament.
   c. Paroophoron of Waldeyer—persistent tubules in broad ligament near uterus.
   d. Gartner's duct—persistent duct in broad ligament, along lateral uterus, or in the vaginal wall.
3. Mullerian (paramesonephric) remnants in males
   a. Appendix testis—persistent cranial end.
   b. Prostatic utricle (utriculus prostaticus)
4. Mullerian (paramesonephric) remnants in females—Morgagni's hydatid

Summary of Homologous Structures

Male	Female
Prostate	Skene's glands
Prostatic utricle	Vagina and uterus
Prostatic urethra	Entire urethra
Vas deferens and ejaculatory duct	Gartner's duct
Scrotum	Labia majora
Penis	Clitoris
Cowper's glands	Bartholin's glands
Gubernaculum	Round ligament and ovarian ligament
Testis	Ovary

Ectopic Ureteral Orifices

1. An ectopic ureter is a ureter that does not insert into the trigone.
2. More common in girls than boys.
3. Most commonly present with UTI.
4. When boys have an ectopic ureteral orifice, they are usually *not* associated with a duplicated system. When girls have an ectopic ureteral orifice, they *are* usually associated with a duplicated system.
5. Girls frequently present with urinary incontinence because some sites of ectopic insertion are distal to the urinary sphincter. Insertion sites include bladder neck, proximal or distal urethra, vestibule, vagina, uterus, cervix, and rarely rectum.
6. Boys never present with urinary incontinence (if the urinary sphincter is functioning) because *all* the sites of ectopic ureteral insertion are proximal to the urinary sphincter. The most common ectopic sites are bladder neck and proximal urethra. Less common sites include seminal vesicle, vas deferens, and rarely rectum.

Complete Duplication of the Collecting System
1. Lateral Orifice
   a. Drains the lower pole of the kidney
   b. Has a shorter intravesical segment
   c. Can reflux
   d. More likely to have UPJ obstruction
2. Medial Orifice
   a. Drains the upper pole of the kidney
   b. Commonly associated with an ectopic ureterocele
   c. Commonly obstructed
   d. More likely to be ectopic

REFERENCES

George FW, Wilson JD: Embryology of the genital tract. Campbell's Urology. 6th Edition. Ed. PC Walsh, AB Retik, TA Stamey, et al. Philadelphia: W. B. Sanders Company, 1992, pp 1496-1508.

Hendren WH: Cloacal malformations. Campbell's Urology. 6th Edition. Ed. PC Walsh, AB Retik, TA Stamey, et al. Philadelphia: W. B. Sanders Company, 1992, pp 1822-1850.

Langman J: Medical Embryology. 4th ed. Baltimore: The Williams and Wilkins Company, 1981.

Maizels M: Normal development of the urinary tract. Campbell's Urology. 6th Edition. Ed. PC Walsh, AB Retik, TA Stamey, et al. Philadelphia: W. B. Sanders Company, 1992, pp 1301-1343.

PREGNANCY: UROLOGIC CONSIDERATIONS

Physiologic Changes During Pregnancy
1. Renal and Urinary
   a. Increased renal blood flow.
   b. Increased glomerular filtration rate (GFR) and creatinine clearance.
   c. Minor decrease in BUN and creatinine.
   d. Increased urinary calcium excretion (hypercalciuria) from increased levels of vitamin D and increased GFR.
   e. Increased urinary excretion of crystal inhibitors (e.g. magnesium and citrate).
   f. *No change in risk of urolithiasis* (the increased urinary calcium is offset by the increased inhibitors of crystallization). There is also no change in the composition of stones formed during pregnancy.
   g. Hydroureteronephrosis—*the most important cause of hydronephrosis is uterine compression of the ureter.* Since the uterus is dextrorotatory (leans to the right), compression and hydronephrosis are more common on the right. Reduced ureteral peristalsis (from hormonal influences) and increased urine production may also contribute to hydronephrosis. Hydronephrosis may begin in the first trimester and resolves postpartum.
   h. Increased risk of urinary tract infection.
2. Hematologic
   a. Increased risk of thromboembolism (especially in the 3rd trimester and postpartum) from
      i. Increased levels of serum clotting factors (hypercoagulable state).
      ii. Decreased venous flow in legs (venous stasis).
   b. Anemia—red blood cell mass increases during pregnancy, but the plasma volume expands to a greater degree; therefore, the hematocrit declines.
3. Gastrointestinal
   a. Increased incidence of gastroesophageal reflux and increased risk of aspiration during sedation/anesthesia from
      i. Decreased gastric motility.
      ii. Decreased gastroesophageal sphincter tone.
   b. Increased absorption of calcium (from increased levels of vitamin D).
   c. Decreased colonic motility—may cause constipation.
4. Cardiovascular
   a. Increased cardiac output.
   b. Vascular compression by the uterus—starting in the second trimester, the uterus can compress both the vena cava and the aorta when the mother is in the supine position. Reduced venous return (from vena cava compression) and reduced arterial blood flow (from aortic compression) may decrease uteroplacental blood flow, resulting in fetal compromise. *This can be prevented by placing the mother in the left lateral position.*
5. Pulmonary
   a. Increased risk of hypoxia during hypoventilation from
      i. Reduced functional residual capacity.
      ii. Increased oxygen consumption.

Pregnancy Induced Hydronephrosis and Obstruction

1. For the cause of gestational hydronephrosis, see Physiologic Changes During Pregnancy, page 214.
2. Hydronephrosis may begin in the first trimester and resolves postpartum.
3. Symptomatic obstruction can be relieved by positioning the patient in the *left lateral decubitus position*. On rare occasions, obstruction may require a ureteral stent or nephrostomy tube.
4. Spontaneous renal rupture (of either the collecting system or renal parenchyma) can occur in severe cases of pregnancy induced ureteral obstruction. However, this is extremely rare. It usually occurs in kidneys that have had prior disease, surgery, or trauma. Sometimes rupture may occur in kidneys with tumors; therefore, a thorough evaluation of the kidney is required. Parenchymal renal rupture has usually been treated with nephrectomy. Rupture of the collecting system has usually been treated with a ureteral stent or nephrostomy tube.

Genitourinary Infections During Pregnancy

Asymptomatic Bacteriuria During Pregnancy

1. For details, see Asymptomatic Bacteriuria in Adults, page 334.
2. *Pregnancy does not increase the risk of bacteriuria.* The incidence of bacteriuria is approximately 5% in both pregnant and nonpregnant women.
3. During pregnancy, asymptomatic bacteriuria increases the risk of developing pyelonephritis by 20-30 fold. Treatment of asymptomatic bacteriuria during pregnancy reduces risk of pyelonephritis, and may reduce the frequency of premature labor and low birth weight. Thus, *pregnant women are screened and treated for asymptomatic bacteriuria to prevent pyelonephritis and the complications associated with it.*
4. 20-40% of women with asymptomatic bacteriuria during the first trimester develop symptomatic pyelonephritis in the third trimester. Thus, *screening should begin in the first trimester.*
5. Asymptomatic bacteriuria is defined as ≥ 100,000 cfu per ml on a clean catch urine culture in a patient without fever or urinary symptoms.
6. Infectious Diseases Society of America (ISDA) recommendations
   a. *Pregnant women should be screened for asymptomatic bacteriuria by urine culture starting early in pregnancy (e.g. in the first trimester).*
   b. When the culture is positive, treat with 3-7 days of antibiotics and then repeat the urine culture. Periodic screening (e.g. monthly) for recurrent bacteriuria should be conducted after therapy.
   c. When the culture is negative, the ISDA made no recommendations regarding continued screening during the rest of pregnancy.

Acute Bacterial Cystitis

1. Symptomatic cystitis should be treated (regardless of the colony count on culture) with 3-7 days of antibiotics. Then, repeat the urine culture.
2. Pyelonephritis increases the risk a premature labor, low birth weight, and intrauterine growth retardation.
3. When infection or bacteriuria are recurrent, persistent, or severe, evaluate the patient for urinary tract obstruction and urolithiasis (see Urolithiasis During Pregnancy, page 221). If there is no obstruction or urolithiasis, the patient should have a complete urologic evaluation after delivery. Suppressive antibiotics may be needed for the duration of pregnancy.

Vaginitis—See page 353

Sexually Transmitted Diseases—See page 373

Safe Antibiotics During Pregnancy (Assuming No Allergy)
1. Penicillins
2. Cephalosporins
3. Erythromycin base and erythromycin ethylsuccinate (erythromycin estolate is contraindicated)
4. Aminoglycosides—monitor BUN, creatinine, and aminoglycoside levels.

Diagnostic Radiology During Pregnancy

Before Diagnostic Imaging of Females
1. Obtain a pregnancy test in fertile females before performing x-rays, computerized tomography (CT) scan, nuclear studies, and magnetic resonance imaging (MRI). A pregnancy test is not necessary for ultrasound and doppler imaging since they are considered safe throughout pregnancy.
2. If possible, use imaging modalities that do not emit ionizing radiation, such as ultrasound or MRI. MRI is often avoided during the first trimester.
3. Use studies that emit ionizing radiation *only* when they are absolutely necessary for the medical well being of the mother. If ionizing radiation is required, concern regarding its effect on the fetus should not delay diagnostic radiographs of the mother.
   • "Diagnostic procedures should not be performed during pregnancy unless the information to be obtained from them is necessary for the cure of the patient and cannot be obtained by other means (especially ultrasound)...There is no contraindication to a diagnostic radiologic procedure that will likely be beneficial to the patient."—American Academy of Pediatrics (AAP) and American College of Obstetricians and Gynecologists (ACOG), 1992.
   • "Concern about possible effects of high-dose ionizing radiation exposure should not prevent medically indicated diagnostic x-ray procedures from being performed on a pregnant woman. During pregnancy, other imaging procedures not associated with ionizing radiation (e.g. ultrasonography, MRI) should be considered instead of x-rays when appropriate."—ACOG, 2004.
   • "If, in the best judgement of the attending physician, a diagnostic examination or nuclear medicine procedure, at that time, is deemed advisable to the medical well-being of the patient, it should be carried out without delay..."—National Council on Radiation Protection and Measurements (NCRP), 1977.
4. The mother should be counseled regarding the risks of fetal exposure to ionizing radiation before an imaging study is performed.
   • See Effects of Ionizing Radiation on the Fetus, page 218.
   • "It is important to discuss the plans of the procedure with the patient so that she understands its necessity and to allay any concerns regarding radiation to her embryo or fetus."—AAP and ACOG, 1992.
   • "Women should be counseled that x-ray exposure from a single diagnostic procedure does not result in harmful fetal effects."—ACOG, 2004.
   • "...the exposure of the fetus to radiation arising from diagnostic procedures would very rarely be cause, by itself, for terminating pregnancy."—NCRP, 1977.
5. Minimize fetal exposure to ionizing radiation. Shield the fetus when possible. However, "Modification of an examination for dose reduction is warranted only if it reasonably can be done without significant jeopardy to the medical care of the patient and/or her unborn child."—NCRP, 1977.
6. "Consultation with an expert in dosimetry calculation maybe helpful in calculating estimated fetal dose when multiple diagnostic x-rays are performed on a pregnant patient."—ACOG, 2004.

Iodine Contrast
1. Iodine based contrast has been shown to cross the placenta.
2. "Radiopaque and paramagnetic contrast agents are unlikely to cause harm and may be of diagnostic benefit, but these agents should be used during pregnancy only if the potential benefit justifies the potential risk to the fetus."—ACOG, 2004.

Non-Ionizing Radiation
1. "Ultrasonography and MRI are not associated with known adverse fetal effects."—ACOG, 2004.
2. Ultrasound and doppler imaging is considered safe throughout pregnancy.
3. Magnetic resonance imaging is considered safe, but it is often avoided during the first trimester.

Ionizing Radiation
1. "Low risk" dose—fetal exposure to a *cumulative* dose of less than 5 rads (5000 millirads) of ionizing radiation has not been shown to increase teratogenesis, growth retardation, or spontaneous abortion. *Therefore, the fetus should not be exposed to more than a cumulative dose of 5 rads*. This recommendation is supported by several advisory boards:
   - "The risk [of fetal abnormality] is considered negligible at 5 rad or less when compared to other risks of pregnancy..."—NCRP, 1977.
   - "It is generally accepted that exposure to less than 5 rads is incapable of producing any detectable teratogenic effect in humans or animal models."—AAP and ACOG, 1992.
   - "...exposure to less than 5 rad has not been associated with an increase in fetal anomalies or pregnancy loss."—ACOG, 2004.
2. Determining Fetal Radiation Exposure
   a. The total dose delivered to the fetus depends on
      i. The amount of radiation generated by the radiographic source.
      ii. The distance of the radiation source from the mother.
      iii. The distance from the mother's skin to the fetus—usually estimated by maternal size and her position relative to the radiation source, e.g. oblique, anterior-posterior (AP), or posterior-anterior (PA).
      iv. Shielding of the fetus.
   b. A radiologist and/or radiation physicist may be helpful for calculating an accurate estimate of fetal radiation exposure at your facility.

Radiographic Study		Approximate Fetal Radiation Exposure (millirads)*
Chest X-ray (AP and lateral)		0.07
KUB (single AP projection)		80-163
Retrograde pyelogram (AP)		109-220
I V P	per AP projection	130-264
	per lateral (oblique) projection	37
	3 shot IVP (AP only)	390-792
	7 shot IVP (5 AP + 2 oblique)	724-1394
Abdominal CT (10 slices)		1700-2600
Renal Scan (DMSA, DTPA, MAG3)		< 500
Ultrasound		0
MRI		0
Exposure from background radiation during gestation		86

* Estimated exposure may be different at your radiologic facility.

Effects of Ionizing Radiation on the Fetus
1. "The risk [of fetal abnormality] is considered negligible at 5 rad or less when compared to other risks of pregnancy..."—NCRP, 1977. However, fetal risk may exist even at low radiation doses.
2. Potential effects of radiation on the fetus include
   a. Carcinogenesis (induces cancer)—the risk of carcinogenesis for the first 14 years of life is estimated to be 0.05% per rad of fetal exposure. Leukemia and solid malignancies have been reported with fetal doses of less than 1 rad. The risk of leukemia increases from 3.6 per 10,000 in the general population to approximately 5 per 10,000 in fetuses exposed to 1-2 rads. To put this into perspective, the risk of leukemia is 13.8 per 10,000 for the sibling of a child with leukemia.
   b. Mutagenesis (induces a heritable change in the chromosomes)—after acute exposure to 1 rad, the chance of a new genetic mutation is estimated to be 0.1% to 0.4%.
   c. Teratogenesis (induces an abnormality, either physical or functional, in a developing organism)—this can occur at doses as low as 10 rads, but usually occurs at doses > 100 rads. Doses 5 rads or less are generally not associated with teratogenesis. Examples of teratogenesis include malformations, growth retardation, and mental retardation.
   d. Spontaneous abortion—the greatest risk occurs with radiation exposure before embryo implantation.
3. The primary determinants of whether these adverse effects occur are
   a. Dose of radiation delivered to the fetus—the most important factor.
   b. Gestational age of the fetus—the gestational age when radiation damage is most likely to occur is $\leq$ 15 weeks gestation.
      i. The probability of inducing malformations and growth retardation is greatest during the period of organogenesis (1-10 weeks gestation).
      ii. The risk of radiation induced mental retardation and low intelligence is greatest between 8 and 15 weeks gestation. The *extrapolated* risk of severe mental retardation may be as high as 0.4% per rad of fetal exposure; however, few cases have been reported below 100 rads.

Summary of Recommendations
Any amount of fetal exposure to radiation may increase the risk of congenital abnormalities, spontaneous abortion, cancer, genetic defects, etc. The goal is to minimize these risks by minimizing fetal exposure to radiation, especially during critical periods.
1. Before performing imaging studies of the abdominal or pelvic region (except for ultrasound), obtain a pregnancy test in fertile females.
2. If possible, use imaging modalities that do not emit ionizing radiation, such as ultrasound or MRI. MRI is often avoided during the first trimester.
3. Use studies that emit ionizing radiation *only* when they are absolutely necessary for the medical well being of the mother. If ionizing radiation is required, concern regarding its effect on the fetus should not delay diagnostic radiographs of the mother.
4. The mother should be counseled regarding the risks of fetal exposure to ionizing radiation before an imaging study is performed.
5. Minimize fetal exposure to ionizing radiation. Shield the fetus if possible.
6. If possible, avoid radiation during critical periods when the fetus appears to be more vulnerable, especially $\leq$ 15 weeks gestation.
7. The fetus should not be exposed to a *cumulative* dose of more than 5 rads of ionizing radiation. When a cumulative fetal dose of more than 5 rads seems possible, consult with a radiologist and/or radiation physicist to calculate a more accurate estimate of fetal radiation exposure.

Nonobstetric Surgery During Pregnancy

General Concepts
1. During pregnancy, surgery should only be performed for emergencies or for surgical problems that pose a significant medical risk to the mother if treatment is delayed until after delivery. Concern regarding the effects of surgery on the fetus should not delay necessary procedures.
2. The most important factor in determining the surgical morbidity and mortality of both the mother and fetus is the *severity of the maternal surgical illness*. The surgery itself appears to be less important.
3. During pregnancy, physiologic changes can result in conditions that increase surgical risk (see Physiologic Changes During Pregnancy, page 214). The mother has an increased risk of
   a. Thromboembolism (especially during the 3rd trimester and postpartum)
   b. Aspiration during anesthesia and sedation
   c. Hypoxia during hypoventilation
4. Starting in the second trimester, the uterus can compress the great vessels when the mother is supine, resulting in reduced uteroplacental blood flow and fetal compromise. Therefore, *beginning in the second trimester, the mother should be placed in the left lateral decubitus position, not supine.*
5. There appears to be a higher risk with general anesthesia compared to other types of anesthesia (e.g. spinal, epidural, local).

Risks to the Fetus
1. Exposure of the human fetus to anesthetics or surgery is not associated with congenital anomalies.
2. *The most important factor in determining the outcome of the fetus, is the severity of the maternal surgical illness.*
3. The risks to the fetus include spontaneous abortion, premature labor, low birth weight, and perinatal mortality. These are all relatively rare events if the mother is not severely ill.
4. Any adverse intraoperative event affecting the mother (e.g. hypotension, hypoxia, etc.) can also effect the fetus.

Optimal Timing of Non-emergent Surgery
1. Based on limited information, *the second trimester appears to be the safest time to perform surgery.*
   a. Studies of surgery during pregnancy, especially appendectomy and cholecystectomy, suggest that there is an increased risk of spontaneous abortion during the first trimester and an increased risk of premature labor during third trimester.
   b. Animal studies have demonstrated that the teratogenic effects of anesthesia may be more profound during certain critical developmental periods, especially during organogenesis (first trimester in humans) and during central nervous system myelination (third trimester in humans). However, there is no evidence that exposing the human fetus to anesthetics causes deleterious long-term effects.
   c. Hypercoagulability and the risk of thromboembolism are greatest during the third trimester.
2. If it does not pose significant risk to the mother, non-emergent surgery can be delayed until after delivery. During the third trimester, if surgery is required and if the fetus is mature enough, labor can be induced and the surgery performed after delivery.

Recommendations for Surgery During Pregnancy
1. During pregnancy, surgery should only be performed for emergencies or for a surgical problem that poses significant medical risk to the mother if treatment is delayed until after delivery. Concern regarding the effects of surgery on the fetus should not delay a necessary procedure.
2. The safest time to operate appears to be during the second trimester.
3. Beginning in the second trimester, position the mother in left lateral decubitus position, not supine, to minimize compression of the great vessels.
4. Consider consulting the following specialists prior to surgery: an obstetrician, a neonatologist, and an anesthesiologist with expertise in pregnancy. It may be helpful to have them available for the procedure.
5. If it does not compromise the sterile surgical field, intraoperative and postoperative fetal monitoring may help detect fetal compromise.

Hematuria During Pregnancy

General Information
1. There is minimal information in the literature regarding the work up of hematuria in pregnant patients.
2. In addition to the hematuria work up, it is prudent to have an obstetrician evaluate the patient.
3. For patients suspected of having hematuria caused by urolithiasis, see Urolithiasis During Pregnancy, page 221.
4. Life-threatening causes of hematuria during pregnancy
   a. Spontaneous renal rupture—see Pregnancy Induced Hydronephrosis and Obstruction, page 215.
   b. Placenta percreta—a potentially life-threatening cause of hemorrhagic hematuria during pregnancy. In this condition, the trophoblastic tissue of the placenta penetrates through the uterus and into surrounding structures, occasionally into the bladder. Most patients with placenta percreta present with hematuria and have had a prior cesarean section. Severe bleeding may occur if this lesion is biopsied; therefore, if a cystoscopy is performed, avoid biopsy. Pelvic ultrasound may help diagnose this condition.

Work Up
1. History and physical
2. Blood pressure measurement
3. Urinalysis and microscopic examination—confirm a positive dipstick with a microscopic examination. If protein is out of proportion to hematuria (i.e. more than 1+ proteinuria with microhematuria), obtain a 24 hour urine for protein and creatinine clearance.
4. Urine culture—if a urine infection exists, treat accordingly and repeat urinalysis and urine culture. If hematuria persists after the infection is eradicated, proceed with further work up.
5. BUN and creatinine
6. Urine cytology or other urothelial tumor markers
7. Renal and bladder ultrasound—if the patient had a prior cesarean section, obtain a transvaginal pelvic ultrasound to check for placenta percreta.
8. Cystoscopy and IVP (or retrograde pyelograms) may be necessary. However, these tests should be delayed until after delivery if possible.
9. Consider CBC with differential, platelet count, PT, PTT, bleeding time.
10. When possible, the hematuria evaluation can be completed after delivery to reduce the risk to the fetus.

Urolithiasis During Pregnancy

General Information

1. *The risk of urolithiasis is not changed by pregnancy.* An elevated level of vitamin D increases urinary calcium excretion (hypercalciuria); however, this is offset by an increase in urinary inhibitors of crystallization (including magnesium and citrate).
2. Most kidney stones occur in the 2nd and 3rd trimesters. 66%-85% of stones diagnosed during pregnancy will pass spontaneously.

Work Up

1. The initial work up in a pregnant patient includes
   a. History and physical examination
   b. Urinalysis and urine culture
   c. BUN, creatinine, and CBC with differential
   d. Renal ultrasound—this is often the initial imaging study, but it usually fails to diagnose the stone. Furthermore, a dilated collecting system may be physiologic hydronephrosis of pregnancy and not from urolithiasis. Ultrasound may detect other causes abdominal and flank pain.
   e. Pelvic ultrasound (trans-abdominal ± trans-vaginal)—this may help identify stones near the ureterovesical junction. Doppler may be used to determine if ureteral jets are present. The absence of a ureteral jet suggests an ipsilateral ureteral obstruction.
2. If ultrasound does not diagnose a suspected kidney stone, a single KUB may be performed to determine the size and location of the stone. Approximately 90% of kidney stones are radio-opaque. The overlapping fetal skeleton can make it difficult to identify kidney stones on KUB.
3. 2 or 3 shot intravenous pyelogram (IVP)
   a. May be indicated when a kidney stone is suspected and any of the following are present:
      i.   Fever
      ii. Massive or worsening hydronephrosis.
      iii. Pain unresponsive to analgesics.
      iv. Impaired oral intake because of persistent nausea or vomiting.
      v.   KUB and ultrasound are not diagnostic.
   b. A 2 or 3 shot IVP includes the following films:
      i.   Scout KUB
      ii. KUB 30-60 minutes after contrast injection
      iii. To help identify the point of obstruction, a third KUB may be taken 1-3 hours post-injection depending on the results of the second KUB.
   c. A 2 or 3 shot IVP is considered very low risk to the fetus.
4. The role of MRI and renal scan are not well-defined.
5. See Diagnostic Radiology During Pregnancy, page 216.

Treatment

1. Some urologists recommend aggressive treatment of fertile non-pregnant females with asymptomatic stones to prevent the stones from becoming symptomatic during pregnancy.
2. ESWL is contraindicated during pregnancy.
3. The criteria for admission/surgical intervention are outlined in Indications for Admission/Surgical Intervention, page 142.
   a. In a patient that is septic or toxic, the initial therapy is broad spectrum antibiotics and ultrasound guided percutaneous nephrostomy of the obstructed side under local anesthesia. The stone can be treated definitively after delivery.

b. In nontoxic patients with any of the criteria below, consider antibiotics and cystoscopic placement of a ureteral stent. If a stent cannot be placed using a cystoscope, perform ultrasound guided percutaneous nephrostomy under local anesthesia. A nephrostomy tube may be preferable in patients presenting early in pregnancy because it avoids the anesthetic required for cystoscopic stent exchanges. The stone can be treated definitively after delivery.
  i.   High grade or complete obstruction.
  ii. Any degree of obstruction in a functionally solitary kidney.
  iii. Renal insufficiency
  iv. Bilateral obstruction
  v.   A stone that is not likely to pass spontaneously (size > 5 mm)
  vi. Inability to tolerate food because of persistent nausea or vomiting.
  vii. Pain unresponsive to analgesics.
c. In patients with a ureteral stent or nephrostomy tube, stent/tube exchange is recommended at least every 6 weeks. Women with persistent urinary infections or a history of frequent stone formation may require a stent/tube change every 3-4 weeks.
d. Consider prophylactic antibiotics in patients with a stent or nephrostomy tube.

4. In patients that do not meet the criteria in # 3 above, expectant management is recommended.
  a. Prophylactic antibiotics may be considered.
  b. Adequate hydration
  c. Ultrasound, BUN, creatinine, and urine culture at least once a month.
  d. Analgesics that should be *avoided* during pregnancy include NSAIDS (can prolong labor and cause constriction of the fetal ductus arteriosus) and codeine (teratogenic).

5. Endoscopic and open surgical stone removal have been performed during pregnancy and are usually reserved for patients that cannot tolerate a stent or nephrostomy tube. Ureteroscopy and stone extraction (with or without holmium laser lithotripsy) is usually the preferred method of treating stones during pregnancy. Ultrasonic lithotripsy and electrohydrolic lithotripsy should probably be avoided because shock waves may damage the fetal inner ear and may induce premature labor.

6. In the third trimester, labor can be induced and stone surgery performed after delivery.

Incontinence and Voiding Symptoms From Pregnancy

Voiding Symptoms During Pregnancy
1. Frequency, urgency, nocturia, and urinary incontinence are more likely during pregnancy. After delivery, these symptoms usually resolve.
2. The chance of having voiding symptoms increases as pregnancy progresses. Most women have urgency, frequency, or nocturia by the third trimester.
3. The cause of urinary symptoms during pregnancy probably arises from increased urine production and compression of the bladder by the enlarging uterus.
4. Temporary urinary retention may occur when an epidural is utilized for pain during delivery.
5. Management usually consists of reassurance (the symptoms usually resolve after delivery), behavioral modification (see page 177), and pelvic floor muscle training (e.g. Kegel exercises).

Urinary Incontinence During Pregnancy

1. Stress urinary incontinence (SUI), urge urinary incontinence (UUI), and mixed incontinence are all more likely during pregnancy.

2. The chance of incontinence increases as pregnancy progresses. Incontinence may begin as early as the first trimester and usually resolves after delivery.

Chance of Urinary Incontinence at 32 Weeks Gestation	
SUI	35%
UUI	15%

3. Management consists of reassurance (symptoms usually resolve after delivery), behavioral modification (see page 177), and pelvic floor muscle training (e.g. Kegel exercises). Pelvic floor muscle training during pregnancy may prevent urinary incontinence in the postpartum period.

4. Incontinence during pregnancy increases the risk of persistent incontinence after delivery.

Persistent Urinary Incontinence After Delivery (Postpartum Incontinence)

1. Etiology of persistent urinary incontinence after delivery.
   a. Pudendal nerve injury—stretching or compression of the pudendal nerve during vaginal delivery can impair innervation of the pelvic sphincters. Pudendal nerve damage may cause urinary and fecal incontinence.
   b. Pelvic floor muscle injury—damage to the pelvic floor muscles (levator ani) during vaginal delivery is associated with SUI.

2. Risk factors for postpartum urinary incontinence
   a. Incontinence during pregnancy—incontinence during pregnancy increases the risk of persistent incontinence after delivery.
   b. Primagravid—postpartum incontinence is more likely in primagravid (first pregnancy) than in multigravid women (more than one pregnancy).
   c. Vaginal delivery—SUI is more likely after a vaginal delivery than after a cesarean section. Vaginal delivery also increases the risk of pelvic organ prolapse.

3. *Urinary incontinence usually resolves within 3 months after delivery.* Persistent incontinence longer than 3 months after delivery is associated with a higher risk of long-term urinary incontinence.

4. Treatment
   a. Pelvic floor muscle training during pregnancy may prevent urinary incontinence after delivery.
   b. Management usually consists of reassurance (the symptoms usually improve with time), behavioral modification (see page 177), and pelvic floor muscle training (see page 178).

Pregnancy After Urologic Surgery

Pregnancies after urologic surgery should be considered *high risk* pregnancies.

Pregnancy After Unilateral Nephrectomy

Women with a single functioning kidney probably have similar outcomes as women with two kidneys. Consider a functional evaluation of the solitary kidney before pregnancy.

Pregnancy After Ureteral Reimplant

1. Pregnancies after ureteral reimplant are usually successful.

2. Women who underwent ureteral reimplantation appear to be at higher risk for pyelonephritis during pregnancy; therefore, the risk of spontaneous abortion may be higher as well.

3. Although uncommon, ureteral obstruction at the ureterovesical junction has been reported.

4. During pregnancy, aggressive screening in these patients is recommended and should include renal ultrasound and urine cultures.

Pregnancy After Renal Transplant

1. Since pregnancy is an immunologically privileged state, rejection in pregnant patients may be less likely.
2. Pregnant patients with a renal transplant have an increased risk of
   a. Low birth weight babies (intrauterine growth retardation)
   b. Premature labor
   c. Infections (because of immunosuppression)
3. *Pregnancy does not substantially alter long-term renal transplant function.*
4. Pregnancy with renal transplant does not appear to increase fetal malformations.
5. Immunosuppressive medications
   a. *Immunosuppressive drugs should be continued during pregnancy to maintain the transplanted kidney.*
   b. Although immunosuppressive agents may be teratogenic, the children of transplant patients do not appear to have more congenital defects. This statement is based on studies of azathioprine, cyclosporine, steroids, and tacrolimus. Minimal information exists on the fetal effects mycophenolate mofetil, OKT3, and antithymocyte globulin.
   c. Steroids, cyclosporine, and tacrolimus may increase the risk of
      i. Gestational diabetes
      ii. Gestational hypertension
      iii. Infection (from immunosuppression)
6. Optimal conditions for pregnancy after renal transplant—adverse pregnancy outcome is less likely if pregnancy occurs with
   a. Creatinine < 2 mg/dl*
   b. Proteinuria < 1 g/day
   c. Absence of rejection*
   d. Well controlled hypertension

   > * These are also associated with a lower risk of transplant loss.

7. Optimal timing for pregnancy after renal transplant
   a. Abortion, premature labor, and low birth weight occurs more often within 2 years of transplant. Therefore, for the best pregnancy outcome, the safest time for pregnancy is > 2 year after transplantation.
   b. The risk of acute rejection is highest within the first year after transplant. Five years or more after transplantation, pregnancy can lead to a permanent reduction in renal function.
   c. Thus, it appears that *the optimal time for pregnancy is 2-5 years after renal transplant.*
8. Normal changes in transplant function during pregnancy
   a. Up to 40% of patients develop proteinuria near term; however, this resolves postpartum. If proteinuria occurs with hypertension, pre-eclampsia must be considered.
   b. GFR may decline in the third trimester; however, a similar decline is seen in non-transplanted women. Although this decline in GFR usually does not indicate a failing transplant, close monitoring is warranted.
   c. Ultrasound of the transplant kidney may reveal mild to moderate hydronephrosis, which tends to become more pronounced as pregnancy progresses. However, when the serum creatinine is > 2 mg/dl, hydronephrosis is usually absent.
9. Delivery
   a. Cesarean section should be performed mainly for obstetric indications. Occasionally the renal transplant can obstruct labor, making cesarean section necessary.
   b. *Vaginal delivery does not appear to harm the transplant kidney.* In fact, normal renal transplant function has been reported after the seven consecutive vaginal deliveries.

10. Recommendations for pregnancy with a renal transplant
    a. For the best pregnancy outcome, the safest time for pregnancy is > 2 years after transplant. Five years or more after transplant, pregnancy can lead to a permanent reduction in renal function. Thus, it appears that *the optimal time for pregnancy is 2-5 years after renal transplant.*
    b. Pregnancy outcome is best when hypertension is controlled, creatinine is normal, rejection is absent, and proteinuria is minimal.
    c. Continue immunosuppressive medications.
    d. Closely monitor for gestational diabetes.
    e. Closely monitor blood pressure—hypertension may be caused by pre-eclampsia, decline in renal function, and transplant medications.
    f. Closely monitor renal function with serial creatinine—if the creatinine increases, check blood pressure, serum levels of immunosuppressants (e.g. cyclosporine level), transplant ultrasound, and glomerular filtration rate. Reasons for creatinine elevation include rejection, dehydration, urinary obstruction, pre-eclampsia, and cyclosporine toxicity. Transplant biopsy may be needed to determine the cause of the elevated creatinine.
    g. Closely monitor the patient for asymptomatic bacteriuria and urinary tract infection with urine cultures.
    h. Closely monitor fetal growth by ultrasound (because of the risk of intrauterine growth retardation).
    i. Consider checking periodically for cytomegalovirus and herpes virus.
    j. Mode of delivery should be based primarily on obstetric factors. Labor obstruction from the renal transplant is uncommon. Vaginal delivery does not appear to harm the transplanted kidney.
    k. If the patient had been taking steroids, consider administering "stress doses" of steroids (regardless of the mode of delivery) starting when labor begins and tapering the dose after delivery.

Pregnancy After Kidney-Pancreas Transplant

Reports indicate that pregnancy is possible after kidney pancreas transplant. Many result in premature labor and low birth weight babies. However, transplant graft losses are uncommon. The information on renal transplant listed above may be helpful in managing these patients.

Pregnancy After Artificial Urinary Sphincter

1. The presence of an artificial urinary sphincter is generally not considered to be an indication for cesarean section. Cesarean section should be performed mainly for obstetric indications.
2. Pregnancy, vaginal delivery, and cesarean section do not appear to influence urinary continence or the function of the artificial sphincter.
3. If cesarean section is required, division of deep tissues (except the uterus) with electrocautery rather than sharp dissection will prevent inadvertent damage to the sphincter tubing. Preoperative abdominal ultrasound may help localize the reservoir and tubing.
4. During labor and delivery
   a. Consider administering broad spectrum antibiotics
   b. Deactivate the sphincter. This keeps the bladder empty and prevents excessive intravesical pressure from being transmitted to the bladder neck and the cuff.
5. Other recommendations that have been suggested
   a. Deactivate the sphincter during the third trimester.
   b. Antibiotic prophylaxis during pregnancy.

Pregnancy After Urinary Diversion/Augmentation

1. Successful pregnancy has been reported in virtually all types of urologic reconstruction including augmentation cystoplasty, conduits, ureterosigmoidostomy, and continent catheterizable diversions.

2. With continent diversions, catheterizing may become difficult because uterine enlargement may compress or alter the course of the catheterizable limb. An indwelling catheter may be needed if catheterizing is difficult.

3. In patients with conduits, the uterus may compress the conduit and obstruct the outflow of urine. Placing a catheter in the conduit may help drain the urine until delivery.

4. Pregnant women with a urinary diversion have a higher risk of

   a. Gestational hydronephrosis—ureteral obstruction has been reported during pregnancy in patients with urinary diversions.

   b. Pyelonephritis—may be related to bacterial colonization of the diversion and outflow obstruction from uterine compression. Some physicians recommend antibiotic prophylaxis during pregnancy.

   c. Metabolic complications—which can occur because of outflow obstruction and increased demands on the kidney. See Use of Intestine in the Urinary Tract, page 414.

5. Mode of delivery should be based primarily on obstetric factors. Most reported deliveries were vaginal. If a cesarean section is required, a urologist should be available for consultation. The vascular pedicle to the diversion must not be injured.

6. It is unclear if amniocentesis is associated with increased risk to the diversion or its vascular pedicle.

7. These patients should be followed closely with renal ultrasound, creatinine, electrolytes, and urine cultures.

REFERENCES

General

Loughlin KR: Management of urologic problems in the pregnant patient. AUA Update Series, Vol. 26, Lesson 2, 1997.

Weiss LP, Hanno PM: Pregnancy and the urologist. AUA Update Series, Vol. 9, Lesson 34, 1990.

Loughlin K, McAleer S: Management of urological problem during pregnancy: a rational strategy. AUA Update Series, Vol. 24, Lesson 5, 2005.

Nicolle LE, et al: Infectious Diseases Society of America guidelines for the diagnosis and treatment of asymptomatic bacteriuria in adults. Clin Infect Dis, 40: 643, 2005.

Urolithiasis During Pregnancy

Medical and surgical complications in pregnancy. Williams Obstetrics, 20th edition. Ed. FG Cunningham, PC MacDonald, NF Gant, et al. Stamford: Appleton and Lange, 1997, pp 1131-3.

Menon M, Parulkar BG, Drach GW: Urinary lithiasis: etiology diagnosis, and medical management. Campbell's Urology. 7th Edition. Ed. PC Walsh, AB Retik, et al. Philadelphia: W. B. Sanders Company, 1998, pp 2661-2733.

Riddell JVB, Denstedt JD: Management of urolithiasis during pregnancy. Contemporary Urology, 12(3): 12, 2000.

Stothers L, Lee LM: Renal colic in pregnancy. J Urol, 148: 1383, 1992.

Incontinence and Voiding Symptoms From Pregnancy

Fitzgerald MP, Graziano S: Anatomic and functional changes of the lower urinary tract during pregnancy. Urol Clin N Am, 34: 7, 2007.

Rogers RG, Leeman LL: Postpartum genitourinary changes. Urol Clin N Am, 34: 13, 2007.

Radiology During Pregnancy

American College of Obstetricians and Gynecologists (ACOG): Guidelines for diagnostic imaging during pregnancy. Committee opinion No. 299. Obstet Gynecol, 104: 647, 2004.

Brent RL, Gorson RO: Radiation exposure in pregnancy. Curr Probl Radiol, 2: 1, 1972.

Guidelines for Prenatal Care. 3rd edition. Elk Grove Village, IL: American Academy of Pediatrics and American College of Obstetricians and Gynecologists, 1992, pp 210-212.

Medical and Surgical Complications in Pregnancy. Williams Obstetrics, 20th edition. Ed. F.G. Cunningham, P.C. MacDonald, N.F. Gant, K.J. Leveno, and L.C. Gilstrap. Stamford: Appleton and Lange, 1997, pp 1045-1057.

National Council on Radiation Protection and Measurements: Considerations regarding the unintended radiation exposure to the embryo, fetus, or nursing child. NCRP commentary No. 9. Bethesda, MD: NCRP, 1994.

National Council on Radiation Protection and Measurements: Medical radiation exposure of pregnant and potentially pregnant women. NCRP report No. 54. Bethesda, MD: NCRP, 1977.

National Council on Radiation Protection and Measurements: Radionuclide exposure of the embryo/fetus. NCRP report No. 128. Bethesda, MD: NCRP, 1998.

National Council on Radiation Protection and Measurements: Recommendations on limits for exposure to ionizing radiation. NCRP report No. 91. Bethesda, MD: NCRP, 1977, pp 29-31.

Toppenberg KS, Hill DA, Miller DP: Safety of radiographic imaging during pregnancy. Am Fam Physician, 59: 1813, 1999.

Surgery During Pregnancy

Barron WM: The pregnant surgical patient: medical evaluation and management. Ann Intern Med, 101: 683, 1984.

Duncan PG, Pope WDB, Cohen MM, et al: Fetal risk of anesthesia and surgery during pregnancy. Anesthesiology, 64: 790, 1986.

Hunt MG, Martin JN Jr, Martin RW, et al: Perinatal aspects of abdominal surgery for nonobstetric disease. Am J Perinatol, 6: 412, 1989

Landers D, Carmona R, Crombeholme W, et al: Acute cholecystitis in pregnancy. Obstet Gynecol, 69: 131, 1987.

Kammerer WS: Nonobstetric surgery in pregnancy. Med Clin North Am, 71(3): 551, 1987.

Mazze RI, Kallen B: Appendectomy during pregnancy: a Swedish registry study of 778 cases. Obstet Gynecol, 77: 835, 1991.

Pedersen H, Mieczyslaw F: Anesthetic risk in the pregnant surgical patient. Anesthesiology, 51: 439, 1979.

Pregnancy After Urologic Surgery: Artificial Urinary Sphincter

Creagh TA, McInerney PD, Thomas PJ, et al: Pregnancy after lower urinary tract reconstruction in women. J Urol, 154: 1323, 1995.

Fishman IJ, Scott FB: Pregnancy in patients with the artificial urinary sphincter. J Urol, 150: 340, 1993.

Pregnancy After Urologic Surgery: Urinary Diversion

Barrett RJ II, Peters WA III: Pregnancy following urinary diversion. Obstet Gynecol, 62: 582, 1983.

Greenberg RE, Vaughan ED Jr., Pitts WR Jr.: Normal pregnancy and delivery after ileal conduit urinary diversion. J Urol, 125: 172, 1981.

Hatch TR, Steinberg RW, Davis LE: Successful term delivery by cesarean section in a patient with a continent ileocecal urinary diversion. J Urol, 146: 1111, 1991.

Kennedy WA II, Hensle TW, Reiley EA, et al: Pregnancy after orthotopic continent urinary diversion. Surg Gynecol Obstet, 177: 405, 1993.

Vordermark JS, Deshon GE, Agee RE: Management of pregnancy after major urinary reconstruction. Obstet Gynecol, 75: 564, 1990.

Pregnancy After Urologic Surgery: Transplant

Armenti VT, McGrory CH, Cater JR, et al: Pregnancy outcomes in female renal transplant recipients. Transplant Proc, 30: 1732, 1998.

Armenti VT, Moritz MJ, Davison JM: Drug safety issues in pregnancy following transplantation and immunosuppression: effects and outcomes. Drug Saf, 19: 219, 1998.

Bar J, Ben-Rafael Z, Padoa A, et al: Prediction of pregnancy outcome in subgroups of women with renal disease. Clin Nephrol, 53: 437, 2000.

Barrou BM, Gruessner AC, Sutherland DE, et al: Pregnancy after pancreas transplantation in the cyclosporine era: report from the International Pancreas Transplant Registry. Transplantation, 65: 524, 1998.

Casciani CU, Pasetto N, Piccione E, et al: Pregnancy in renal transplantation: clinical aspects. Clin Exp Obst Gyn, 11: 136, 1984.

Crowe AV, Rustom R, Gradden C, et al: Pregnancy does not adversely affect renal transplant function. QJM, 92: 631, 1999.

Davison JM, Lindheimer MD: Pregnancy in renal transplant recipients. J Repr Med, 27: 613, 1982.

First MR, Combs CA, Weiskittel P, et al: Lack of effect of pregnancy on renal allograft survival or function. Transplantation, 59: 472, 1995.

Haugen G, et al: Pregnancy outcome in renal allograft recipients in Norway. The importance of immunosuppressive drug regimen and health status before pregnancy. Acta Obstet Gynecol Scand, 73: 541, 1994.

Kuvacic I, Sprem M, Skrablin S, et al: Pregnancy outcome in renal transplant recipients. Int J Gynecol Obstet, 70: 313, 2000.

Levine D, Filly RA, Graber M: The sonographic appearance of renal transplants during pregnancy. J Ultrasound Med, 14:291, 1995.

Little MA, Abraham KA, Kavanagh J, et al: Pregnancy in Irish renal transplant recipients in the cyclosporine era. Ir J Med Sci, 169: 19, 2000.

McGrory CH, Radomski JS, Moritz MJ, et al: Pregnancy outcomes in 10 female pancreas-kidney recipients. J Transpl Coord, 8: 55, 1998.

Owda AK, Abdalla AH, Al-Sulaiman MH, et al: No evidence of functional deterioration of renal graft after repeated pregnancies-a report on three women with 17 pregnancies. Nephrol Dial Transplant, 13: 1281, 1998.

Sturgiss SN, Davison JM: Effect of pregnancy on the long-term function of renal allografts: an update. Am J Kidney Dis, 26: 54, 1995.

Willis FR, Findlay CA, Gorrie MJ, et al: Children of renal transplant recipient mothers. J Paediatr Health, 36: 230, 2000.

Pregnancy After Urologic Surgery: Other

Mansfield JT, Snow BW, Cartwright PC, et al: Complications of pregnancy in women after childhood reimplantation for vesicoureteral reflux: an update with 25 years of follow up. J Urol, 154:787, 1995.

Medical and Surgical Complications in Pregnancy. Williams Obstetrics, 20th edition. Ed. FG Cunningham, PC MacDonald, NF Gant, et al. Stamford: Appleton and Lange, 1997, pp 1126, 1138-9.

VESICOURETERAL REFLUX (VUR)

General

1. Ureterovesical junction competence depends on trigone tone and is independent of detrusor action. If the trigone is weak, the ureteral orifice migrates towards the ureteral hiatus (i.e. where the ureter penetrates the outer surface of the bladder) which decreases the length of the submucosal tunnel. A congenital 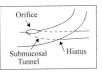 defect can also cause a short submucosal tunnel. *A shorter submucosal tunnel is more likely to result in VUR.*

2. Characteristics of ureters with congenital primary reflux
   a. Distal ureteral muscle weakness
   b. Ureteral orifice located more lateral than normal
   c. A short intravesical segment (i.e. a short submucosal tunnel)

3. Reflux is prevented by
   a. Trigone contraction—moves the ureteral orifice away from the ureteral hiatus and lengthens the submucosal tunnel.
   b. Filling of bladder—stretches the trigone and increases the length of the submucosal tunnel.
   c. A submucosal ureteral tunnel of adequate length.

4. Ureteral orifice appearance during cystoscopy often correlates with the degree of ureteral orifice incompetence. From most to least competent:
   a. Cone (normal appearance)
   b. Stadium
   c. Horseshoe
   d. Golf hole

Etiology

1. Congenital
   a. Primary reflux (trigonal weakness)—*most common cause of VUR.* It occurs because of improper development of the ureteral bud on the mesonephric duct. Most kids "outgrow" it.
      i. The ureter acquires its musculature from the cephalad to caudad; therefore, if a segment is deficient in musculature, it will be the most caudal part, i.e. the ureterovesical junction (UVJ).
      ii. If the ureteric bud is close to the urogenital sinus, it will join the urogenital sinus too early; therefore, it will not acquire adequate mesenchymal tissue and the trigone musculature will fail to develop.
      iii. Siblings of children with congenital VUR are at higher risk for VUR.
   b. Complete ureteral duplication—the majority of these do not reflux; however, in those that do reflux, it generally occurs in the ureter that drains the lower pole (Weigert-Meyer law).
   c. Ectopic ureteral orifice
   d. Multicystic dysplastic kidney—contralateral VUR is present in 20-40%.

2. Contracted or poorly compliant bladder—a contracted bladder causes high pressure reflux that may damage the kidney even if the urine is sterile.

3. Bladder wall edema from cystitis

4. Prune belly syndrome (Eagle-Barrett)

5. Iatrogenic

6. Posterior urethral valves—50% with posterior urethral valves have VUR.

Presentation
1. Most cases of VUR present with urinary tract infection (UTI).
2. The peak age of diagnosis is 3-6 years.
3. 85% of cases of VUR occur in females.
4. Compared with girls, VUR in boys typically presents
   a. Earlier in life.
   b. With higher grade VUR.
   c. Less commonly associated with voiding dysfunction.
5. VUR is more common in whites than in blacks.
6. The siblings of children with VUR will also have VUR in 30% of cases; therefore, siblings should be screened for VUR with a VCUG or nuclear cystogram.
7. VUR is graded using the classification by the International Reflux Study Committee.

Reflux Grade	Reflux into These Structures	Dilation of the Affected Structures	Tortuous Ureter
Grade 1	Ureter	No	No
Grade 2	Ureter, Pelvis	No	No
Grade 3	Ureter, Pelvis, Infundibulum	Mild	No
Grade 4	Ureter, Pelvis, Infundibulum, Calyces	Moderate	Mild
Grade 5	Ureter, Pelvis, Infundibulum, Calyces	Severe	Severe

Complications
1. UTI/pyelonephritis—*the most common complication of VUR is infection.*
2. Hydroureteronephrosis—reasons for hydronephrosis include
   a. Congenital ureteral muscle weakness.
   b. Decompensation of ureteral musculature from increased workload (i.e. the ureter is attempting to move more and more urine).
   c. Elevated hydrostatic pressure transmitted from bladder through the incompetent ureteral orifice, especially during voiding.
3. Renal scarring—occurs from VUR associated with *urinary tract infection and intrarenal reflux.* Some general principles of scarring are
   a. The higher the grade of reflux, the more likely that scarring will occur.
   b. Some say the initial infection is the most devastating in producing renal scarring (the "Big Bang" effect of the initial UTI).
   c. The infection is more important in producing scarring than the mechanical forces of intrarenal VUR. In fact, it is unlikely that reflux of sterile urine causes renal scarring unless high pressure reflux exists.
   d. The neonatal/infant kidney is more susceptible to scarring than the adult kidney.
   e. Scaring is more likely to occur at the *poles of the kidney* because these areas have *confluent papillae* that allow intrarenal reflux.
   f. Scarring is more likely if there is a delay in treating pyelonephritis.
   g. *Renal scarring increases the risk of developing hypertension.*
4. Reflux Nephropathy—renal damage resulting from renal scarring.
5. Hypertension—from severe renal scarring and reflux nephropathy.

Work Up

1. VUR almost always presents with UTI; therefore, these children undergo the work up for pediatric UTI.
   a. History and physical exam (including blood pressure measurement).
   b. Voiding cystourethrogram (VCUG)—urine culture should be negative before performing the VCUG. Therefore, obtain a urine culture and treat any UTI before proceeding. In addition, all children should be placed on prophylactic antibiotics for this procedure. A catheterized urine culture can be obtained at the time of the VCUG.
   c. Renal and bladder ultrasound—to look for hydronephrosis, renal abnormalities, and bladder abnormalities (e.g. ureterocele). If the ultrasound shows hydronephrosis, obtain a renal scan to rule out obstruction and to check for renal scarring.
   d. Consider BUN and creatinine, especially if hydronephrosis, obstruction, or renal scarring are present.
2. If VUR is present, siblings should be screened with a VCUG or nuclear cystogram.

Treatment—General Principles

1. In general, VUR is less likely to resolve spontaneously if any of the following are present: older age at presentation, higher grade VUR, bilateral VUR, presence of voiding dysfunction, and associated urinary tract anatomic abnormalities.
2. 30% of VUR that resolves spontaneously will recur.
3. Spontaneous resolution rate for primary VUR

VUR Grade	Laterality	Age at Presentation (years)	Spontaneous Resolution Rate at 5 Years
Grade I	Unilateral or Bilateral	< 10	90%
Grade II	Unilateral or Bilateral	< 10	80%
Grade III	Unilateral	1-2	70%
		3-5	50%
		6-10	44%
	Bilateral	1-2	60%
		3-5	32%
		6-10	12%
Grade IV	Unilateral	< 10	60%
	Bilateral	< 10	10%

4. Treat the underlying cause if one is identified, e.g. distal urethral stenosis (girls), posterior urethral valves (boys), cystitis, voiding dysfunction, etc.
5. Surgical versus medical treatment in patients with grade III or IV VUR— the incidence of pyelonephritis is 2.5 times higher in patients managed medically compared to those treated surgically; however, renal scarring is similar in patients managed medically or surgically There is no difference in DMSA scan findings (with 5 years of follow up) or in renal growth (with 10 years follow up) between children managed by surgical or medical therapy.

6. Initial therapy recommendations in children age ≤ 10 years with primary VUR without voiding dysfunction and without functional/anatomic abnormalities (Based on VUR Guidelines Panel, J Urol, 157: 1846, 1997). In general, antibiotic prophylaxis is the initial management except in
   • Grade III-IV reflux in children age 6-10 that is bilateral.
   • Grade V reflux in children age 1-5 with renal scarring or bilateral VUR.
   • Grade V reflux in children age 6-10.

VUR Grade	Age at Presentation (years)	Laterality	Renal Scarring	Preferred Initial Therapy	Reasonable Alternative Therapy
I or II	< 10	Unilateral or Bilateral	Yes or No	Antibiotic prophylaxis	—
III-IV	< 1	Unilateral or Bilateral	Yes or No	Antibiotic prophylaxis	—
	1-5	Unilateral	Yes or No	Antibiotic prophylaxis	—
		Bilateral	No	Antibiotic prophylaxis	—
			Yes	Antibiotic prophylaxis	Surgery
	6-10	Unilateral	Yes or No	Antibiotic prophylaxis	—
		Bilateral	No	Surgery	Antibiotic prophylaxis
			Yes	Surgery	—
V	< 1	Unilateral or Bilateral	No	Antibiotic prophylaxis	—
			Yes	Antibiotic prophylaxis	Surgery
	1-5	Unilateral	No	Antibiotic prophylaxis	Surgery
			Yes	Surgery	—
		Bilateral	No	Surgery	Antibiotic prophylaxis
			Yes	Surgery	—
	6-10	Unilateral or Bilateral	Yes or No	Surgery	—

Treatment—Medical Management
1. Antibiotic prophylaxis—mandatory prophylaxis to prevent UTI. Prophylactic antibiotics are given *continuously* until the reflux resolves. In the first two months of life, ampicillin may be used (nitrofurantoin can cause hemolytic anemia and trimethoprim/sulfamethoxazole can cause kernicterus if used during this time). Trimethoprim/sulfamethoxazole and nitrofurantoin do not alter intestinal flora; therefore, they are preferred over penicillin (which does alter intestinal flora) for prophylaxis after the first two months of life.
2. Triple voiding (the least effective treatment).
3. Void by the clock for those without appropriate bladder sensation.

Treatment—Surgical Management

1. Absolute indications for surgery
   a. If it is not possible to keep the urine sterile with antibiotics.
   b. If a febrile UTI or pyelonephritis occur on antibiotics.
   c. Progressive renal damage or hydronephrosis despite medical therapy.
2. Relative indications for surgery
   a. Persistent reflux
   b. Anatomic abnormality (e.g. ectopic ureter, ureteral duplication, etc.)
   c. Age > 10
   d. Poor compliance or inability to tolerate medical treatment.
3. Surgical options include
   a. Ureteroneocystostomy (ureteral reimplant).
   b. Subureteric injection of a bulking agent.
   c. In males, circumcision should be considered.
   d. In a child who fails medical therapy and who is too young to have a
      reimplant or submucosal injection, vesicostomy may be performed. A
      definitive procedure may be performed when the child is older.
4. Success rate of treatments.

	Success Rate† (%)		
	All Grades	**Grade I-IV**	**Grade V**
Ureteral Reimplant	95%	>98%	80%
Subureteric Injection	70%*	–	32%

* 70% after one procedure. Success increases to 85% with repeat procedures.
† Success for reimplant is defined as no VUR postoperatively. Success for
  subureteric injection is defined as no VUR or Grade 1 VUR
  postoperatively.

Ureteroneocystostomy (Ureteral Reimplant)

1. Principles of repair
   a. Resect the lower 2-3 cm of ureter because its muscle is underdeveloped.
   b. Put the intravesical portion of the ureter into a submucosal tunnel.
   c. The submucosal tunnel should be 3 times as long as the ureter diameter.
   d. Create a *tension-free* anastomosis between bladder and ureter.
   e. Taper megaureters before implantation.
2. Reimplant types—intravesical (Politano-Leadbetter, Cohen cross trigonal,
   Glenn-Anderson advancement), extravesical (Lich-Gregoir), etc.
3. Complications
   a. Ureteral obstruction—occurs in 2% of cases and usually presents 1-2
      weeks after surgery with abdominal pain, nausea, and vomiting.
      i. Obstruction in the perioperative period usually resolves
         spontaneously and is often caused by ureteral edema.
      ii. Persistent obstruction or obstruction after the perioperative period is
         usually caused by an ischemic stricture. A ureteral stent or
         nephrostomy tube may be required to relieve obstruction.
   b. Persistent reflux
      i. *The most common cause of persistent reflux after surgical repair is
         unrecognized voiding dysfunction.*
      ii. VUR can persist in the reimplanted ureter in up to 3% of cases.
      iii. After unilateral reimplant, VUR develops in the contralateral ureter
         in 10% of cases. In these cases, the contralateral VUR usually
         resolves within 1 year; therefore, wait at least one year before
         considering surgical repair.
   c. Reoperation rate is approximately 2%.

Subureteric Injection of a Bulking Agent

1. An endoscopic needle is inserted under direct vision in the 6 o'clock position 4-6 mm distal to the ureteral orifice and the bulking agent is injected slowly into the subureteric space.
2. Bulking agents
   a. Teflon and silicone can migrate to distant sites and are not FDA approved for this procedure.
   b. Collagen can cause anaphylaxis and it loses its volume over time (which causes VUR to recur).
   c. Dextranomer/hyaluronic acid copolymer (Deflux®) does not migrate, does not cause anaphylaxis, and is biodegradable.

Follow Up

1. While on antibiotic prophylaxis
   a. Urinalysis every month for 1 year, then less often.
   b. Urinalysis, blood pressure, BUN, creatinine, and cystogram every 12 months. Some physicians required 2 consecutive negative cystograms to confirm resolution of reflux.
   c. Consider nuclear renal scan to check for renal scarring if indicated.
2. After surgical repair
   a. Prophylactic antibiotics should be continued after surgery.
   b. Perform a renal ultrasound 4-6 weeks after surgery and a VCUG 3 months after surgery.
   c. If hydronephrosis is present, a renal scan should be performed to check for obstruction.
   d. If the ultrasound shows no hydronephrosis and the VCUG shows no reflux, the prophylactic antibiotic may be stopped.
3. After VUR has resolved, long-term follow up should include blood pressure and urinalysis (especially for proteinuria).

REFERENCES

Belman AB: A perspective on vesicoureteral reflux. Urol Clin North Am, 22(1): 139, 1995.

Connolly LP, Treves ST, Zurakowski D, et al: Natural history of vesicoureteral reflux in siblings. J Urol, 156: 1805, 1996.

Elder JS, Peters CA, Arant Jr BS, et al: Pediatric vesicoureteral reflux guidelines panel summary report on the management of primary vesicoureteral reflux. J Urol, 157: 1846, 1997.

Erhard M, et al: Management of vesicoureteral reflux in adolescents and adults. AUA Update Series, Vol. 27, Lesson 5, 1998.

International Reflux Study Committee: Medical versus surgical treatment of primary vesicoureteral reflux: a prospective international reflux study in children. J Urol, 125: 277, 1981.

King LR: Vesicoureteral reflux, megaureter, and ureteral reimplantation. Campbell's Urology. 6th Edition. Ed. PC Walsh, AB Retik, TA Stamey, et al. Philadelphia: W. B. Saunders Company, 1992, pp 1689-1742.

Lackgren G, et al: Endoscopic treatment of vesicoureteral reflux and urinary incontinence in children. AUA Update Series, Vol. 22, Lesson 5, 2003.

Olbing H, Hirche H, Koskimies O, et al: Renal growth in children with severe vesicoureteral reflux: 10 year prospective study of medical and surgical treatment. Radiology, 216: 731, 2000.

Piepz A, Tamminen-Mobius T, Reiners C, et al: Five year study of medical or surgical treatment in children with severe vesico-ureteral reflux, dimercaptosuccinic acid findings. Eur J Pediatr, 157: 753, 1998.

Walker RD, Weiss RA: Vesicoureteral reflux 2000. AUA Update Series, Vol. 19, Lesson 37, 2000.

ERECTILE DYSFUNCTION (ED)

Physiology of Erections

1. Erections require two main processes
    a. Cavernosal artery smooth muscle relaxation—an *active* process that is *the initial event of an erection* (see page 168) Parasympathetic nerves release nitric oxide, leading to increased cyclic GMP (cGMP), decreased intracellular calcium, and greater smooth muscle relaxation. Cyclic AMP (cAMP) also causes smooth muscle relaxation. Smooth muscle relaxation leads to arterial dilation, increased penile blood flow, increased intracavernosal pressure, and cavernosal expansion.
    b. Increased venous outflow resistance—a *passive* process occurring when the cavernosa expand and compress sub-tunic venous sinuses.
2. High arterial inflow and low venous outflow sustains the pressure required to maintain an erection. The intracavernosal pressure during a normal erection is equal to the systemic *mean arterial pressure* (MAP).
3. Sympathetic nerves release norepinephrine, which stimulates α-adrenergic receptors, resulting in smooth muscle contraction and detumescence.

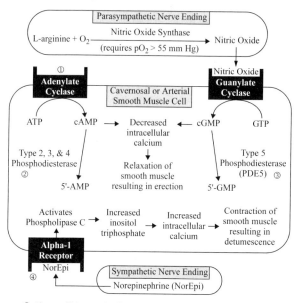

① Alprostadil (prostaglandin E1) stimulates this receptor.
② & ③ Papaverine inhibits phosphodiesterases.
③ Sildenafil, tadalafil, and vardenafil inhibit PDE5.
④ Phentolamine and other α-adrenergic antagonists inhibit this receptor.

General Information
1. Erectile dysfunction (ED) is defined as "the inability to attain and/or maintain penile erection sufficient for satisfactory sexual performance." (NIH Consensus Conference on Impotence 1993, AUA Guidelines 2005)
2. The prevalence of ED increases with age. 52% of men older than 40 have some degree of erectile dysfunction.
3. Testosterone decreases as age increases.
4. Treated hypertension has a higher rate of erectile dysfunction than untreated hypertension (mainly from the side effects of the antihypertensive medications). However, alpha-blockers do *not* cause erectile dysfunction, and may actually cause priapism.

Etiology of Erectile Dysfunction
1. Vasculogenic
   a. Arteriogenic (arterial insufficiency)
   b. Veno-occlusive dysfunction (venous leak)
2. Neurogenic
3. Psychogenic—depression, stress, anxiety, psychiatric disorder.
4. Endocrinologic–hyperprolactinemia, thyroid disorder, hypogonadism, etc.
5. Medication induced (see below)

Medications That Can Cause Erectile Dysfunction
1. Antihypertensives—especially beta-blockers, thiazides, clonidine, and methyldopa. *α–1 blockers and ACE inhibitors rarely cause impotence.*
2. Antidepressants and antipsychotics—especially tricyclic antidepressants, MAO inhibitors, lithium, and phenothiazines.
3. Medications that block or reduce testosterone—cimetidine, spironolactone (see also Androgen Deprivation, page 102).
4. Other medications/drugs—sedatives, phenytoin, anticholinergics, alcohol, tobacco smoking.

Disease States That Can Cause Erectile Dysfunction
1. Medical—chronic renal failure, diabetes mellitus, chronic liver failure, alcoholism, neurologic disease, thyroid disorders, atherosclerosis (see Major Risk Factors for CAD and Atherosclerosis, page 237).
2. Surgical—radical prostatectomy, radical cystectomy, proctocolectomy, aorto-iliac vascular surgery, aortic aneurysm repair, pituitary surgery, penile surgery, etc.
3. Traumatic—pelvic fracture, penile fracture, perineal trauma, priapism, spinal cord injury, neuropathy from bicycle riding, pelvic radiation.

Work Up

History and Physical
1. History
   a. Medical, surgical, psychologic, social, trauma, and medication history.
   b. Sexual history—onset and duration of ED, maximum rigidity, sustaining capability, penetration capability, nocturnal/morning erections, erections with masturbation, last successful intercourse, frequency of intercourse currently and one year prior, libido, ejaculatory dysfunction, orgasmic dysfunction, ability to achieve sexual satisfaction, penile curvature, relationship problems, performance anxiety, stress.
2. Physical exam—includes peripheral pulses, external genitalia, presence of testes and their size, prostate, bulbocavernosus reflex, perianal sensation, anal sphincter tone, secondary sexual characteristics. Note the presence of penile plaques, gynecomastia, galactorrhea, and visual field defects.

Cardiovascular Risk Assessment of Men Resuming Sexual Activity

1. Major risk factors for coronary artery disease (CAD) and atherosclerosis.

Older age	Hypertension (HTN)
Male	Diabetes mellitus
Family history of premature CAD	Cigarette smoking
Sedentary lifestyle	Dyslipidemia

2. *ED may serve as an early indicator for underlying cardiovascular disease because it shares risk factors with atherosclerosis. Therefore, an evaluation for cardiovascular risk factors should be performed in men presenting with ED* (e.g. blood pressure measurement, fasting serum glucose or A1c, and lipid panel).

3. Sexual activity increases the risk of myocardial infarction (MI) by 2 to 3 fold; however, sexual activity causes < 1% of MIs and the absolute risk of MI within 2 hours of sexual activity is < 0.01%. Nonetheless, the exertion of sexual activity may be too risky for some patients.

4. Cardiovascular medications in men with ED
   a. Nitrates—type 5 phosphodiesterase (PDE5) inhibitors are contraindicated in men taking nitrates.
   b. Anti-arrhythmics—vardenafil is contraindicated in men on anti-arrhythmics that prolong the QT interval (such as procainamide, quinidine, sotalol, and amiodarone).
   c. α-blockers—use caution when coadministering an α-blocker with a PDE5 inhibitor because hypotension may occur when they are taken together (see page 247).
   d. Antihypertensive agents—PDE5 inhibitors rarely cause adverse effects in men taking one or more antihypertensive agents (although α-blockers may be associated with hypotension; see above).
   e. Anticoagulants—the vacuum erection device is contraindicated in men taking anticoagulants. Intracavernosal injections and MUSE should be used with caution in men on anticoagulants.

5. ED medications in men with cardiovascular disease
   a. Patients with known coronary artery disease or heart failure receiving PDE5 inhibitors did not exhibit coronary vasoconstriction, worse cardiac ischemia, or worse hemodynamics during exercise testing or cardiac catheterization.
   b. Vardenafil is contraindicated in men with congenital QT prolongation and in men on medications that prolong QT interval (including anti-arrhythmics; see above). Statistically significant QTc interval changes have not been observed with sildenafil or tadalafil.
   c. Patients with left ventricular outflow obstruction (e.g. aortic stenosis, idiopathic hypertrophic subaortic stenosis) can be sensitive to the action of vasodilators, including PDE5 inhibitors.
   d. Testosterone may be used in hypogonadal men with cardiovascular disease. However, testosterone is contraindicated in men with significant risk of volume overload and in men with inadequately treated congestive heart failure or pulmonary edema.
   e. Yohimbine has been associated with cardiac dysfunction, hypertension, and cardiac arrhythmia. The AUA guidelines recommend not using yohimbine for treating ED.

6. *All patients with ED that want to resume sexual activity should be assessed for cardiovascular risk before ED therapy is administered.* See Cardiovascular Risk Assessment in Men Resuming Sexual Activity, page 238.

Cardiovascular Risk Assessment in Men Resuming Sexual Activity
(based on the Princeton Consensus Conference)

History & Physical Exam

Low Risk
- Asymptomatic CAD
- < 3 CAD risk factors (excluding gender)
- Controlled HTN with ≥ 1 medications
- Mild stable angina (evaluated & treated)
- Successful coronary revascularization
- Uncomplicated MI > 6-8 weeks ago
- Mild valvular heart disease

1. Treat ED.
2. The patient may resume sexual activity.

Follow-up and assessment at regular intervals

Indeterminate or Intermediate Risk
- ≥ 3 CAD risk factors (excluding gender)
- Moderate stable angina
- Recent MI 2-6 weeks ago
- LVD/CHF NYHA class II
- Non-cardiac sequela of atherosclerosis *
- Cardiac condition uncertain
- Murmur of unknown significance

1. Refer to internist or cardiologist for cardiovascular testing.
2. Defer sexual activity until cardiovascular testing is complete.
3. Reclassify as low or high risk based on cardiovascular testing.

Follow-up and assessment at regular intervals

High Risk
- Unstable or refractory angina
- Uncontrolled HTN
- LVD/CHF NYHA class III or IV
- Recent MI < 2 weeks ago
- High risk arrhythmias
- Obstructive hypertrophic cardiomyopathy
- Moderate or severe valvular disease

1. Refer to cardiologist.
2. Defer sexual activity until the cardiac condition stabilizes & the patient is cleared by a cardiologist.

Follow-up and assessment at regular intervals

* Peripheral vascular disease, history of stroke, history of transient ischemic attack.   LVD = left ventricular dysfunction; HTN = hypertension.
CHF = congestive heart failure; NYHA = New York Heart Association; CAD = coronary artery disease; MI = myocardial infarction.
NOTE: A given risk category is assigned if the patient has any of the risk factors within the category. If the patient has risk factors in more than one category,
then the higher risk category is assigned.

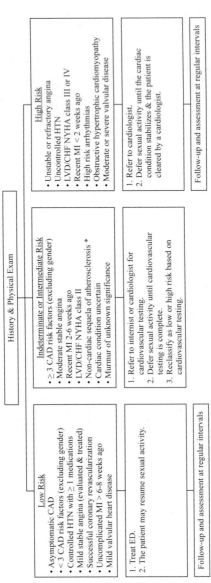

Tests to Assess ED
1. Testosterone
   a. Methods to assess serum testosterone
      i. Total testosterone—the entire amount of circulating testosterone. A portion is unbound (free), a portion is "weakly" bound to proteins such as albumin, and a portion is "tightly" bound to a protein called steroid hormone binding globulin (SHBG). Most testosterone is bound to proteins.
      ii. SHBG—a protein that binds "tightly" to testosterone; therefore, testosterone cannot dissociate from SHBG, does not diffuse into tissues, and does not exert a biological effect. Hyperthyroidism, liver disease, elevated estrogen, and older age can increase SHBG. As SHBG increases, free testosterone decreases.
      iii. Free testosterone—unbound testosterone that can diffuse into tissues and exert a biologic effect.
      iv. Weakly bound testosterone—testosterone that can dissociate from albumin and other proteins, diffuse into tissues, and exert a biologic effect.
      v. Bioavailable testosterone—the sum of free and weakly bound testosterone (a measure of all biologically active testosterone). It is a more accurate measure of androgen effect than total testosterone.
   b. Random testosterone levels are often drawn, but a morning testosterone is most accurate.
   c. *Morning testosterone is the minimum initial hormone evaluation for ED.* Some urologists also obtain either a free or a bioavailable testosterone with the initial test, while others reserve these tests for men with signs and symptoms of hypogonadism or in men with a low total testosterone.
   d. If the initial testosterone is low, obtain a prolactin, LH, FSH, and a repeat testosterone in the morning to confirm hypogonadism and to help determine its underlying cause.
2. Prolactin—some urologists check prolactin routinely, while others check prolactin only when any of the following are present: low testosterone, visual field defect, headaches, gynecomastia, or decreased libido.
3. Nocturnal penile tumescence and rigidity (NPTR)
   a. NPTR detects erections (and may also measure rigidity) during REM sleep. Examples include Rigiscan, strain gauge, and plethysmography (a blood pressure cuff that measures intracavernosal pressure).
   b. NPTR may help distinguish psychogenic ED from organic causes. NPTR can be confounded by non-psychogenic factors including dream content, sleep disturbances, neurologic conditions, medications, etc. Erections during sleep do not always correlate with erections during sexual activity. NPTR correlates poorly with sexual performance.
   c. NPTR is neither sensitive nor specific enough to use as a single diagnostic evaluation.
4. Combined intracavernosal injection and stimulation
   a. This test is used as an initial test to evaluate the functional status of the erectile mechanism. The patient undergoes intracavernosal injection and stimulates himself to achieve erection.
   b. The optimal intracavernosal medication and its dosage have not been established. Furthermore, standard criteria of what constitutes a normal test have not been established.
   c. *A good erection rules out veno-occlusive disease, but does not rule out arterial insufficiency.*
   d. A poor response can be caused by inadequate dosing or administration, veno-occlusive disease, arterial insufficiency, or extreme anxiety.

5. Penile duplex Doppler sonography
   a. Uses a 5-10 Hz transducer to image the penis 5-10 minutes after intracavernosal injection of an erectogenic medication.
   b. Arterial flow—this is examined in each of the cavernous arteries.
      • Cavernous artery peak systolic velocity (PSV)—normal > 30 cm/s, severe arterial insufficiency < 25 cm/s. The sum of the right and left PSV should be > 50-60 cm/s to rule out arteriogenic ED. PSV is measured with the probe-vessel doppler angle at 60°.
      • Cavernous artery diameter—normal flaccid diameter = 0.3-0.4 mm, normal erect diameter = 0.7-1.2 mm. Arteriogenic insufficiency is suspected if erect cavernous artery diameter is < 0.7 mm. In some studies, artery diameter correlates poorly with arterial insufficiency.
      • Cavernous artery end diastolic velocity (EDV)—normal ≤ 3 cm/s. With isolated veno-occlusive disease, PSV is normal and EDV > 3 cm/s.
   c. Venous outflow—deep dorsal vein flow will persist during erection and should not be misinterpreted as veno-occlusive dysfunction.
6. Cavernosometry
   a. *This is the most sensitive test to detect veno-occlusive dysfunction.*
   b. Two needles are placed into the corpora. One needle is used to measure intracavernosal pressure. The other needle is used to infuse heparinized saline. An erectogenic medication is injected into the corpora to achieve maximum cavernosal artery dilation (and thus maximum erection).
   c. Saline is infused into the corpora to generate each of these intracavernosal pressures: 30, 60, 90, 120, and 150 mm Hg. The saline flow rate required to maintain these pressures is measured. Maximal cavernosal artery dilation is confirmed by demonstrating a linear relationship between intracavernosal pressure and saline flow (as pressure increases, flow decreases). If this relationship is not linear, continue administering erectogenic injections until maximum arterial dilation is achieved. When a linear relationship exists, the flow required to maintain an intracavernosal pressure of 150 mm Hg is measured (flow to maintain). Then, the flow is stopped and the intracavernosal pressure decay is measured.
   d. Flow to maintain—when veno-occlusive dysfunction is present, blood flows out of the corpora and the intracavernosal pressure begins to fall. To sustain intracavernosal pressure, saline must be infused into the corpora. The flow of saline required to maintain an intracavernosal pressure of 150 mm Hg is called "flow to maintain." Veno-occlusive dysfunction is present when flow to maintain is > 3 ml/minute.
   e. Intracavernosal pressure decay—when the intracavernosal pressure is 150 mm Hg, the saline infusion is stopped and the intracavernosal pressure is monitored. Veno-occlusive dysfunction is present when intracavernosal pressure declines by ≥ 45 mm Hg in 30 seconds.
   f. In some cases, the intracavernosal pressure cannot be increased to the desired level, even at very high flow rates. Veno-occlusive dysfunction is present when the intracavernosal pressure cannot be increased to the mean arterial pressure.
7. Cavernosography
   a. This is usually performed at the same time as cavernosometry. After an intracavernosal injection with an erectogenic medication, radiographic contrast is infused into the corpora to maintain flow. Both AP and oblique images are obtained. This test is used to *visualize the location of the venous leak.*
   b. With normal veno-occlusive function, minimal or no venous drainage from the corpora is seen on cavernosography (i.e. only the corpora are visualized during erection).

8. Bilateral internal pudendal and inferior epigastric arteriography
   a. *This is the gold standard for demonstrating arterial insufficiency.*
   b. Indicated in young men with suspected arterial insufficiency who are candidates for a revascularization procedure.
   c. Note the following: Are the inferior epigastric vessels patent? (these vessels are used for revascularization) Is there a stenosis in the penile arterial blood supply? Can the arterial stenosis be bypassed?
9. Cavernous arterial systolic occlusion pressure (CASOP)—after an erectogenic medication is injected intracavernosally, a penile blood pressure cuff determines the pressure at which the cavernous artery flow becomes detectable. Arteriogenic ED is probably present when this equation is true: CASOP < Brachial systolic pressure - 35 mm Hg. This test can be performed with cavernosometry.
10. Penile brachial index (PBI)—similar to CASOP except measured in the flaccid state. A blood pressure cuff is used to measure the penile systolic pressure (while flaccid) and the brachial systolic pressure. PBI = penile systolic blood pressure ÷ brachial systolic blood pressure. PBI ≤ 0.7 implies arteriogenic ED.
11. Self administered questionnaires—the International Index of Erectile Function (IIEF), the Erectile Dysfunction Intensity Scale, etc.
12. Other tests—psychological testing, neurologic testing, etc.

Tests to Assess for Medical Diseases that Cause ED

1. Testosterone ± prolactin—see page 239.
2. Tests to assess cardiovascular risk factors
   a. Blood pressure measurement to check for hypertension.
   b. Fasting glucose or A1c to check for diabetes mellitus.
   c. Lipid profile to check for hyperlipidemia.
3. Complete blood count (CBC) to check for anemia.
4. Creatinine to check for renal insufficiency.
5. In patients with symptoms of thyroid dysfunction, obtain a thyroid profile.

Indicators of Arteriogenic ED (Arterial Insufficiency)

1. Cavernous artery PSV < 25 cm/s (or sum of right and left cavernous artery PSV < 50 cm/s)
2. Dilation of cavernosal artery to < 0.7 mm
3. CASOP < Brachial systolic pressure - 35 mm Hg.
4. Arterial occlusion or stenosis identified on internal pudendal arteriography.
5. PBI ≤ 0.7

Indicators of Veno-occlusive ED (Venous Leak)

1. On cavernosometry
   a. Flow to maintain > 3 ml/min (at intracavernosal pressure of 150 mm Hg)
   b. Intracavernosal pressure decay ≥ 45 mm Hg in 30 seconds.
   c. Inability to increase intracavernosal pressure to mean arterial pressure.
2. Venous leak seen on cavernosography.
3. Cavernous artery EDV > 3 cm/s.

Indicators That Suggest Psychogenic ED

1. Rigid erections with NPTR.
2. Good erection with combined intracavernosal injection and stimulation.
3. Normal arterial and veno-occlusive function.

Evaluation and Treatment of ED - Part 1

History and Physical Exam (including BP measurement)

Cardiovascular Risk Assessment (see page 237)

Consider Self Administered Questionnaire & NPTR testing

Presence of any of the following:
- Poorly controlled diabetes
- Inadequately treated thyroid disorder
- Inadequately treated neurologic disorder
- Psychiatric disorder
- Urinary tract infection
- Prostatitis
- Sleep disorder

Yes | **No**

Treat the above medical problems, then reassess. Offer non-surgical erection therapies during treatment.

- Morning testosterone level* ± prolactin level**
- Glycohemoglobin (A1c) or fasting serum glucose
- Serum lipids and cholesterol
- Complete blood count (CBC)
- Creatinine
- Thyroid function tests (TFTs) if indicated

Abnormal | **Normal**

- If the initial testosterone level is low, obtain a morning testosterone* and prolactin level.
- If abnormal TFTs, A1c, glucose, cholesterol, lipids, CBC, or creatinine, refer to internist.
- Offer non-surgical erection therapies and reassess after treatment by internist.

See Evaluation and Treatment of ED Part 2

Low testosterone and elevated prolactin | Low testosterone and normal prolactin | Normal Testosterone

MRI to rule out pituitary tumor‡ | Prostate exam, breast exam, PSA, LFTs, lipids, cholesterol, hematocrit (± FSH & LH §)

The patient has any of the following: presence or significant risk for prostate or breast cancer, fertility concerns, significant risk for congestive heart failure or pulmonary edema, or severe forms of any of the following: hyperlipidemia†, bladder outlet obstruction†, liver dysfunction†, polycythemia†, or sleep apnea†

No | **Yes**

Give testosterone replacement and draw a testosterone level in 4 weeks | See Evaluation and Treatment of ED - Part 2

If testosterone is low, increase the dose of testosterone | If testosterone is normal, follow PSA, prostate exam, hematocrit, cholesterol, lipid profile, LFTs and testosterone at least every 6 months°

If the patient is not satisfied with his erections, See Evaluation and Treatment of ED - Part 2 | The patient is satisfied with his erections

NPTR = nocturnal penile tumescence and rigidity; LFTs = liver function tests

* Morning total testosterone (with or without free or bioavailable testosterone).

** Some urologists recommend measuring prolactin only when any of the following are present: low testosterone, a visual field defect, headaches, gynecomastia, or significantly decreased libido.

§ FSH and LH help determine the primary abnormality causing low testosterone and may be helpful in investigating infertility.

† Consider delaying testosterone replacement until the patient is adequately treated for mild or moderate forms of these syndromes.

° If the patient is on anticoagulants, PT/PTT should also be measured.

‡ MRI of brain and pituitary with gadolinium.

Evaluation and Treatment of ED - Part 2

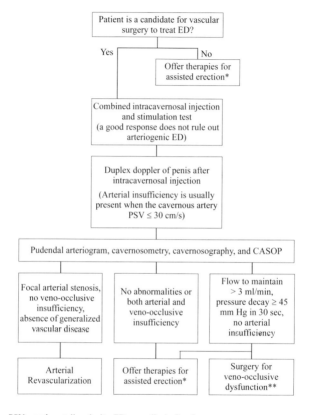

PSV = peak systolic velocity; ED = erectile dysfunction
CASOP = cavernous arterial systolic occlusion pressure
* The 2005 AUA guidelines recommend a type 5 phosphodiesterase (PDE5)
  inhibitor as first-line therapy (unless it is contraindicated). Other therapies
  include vacuum erection device, MUSE, intracavernosal injections, and
  penile prosthesis. The AUA guidelines do not recommend herbal therapies,
  yohimbine, or trazodone.
** The 2005 AUA guidelines do not recommend surgeries to limit the venous
   outflow of the penis.

Treatment for Erectile Dysfunction

NOTE: All patients with ED should be assessed for cardiovascular risk before erectile dysfunction therapy is administered (see page 237).

General Recommendations
1. Avoid smoking
2. Maintain an ideal body weight (avoid obesity)
3. Stop alcohol abuse
4. If the patient takes a prescription medication that may contribute to ED, consider changing to another medication.
5. Optimize management of diabetes, hypertension, and heart disease.

Psychogenic ED
1. Suggest counseling
2. Any of the therapies for assisted erection may be tried (start with the least invasive therapies). Sometimes these may be used temporarily until the psychogenic cause has been overcome.

Neurogenic ED
Pharmacologic treatments in men with neurogenic impotence should be started a lower dose than the initial dose used in men with other types of ED.

Arteriogenic ED (Arterial Insufficiency)
1. Arterial revascularization
   a. Men with generalized atherosclerosis are not candidates for revascularization.
   b. Indicated in young men with a focal arterial defect on internal pudendal arteriogram, no veno-occlusive dysfunction, and cessation of tobacco use. The success rate in these men is 60%-70% at 5 years.
   c. The inferior epigastric arteries are rarely affected by atherosclerosis.
   d. Revascularization is achieved by anastomosing the inferior epigastric artery to the dorsal penile artery or to the deep dorsal penile vein. Anastomosis to the deep dorsal vein may cause *glans hyperemia*, which is uncomfortable for the patient.
2. If the patient is not a candidate for revascularization, any of the therapies for assisted erection may be tried.

Veno-occlusive ED (Venous Leak)
1. Venous constriction band—a circular band that fits around the base of the penis. It can be used alone or in combination with other erection therapies (except penile prostheses). Use the least constrictive tension that will maintain an erection. Maximum duration of each use = 20-30 minutes. Wait at least one hour after removing the band before using it again.
2. Surgery for veno-occlusive disorders
   a. Indicated in men who meet all of the following criteria: short duration erections, failure to maintain or obtain erection with intracavernosal injections, normal cavernous artery flow, faulty veno-occlusive mechanism by cavernometry, venous leak on cavernosography, and cessation of tobacco use. Long-term success rate is 50-60%.
   b. Surgery for veno-occlusive dysfunction is accomplished by ligation of the deep dorsal vein.
   c. This surgery was not recommended by the 2005 AUA guidelines.
3. If the patient is not a candidate for veno-occlusive surgery, therapies for assisted erection ± venous constriction band may be tried.

ED with Renal Failure or Renal Transplant

1. The cause of ED in men with renal insufficiency is multi-factorial. Renal insufficiency can increase prolactin (and thus decrease testosterone). In some patients, bromocriptine can reduce prolactin and improve erections.
2. In men with end stage renal disease, ED may resolve after renal transplant; therefore, avoid placing a penile prosthesis prior to transplant. If a penile prosthesis is placed, use a scrotal reservoir, not an abdominal reservoir.
3. For patients with severe renal insufficiency (including men on dialysis)
   a. The maximum recommended dose of vardenafil is 5 mg per 24 hours.
   b. The maximum recommended dose of tadalafil is 5 mg per 24 hours.
   c. The recommended starting dose for sildenafil is 25 mg per 24 hours.
4. The internal iliac arteries supply blood to the penis. If both internal iliac arteries are used for kidney transplant, ED is highly likely. When a second renal transplant is required, it should be anastomosed to the contralateral common or external iliac artery to help preserve erections.
5. Sildenafil appears to be safe and effective in renal transplant recipients and did not appear to affect the serum levels of the immunosuppressive drugs. Data are lacking for other PDE5 inhibitors.

ED After Radical Prostatectomy

1. Radical prostatectomy may cause shortening of the penis (mean loss of length = 1 cm, range = 0 to 5 cm).
2. Potency after radical prostatectomy (RP) is better when
   a. Preoperative erectile function is good.
   b. Age is less than 60.
   c. Nerve sparing is performed—the neurovascular bundles (NVB) course posterior-lateral to the prostate and contain cavernous vessels and nerves (which are vital for erections). Bilateral nerve sparing results in better erections after RP than unilateral nerve sparing. Unilateral nerve sparing results in better erections after RP than non-nerve sparing.
3. Causes of ED after RP
   a. Nerve compromise—the cavernous nerves in the NVB are crucial for erections. During non-nerve sparing RP, these nerves are removed and ED is inevitable. After nerve sparing RP, erections recover slowly over the first 24 months postoperatively, probably because nerve function is temporarily impaired from surgical trauma (neuropraxia).
   b. Vascular compromise—ligation or injury to the penile vascular supply, including the cavernous arteries in the NVB and accessory pudendal arteries, may impair blood flow to the penis and contribute to ED.
   c. Fibrosis of the erectile tissue—vascular and nerve compromise after RP appear to induce hypoxia, which then causes fibrosis of the corporal tissue. *Corporal fibrosis begins within 2 months after RP and may progress during the postoperative period.*
4. Penile rehabilitation after RP
   a. Rationale—inducing erections after RP may reduce hypoxia, prevent corporal fibrosis, and promote nerve and vascular function.
   b. The FDA has not approved any therapy for penile rehabilitation. Limited data suggests that rehabilitation may improve spontaneous erections. The optimal regimen is unknown. Example regimens (one of the agents listed below may be titrated to the maximum well-tolerated dose):
      i. Intraurethral alprostadil (MUSE®)—3 times a week.
      ii. Intracavernosal alprostadil—3 times a week.
      iii. Type 5 phosphodiesterase inhibitor—every night.
   c. The vacuum erection device does not appear to improve spontaneous erections after RP, but it may prevent penile shortening.
   d. Penile rehabilitation should be initiated within 2 months after RP.

Low Testosterone/Hypogonadism

1. *Testosterone is not indicated for the treatment of erectile dysfunction in men with normal serum testosterone* (2005 AUA Guidelines).
2. For testosterone testing, see Testosterone page 239.
3. There are no universally accepted guidelines for the level of testosterone that defines hypogonadism nor what level is low enough to warrant treatment. The AACE 2002 guidelines suggest "Men with symptomatic hypogonadism and a total testosterone level of less than 200 ng/dl may be potential candidates for therapy."
4. Low testosterone can cause ED, decreased libido, infertility, fatigue, altered masculine features (gynecomastia, reduced facial and body hair, reduced muscle mass), osteoporosis, and mood disturbances (increased levels of anger, confusion, and depression).
5. Testosterone replacement therapy
   a. Indications for testosterone replacement may include improving any of the following: masculinization, muscle strength, mood, energy, libido, erectile function, or osteoporosis. Perform a complete endocrine evaluation to ensure that testosterone replacement is indicated.
   b. Contraindications
      i. Absolute contraindications to testosterone replacement include prostate or breast cancer, inadequately controlled congestive heart failure, significant risk of pulmonary edema or volume overload, and severe forms of bladder outlet obstruction from the prostate, liver dysfunction, polycythemia, sleep apnea, or dyslipidemia.
      ii. Relative contraindications to testosterone replacement include risk of prostate or breast cancer, fertility concerns, and mild forms of bladder outlet obstruction from the prostate, liver dysfunction, polycythemia, sleep apnea, or dyslipidemia.
   c. Before therapy and periodically thereafter (e.g. at least every 6 months) perform prostate exam, serum testosterone, liver function tests, PSA, hematocrit, triglycerides, HDL, and LDL (PT/PTT for men on coumadin).
   d. Dose—adjust the dose based on testosterone levels and response.
      i. Intramuscular—testosterone enanthate or testosterone cypionate 50-400 mg IM q 2-4 weeks. This route causes large fluctuations in testosterone with a high peaks and low troughs.
      ii. Oral—oral testosterone has a high rate of hepatotoxic side effects and is not a favored route of administration.
      iii. Buccal—absorbed through the mucosa of the mouth. See page 421.
      iv. Transdermal—absorbed through the skin. See page 421.
   e. Buccal and transdermal routes produce more stable testosterone levels than the IM route (which has high peaks and low troughs).
   f. Side effects—growth of prostate and breast cancer, bladder outlet obstruction from benign prostate growth, hepatitis, hepatic tumors, acne, fluid retention, weight gain, worse sleep apnea, dyslipidemia (high LDL, high triglycerides, low HDL), polycythemia, testicular atrophy, infertility, and priapism. *Testosterone can cause infertility* by lowering luteinizing hormone, which results in lower intratesticular androgens and impaired spermatogenesis.
   g. Testosterone replacement does not alter total PSA or PSA velocity beyond established norms. Abnormal PSA should not be attributed to testosterone replacement and should be worked up in the usual fashion.
   h. Testosterone may induce hypoglycemia in diabetics taking insulin.
   i. Testosterone can prolong coumadin activity.

<u>Therapies for Assisted Erections</u>

Important Considerations
1. Avoid ED therapies when sexual activity is inadvisable or contraindicated.
2. ED therapies may cause priapism. The patient must seek immediate medical attention if priapism occurs.
3. ED therapies should not be used in patients with penile tumors, phimosis, paraphimosis, or recent penile surgery until these problems have resolved.

Type 5 Phosphodiesterase (PDE5) Inhibitors
1. Examples—sildenafil (Viagra®), vardenafil (Levitra®), tadalafil (Cialis®)
2. PDE5 is located primarily in the cavernosal smooth muscle.
3. PDE5 inhibitors do not initiate an erection, but once an erection is present, these drugs make the erection stronger. *Therefore, physical stimulation is required to initiate an erection before these medications have an effect.*
4. *The 2005 AUA guidelines recommend an oral PDE5 inhibitor as first-line therapy for erectile dysfunction (unless they are contraindicated).*
5. Contraindications—*PDE5 inhibitors are contraindicated in patients taking nitrates or nitric oxide donors.* PDE5 inhibitors potentiate nitrates and may cause life-threatening hypotension.
6. α-blockers—use caution when coadministering an α-blocker with a PDE5 inhibitor because hypotension may occur when they are taken together.
   a. Men should be hemodynamically stable on an α-blocker before starting a PDE5 inhibitor. When stable on an α-blocker, the PDE5 inhibitor should be started at the lowest recommended starting dose.
   b. In men already taking an optimized dose of PDE5 inhibitor, an α-blocker should be started at the lowest dose.
   c. Increasing the dose of the α-blocker or the PDE5 inhibitor may be associated with further lowering of blood pressure.
   d. Sildenafil > 25 mg should not be used within 4 hours of taking an α-blocker.
   e. Safe use of an α-blocker and a PDE5 inhibitor may be affected by other factors such as hypovolemia and use of other anti-hypertensive drugs.
7. Consider avoiding PDE5 inhibitors in men with any of the following:
   a. Resting hypotension (BP < 90/50) or hypertension (BP > 170/110),
   b. Taking drugs that prolong the half life of PDE5 inhibitors.
   c. Retinitis pigmentosa or inherited disorders of retinal phosphodiesterase.
   d. Significant cardiovascular disease (see page 237).
8. Patients with stable coronary artery disease or heart failure receiving PDE5 inhibitors do not exhibit coronary vasoconstriction, worse cardiac ischemia, or worse hemodynamics during exercise testing or cardiac catheterization. The rate of heart attack other cardiovascular events (excluding flushing) is similar in men taking PDE5 inhibitors and placebo.
9. Side effects—include headache, flushing, dyspepsia, back pain/myalgia, nasal congestion, abnormal vision (e.g. blue tint), and priapism (very rare).
   a. Back pain and myalgia are more common with tadalafil, while visual changes are more common with vardenafil and sildenafil.
   b. Side effects tend to lessen (and often resolve) after several weeks of use.
   c. Non-arteritic anterior ischemic optic neuropathy (NAION), a stroke of the optic nerve that causes a sudden loss of vision, rarely occurs in men taking PDE5 inhibitors. There is no evidence that PDE5 inhibitors increase the risk of NAION. ED and NAION have similar risk factors (e.g. age > 50, HTN, elevated cholesterol, diabetes). Vasodilators may adversely affect patients with NAION; therefore, caution should be used when prescribing PDE5 inhibitors to patients with NAION. Patients who experience a sudden loss of vision should stop using PDE5 inhibitors.

10. Poor patient education is a common cause of why men have a poor response to PDE5 inhibitors. In men who report a poor response to PDE5 inhibitors, determine whether the patient is taking the medication in a manner that achieves maximal effect. Re-educate the patient regarding titration to maximum dose, timing of administration, need for stimulation, effect of a recent meal, and side effect profile.

11. Dose

a. Sildenafil (Viagra®)—initial dose is 50 mg po before sex. Adjust the dose from 25 to 100 mg. Maximum dose = 100 mg. Maximum dosing frequency is once per day. [Tabs: 25, 50, 100 mg]

b. Tadalafil (Cialis®)—initial dose is 10 mg po before sex. Adjust the dose from 5 to 20 mg. Maximum dose = 20 mg; Maximum dosing frequency is once per day. [Tabs: 5, 10, 20 mg]

c. Vardenafil (Levitra®)—initial dose is 10 mg po before sex. Adjust the dose from 5 to 20 mg. Maximum dose = 20 mg; Maximum dosing frequency is once per day. [Tabs: 2.5, 5, 10, 20 mg]

d. PDE5 inhibitors are most effective starting 60 minutes after an oral dose, but can be effective in as little as 20 minutes.

e. Reduce the dose in men taking cytochrome P450 3A4 inhibitors (e.g. ritonavir, indinavir, erythromycin, ketoconazole, grapefruit juice) because these substances increase serum PDE5 inhibitor levels.

f. Dose adjustment may be required in patients with hepatic dysfunction, renal dysfunction, or age >65 years.

PDE5 Inhibitor	Absorption Reduced by Fatty Food	QT Interval Warning	Approximate Half Life	Approximate Duration of Action	Also Has Significant Affinity For
Sildenafil	Yes	No	4 hrs	6-8 hrs	PDE-6 *
Vardenafil	Yes	Yes ‡	4 hrs	6-8 hrs	PDE-6 *
Tadalafil	No	No	17.5 hrs	36 hrs	PDE-11 †

* PDE-6 is in the retina and is responsible for visual side effects.

† PDE-11 is in the muscle, testicles, prostate, and kidney. PDE-11 inhibition may cause back pain and myalgia, but its long-term effects are unknown. Testosterone, LH, FSH, and semen analysis are not affected after 6 months of tadalafil use.

‡ Vardenafil should not be used by men on drugs that prolong the QT interval or in men with congenital prolonged QT interval because of the theoretical risk of torsades de pointes and sudden cardiac death.

Yohimbine

1. An oral inhibitor of presynaptic alpha-2 adrenergic receptors. It probably acts on the central nervous system to increase libido and erection.

2. It is *not* significantly better than placebo in patients with organic ED. It may be of some benefit in patients with psychogenic ED.

3. Contraindications—renal insufficiency, cardiac dysfunction, arrhythmia, peptic ulcer disease, hypertension, concomitant use with other mood modifying drugs (see also Important Considerations, page 247).

4. Side effects—include anxiety, tremor, nausea/vomiting, hypertension, tachycardia, dizziness, headache, flushing, sweating, and anti-diuresis.

5. Initial dose—yohimbine 5.4 mg po TID [Tabs: 5.4 mg]. The dose can be reduced to 2.7 mg po TID. It may take several weeks before a clinical response is observed.

6. The use of yohimbine was not recommended by the 2005 AUA guidelines.

7. Yohimbine is one of the active ingredients in many non-prescription and "all natural" formulas for "male enhancement."

Vacuum Erection Device (VED)

1. A cylindrical vacuum pump is placed over the penis. Air is drawn from the cylinder, causing blood to flow into the penis. When erection is achieved, an occlusive ring is placed around the penile base to maintain the erection.
2. *Vacuum erection devices should be used only if they have a vacuum limiter.* Vacuum limiters reduce the risk of penile injury by preventing the VED from generating high negative pressures.
3. Contraindications—predisposition to priapism, penile implant, significant angulation or fibrosis of the penis, bleeding disorder or anticoagulation (see also Important Considerations, page 247).
4. Side effects—hematoma, penile buckling/pivoting at the ring, retarded ejaculation, cold penis, numb penis, penile pain.
5. Maximum duration of use—20-30 minutes.
6. Maximum frequency of use—wait at least one hour after removing the occlusive band before using the VED again.

MUSE® (Medicated Urethral System for Erection)

1. MUSE® is an intraurethral formulation of alprostadil (prostaglandin E1).
2. Alprostadil binds to a membrane receptor, activates adenylate cyclase, and increases intracellular cyclic AMP. It also inhibits platelet aggregation.
3. Erection begins 5-20 minutes after administration.
4. Contraindications—predisposition to priapism, distal urethral stricture, significant penile angulation or fibrosis, balanitis, and urethritis (see also Important Considerations, page 247). Do not use MUSE during sexual activity with a pregnant female unless a condom barrier is used.
5. Side effects—burning in the genitals or urethra (in up to 36%), urethral bleeding, priapism, hypotension, headache, dizziness. Men with significant venous leakage may be at higher risk for hypotension.
6. Dose—[urethral suppository: 125, 250, 500, 1000 mcg]
   • Initial dose—for neurogenic ED, start alprostadil 125 mcg intraurethral and increase the dose in increments of 125 mcg as needed. For mixed or non-neurogenic ED, start alprostadil 125 or 250 mcg intraurethral and increase the dose as needed.
   • Maximum Dose = 1000 mcg; Maximum dosing frequency = 2 times per 24 hours. An erection should completely detumescence before another dose is administered.
7. The 2005 AUA guidelines recommend that the first dose of MUSE be administered under the supervision of a health care provider because hypotension has been reported in 3% of patients after the first dose.

Intracavernosal Injections (ICI)

1. Contraindications–predisposition to priapism, significant penile angulation or fibrosis, penile implant (see also Important Considerations, page 247).
2. Alprostadil has a lower incidence of priapism (2% vs. 10%) and penile fibrosis (1% vs. 12%) than papaverine. *Papaverine has a lower incidence of penile pain than alprostadil.*
3. Men with significant venous leakage may be at higher risk for hypotension and systemic side effects from ICI.
4. The 2005 AUA guidelines recommend that the first dose of ICI therapy should be administered under the supervision of a health care provider.

5. Alprostadil (prostaglandin E1)
   a. Alprostadil binds to a membrane receptor, activates adenylate cyclase, and increases intracellular cyclic AMP. It inhibits platelet aggregation.
   b. Side effects—include penile pain/burning (in up to 37%), priapism, penile fibrosis (up to 8%), hypotension, and headache.
   c. Dose—dose titration should be supervised by a health care professional.
      • Initial dose—in neurogenic ED, start with alprostadil 1.25 mcg ICI. If response is insufficient, increase the dose in increments of 1.25 mcg. In mixed or non-neurogenic ED, start with 2.5 mcg ICI. If response is insufficient, increase the dose in increments of 5 mcg.
      • Maximum Dose = 60 mcg; Maximum dosing frequency = 3 times per week with at least 24 hours between each dose.
6. Papaverine (not FDA approved for intracavernosal injection)
   a. Papaverine is a nonspecific inhibitor of phosphodiesterases.
   b. Side effects—priapism, penile fibrosis, elevated liver function tests (LFTs). If high doses are used or venous leak is present, check LFTs.
   c. Dose—dose titration should be supervised by a health care professional.
      • Initial dose—in neurogenic ED, start with papaverine 3 mg ICI. In mixed or non-neurogenic ED, start with papaverine 5-10 mg ICI. If response is insufficient, increase the dose in small increments. The effective dose range is usually 20-80 mg.
      • Maximum dosing frequency should probably be 3 times per week with at least 24 hours between each dose.
7. Phentolamine—inhibits α-adrenergic receptors. *Phentolamine inhibits detumescence, but it does not induce an erection.* Therefore, it is only used in combination with other ICI agents to help potentiate an erection.
8. Combinations of intracavernosal medications
   a. The efficacy of combination therapy is better than papaverine alone and phentolamine alone, but is similar to alprostadil alone.
   b. Combination therapy is useful in men failing alprostadil ICI or in men who have significant penile pain from alprostadil ICI.
   c. Bi-mix or Tri-mix (triple therapy)—refers to a mixture containing 2 or 3 of the following agents: papaverine, phentolamine, alprostadil.
   d. Initial dose—start at a low dose, then increase the dose slowly if needed. In neurogenic impotence, start with the lowest possible dose.

Penile Prosthesis (Penile Implant)

1. Penile prosthesis requires surgical implantation. Some patients use MUSE with a penile implant to help make the glans more rigid during intercourse.
2. Penile implants are either non-inflatable (also called semi-rigid or malleable) or inflatable. Erosion is more common with non-inflatable prostheses. More manual dexterity is required for an inflatable prosthesis.
3. Satisfaction is high for the patient (60-80%) and the patient's partner (60-80%). Men requiring additional operations are least satisfied.
4. Complications include hematoma, infection, mechanical failure, erosion, and penile shortening.
   a. The chance of prosthesis malfunction requiring reoperation is approximately 6-16% at five years postoperatively.
   b. Infection rate in primary implants is 0-3%. *Staphylococcus is the most common organism cultured.* Antibiotic impregnated implants decrease the risk of infection. Infection rates are higher for immunosuppressed men, poorly controlled diabetes mellitus, and existing cutaneous, systemic, or urinary infection. Infection rates are higher when multiple implants are placed at once or with replacement penile prosthesis. Preoperative antibiotics should cover gram negative and gram positive organisms.

Peyronie's Disease

General Information

1. Peyronie's causes an inelastic scar (called a plaque) in the *tunica albuginea* of the corpora cavernosa. The plaque is usually located on the *dorsal penis.*
2. The cause of Peyronie's disease is unknown. One possible cause is trauma.
3. Peyronie's disease can present with any of the following:
   a. Penile pain—especially with erection.
   b. Penile shortening or deformity—deformities include mild penile curvature, severe angulation, and corporal narrowing ("hourglass deformity"). Penile deformity may prevent penetration during sex.
   c. Penile induration or plaque—many patients do not notice the plaque.
   d. Erectile dysfunction (ED)—ED may occur with Peyronie's. The most common cause of ED in these men is *veno-occlusive dysfunction*. It is unclear if Peyronie's is the cause of ED or simply occurs with ED.
4. Peyronie's is associated with Dupuytren's contracture, Ledderhose's disease of the plantar fascia, and tympanosclerosis of the eardrum.
5. During the acute phase, inflammation peaks, penile deformity and pain may occur, and the plaque is remodeled. After approximately 1 year, pain resolves, remodeling stops, plaque and deformity stabilize, and the chronic phase begins. Plaque calcification indicates that remodeling is complete.
6. Curvature resolves spontaneously in 14%, stabilizes in 46%, and progresses in 40% of men.
7. Evaluation—history and physical exam (note plaques). Penile deformity can be revealed using a patient's photo/drawing of the erection or by direct visualization after intracavernosal injection (ICI). Ultrasound may be used to visualize the plaque.

Treatment—Medical Therapy

1. During the acute phase, treatment is aimed at preventing progression and relieving pain.
2. The 2nd International Consultation on Erectile Dysfunction (2nd ICED) states "The combination of vitamin E and colchicine would appear to be a simple, well-tolerated, evidence based option." Therefore, a combination of vitamin E and colchicine is a reasonable first line treatment.
3. The 2nd ICED reviewed the following medical therapies for Peyronie's disease; however, the efficacy of these therapies is not well-defined.
   a. Surveillance
   b. Vitamin E—2nd ICED conclusion: "...there is no evidence as to the effectiveness of vitamin E, but the drug has been widely used, is free of side effects, and cheap." Some urologists utilize 600-1200 IU po q day, but recent evidence suggests that long-term use (> 1 year) of more than 400 IU per day may increase the risk of heart failure and mortality.
   c. Aminobenzoate potassium (Potaba®) 3 g po q 6 hrs or 2 g po q 4 hrs. Gastrointestinal symptoms can be reduced by dissolving the tablets in liquid and gradually increasing the dose. Benefits may be observed after 2-3 months of therapy. Potaba® is expensive. Initial reports suggested that Potaba® reduced penile pain, but subsequent data showed no improvement in pain. 2nd ICED conclusion: "It would seem that paraaminobenzoate has little benefit in the treatment of Peyronie's disease."
   d. Colchicine 0.6 mg po TID or 1.2 mg po BID after meals—side effects include nausea, vomiting, diarrhea, abdominal pain, thrombocytopenia, anemia, and leukopenia. Monitor complete blood count during therapy. Colchicine is inexpensive. Colchicine appears to improve pain and deformity.

    e. Tamoxifen 20 mg po BID—side effects include alopecia. Some data suggests that tamoxifen may be beneficial in early stage disease. 2nd ICED conclusion: "...there is no evidence for the benefit of tamoxifen in late stage Peyronie's disease."

    f. Intralesional verapamil—other agents (e.g. collagenase, interferon, etc.) have been used, but only verapamil appears to achieve benefit. Verapamil may decrease plaque volume and improve penile deformity. 2nd ICED conclusion: "...studies suggest that there is some benefit from verapamil injection but there is no evidence to suggest that it is superior to other forms of treatment..." The dose is verapamil 10 mg intralesional q 2-4 weeks for 12 weeks.

4. Other therapies that have been used

    a. Pain or anti-inflammatory medications may help.

    b. Penile radiation—appears to be no better than surveillance. 2nd ICED conclusion: "Radiotherapy should probably be avoided because of the possible risk of malignancy and increased risk of erectile dysfunction..."

    c. Extracorporeal shock wave lithotripsy (ESWL) of the plaque—inconsistent data makes conclusions difficult. 2nd ICED conclusion: "There have been no controlled trials but one case controlled study was favorable." ESWL was not recommended by the 2nd ICED.

    d. Topical therapy—an example is topical verapamil. Transdermal therapy alone does not appear to be effective. Electromotive therapy (EMT) has been used to help enhance transdermal delivery. EMT may improve deformity and plaque size; the 2nd ICED concluded that EMT "merits further study."

5. After the acute phase resolves, treatment is based on sexual function. If the patient's sexual function is satisfactory, no therapy is required. If it is not satisfactory, surgery may be indicated.

Treatment—Surgical Therapy

1. *Surgery is performed only after the acute phase resolves* (> 1 year from symptom onset and stable curvature for at least 3-6 months). If remodeling has not finished, the plaque may progress after surgery.

2. ESWL of the plaque—not recommended by the 2nd ICED.

3. In men with satisfactory erections (with or without ED therapy), surgical options for Peyronie's disease include procedures that shorten the contralateral corpora or plaque incision/excision with grafting.

4. Procedures that shorten the contralateral corpora—by shortening the corpora that is contralateral to the plaque, these procedures straighten the penis. They cause less postoperative ED than grafting procedures (2% versus 10%, respectively), but they always cause penile shortening. These procedures are best for men with adequate erections, ample penile length, and a minor penile curvature without significant corporal deformity (e.g. no "hourglass deformity").

    a. Nesbit—an elliptical piece of tunica albuginea is excised from the contralateral (unaffected) corporal body and the defect is closed in the transverse direction. *The Nesbit procedure has a higher long-term success rate than plication and a lower rate of postoperative ED than grafting; therefore, it is usually the procedure of choice.*

    b Corporoplast—a longitudinal incision is made in the tunica albuginea of the contralateral (unaffected) corporal body and the defect is closed in the transverse direction. There is minimal data on this technique.

    c. Plication—the tunica albuginea of the contralateral (unaffected) corporal body is imbricated (folded) in the transverse direction sutured in place.

5. Plaque excision/incision and grafting—with this technique, the defect created by excising or incising the plaque is covered using a graft. Grafting is more likely to cause ED than procedures that shorten the contralateral corpora, but it is less likely to cause penile shortening. This technique is best for men with adequate erectile function and either significant penile shortening or severe corporal deformity.

6. In men with ED not responsive to less invasive erection therapies, penile prosthesis placement can be combined with molding, Nesbit type procedure, or plaque incision/excision with grafting.

REFERENCES

<u>General</u>

AACE medical guidelines for clinical practice for the evaluation and treatment of male sexual dysfunction: a couple's problem - 2003 update. Endocrine Practice, 9(1): 77, 2003.

AACE medical guidelines for clinical practice for the evaluation and treatment of hypogonadism in adult male patients - 2002 update. Endocrine Practice, 8(6): 439, 2002.

Bhasin S, et al: Testosterone therapy in adult men with androgen deficiency syndromes: and Endocrine Society clinical practice guideline. J Clin Endocrinol Metab, 91(6): 1995, 2006.

Broderick, GA: Color duplex Doppler ultrasound: penile blood flow study. Male Infertility and Sexual Dysfunction. Ed. WJG Hellstrom. New York: Springer-Verlag New York, Inc., 1997, pp 367-395.

Broderick GA, Lue TF: Evaluation and nonsurgical management of erectile dysfunction and priapism. Campbell's Urology. 8th Edition. Ed. PC Walsh, et al. Philadelphia: W. B. Sanders Company, 2002, pp 1619-1671.

Kostis JB et al: Sexual dysfunction and cardiac risk (The Second Princeton Consensus Conference). Am J Cardiol, 96: 313, 2005 [update of Am J Cardiol, 86: 175, 2000].

Feldman HA, et al: Impotence and its medical and psychological correlates: results of the Massachusetts male aging study. J Urol, 151: 54, 1994.

Jackson G, Betterridge J, et al: A systematic approach to erectile dysfunction in the cardiovascular patient: a consensus statement. Int J Clin Pract, 53(6): 445, 1999.

Manning M, Juenemann KP: Pharmacotherapy of erectile dysfunction. Male Infertility and Sexual Dysfunction. Ed. WJG Hellstrom. New York: Springer-Verlag New York, Inc., 1997, pp 440-451.

Montague DK, and the AUA guidelines panel: The management of erectile dysfunction: an update. AUA Education and Research, Inc., 2005 (http://www.auanet.org).

Morales A, et al for the Second International Consultation on Erectile Dysfunction: Endocrine aspects of sexual function in men. J Sex Med, 1: 69, 2004.

NIH consensus development panel on impotence: NIH consensus conference – Impotence. JAMA, 270(1): 83, 1993.

Pryor, J, et al: Sexual Dysfunctions in Men and Women. Second International Consultation on Erectile Dysfunction. Ed. TF Lue, et al. Plymouth, United Kingdom: Health Publication Ltd., 2004, pp 391-400.

Svetec DA, Canby ED, Thompson IM, et al: The effect of parenteral testosterone replacement on prostate specific antigen in hypogonadal men with erectile dysfunction. J Urol, 158: 1775, 1997.

The Process of Care Consensus Panel: The process of care model for evaluation and treatment of erectile dysfunction. Int J Impot Res, 11(2): 59, 1999.

PDE5 Inhibitors

Brock, GB, et al: Efficacy and safety of tadalafil for the treatment of erectile dysfunction: results of an integrated analysis. J Urol, 168: 1332, 2002.

Cheitlin MD, et al: ACC/AHA expert consensus document: use of sildenafil (Viagra®) in patients with cardiovascular disease. J Am Coll Cardiol, 33: 273, 1999.

Conti RC, Pepine CJ, Sweeney M: Efficacy and safety of sildenafil citrate in the treatment of erectile dysfunction in patients with ischemic heart disease. Am J Cardiol, 83: 29C, 1999.

Hellstrom WJ, Overstreet JW, et al: Tadalafil has no detrimental effect on human spermatogenesis or reproductive hormones. J Urol, 170: 887, 2003.

Padma-Nathan H, et al: Sildenafil Citrate (Viagra®) and erectile dysfunction: a comprehensive four year update. Urology, 60 (2B): 1-90, 2002.

Porst H, et al: Efficacy and tolerability of vardenafil for treatment of erectile dysfunction in patient subgroups. Urology, 62: 519, 2003.

Zusman RM, Morales A, Glasser DB, et al: Overall cardiovascular profile of sildenafil citrate. Am J Cardiol, 83: 35C, 1999.

Renal Failure and Transplant

Barrou B, et al: Early experience with sildenafil for the treatment of erectile dysfunction in renal transplant recipients. Nephrol Dial Transplant, 18(2): 411, 2003.

Burns JR, Houttuin E, Gregory JG, et al: Vascular-induced erectile impotence in renal transplant recipients. J Urol, 121(6): 721, 1979.

Gittes RF, Waters WB: Sexual impotence: the overlooked complication of a second renal transplant. J Urol, 121(6): 719, 1979.

Salvatierra O Jr, Fortmann JL, Belzer FO: Sexual function of males before and after renal transplantation. Urology, 5: 64, 1975.

Sharma RK, et al: Treatment for erectile dysfunction with sildenafil citrate in renal allograft recipients: a randomized, double blind, placebo controlled, cross over trial. Am J Kidney Dis, 48(1): 128, 2006.

Wieder J: Hormonal politics. Contemporary Urology, 15(9): 12, 2003.

ED after Radical Prostatectomy

Dall'Era JE, et al: Penile rehabilitation after radical prostatectomy: important therapy or wishful thinking? Rev Urol, 8(4): 209, 2006.

Goldstein I: Early penile rehabilitation following radical prostatectomy - overview and rationale. Contemporary Urology, 18 (suppl 1): 1, 2006.

Tsao AK, Nehra A: Early penile rehabilitation following radical prostatectomy - evaluation and treatment strategies. Contemporary Urology, 18 (suppl 1): 1, 2006.

Surgical Treatment of ED

Govier FE: The surgical management of erectile dysfunction utilizing inflatable prosthetic devices. AUA Update Series, Vol. 15, Lesson 10, 1996.

Lewis RW: Venous surgery for impotence. Male Infertility and Sexual Dysfunction. Ed. WJG Hellstrom. New York: Springer-Verlag New York, Inc., 1997, pp 503-513.

Lewis RW, Jordan GH: Surgery for erectile dysfunction. Campbell's Urology. 8th Edition. Ed. PC Walsh, et al. Philadelphia: W. B. Sanders Company, 2002, pp 1673-1709.

Mulhall J, Goldstein I: Arterial surgery for erectile dysfunction. Male Infertility and Sexual Dysfunction. Ed. WJG Hellstrom. New York: Springer-Verlag New York, Inc., 1997, pp 514-528.

Peyronie's Disease

Gholami SS, et al: Peyronie's disease–a review. J Urol, 168: 1234, 2003.

Hellstrom WJG, Bryan WW: Treatment of Peyronie's disease. Male Infertility and Sexual Dysfunction. Ed. WJG Hellstrom. New York: Springer-Verlag New York, Inc., 1997, pp 481-491.

Levine LA, Elterman L: Peyronie's disease and its medical management. Male Infertility and Sexual Dysfunction. Ed. WJG Hellstrom. New York: Springer-Verlag New York, Inc., 1997, pp 474-480.

Lonn E, et al: Effects of long term vitamin E supplementation on cardiovascular events and cancer: a randomized controlled trial. JAMA, 293(11): 1338, 2005.

Miller ER, et al: Meta-analysis: high dosage vitamin E supplementation may increase all cause mortality. Ann Intern Med, 142: 37, 2005.

Pryor J, et al for the Second International Consultation on Erectile Dysfunction: Peyronie's disease. J Sex Med, 1: 110, 2004.

EJACULATORY DISORDERS

Physiology of Ejaculation
1. The normal male physiologic sexual response consists of
   a. Erection—under parasympathetic control (see page 235).
   b. Ejaculation—this is dependant of the following events:
      i. Emission—semen is pushed into the urethra by contraction of the prostate, seminal vesicles, and vas. Emission is induced by sympathetic stimulation of α-adrenergic receptors.
      ii. Bladder neck contraction—closes the bladder neck so semen is not pushed into the bladder. Bladder neck contraction is induced by sympathetic stimulation of α-adrenergic receptors.
      iii. Expulsion of semen out of the urethra by rhythmic contractions of the bulbospongiosus and ischiocavernosus muscles. Semen expulsion is induced by somatic (pudendal nerve) stimulation of nicotinic cholinergic receptors.
   c. Orgasm—the pleasurable sensation associated with ejaculation.
   d. Detumescence—under sympathetic control (see page 235).
2. See page 168 for the neurologic pathways that control these processes.
3. *Most of the semen volume derives from the seminal vesicles.* The prostate, epididymis, vas deferens, and Cowper's glands also contribute fluid.

Classification of Ejaculatory Disorders
1. Unsatisfactory timing of ejaculation
   a. Premature ejaculation (rapid ejaculation)
   b. Delayed ejaculation (retarded ejaculation)
2. Unsatisfactory sensation of ejaculation
   a. Painful ejaculation
   b. Ejaculatory anhedonia
3. Absent ejaculate (Aspermia)
   a. Retrograde ejaculation
   b. Anejaculation
4. Low volume ejaculate
5. Hematospermia

Unsatisfactory Timing of Ejaculation

Delayed (Retarded) Ejaculation
1. Delayed ejaculation is defined as prolonged time to ejaculation despite desire, stimulation, and erection.
2. Causes include psychological, medications (selective serotonin reuptake inhibitors, clomipramine), and sensory neuropathy (e.g. from diabetes).
3. Treatment
   a. Medication induced—switch to a different medication. If the patient requires an antidepressant, nefazodone, citalopram, and fluvoxamine are less likely to cause delayed ejaculation.
   b. Psychologically induced—consider counselling.
   c. Neuropathy—control diabetes.
   d. If the above measures do not work, penile vibratory stimulation using a handheld vibrator, or sensate focus therapy may be tried.

Premature Ejaculation (Rapid Ejaculation)
1. The 2003 AUA guideline defines premature ejaculation as "ejaculation that occurs sooner than desired, either before or shortly after penetration, causing distress to either one or both partners."
2. The etiology of premature ejaculation may include congenital, psychological, and chemical substances (e.g. opioid withdrawal).
3. The diagnosis of premature ejaculation is based on sexual history.
4. Work up—history and physical examination.
5. In men with erectile dysfunction (ED) and premature ejaculation, treat ED first. Premature ejaculation often resolves after treating ED.
6. Treatment—behavioral/psychological therapies
   a. Behavioral/psychological therapies have a high short-term success rate, but long-term success rates are poor.
   b. Squeeze (pause-squeeze) technique—when ejaculation approaches, the male stops sexual activity and squeezes the glans penis until the urge to ejaculate ceases. He then resumes sexual activity.
   c. Start-stop technique—penile stimulation is stopped when ejaculation approaches. Stimulation is resumed when the urge to ejaculate ceases.
   d. Quiet vagina—during intercourse, the female stops moving when her partner approaches ejaculation. Movement is resumed when the urge to ejaculate ceases.
   e. Sensate focus—a technique used to heighten sexual self-awareness by gradually progressing from non-sexual touching to sexual touching to vaginal penetration.
7. Treatment—pharmacological therapies (based on 2003 AUA guidelines)
   a. These therapies are not approved by the FDA for premature ejaculation.
   b. Topical therapy—2.5% Prilocaine + 2.5% lidocaine (EMLA™) cream [Tubes: 5, 30 g]. Apply 2.5 grams of cream to the glans and shaft and cover the penis with a condom. After 20-30 minutes, remove the condom, wipe off the cream, and then initiate sexual relations. The data on this treatment is sparse, but results are encouraging. Side effects include temporary numbness of the penis.
   c. Oral antidepressants—clomipramine seems to generate the longest latency period, but has the most side effects. Paroxetine may be the best initial choice since it is efficacious and has the fewest side effects. If one medication is not working, consider switching to another medication.
      i. Clomipramine—an antidepressant that inhibits serotonin reuptake.
         • Do not use clomipramine with monoamine oxidase inhibitors (MAOI) because this can cause fatal reactions. The patient should be off MAOIs for at least 5 weeks before starting clomipramine.
         • Clomipramine can lower the seizure threshold; therefore, clomipramine should be avoided in patients with a history of seizures or at risk for seizures (e.g. brain lesion, brain damage, alcoholism, or use of other drugs that lower seizure threshold).
         • Side effects include dry mouth, constipation, sleep disturbances, nausea, fatigue, hot flashes, and seizures.
      ii. Selective serotonin reuptake inhibitors (SSRIs)
         • Do *not* use SSRIs in combination with MAOIs because this can cause fatal reactions. The patient should be off MAOIs for at least 5 weeks before starting SSRIs.
         • Side effects of SSRIs include nausea, diarrhea, anorexia, tremor, nervousness, dizziness, sleep disturbances, increased sweating, decreased libido, and dry mouth.
         • Examples—sertraline, fluoxetine, paroxetine.

Oral Therapy For Premature Ejaculation			
Medication	Dose Daily		prn Dose
	Initial Dose	Dose Range	
Clomipramine* (Anafranil)	25 mg po q day	25-50 mg	25 mg po 4-24 hours before intercourse
Sertraline** (Zoloft)	50 mg po q day	25-200 mg	50 mg po 4-8 hours before intercourse
Fluoxetine† (Prozac)	20 mg po q day	5-20 mg	—
Paroxetine†† (Paxil)	20 mg po q day	10-40 mg	20 mg po 3-4 hours before intercourse

   * clomipramine [Caps: 25, 50 mg]
  ** sertraline [Tabs: 25, 50, 100 mg]—at least one week must pass before each
     dose increase. Maximum dose = 200 mg/day.
   † fluoxetine [Caps: 10, 20 mg]—maximum dose = 80 mg/day.
  †† paroxetine [Tabs: 10, 20, 30, 40 mg]—if needed, the dose may be increased
     by 10 mg to a maximum of 60 mg/day. At least 1 week must pass before
     each increase in dose.

Unsatisfactory Sensation of Ejaculation

Painful Ejaculation

1. Complaints often consist of perineal, scrotal, or testicular pain during or shortly after ejaculation.
2. Etiology
   a. Infection/inflammatory–orchitis, epididymitis, prostatitis, urethritis, etc.
   b. Urethral stricture
   c. Obstruction of the vas
      i. After vas ligation—e.g. after vasectomy or radical prostatectomy.
      ii. After hernia repair—may cause scarring and/or kinking of the vas.
   d. Ejaculatory duct obstruction
   e. Seminal vesicle calculi
   f. Psychological
3. Work up
   a. History and physical (including exam of external genitals and prostate).
   b. Urinalysis $\pm$ urine culture.
   c. After inflammatory/infectious causes have been adequately treated, consider obtaining a PSA in patients at risk for prostate cancer.
   d. Consider transrectal ultrasound to check for ejaculatory duct obstruction (e.g. dilated seminal vesicles) and seminal vesicle calculi.
   e. Consider cystoscopy to check for urethral stricture.
4. Treatment
   a. Treat potential inflammatory, infectious, and obstructive causes.
   b. When the above fails, consider non-steroidal inflammatory drugs (NSAIDs).
   c. Other therapies that have been suggested include α-blockers, muscle relaxants, acupuncture, and counselling.
   d. When hernia repair appears to be the cause, pain relief may be achieved by surgical exploration with untethering of the vas and excision of the ilioinguinal nerve.
   e. When seminal vesicle stones are symptomatic, transurethral endoscopic stone removal or seminal vesiculectomy may relieve the pain.

Ejaculatory Anhedonia
 1. Ejaculatory anhedonia is normal ejaculation without pleasure or orgasm.
 2. Possible causes include
   a. Diminished libido
   b. Hormonal or metabolic imbalances (e.g. pituitary, thyroid, or testicular)
   c. Psychological
   d. Medications
 3. Work up
   a. History and physical (including stigmata of testosterone deficiency and prolactin elevation).
   b. Consider obtaining serum testosterone, prolactin, and thyroid function tests. If testosterone is abnormal, consider obtaining LH and FSH.
 4. Treatment—consists primarily of treating any underlying disorder. Consider counselling if a psychologic cause is likely.

Absent Ejaculate (Aspermia)

General Information
 1. Aspermia is when there is no semen expelled from the penis.
 2. Work up of aspermia—see Work Up of Male Infertility, Parts 1 & 2.
 3. Aspermia may be caused by
   a. Anejaculation—failure of emission or failure of the rhythmic contractions of the bulbospongiosus and ischiocavernosus muscle.
   b. Retrograde ejaculation—semen goes into the bladder, not out the penis.
   c. Obstruction
     i. Ejaculatory duct obstruction (see page 276)
     ii. Urethral obstruction distal to the ejaculatory ducts (e.g. stricture)
   d. Hypogonadism

Anejaculation
 1. Anejaculation is failure of emission or failure of the rhythmic contractions of the bulbospongiosus and ischiocavernosus muscle.
 2. Causes
   a. Medications
     i. Alpha blockers—tamsulosin, terazosin, doxazosin, alfuzosin, etc.
     ii. Beta blockers
     iii. Antidepressants—SSRIs, MAOIs, tricyclics such as clomipramine.
     iv. Benzodiazepines
     v. Antipsychotics (α-antagonist activity)—chlorpromazine, haloperidol
     vi. Aminocaproic acid (Amicar®)
   b. Diabetes mellitus—autonomic and somatic neuropathy may impair pathways responsible for erection, emission, and ejaculation.
   c. Sympathetic nerve injury—retroperitoneal lymph node dissection, spinal cord injury, colorectal surgery, abdominal vascular surgery, etc.
   d. Surgical disruption of ejaculatory organs—e.g. radical prostatectomy.
 3. Treatment
   a. If caused by a medication, consider switching to a different medication.
   b. If caused by urethral obstruction, relieve the obstruction.
   c. Control diabetes.
   d. If the above do not resolve the problem, consider either of the following.
     i. Alpha agonist—see Retrograde Ejaculation, Treatment, page 260 for dosage and warnings. Alpha agonists may convert anejaculation to retrograde ejaculation, which allows sperm retrieval from the bladder.
     ii. Penile vibratory stimulation or electroejaculation—see page 285.

Retrograde Ejaculation
1. Defined as partial or complete ejaculation of the semen into the bladder. It is usually caused by failure of the bladder neck to contract adequately. This may result in either low volume ejaculate or absent ejaculate.
2. Causes
   a. Medications
      i. α-blockers—tamsulosin, terazosin, doxazosin, alfuzosin, etc.
         Retrograde ejaculation seems to occur most often with tamsulosin.
      ii. Ganglion Blockers—methyldopa, guanethidine, reserpine.
      iii. Antipsychotics (α-antagonism)—chlorpromazine, haloperidol.
   b. Partial prostate resection/ablation (TURP, TUIP, TUNA, etc.)
   c. Diabetes mellitus—autonomic neuropathy may impair the sympathetic pathways responsible for bladder neck contraction.
   d. Sympathetic nerve injury—retroperitoneal lymph node dissection, spinal cord injury, colorectal surgery, abdominal vascular surgery, etc.
   e. Urethral stricture—may prevent antegrade expulsion of semen.
3. Diagnosis—requires post-ejaculate urinalysis. See page 269 for details.
4. Treatment
   a. If caused by a medication, consider switching to a different medication.
   b. If caused by urethral obstruction, relieve the obstruction.
   c. Control diabetes.
   d. If the above do not resolve the problem, an α-agonist may be tried.
      i. These agents may cause hypertension, cardiac arrhythmias, and urinary retention. They must be used with extreme caution in patients with heart disease.
      ii. α-agonists are not FDA approved for ejaculatory disorders.
      iii. Contraindications—narrow angle glaucoma, severe or uncontrolled hypertension, cardiovascular disease (e.g. coronary artery disease, angina, congestive heart failure, arrhythmia, and recent myocardial infarction), urinary retention, diabetes mellitus, hyperthyroidism or on thyroid replacement, patients on a monoamine oxidase inhibitor (MAOI) or within 14 days of stopping an MAOI, and seizures.
      iv. Doses
         • Pseudoephedrine—60 mg po q day to QID [Tabs: 30, 60 mg]; extended release 120 mg po BID [Tabs: 120 mg]; extended release 240 mg po q day [Tabs: 240 mg].
         • Imipramine 25 mg po BID [Tabs: 10, 25, 50 mg]
         • Ephedrine sulfate 50 mg po QID [Caps: 25, 50 mg]
         • Phenylpropanolamine 25-75 mg po BID—no longer available in the United States. The FDA removed it from the market because of the risk of hemorrhagic stroke.

Low Volume Ejaculate
1. Usually defined as semen volume < 2 cc.
2. Causes
   a. Inadequate semen collection—the most common cause.
   b. Ejaculation within 72 hours of collection—abstinence for ≥ 72 hours before collection is required for an adequate semen sample.
   c. Retrograde ejaculation
   d. Hypogonadism
   e. Finasteride, dutasteride, and other androgen inhibitors
   f. Urethral stricture—may prevent expulsion of semen from the urethra.
   g. Ejaculatory duct obstruction
   h. Congenital bilateral absence of the vas deferens (CBAVD)
3. Work up—see Work Up of Male Infertility, Parts 1 & 2

Hematospermia

1. Hematospermia is blood in the ejaculate.
2. *Hematospermia is almost always benign and self-limiting.*
3. Etiology
   a. Inflammation/infection—prostatitis, seminal vesiculitis, urethritis, epididymo-orchitis, sexually transmitted disease, etc.
   b. Calculi—e.g. stones in the seminal vesicle, prostate, bladder, or urethra.
   c. Trauma to perineum, prostate, or genitals—e.g. cycling, constipation.
   d. Obstruction—urethral stricture, ejaculatory duct obstruction.
   e. Cysts—cysts of the seminal vesicle, ejaculatory duct, prostate, or utricle.
   f. Tumor—e.g. prostate, seminal vesicle, epididymis, or testicular tumors.
   g. Vascular abnormalities—e.g. arteriovenous malformation.
   h. Iatrogenic—after prostate biopsy, vasectomy, TUNA, etc.
   i. Uncontrolled hypertension
4. Evaluation—in most cases a limited evaluation is sufficient.
   a. History and physical examination (especially blood pressure, genital exam, and prostate exam).
   b. Urinalysis $\pm$ urine culture. When indicated, test for sexually transmitted diseases (see page 373) and for tuberculosis (semen and 3 morning urine samples for acid-fast staining and mycobacterial culture).
   c. Evaluate for prostatitis (see page 365).
   d. In men at risk for prostate cancer, consider obtaining a PSA.
5. If hematospermia is persistent, particularly severe, or a significant abnormality is suspected, considered performing transrectal ultrasound, semen culture, cystoscopy, and pelvic or endorectal MRI with gadolinium.
6. Treatment—*in most cases, hematospermia resolves spontaneously and no intervention is required.* When indicated, treat the underlying abnormality.
   a. Cysts of the genital glands or ducts may be aspirated. When the cyst is close to the urethra, transurethral unroofing may be attempted.
   b. Seminal vesicle or prostate stones may be removed by transurethral endoscopic stone removal.
   c. Cases of severe intractable hematospermia may be treated by either embolization or excision of the bleeding structure (e.g. seminal vesiculectomy, excision of embryologic remnants).

REFERENCES

Berkovitch M, Keresteci AG, Koren G: Efficacy of prilocaine-lidocaine cream in the treatment of premature ejaculation. J Urol, 154: 1360, 1995.

Butler JD, et al: Painful ejaculation after inguinal hernia repair. J R Soc Med, 91: 432, 1998.

Munkelwitz R, et al: Current perspectives on hematospermia: a review. J Androl, 18(1): 6, 1997.

Guideline on the pharmacologic management of premature ejaculation. AUA Education and Research, Inc., 2003 (http://www.auanet.org).

Ozgok Y, et al: Endoscopic seminal vesicle stone removal. Urology, 65: 591, 2005. (http://www.goldjournal.net).

Sandlow JI, Williams RD: Surgery of the seminal vesicles. Campbell's Urology. 8th Ed. Ed. PC Walsh, et al. Philadelphia: W. B. Sanders Co., 2002, pp 3876.

Seftel AD, Althof SE: Premature ejaculation. Male Infertility and Sexual Dysfunction. Ed. WJG Hellstrom. New York: Springer-Verlag New York, Inc., 1997, pp 356-361.

Shenassa B, Hellstrom WJG: Understanding ejaculatory disorders. Contemporary Urology, 13(4): 51, 2001.

Wang LJ, et al: Arterial bleeding in patients with intractable hematospermia and concomitant hematuria: a preliminary report. Urology, 68: 938, 2006.

MALE INFERTILITY

Normal Reproductive Physiology
1. Spermatogenesis—transformation of germ cells into spermatozoa.
   a. The terms sperm and spermatozoa are interchangeable.
   b. Spermatogenesis occurs in the *seminiferous tubules* of the testicles and takes *74 days* to complete.
   c. Spermatogenesis consists of 3 steps (2n = diploid; 1n = haploid)
      ① Mitosis (2n → 2n): converts spermatogonia to spermatocytes.
      ② Meiosis (2n → 1n): consists of two sub-steps:
      • 1st meiotic division:
         primary spermatocytes (2n) → secondary spermatocytes (2n)
      • 2nd meiotic division:
         secondary spermatocytes (2n) → spermatids (1n)
      ③ Spermiogenesis (1n → 1n): converts spermatids to spermatozoa.

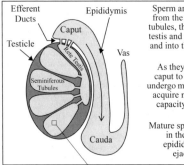

Sperm are transported from the seminiferous tubules, through the rete testis and efferent ducts, and into the epididymis
↓
As they travel from caput to cauda, sperm undergo maturation (they acquire motility & the capacity to fertilize)
↓
Mature sperm are stored in the cauda of epididymis until ejaculation

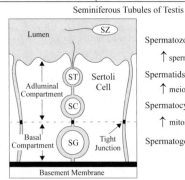

Seminiferous Tubules of Testis

SG = spermatogonia; SC = spermatocyte; ST = spermatid, SZ = spermatozoa; 1n = haploid; 2n = diploid

    d. Spermatogenesis requires
       i. Follicle stimulating hormone (FSH)—stimulates Sertoli cells to maintain normal spermatogenesis.
      ii. High intraluminal levels of testosterone in the seminiferous tubules (circulating testosterone are less important).
     iii. Sertoli cells—Sertoli cells support spermatogenesis. Tight junctions between Sertoli cells form the *blood-testis barrier* and separate the basal compartment from the adluminal compartment. The blood-testis barrier isolates the tubular environment and protects the haploid ("non-self") germ cells from the immune system.
     iv. Testis temperature approximately 34°C—this temperature, which is lower than the core body temperature of 37°C, is achieved by locating the testes outside the abdomen and in the scrotum.
    e. As spermatogenesis progresses, germ cells move from the basal compartment to the adluminal compartment. When spermatogenesis is complete, spermatozoa are shed into the lumen and transported toward the caput (head) of the epididymis.
  2. Sperm maturation—*as spermatozoa travel through the epididymis, they acquire motility and the capacity to fertilize (a process called maturation).* When sperm reach the cauda (tail) of the epididymis, maturation is complete. *The epididymis is the earliest location where one finds sperm with motility and the capacity to fertilize.*
  3. Sperm storage—mature sperm are stored in the tail of the epididymis until ejaculation.
  4. Ejaculation—see Physiology of Ejaculation, page 256.
  5. Capacitation—although sperm in the tail of the epididymis have the capacity to fertilize, their activity is inhibited by factors in the male genital tract. *Capacitation is activation of the sperm's fertilizing capacity and it occurs in the female genital tract (uterus or fallopian tube).*
  6. Hyperactivation (hyperactivated motility)—hyperactivation is triggered by capacitation and results in a sudden increase in sperm motility. Thus, *the greatest sperm motility occurs in the female genital tract.*
  7. Acrosome reaction—when a sperm reaches the ovum, the sperm head releases enzymes that clear a path through the outer layers of the ovum, This allows the sperm to enter the ovum and fertilize it.
  8. Fertilization—fusion of gametes. During the normal reproductive process, *fertilization occurs in the fallopian tube.*
  9. Zona reaction—upon fertilization, this reaction alters the permeability of the zona pellucida so that another sperm cannot enter the ovum.
 10. Implantation—after being transported from the fallopian tube, *the fertilized egg implants onto the endometrium of the uterus.*

General Information About Infertility
  1. Infertility is usually defined as the *inability of a couple to achieve pregnancy after one year of regular unprotected intercourse.*
  2. Primary infertility affects approximately 15% of couples.
  3. Male factor infertility is present in 50% of infertile couples.

Source of Infertility in an Infertile Couple	
Female Only	50%
Male Only	30%
Male & Female	20%
Total	100%

Male factor present in 50% of infertile couples

4. Indications for infertility evaluation
   a. For a couple—evaluation is warranted if the couple does not achieve pregnancy after 1 year of regular unprotected intercourse. The evaluation should be conducted earlier if
      i. The male partner has risk factors for infertility.
      ii. The female partner has risk factors for infertility.
      iii. The couple questions their fertility.
   b. For a male without a current partner—evaluate a male who questions his fertility or who is at risk for infertility.
5. Risk factors for infertility
   a. Male—See Etiology and Risk Factors for Male Infertility, page 265.
   b. Female
      i. *One of the most important factors is maternal age > 35* (fertility declines after age 35 and is limited after age 40). All of the following factors decline as maternal age increases: fertility, the chance of retrieving oocytes, and the pregnancy rate with ICSI.
      ii. Other risks factors—endometriosis, pelvic inflammatory disease, tubal ligation, polycystic ovarian syndrome, etc.
6. *The most common cause of male infertility is a varicocele.*
7. The most common cause of low ejaculate volume is incomplete collection.
8. If cancer patients are interested in having children in the future, they are encouraged to cryopreserve sperm before beginning cancer therapy (e.g. chemotherapy, radiation, etc.)

Classification of Male Infertility

1. Primary or secondary
   a. Primary—the man was never fertile.
   b. Secondary—the man was fertile, but became infertile.
2. Location of the abnormality
   a. Pre-testicular (hormonal)—hypogonadal hypogonadism, see page 273.
   b. Testicular (abnormal sperm production)—see page 274.
   c. Post-testicular (impaired delivery of sperm from testis to female)
      i. Obstruction or agenesis of the genital ducts—see page 276.
      ii. Ejaculatory disorders—see Ejaculatory Disorders, page 256.
      iii. Improper placement of semen into the vaginal vault—causes include penile curvature, hypospadias, and improper coital technique.
3. Sperm parameters
   a. Normospermia—normal semen parameters.
   b. Azoospermia—no sperm in the ejaculate (must be confirmed by examining 2 centrifuged semen samples). See Azoospermia below.
   c. Oligospermia—sperm concentration < 20 million/ml.
   d. Asthenospermia—impaired sperm motility.
   e. Teratospermia—abnormal sperm morphology.
   f. Aspermia—no ejaculate (semen volume = 0 ml).
4. Obstructive or non-obstructive
   a. Obstructive—partial or complete obstruction of the genitourinary tract.
   b. Non-obstructive—all portions of the genitourinary tract are patent.

Azoospermia

1. Two separate semen specimens must be centrifuged at maximum speed (preferably at $\geq 3000g$) for 15 minutes and the pellets examined. Azoospermia is diagnosed if sperm are absent from both pellets.
2. Causes of azoospermia
   a. Pre-testicular—see page 273.
   b. Testicular—see page 274.
   c. Post-testicular—see page 276 and page 256.

3. Pre-testicular and post-testicular causes of azoospermia can often be rectified. Testicular causes are usually irreversible (although azoospermia from a varicocele can sometimes be corrected).
4. Azoospermia is often classified as obstructive (ductal defect) or non-obstructive (testicular defect).
5. Obstructive azoospermia
   a. Risk factors—inguinal surgery, prolonged catheterization, sexually transmitted diseases, genitourinary infections, prostatitis, urethral instrumentation, cystic fibrosis, and congenital absence of the vas.
   b. Physical findings—normal size testis. Absent vasa, epididymal induration, or inguinal scars may be identified.
   c. Common causes—ejaculatory duct obstruction, congenital bilateral absence of the vas deferens (CBAVD), and cystic fibrosis.
   d. In azoospermic men with normal testis size, palpable vasa, and low volume ejaculate, obtain a transrectal ultrasound. These men probably have ejaculatory duct obstruction.
6. Non-obstructive azoospermia
   a. Risk factors—gonadotoxin exposure, cryptorchidism, testicular torsion, and mumps orchitis.
   b. Physical findings—atrophic testes and normal vasa.
   c. Common causes—maturation arrest, hypospermatogenesis, Sertoli only syndrome, and Klinefelter's syndrome.
   d. Patients with non-obstructive azoospermia or severe oligospermia should be informed that they may have chromosomal abnormalities or Y microdeletions that can be passed on to their children.

Coital Technique to Achieve Pregnancy

1. Lubricants
   a. Most lubricants impair sperm motility (including K-Y jelly, Lubrifax, Keri lotion, petroleum jelly, and saliva)
   b. Lubricants that do not impair sperm motility include safflower oil, vegetable oil, peanut oil, and raw egg white.
2. Frequency—the optimum frequency of intercourse is *every other day* around the time of ovulation (based on the fact that sperm survival in normal cervical mucus is approximately 2 days).
3. Timing—the highest likelihood of conception occurs when intercourse is performed within 48 hours of ovulation. Thus, it is best to engage in intercourse every other day starting 2 days before ovulation. Monitoring the female's ovulatory cycle helps ensure optimal timing.
4. Avoid spermacides and contraceptives.

Etiology and Risk Factors for Infertility

Medical Conditions That May Cause Male Infertility

1. Varicocele—see page 275.
2. Ejaculatory disorders—see page 256.
3. Prostatitis
4. Hormonal disorders
   a. Hypogonadotropic hypogonadism—see page 273.
   b. Hypergonadotropic hypogonadism—see page 274.
5. Febrile illness—may impair spermatogenesis for up to 3 months.
6. Thyroid disorders—hypothyroidism can increase prolactin. Hyperthyroidism can cause pituitary abnormalities, testicular abnormalities, and elevated estradiol.

7. Cirrhosis
8. Diabetes mellitus—autonomic neuropathy can cause anejaculation, retrograde ejaculation, and erectile dysfunction. Vascular insufficiency may also contribute to erectile dysfunction.
9. Post-puberty mumps orchitis—mumps orchitis does not affect fertility when contracted before puberty. If contracted after puberty, mumps orchitis can cause infertility by damaging the seminiferous tubules (impairs spermatogenesis) and the Leydig cells (causes testosterone deficiency). Orchitis usually develops a few days after the parotiditis. Mumps and mumps orchitis are prevented mainly by the mumps vaccine.
10. Myotonic dystrophy
11. Young's syndrome—thick epididymal secretions cause obstructive azoospermia. Bronchiectasis, sinusitis, and normal vasa are present.
12. Cystic fibrosis—obstructive azoospermia from congenital bilateral agenesis of the vas. Bronchiectasis, sinusitis, and pancreatic disease are present. For genetic aspects of cystic fibrosis and CBAVD, see Genetic Abnormalities, CFTR Mutation, page 267.
13. Congenital bilateral absence of the vas deferens (CBAVD)—obstructive azoospermia from congenital bilateral agenesis of the vas. Lung and pancreatic disease are absent. For genetic aspects of cystic fibrosis and CBAVD, see Genetic Abnormalities, CFTR Mutation, page 267.
14. Immotile cilia syndrome—there are several variants of this syndrome, but the most well known is Kartagener's syndrome.
15. Kartagener's syndrome—bronchiectasis, sinusitis, *situs inversus*, and *immotile spermatozoa* with a normal sperm concentration. The diagnosis can be confirmed by electron microscopy of the axoneme.

Syndrome	Cilia	Vas Deferens	Bronchiectasis & Sinusitis
Young's	Motile	Normal but obstructed by secretions	Yes
Cystic Fibrosis	Motile	Absent	Yes
CBAVD	Motile	Absent	No
Kartagener's	Immotile	Normal & Patent	Yes

Gonadotoxins
1. Pharmacologic and therapeutic agents
   a. Antibiotics—nitrofurantoin, ofloxacin, tetracycline (can lower testosterone by 20%), erythromycin.
   b. Drugs of abuse—cigarettes, marijuana, alcohol, steroids, opiates, heroin, methadone, cocaine.
   c. Other drugs—cimetidine, spironolactone, allopurinol, dilantin, tricyclic antidepressants (increase prolactin), colchicine, LHRH agonists, androgens, sulfasalazine.
   d. Chemotherapy (often has a dose dependant effect)—nitrogen mustards, cyclophosphamide, and chlorambucil are particularly damaging.
   e. Radiation
2. Occupational or environmental agents
   a. Heavy metals—lead, mercury, cadmium, boron, and boric acid.
   b. Agricultural chemicals—DDT, DBCP, methyl chloride, etc.
   c. Hyperthermia—hot tub, sauna, warm baths.
   d. Cigarette smoke
3. Biological or physiological agents
   a. Genital infection/inflammation—tuberculosis, epididymo-orchitis, etc.
   b. Genital ischemia—torsion, trauma.
   c. Hyperthermia—fever, varicocele.

Genetic Abnormalities
1. The three most common genetic causes of male infertility are
   a. Mutations of the cystic fibrosis transmembrane conductance regulator (CFTR) gene.
   b. Y chromosome microdeletions.
   c. Karyotypic abnormalities resulting in impaired testicular function.
2. CFTR mutation
   a. CFTR is located on chromosome 7.
   b. Cystic fibrosis, CBAVD, and unilateral absence of the vas may be associated with CFTR mutations.
   c. Almost all men with cystic fibrosis have CBAVD and the CFTR mutation. Approximately 60% of men with CBAVD have known mutations in CFTR. In unilateral absence of the vas, CFTR mutations are infrequent. Since there may be CFTR mutations that we cannot detect yet, it is best to assume that men with CBAVD have a CFTR mutation and may be carriers for cystic fibrosis.
3. Y chromosome microdeletions
   a. Approximately 10-15% of men with azoospermia or severe oligospermia have Y chromosome microdeletions.
   b. Most microdeletions occur in the *AZF regions on the long arm of the Y chromosome (Yq11)*. The AZF regions (AZFa, AZFb, and AZFc) contain genes that are necessary for normal spermatogenesis. The *DAZ gene* is an example of a gene in the AZFc region that is necessary for normal fertility. (AZF = AZoospermia Factor, DAZ = Deleted in AZoospermia)
   c. Y microdeletions have been found in fertile and subfertile men who have fathered children. Thus, a Y microdeletion does not always result in infertility.
   d. If a man has a Y chromosome microdeletion, all of his sons will inherit the abnormality; therefore, the sons may be infertile. It is unclear if the Y microdeletion can cause additional health problems.
   e. The assay for Y chromosome microdeletions does not necessarily detect all Y chromosome abnormalities. If a genetic defect is suspected, the patient should be offered genetic counseling.
4. Karyotypic abnormalities
   a. *The most common karyotypic abnormality in infertile men is Klinefelter's syndrome,* which accounts for 66% of chromosomal abnormalities (see page 274).
   b. Approximately 7% of infertile men have karyotypic abnormalities. A lower sperm count correlates with a higher rate of karyotypic abnormalities.

Frequency of Karyotypic Abnormalities in Infertile Men	
Azoospermia	10-15%
Oligospermia	5-7%
Normospermia	1%
All Infertile Men	7%

5. Patients with a known or suspected genetic defect should be warned that they might transmit genetic abnormalities to their children.
   a. Men with non-obstructive azoospermia or severe oligospermia should be informed that they might have a chromosomal abnormality.
   b. Men with CBAVD should be informed that they probably have a CFTR mutation; therefore, they may be carriers of cystic fibrosis.
   c. All patients with a known or suspected genetic abnormality should be offered genetic counseling.

Work Up

1. History
   a. Prior episodes, evaluation, or treatment for infertility.
   b. Duration of infertility—how long have they been trying to conceive?
   c. Did the male get someone pregnant before? Has the female partner ever been pregnant? Has the female partner had a miscarriage?
   d. Coital timing, frequency, lubrication, etc.
   e. Febrile illness within 1-3 months or recent stressful condition.
   f. Genitourinary infections—sexually transmitted diseases (STDs), post-puberty mumps orchitis, epididymitis, orchitis, prostatitis, etc.
   g. Sexual history—STDs, erections, ejaculation, libido, orgasm, etc.
   h. Hormone related symptoms—gynecomastia, galactorrhea, hot flashes, loss of libido, loss of facial and body hair, etc.
   i. Age of puberty—precocious puberty may indicate adrenogenital syndrome; delayed puberty may indicate Klinefelter's or hypogonadism.
   j. Cryptorchidism or testicular torsion
   k. Trauma to the genitals, pelvis, or perineum.
   l. Current medical illness—diabetes mellitus, cystic fibrosis, etc.
   m. Recurrent respiratory infections—as with Kartagener's syndrome, Young's syndrome, and cystic fibrosis.
   n. Prior surgery—vasectomy, vasectomy reversal, inguinal hernia repair, orchiectomy, orchiopexy, prostate surgery, RPLND, etc.
   o. Hyperthermia—febrile illness, sauna, hot tub, warm baths.
   p. Gonadotoxin exposure—radiation, chemotherapy, pesticides, etc.
   q. Medications—prescription and non-prescription.
   r. Social history—tobacco, drug abuse, occupational exposures.
   s. Family history
   t. Other—chronic headaches (pituitary tumor), anosmia (Kallmann's syndrome), symptoms of thyroid disorder.
2. Physical Examination
   a. Genitals—Tanner stage, presence of vasa, testis size and location, penile plaques or curvature, location of the meatus, varicocele, etc.
      Seminiferous tubules comprise most of the testis volume; therefore, atrophy or damage to the tubules causes atrophy of the testicles.
   b. Prostate—especially signs of prostatitis.
   c. Secondary sexual characteristics
   d. Evidence of endocrine dysfunction—gynecomastia, galactorrhea, etc.
   e. Neurologic—visual fields, anal sphincter tone, neuropathy, etc.
   f. General—abnormal skin pigmentation (may be related to adrenal disease), thyroid exam, abdominal exam (especially liver), etc.
3. Semen Analysis
   a. Proper collection
      i. Obtain semen at least 3 months after a febrile illness or extremely stressful event.
      ii. Obtain at least 2 specimens with 7 to 21 days between specimens. If semen parameters vary considerably between specimens, consider obtaining additional specimens.
      iii. Masturbation is the preferred method for obtaining sperm. For specimens obtained by intercourse, special collection condom must be used to prevent damage to the sperm. Avoid lubricants.
      iv. Ensure complete collection of the ejaculate.
      v. Abstinence of > 48 hours but ≤ 7 days before ejaculation.
      vi. Avoid gonadotoxins, especially alcohol.
      vii. Once the specimen is obtained, store it at body temperature (by keeping it in a pocket close to the body) and analyze it within 1 hour.

b. Liquefaction—normal semen liquefies at room temperature within 60 minutes. Semen parameters are usually measured after liquefaction.

c. Reference values for semen analysis (based on World Health Organization 1999 & AUA Best Practice Policy 2001)

Semen Analysis Reference Values	
Ejaculate Volume	≥ 2 ml
pH	≥ 7.2
Sperm Concentration	≥ 20 million/ml
Total Sperm Count	≥ 40 million/ejaculate
Motility	$\geq 50\%$
Forward Progression	> 2 (scale = 0 - 4)
Normal Morphology	$> 50\%$ (WHO 1987) $> 30\%$ (WHO 1992) $> 14\%$ (WHO 1999)
Sperm Agglutination	< 2 (scale = 0 - 3)
Viscosity (Consistency)	< 3 (scale = 0 - 4)
Leukocytes (WBCs)	< 1 million/ml
Immunobead Test or MAR test	$< 50\%$ motile sperm bound to particles
Vitality	$\geq 50\%$ alive
Fructose content	≥ 13 μmol/ejaculate

d. Selected aspects of semen analysis abnormalities
   i. Men may be infertile when their semen parameters are normal and men may be fertile when their semen parameters are abnormal.
   ii. Sperm agglutination refers to sperm stuck or bound together and may indicate the presence of antisperm antibodies.
   iii. Semen WBCs imply the presence of a genitourinary infection.

4. Endocrine evaluation
   a. Endocrine evaluation is indicated when any of the following are present:
      i. Low sperm concentration, especially < 10 million/ml.
      ii. Erectile dysfunction or decreased libido.
      iii. Other findings that suggest an endocrinopathy.
   b. *The minimum endocrine evaluation is serum testosterone and follicle stimulating hormone (FSH).* If the testosterone is abnormal, obtain total and bioavailable testosterone, prolactin, and luteinizing hormone (LH). When the values are inconclusive, a repeat measurement may be helpful.
   c. Hormone profiles should be drawn in the morning.
   d. Marked elevation of FSH suggests abnormal spermatogenesis, but abnormal spermatogenesis can occur when FSH is normal. *Primary testicular failure is usually present when FSH is ≥ 2 times normal.*

5. Scrotal ultrasound—indicated when the physical examination of the scrotum is inadequate, ambiguous, or suspicious. Scrotal ultrasound should not be used to screen for non-palpable varicoceles.

6. Post-ejaculation urinalysis
   a. Indicated if semen volume is < 2 cc in the absence of CBAVD.
   b. After centrifuging the urine for 10 minutes at a minimum of 300g, examine the pellet under the microscope to see if sperm are present.
   c. There is no consensus on the number of sperm required to diagnose retrograde ejaculation. However, the following guidelines may be used:
      i. The presence of *any* sperm in patients with azoospermia or aspermia suggests retrograde ejaculation.
      ii. In patients with low volume ejaculate and oligospermia, a *significant number* of sperm must be present.

7. Transrectal ultrasound (TRUS)
   a. TRUS is indicated in infertile men with low sperm count (azoospermia or oligospermia), low volume ejaculate, and palpable vasa.
   b. Abnormal findings that suggest ejaculatory duct obstruction
      i. Seminal vesicle diameter ≥ 15 mm in the anterior-posterior plane.
      ii. Dilated ejaculatory ducts.
      iii. Calcifications in the ejaculatory duct.
      iv. Midline cystic structure(s) in the prostate.
8. Genetic screening
   a. All patients with a known or suspected genetic abnormality should be offered genetic counseling and genetic testing.
   b. Indications for genetic screening
      i. Before utilizing sperm from a man with CBAVD, CFTR mutation testing should be offered to the male and female.
      ii. Before undergoing assisted reproductive technologies (ART), a man with non-obstructive azoospermia or severe oligospermia should be offered karyotyping and Y chromosome analysis.
      iii. Perform genetic tests when the clinical findings suggest the presence of a genetic disorder (ambiguous genitalia may indicate intersex, small testis and gynecomastia may indicate Klinefelter's, etc.).
9. Testis Biopsy
   a. Testis biopsy for infertility usually consists of two elements: diagnostic biopsy and sperm harvesting for assisted reproduction.
   b. Testis biopsy is usually an open procedure, but may be performed percutaneously. Percutaneous biopsy seems best suited for verifying the presence of spermatogenesis before performing an open testis biopsy and can be used to "map" the location of spermatogenesis within the testis so that open biopsies can be directed toward these locations.
   c. There is no consensus regarding whether testis biopsies should be unilateral or bilateral. In most cases, unilateral biopsy is adequate (especially when a symmetric process is anticipated). Bilateral biopsy may be considered when an asymmetric process is suspected.
   d. Ways of identifying the presence of sperm intraoperatively
      i. Touch prep cytology—fresh testis tissue is touched to and moved across a slide. The slide is placed in cytofixative and stained (e.g. H&E, Papanicolaou). Touch prep cytology allows immediate intraoperative identification of mature sperm.
      ii. Wet prep—after fresh testis tissue is placed on a slide, a drop of Ringer's lactate and a cover slip are applied. Since no fixative is used, motile sperm can be identified. Even if the wet prep shows no sperm, send the tissue to the embryologist for sperm extraction because sperm can be still be found 30% of the time.
   e. What should be done with the biopsy specimens?
      i. Send a specimen to pathology for diagnosis—place the tissue in Bouin's or Zenker's solution. Formalin should not be used.
      ii. Send a specimen to the embryologist for sperm harvesting—place the tissue in sperm washing media.
      iii. Cryopreserve testicular tissue for use in future IVF/ICSI cycles.
   f. When sperm harvesting is indicated, this is one method of conducting the biopsy—*start with the testis that is more normal in size, shape, and consistency.* If normal spermatogenesis or mature sperm are identified on the touch prep or wet prep, no further sampling is needed. If no sperm are found on the initial sample, additional biopsies on the same side may be obtained. If sperm are still not present, consider performing a biopsy of the other testis.

   g. Indications for testis biopsy
      i. Harvesting sperm for ICSI.
      ii. Distinguishing obstructive from non-obstructive azoospermia—testis
          biopsy is indicated in patients with azoospermia or severe
          oligospermia (< 1 million sperm/ml), normal testis size, at least one
          palpable vas, and normal or near normal FSH. If the biopsy shows
          normal spermatogenesis, then obstructive azoospermia is present.
10. Vasography
   a. Identifies obstruction in the vas and ejaculatory ducts.
   b. It should not used to determine the presence epididymal obstruction.
      Epididymal obstruction is diagnosed by surgical exploration.
   c. Vasography should only be performed if you are prepared to repair
      ductal obstruction during the same procedure.
   d. Indications—men with azoospermia or severe oligospermia, normal
      FSH, and spermatogenesis on testis biopsy or epididymal aspiration.
   e. Technique
      i. Do not inject into the proximal vas (toward the testicle) because it
         can injury the epididymis and testicle.
      ii. Use a 24 gauge angiocath or blunt tip needle to gently inject contrast
          into the distal vas (toward the abdomen) during fluoroscopy.

Specialized Semen and Sperm Tests

   NOTE: These tests are indicated only when identifying the cause of male
   infertility will determine treatment.
1. Semen fructose—fructose is produced by the seminal vesicles. When
   semen fructose is low, an ejaculatory duct or seminal vesicle abnormality
   may be present (e.g. obstruction, agenesis, hypoplasia). Normal semen
   fructose is ≥ 13 μmol per ejaculate.
2. Semen leukocytes (WBCs)
   a. To differentiate WBCs from immature germ cells, special assays should
      be performed (rather than only microscopic inspection).
   b. If more than 1 million WBCs/ml are found in the semen, the patient
      should be evaluated for infection of the genitourinary tract. Consider
      cultures of the urethra, urine, semen, and expressed prostatic sections.
   c. Elevated semen WBCs are associated with impaired sperm function and
      reduced motility.
3. Anti-sperm antibodies
   a. Anti-sperm antibodies in the serum or seminal plasma are not clinically
      significant. *Antibodies bound to sperm are clinically significant.*
   b. *IgG and IgA antibodies are present in the male genital tract,* whereas
      IgM antibodies are not present. Therefore, anti-sperm antibody testing
      should detect IgG and IgA. *Testing for IgM is unnecessary.*
   c. Risks for anti-sperm antibodies
      i. Genital duct obstruction
      ii. History of genital infection
      iii. Traumatic or surgical disruption of the testis or genital tract (e.g.
          vasectomy, vasectomy reversal, ruptured testis, testis biopsy)
   d. Testing for antibodies is indicated when any of the following are present.
      i. Abnormal post-coital test (especially the presence of shaking sperm)
      ii. Impaired sperm motility with normal sperm concentration
      iii. Sperm agglutination
      iv. Unexplained infertility
   e. The immunobead test or the mixed antiglobulin reaction (MAR) test can
      be used to detect antibodies bound to sperm. These tests are normal
      when < 50% of motile sperm are bound to particles/beads.

4. Sperm vitality

   a. *These tests determine if sperm are alive by assessing the integrity of the cell membrane.* Live sperm have an intact cell membrane.

   b. Vitality testing is especially helpful when immotile sperm are present because it distinguishes between live sperm (immotile because of a motility defect) and dead sperm (immotile because they are dead).

   c. Viability testing can be done by the *hypo-osmotic swelling test* (live sperm undergo tail swelling) or using *special dyes* such as eosin (live sperm do not stain).

5. Post-coital test

   a. This test examines for the *presence and motility of sperm in the cervical mucus* after intercourse and is dependant on the *sperm-cervical mucus interaction.*

   b. Abnormal cervical mucus or abnormal sperm-cervical mucus interaction is rarely a cause of infertility.

   c. This test may be indicated when both the male and female have a normal infertility work up.

   d. Intercourse is performed just before the expected time of ovulation. The cervical mucus is collected within 9-24 hours thereafter (using a non-lubricated speculum) and examined under the microscope. A sample of fluid is also obtained from the posterior vagina to verify that sperm were deposited in the vagina.

   e. The most important finding on the post-coital test that indicates normal sperm-cervical mucus interaction is the *presence of sperm with rapidly progressive motility*; therefore, this finding argues against cervical factors as a possible cause of infertility.

   f. Causes of an abnormal test

      i. Poor timing (not performing the test just before ovulation)—*poor timing is the most common cause of an abnormal test.*

      ii. Abnormal semen—infection, high viscosity, abnormal sperm, etc.

      iii. Antisperm antibodies—"shaking" sperm on post-coital test may indicate the presence of antibodies bound to the sperm.

      iv. Abnormal cervical mucus

      v. Abnormal vaginal environment—infection, lubricants, spermacides.

      vi. Sperm were not deposited in the vagina—absence of sperm indicates that the ejaculate was not deposited in the vagina. This may occur with hypospadias, penile curvature, and improper coital technique.

   g. There is no standard method for conducting the post-coital test or for interpreting its results. Thus, the use of this test is controversial.

6. Sperm penetration assay (zona free hamster oocyte test)

   a. Human sperm can penetrate into hamster oocytes when the zona pellucida of the oocyte is removed.

   b. *A low rate of sperm penetration into hamster ova suggests that infertility is caused by a sperm defect* that impairs one of the following processes: capacitation, acrosome reaction, fusion with oolemma, or incorporation into the ooplasm.

   c. This test may be indicated when the male has a normal semen analysis and the female is normal.

   d. This test does not consistently predict the success of IVF; therefore, its clinical usefulness is limited.

7. Acrosome reaction assay—these assays typically measure the number of sperm that undergo spontaneous acrosome reaction and the number of sperm in which the acrosome reaction can be induced. However, the clinical relevance of these assays has not been established.

Hormone Profiles

	Testosterone	LH	FSH	Prolactin
Hypogonadotropic hypogonadism	↓	↓	↓	N
Hypergonadotropic hypogonadism	↓	↑	↑	N
Prolactinoma	↓	N/↓	N/↓	↑
Germ cell failure (e.g. Sertoli only)	N	N	↑	N
Androgen resistance	↑	↑	N/↑	N

↓ = below normal; ↑ = above normal; N = Normal

Pretesticular Causes of Infertility

Hypogonadotropic Hypogonadism (Secondary Testicular Failure)
1. Low testosterone caused by low gonadotropins—see table above.
2. When hypogonadism is present early in life, the patient may have undescended testes, micropenis, and absent puberty.
3. Causes
   a. Kallmann's syndrome—*the most common cause of hypogonadotropic hypogonadism*. This X-linked defect causes hypothalamic dysfunction and absent GnRH secretion. Clinical manifestations include *hypogonadotropic hypogonadism, anosmia, and absent puberty.*
   b. High prolactin—from prolactinoma, renal failure, hypothyroidism, antipsychotic drugs (especially phenothiazines), stress, estrogens, etc.
   c. Pituitary or hypothalamic damage (from tumor, trauma, prior surgery).
   d. Prader-Willi syndrome—absent GnRH secretion, hypogonadotropic hypogonadism, obesity, small hands and feet, mental retardation, hypotonic musculature, and short stature.
   e. Laurence-Moon-Bardet-Biedl syndrome—hypogonadotropic hypogonadism, polydactyly, and retinitis pigmentosa.
   f. Medications—LHRH agonists or antagonists, exogenous androgens (exogenous androgens suppress intratesticular androgen production and reduce gonadotropins, but serum testosterone may be normal or high).
4. Evaluation includes a serum prolactin level to rule out prolactinoma.
5. Treatment of men with elevated prolactin—see Prolactinoma below.
6. Treatment of men with normal prolactin—testosterone replacement may improve hypogonadism (see page 246), but it suppresses spermatogenesis and intratesticular testosterone production. Gonadotropins are required to initiate spermatogenesis (see page 279).

Prolactinoma
1. Prolactinoma is a prolactin secreting pituitary tumor. These patients usually have hypogonadotropic hypogonadism and high prolactin. When prolactin is minimally elevated, gonadotropins may be normal.
2. Symptoms—decreased libido, erectile dysfunction, infertility, visual field defects, headache, galactorrhea, and gynecomastia. *The most common presenting symptoms in men are decreased libido and erectile dysfunction.*
3. If hypogonadotropic hypogonadism is present or symptoms suggest prolactinoma, obtain serum prolactin. If prolactin is elevated, obtain a brain & pituitary MRI. See Work Up of Male Infertility Part 2.
4. Men usually present with macroadenomas (tumors > 10 mm in size), whereas women usually present with microadenomas (< 10 mm in size).
5. A prolactin antagonist (e.g. bromocriptine) is usually the initial treatment. If response to medication is inadequate, consider radiation or surgery.
6. Testosterone may not normalize after prolactinoma treatment. If symptoms of hypogonadism persist, check a serum testosterone. If it is low, consider testosterone (see page 246) or gonadotropin (see page 279) replacement.

Testicular Causes of Infertility

Hypergonadotropic Hypogonadism (Primary Testicular Failure)
1. Low testosterone is caused by a testis defect.
2. Hormone profile—see table on page 273.
3. When hypogonadism presents early in life, the patient may have undescended testes, micropenis, and absent puberty.
4. Causes
   a. Klinefelter's syndrome—see below.
   b. Noonan syndrome (male Turner's syndrome)—short stature, webbed neck, low set ears, cubitus valgus, and undescended testis. Their karyotype is usually 46, XY.
   c. Absent testes (e.g. orchiectomy, testes never developed)
   d. Non-functioning testes (e.g. cryptorchidism, atrophy, torsion, etc.)

Klinefelter's Syndrome
1. These patients have an *extra X chromosome (47 chromosomes, XXY)*, which can arise from chromosomal non-disjunction in either parent.
2. Characteristics of patients with Klinefelter's syndrome
   a. *Small firm testes, gynecomastia, azoospermia, and hypogonadism.*
   b. Elevated serum estradiol levels, which causes gynecomastia.
   c. Sclerosis of the seminiferous tubules, which typically results in azoospermia and small testicles. However, sperm with normal karyotype may be found on testis biopsy. These sperm can be extracted for ICSI.
   d. Hormone profile usually shows low testosterone, high FSH, normal or high LH, and high estradiol.
3. There is no therapy to improve sperm quality in these patients. Testosterone replacement may worsen their infertility, but may alleviate symptoms of hypogonadism.
4. Klinefelter's has an increased risk of *extra-gonadal* germ cell tumors.

Sertoli Cell Only Syndrome (Germ Cell Aplasia)
1. Germ cells (sperm and their precursors) are absent. In other words, there are only Sertoli cells in the seminiferous tubules. Normal numbers of Leydig cells are present outside the tubules in the interstitium.
2. Sperm can be retrieved during a testis biopsy in 25-50% of patients with Sertoli-cell only syndrome; therefore, they are candidates for sperm retrieval and intracytoplasmic sperm injection (SR + ICSI).
3. These men have azoospermia. They may have small testes and high FSH.

Maturational Arrest
1. Maturation arrest is present when spermatogenesis is halted at a particular stage, resulting in failure to complete spermatogenesis. The point of arrest is constant within a patient, but varies between patients. The most common points of arrest are at the primary spermatocytes and late spermatids.
2. These patients present with oligospermia or azoospermia.
3. Sperm can be retrieved during a testis biopsy in 50-75% of patients with maturational arrest; therefore, they are candidates for SR + ICSI.

Gonadotoxin Exposure—see page 266

Genetic Abnormalities—see page 267.

Cryptorchidism—Oligospermia occurs in 25% of men with unilateral cryptorchidism and in 50% of men with bilateral cryptorchidism. The higher the cryptorchid testis, the more severe the testicular dysfunction.

Ultrastructural Sperm Defects—see Immotile Cilia Syndromes, page 266.

Testis Infection—(e.g. mumps orchitis, see page 266).

Varicocele

1. A varicocele is a group of dilated veins in the pampiniform plexus.
2. Varicoceles are more common on the *left side.*
3. In the general population, 15% of men have a left varicocele. In subfertile men, 40% have a left varicocele. *Varicocele is the most common finding in subfertile men.* However, not all varicoceles cause infertility.
4. Non-palpable varicoceles have not been shown to cause infertility. Thus, screening for non-palpable varicoceles (with ultrasound) is not indicated.
5. *A unilateral varicocele can affect both testicles,* causing bilateral testis atrophy and damage.
6. A varicocele may indicate the presence of a renal tumor, especially when the varicocele is right sided or had a rapid or recent onset. When this is the case, consider obtaining imaging to look for a renal mass.
7. Effects of varicocele
   a. Varicoceles can cause pain.
   b. Testis damage—manifestations include
      i. Infertility—the classic semen abnormalities (called a *"stress pattern"*) include *decreased motility, low sperm count, and increased abnormal forms* (especially increased tapered forms and immature cells). However, *the most common finding is decreased motility.*
      ii. Testicular atrophy
      iii. Biopsies may show hypospermatogenesis, incomplete maturational arrest, and peritubular fibrosis.
8. Physical examination
   a. Examine the scrotum with the patient in the supine and upright positions and while he performs a Valsalva maneuver in the standing position.
   b. A varicocele feels like a *"bag of worms"* and should become more prominent when the patient is standing or performing a Valsalva.
   c. Grade—Grade I is small, not grossly visible, and palpated only during Valsalva. Grade II is moderate size, not grossly visible, but easily palpable in the standing position. Grade III is large and grossly visible.
9. Indications for considering varicocele repair
   a. Symptomatic varicocele
   b. Palpable varicocele and abnormal semen analysis—when evaluating an an infertile couple, varicocele repair should be considered when the female is normal or has a potentially correctable cause of infertility.
   c. Adolescents with a varicocele and ipsilateral small testis—repairing a varicocele in adolescents has been shown to reverse testis atrophy, but it does not seem to prevent fertility problems.
   d. For varicocele repair versus assisted reproduction, see page 287.
10. Surveillance
    a. Young men with a palpable varicocele and normal semen analysis should have a semen analysis every 1-2 years to see if semen parameters decline.
    b. Children (or adolescents who are not sexually active) with a varicocele and normal testis size should have annual objective measurements of testis size to detect a decrease in testis size.
11. Varicocele repair (varicocelectomy)
    a. Surgical approaches
       i. Open surgery ± magnification—inguinal, subinguinal, or retroperitoneal.
       ii. Laparoscopic surgery (ligation of retroperitoneal spermatic vein)
       iii. Percutaneous embolization

b. *The microsurgical inguinal or subinguinal approach has the lowest recurrence rate.*

Approach	Recurrence Rate	Hydrocele
Retroperitoneal	15%	7%
Inguinal	≤ 15%	≤ 30%
Laparoscopic	≤ 11%	12%
Radiographic embolization	≤ 25%	0%
Microsurgical (inguinal or subinguinal)	≤ 0.6%	0%

c. Side effects
   i. In the retroperitoneal, inguinal, and laparoscopic approaches, *the most common complication is hydrocele.* In the microsurgical approaches, the most common complication is *hematoma* (hydrocele is rare). Hydrocele is also rare with radiographic embolization.
   ii. Scrotal edema, recurrent varicocele, testis atrophy, infection, etc.
d. *Varicocele repair improves semen quality in approximately 70% of men and appears to improve fertility.* Semen quality should improve by 3-6 months after varicocele repair.
e. After varicocele repair in an infertile male, perform semen analysis every three months until either one year has passed or pregnancy occurs.

Posttesticular Causes of Infertility

Ejaculatory Duct Obstruction (EDO)
1. TRUS findings of a dilated seminal vesicle (SV), dilated ejaculatory duct, or a midline prostate cyst suggests partial or complete EDO.
2. EDO can exist with normal appearing seminal vesicles. If the seminal vesicles are normal by ultrasound but EDO is suspected, do #3 below.
3. TRUS guided SV aspiration and seminal vesiculography can definitively diagnose obstruction and identify its location. *Normally, the SV contains no sperm. If the SV aspirate contains sperm, EDO is probably present.*
4. Semen analysis in patients with EDO may show
   a. Low semen volume (most of the semen volume comes from the SVs)
   b. Low fructose content—see Semen Fructose, page 271.
   c. pH < 7.0—fluid from the SV is basic.
   d. Low number of sperm in ejaculate.
   e. Reduced coagulation and thin watery consistency—proteins responsible for coagulation are made by the seminal vesicles.
5. Treatment
   a. Transurethral resection of the ejaculatory ducts (TURED)
      i. Improved semen quality occurs in approximately 52%. The pregnancy rate is 29%.
      ii. Complications—epididymitis (urine refluxes into epididymis), worse genital duct obstruction (unilateral obstruction becomes bilateral), hematuria, post void dribbling (urine refluxes in and out of SVs), etc.
   b. Ejaculatory duct dilation

Other Ejaculatory Disorders—see page 256.

Epididymal Obstruction
1. Diagnosis requires surgical exploration (whereas absence of the vas is diagnosed by physical exam and does not require surgical exploration).
2. In men who have *not* undergone vasectomy, the epididymis is the *most common location of genital duct obstruction*
3. In men who have undergone vasectomy, a secondary epididymal obstruction may develop from back-pressure in the ductal system.
4. Treatment includes vasoepididymostomy or assisted reproduction.

Vasectomy

1. Vasectomy is surgical ligation of the vas, usually for birth control. It is less expensive and less risky than tubal ligation in the female.
2. Recommendations from the British Andrology Society (BAS):
   a. The couple should use other forms of birth control until 2 consecutive ejaculates show azoospermia.
   b. Semen testing should begin 4 months after vasectomy *and* after at least 24 ejaculations.
3. Recent data suggests that it may be sufficient to start semen testing 3-4 months after vasectomy and to use at least one azoospermic ejaculate as criteria for stopping birth control.
4. Results of the semen analysis at 4 months after vasectomy
   a. Azoospermia (~80% of men)
   b. Non-motile sperm (~20% of men)—these are usually sperm that were down-stream of the vasectomy site and they often clear with more ejaculations. The BAS recommends that when there is a persistent low number of non-motile sperm by ≥ 7 months after vasectomy and after ≥ 24 ejaculations, the patient may be informed that the risk of pregnancy is low and the couple may stop using other forms of birth control.
   c. Motile sperm (< 1%)—if *motile sperm* are present 3 or more months after vasectomy, then the procedure failed. Vasectomy may be repeated.
5. Complications—the most common complication is *scrotal hematoma or hematocele* (see page 311). Uncommon complications include infection, chronic pain (see page 361), spermatocele, and vasectomy failure (< 1%). Recanalization (re-connection) is rare (< 1%) and usually occurs within a few months after vasectomy (but can occur years later). *Interposition of the vasal fascia between the cut vasal ends can reduce recanalization.*
6. Vasectomy does not increase the risk of prostate cancer.

Congenital Absence of the Vas (Vasal Agenesis)

1. Diagnosed by physical examination. Surgical exploration is not necessary.
2. When a vas is absent, other ipsilateral Wolffian duct structures, such as the seminal vesicle and ureter, may be absent. If the ureter is absent, the kidney fails to develop. Therefore, *these patients may have ipsilateral agenesis of the seminal vesicle, ureter, and kidney.* If they have a solitary kidney, they should be warned about the risk of contact sports.
3. Unilateral vasal agenesis—these patients should undergo
   a. Renal ultrasound—25% have ipsilateral renal agenesis.
   b. If they are azoospermic, perform transrectal ultrasound to rule out agenesis of the contralateral seminal vesicle and abdominal vas (which has been associated with unilateral vasal agenesis).
   c. Testing for the CFTR mutation (mutations are rarely found in these men)
4. Bilateral Vasal Agenesis
   a. Bilateral vasal agenesis occurs in the following syndromes.
      i. Congenital bilateral absence of the vas deferens (CBAVD)
      ii. Cystic fibrosis (CF)—most men with CF have absent vasa.
   b. Both CF and CBAVD are associated with mutations of CFTR.
   c. 60% of men with CBAVD have known mutations in CFTR. Since there may be CFTR mutations that we cannot detect yet, it is best to assume that men with CBAVD have a CFTR mutation and are carriers of CF.
   d. Men with absent vasa may have absent or atrophic seminal vesicles; thus, they may have a similar presentation to EDO (see page 276).
   e. These patients should undergo
      i. Renal ultrasound—10% have unilateral renal agenesis.
      ii. The female should be offered testing for CFTR mutations.
      iii. The couple should undergo genetic counseling.

Selected Treatments for Infertility

General Recommendations for Improving Fertility
1. Avoid smoking, alcohol, and drugs (cocaine, marijuana, steroids, etc.)
2. Intercourse every other day starting 2 days before ovulation.
3. Avoid spermacides and lubricants
4. Avoid hyperthermia (hot tub, sauna, etc.)

Options for Having Children
1. Normal intercourse
2. Adoption
3. Assisted reproductive technologies (ARTs)—ARTs manipulate gametes to induce pregnancy. See page 287.
4. Donor insemination (DI)—when male factor infertility is present or the genetic risks associated with the male are too great, another male may donate sperm for insemination.

Vasectomy Reversal
1. Preoperative factors that predict a successful vasectomy reversal
   a. First attempt at reversal (repeated attempts are less successful).
   b. Short interval from vasectomy to reversal (especially < 15 years). *Time since vasectomy is the most important predictive factor.* A long interval from vasectomy to reversal results in a lower chance of pregnancy.

Primary Vasovasostomy

Years Since Vasectomy	Sperm in Semen	Pregnancy Rate
< 3	97%	76%
3-8	88%	53%
9-14	79%	44%
≥ 15	71%	30%

From Belker et al: J Urol 145: 505, 1991

All Forms of Vasectomy Reversal

Procedure	Sperm in Semen	Pregnancy Rate
Primary VV	71-97%	30-76%
Primary VE	37-86%	20-40%
Repeat (VV or VE)	75%	20-40%

VV = vasovasostomy;
VE = vasoepididymostomy

2. Intraoperative factors that predict a successful vasectomy reversal
   a. Presence of sperm in the vasal fluid
   b. Higher sperm quality in the vasal fluid
   c. Clear vasal fluid—cloudy, thick, or creamy fluid has a worse outcome.
   d. Presence of a sperm granuloma at the vasectomy site.
   e. Long distance from epididymis to vasectomy site (especially >2.7 cm)
3. For vasectomy reversal versus assisted reproduction, see page 287.
4. Technique
   a. Consider sperm retrieval & cryopreservation during vasectomy reversal.
   b. Fluid from the proximal vas (side closest to testis) is examined. If sperm are present, perform vasovasostomy (VV). If sperm are absent, explore the epididymis. If epididymal obstruction is present, perform VE.
   c. Inguinal VV can be performed for vasal injury caused by hernia repair.
5. Postoperatively
   a. After vas reversal, avoid ejaculation for approximately 3 weeks.
   b. *Motile sperm are usually seen within 6 months after VV. Motile sperm may take up to 15 months to appear after VE.* If azoospermia is still present after these intervals, a repeat reconstruction should be offered.
   c. Semen analysis is performed 6-8 weeks postoperatively and then every 2-3 months until the semen parameters are stable. Semen analysis can be continued every 3-6 months until pregnancy.
6. Success rate—see charts above. *On average, pregnancy occurs 12 months after vasectomy reversal.*

Hormonal Therapies for Idiopathic Oligospermia

1. Gonadotropin releasing hormone (GnRH)—GnRH is best suited for men with hypogonadotropic hypogonadism. In men with oligospermia, there is no proven benefit; therefore, its use is best confined to clinical trials.
2. Gonadotropic agents—these agents are best suited for men with hypogonadotropic hypogonadism to help restore spermatogenesis. In men with oligospermia, there is no proven benefit; therefore, their use is best confined to clinical trials. Examples include FSH, human chorionic gonadotropin (HCG), and human menopausal gonadotropin (HMG).
3. Anti-estrogens—by blocking estrogen receptors, these drugs prevent estrogen from exerting negative feedback on the pituitary and hypothalamus, which ultimately increases GnRH, LH, FSH, and testosterone. Anti-estrogens may improve spermatogenesis. The desired hormonal effect is maximal FSH and LH without increasing testosterone above normal. After 3 weeks of therapy, obtain a hormone profile. If the desired effect is not achieved, consider increasing the anti-estrogen dose or changing to another drug. If the desired effect is achieved, check a semen analysis in 3 months. Most studies show that anti-estrogens do not improve pregnancy rates.
   a. Clomiphene—initial dose: Clomiphene 25 mg po q day (may increase to 50 mg/day) [Scored Tabs: 50 mg]. Side effects include dermatitis, impaired libido, and rarely gynecomastia.
   b. Tamoxifen—initial dose: 10 po mg BID (may increase to 20 mg po BID)
4. Aromatase inhibitors—aromatase, an enzyme in fat, converts testosterone to estrogen. Thus, obese men may have estrogen-induced infertility. Studies show conflicting results regarding the efficacy of these drugs. Testolactone is an example of this type of drug.
5. Testosterone rebound therapy—large doses of parenteral testosterone are used to inhibit the pituitary gland, intratesticular testosterone production, and spermatogenesis. When the testosterone is stopped, the system rebounds and spermatogenesis may improve over baseline. This treatment is usually not used anymore because it can cause permanent azoospermia.

Non-hormonal Therapies for Idiopathic Infertility

1. Pentoxyphylline—a phosphodiesterase inhibitor that improves sperm motility and the acrosome reaction in vitro. It is unclear if pentoxyphylline improves sperm quality in vivo or if it alters pregnancy rates.
   Dose: pentoxyphylline 400 mg po TID for 3-6 months.
2. Non-steroidal anti-inflammatory drugs (NSAIDs)—prostaglandins may inhibit spermatogenesis and sperm motility. NSAIDS are inhibitors of prostaglandin synthesis; and therefore, may improve semen quality. Example: indomethacin 150 mg/kg/day po for 3-6 months.
3. Alpha blockers—may improve spermatogenesis by chemical sympathectomy. Treat for at least 6 months. See page 113.
4. Proxeed™—this is a dietary supplement that contains L-carnitine fumarate, acetyl-L-carnitine HCl, fructose, and citric acid. These substances appear to be important for sperm maturation and motility. Improvements in semen quality may occur after at least 74 days of treatment. Dose: Proxeed™ one packet (mixed in at least 4 ounces of juice) po BID.

Work Up Of Male Infertility - Part 1

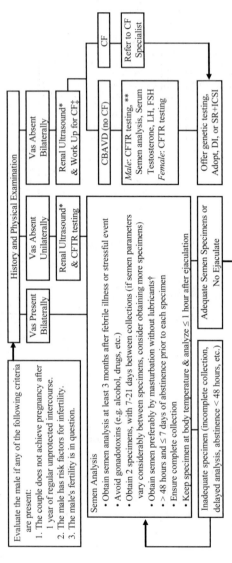

Evaluate the male if any of the following criteria are present:
1. The couple does not achieve pregnancy after 1 year of regular unprotected intercourse.
2. The male has risk factors for infertility.
3. The male's fertility is in question.

History and Physical Examination

Vas Present Bilaterally

Vas Absent Unilaterally
Renal Ultrasound* & CFTR testing

Vas Absent Bilaterally
Renal Ultrasound* & Work Up for CF‡

CF
Refer to CF Specialist

CBAVD (no CF)
Male: CFTR testing, **
Semen analysis, Serum Testosterone, LH, FSH
Female: CFTR testing

Offer genetic testing, Adopt, DI, or SR+ICSI

Semen Analysis
• Obtain semen analysis at least 3 months after febrile illness or stressful event
• Avoid gonadotoxins (e.g. alcohol, drugs, etc.)
• Obtain 2 specimens, with 7-21 days between specimens (if semen parameters vary considerably between specimens, consider obtaining more specimens)
• Obtain semen preferably by masturbation without lubricants†
• > 48 hours and ≤ 7 days of abstinence prior to each specimen
• Ensure complete collection
• Keep specimen at body temperature & analyze ≤ 1 hour after ejaculation

Adequate Semen Specimens or No Ejaculate

Inadequate specimen (incomplete collection, delayed analysis, abstinence < 48 hours, etc.)

DI = donor insemination
CF = cystic fibrosis
CFTR = CF transmembrane conductance regulator gene (testing looks for a mutation)
SR+ICSI = sperm retrieval & intracytoplasmic sperm injection
CBAVD = congenital bilateral absence of vas deferens

* Check for unilateral renal agenesis (occurs in 25% of men with unilateral vasal agenesis and in 10% with bilateral vasal agenesis)
‡ Work up includes sweat test.
† When masturbation is objectionable, semen should be obtained by intercourse using a special condom.
** If the female is CFTR negative, testing in the male is optional.

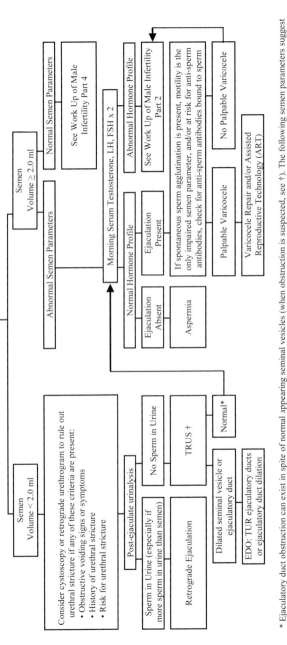

* Ejaculatory duct obstruction can exist in spite of normal appearing seminal vesicles (when obstruction is suspected, see †). The following semen parameters suggest obstruction: volume < 2.0 cc, pH < 7, reduced fructose, reduced semen coagulation (watery consistency), and reduced sperm count.

† TRUS guided seminal vesicle aspiration and seminal vesiculography can help make a more definitive diagnosis and determine the site of obstruction.

FSH = follicle stimulating hormone; LH = luteinizing hormone; TRUS = transrectal ultrasound; TUR = transurethral resection; EDO = ejaculatory duct obstruction

The following text appears within the flowchart (image):

Semen Volume < 2.0 ml

Consider cystoscopy or retrograde urethrogram to rule out urethral stricture if any of these criteria are present:
• Obstructive voiding signs or symptoms
• History of urethral stricture
• Risk for urethral stricture

Post-ejaculate urinalysis

Sperm in Urine (especially if more sperm in urine than semen)

No Sperm in Urine

Retrograde Ejaculation

TRUS †

Dilated seminal vesicle or ejaculatory duct

Normal*

EDO: TUR ejaculatory ducts or ejaculatory duct dilation

Semen Volume ≥ 2.0 ml

Abnormal Semen Parameters

Normal Semen Parameters

See Work Up of Male Infertility Part 4

Morning Serum Testosterone, LH, FSH x 2

Normal Hormone Profile

Abnormal Hormone Profile

See Work Up of Male Infertility Part 2

Ejaculation Absent

Ejaculation Present

Aspermia

If spontaneous sperm agglutination is present, motility is the only impaired semen parameter, and/or at risk for anti-sperm antibodies bound to sperm

Palpable Varicocele

No Palpable Varicocele

Varicocele Repair and/or Assisted Reproductive Technology (ART)

Work Up of Male Infertility - Part 2

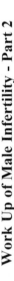
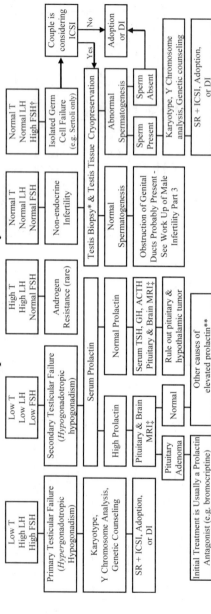

* Vasogram should not be done during the testis biopsy unless you are prepared to fix a vasal obstruction at the same time.

** Conditions that can increase prolactin include renal failure, antipsychotic drugs (especially phenothiazines), hypothyroidism, estrogen exposure, and stress.

† Especially FSH ≥ 2 times normal.

‡ With and without gadolinium.

SR = sperm retrieval; ICSI = intracytoplasmic sperm injection; DI = donor insemination; T = testosterone; LH = luteinizing hormone; GH = growth hormone
FSH = follicle stimulating hormone; TSH = thyroid stimulating hormone; ACTH = adrenocorticotropic hormone; MRI = magnetic resonance imaging

Work Up of Male Infertility - Part 3

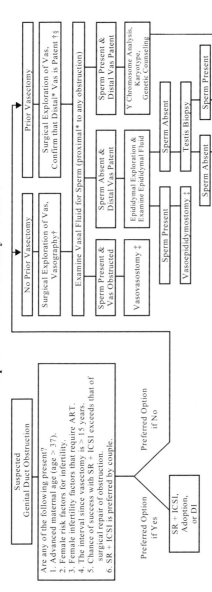

SR = sperm retrieval; ICSI = intracytoplasmic sperm injection;
DI = donor insemination; ART = artificial reproductive technologies
‡ Offer cryopreservation of sperm during these procedures.

* Proximal refers to the portion of vas that is closest to the testicle. Distal refers to the portion of vas that is closest to the abdomen.

† Inject gently into the distal vas using a 24 gauge angiocath or blunt tip needle. Do not inject the proximal vas because it can injure the epididymis and testicle. If the saline flows freely, the distal vas is patent.

§ To confirm a patent vas, inject 5 cc of saline into the distal vas. Alternatively, inject methylene blue into the distal vas when a catheter is in the bladder. If the urine turns blue, the distal vas is patent. If obstruction exists, vasography can identify the site of obstruction.

Work Up of Male Infertility - Part 4

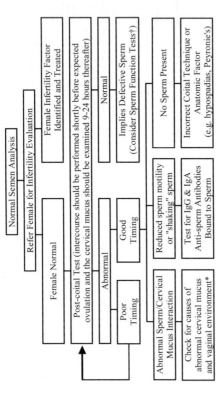

* Potential causes include vaginal infection, lubricant use, female hormone imbalance, and medications that affect mucus (e.g. decongestants).
† Examples include sperm penetration assay and acrosome reaction assay.

Steps of Assisted Reproduction

Ovarian Stimulation (Superovulation or Ovulation Induction)
1. Ovarian stimulation is hormonal stimulation of the ovaries to *produce multiple follicles per ovulatory cycle*. Stimulation is achieved with human menopausal gonadotropin (HMG) or clomiphene citrate.
2. Complications
   a. *Multiple gestations*, ectopic pregnancy, and spontaneous abortion.
   b. May increase the risk of ovarian cancer.
   c. Ovarian hyperstimulation syndrome (OHSS)—manifestations include ovarian enlargement, ascites, abdominal distension and pain, diarrhea, nausea/vomiting, dyspnea, peritonitis and hemorrhage from follicle rupture, thrombosis, and death. OHSS occurs in a moderate form ($\leq 4\%$ of cases) and a severe form ($\leq 0.2\%$ of cases).

Oocyte Retrieval
1. Oocytes are retrieved by ultrasound guided transvaginal follicle aspiration.
2. Complications include bleeding, infection, bowel perforation, etc.

Sperm/Semen Retrieval
Consider sperm cryopreservation during retrieval. Retrieval methods include
1. Masturbation/normal ejaculation—the preferred method of sperm retrieval.
2. Retrieval from bladder after retrograde ejaculation—catheterize the patient, empty the bladder, instill sperm washing media, and remove the catheter. After ejaculation, catheterize the patient to retrieve the sperm.
3. Penile vibratory stimulation (PVS)
   a. PVS permits sperm retrieval from men who are anejaculatory.
   b. A vibrator, which is applied to the penis, stimulates normal ejaculation reflexes, including sympathetic emission pathways (T10-L2) and somatic ejaculation pathways (S2-S4). Therefore, *the ejaculation reflex pathways must be intact for PVS to induce ejaculation*. In men who are anejaculatory from RPLND or spinal cord injury below T10, PVS usually does not work because the reflex pathways are disrupted.
   c. *PVS is well suited for anejaculatory men with spinal cord injury above T10.* In spinal cord injured men, PVS can cause autonomic dysreflexia.
4. Electroejaculation (EEJ)
   a. EEJ permits sperm retrieval from men who are anejaculatory.
   b. Using a transrectal probe, an electrical current is delivered to the pelvis. EEJ often induces retrograde ejaculation, although antegrade ejaculate may be observed. Retrieve the sperm from the bladder.
   c. EEJ is not dependant on the ejaculation reflex. Thus, EEJ can be used successfully after RPLND or spinal cord injury below T10.
   d. EEJ is painful; therefore, men with intact pelvic sensation may require anesthesia (spinal or general).
   e. In spinal cord injured men, EEJ can induce autonomic dysreflexia.
   f. EEJ is best for men who fail PVS or who are anejaculatory from RPLND.
5. Seminal vesicle aspiration—can be used for ejaculatory duct obstruction.
6. Vas aspiration—this is usually done during vasectomy reversal.
7. Epididymal sperm retrieval—used primarily for *obstructive azoospermia.*
   a. PESA (percutaneous epididymal sperm aspiration)—percutaneous aspiration of fluid from the epididymis. Since PESA yields less fluid that MESA, less sperm are available for cryopreservation.
   b. MESA (microsurgical epididymal sperm aspiration)—aspiration of fluid from the epididymis during an open surgery. MESA yields enough sperm to permit cryopreservation.

8. Testicular sperm retrieval–used for *non-obstructive azoospermia.*
   a. TESA (percutaneous testicular sperm aspiration)—percutaneous aspiration of fluid from the testis.
   b. TESE (testicular sperm extraction)—percutaneous or open biopsy is used to obtain testicular tissue, from which sperm is extracted.

Semen Processing
1. If semen is retrieved, it must be processed before using it for ART. Semen processing removes the seminal plasma and yields concentrated motile sperm.
2. The yield of sperm from semen processing may determine which ART can be used.
3. The two most common methods for semen processing are
   a. Swim up method
      i. A culture medium is layered over the liquefied semen. Motile sperm swim up into the culture medium. These motile sperm can be collected and used for ART.
      ii. Swim up has a high yield of motile sperm in men with adequate sperm motility; however, it has a low yield in men with poor motility.
   b. Density gradient method
      i. Semen is placed into a gel suspension and centrifuged. Motile sperm migrate to a layer of the suspension and are collected for ART.
      ii. *In cases of severe oligospermia and/or poor sperm motility, the density gradient method is preferred over the swim up method because it yields more sperm, higher quality sperm, and sperm with a greater fertilizing capacity.*

Fertilization (In Vitro)
1. In vitro fertilization (IVF) can be accomplished by
   a. Conventional method (incubation)—incubating sperm with oocytes. Lower pregnancy rates occur with poor sperm quality and low sperm count. For optimal results, the minimum recommended sperm counts are
      • 25,000-50,000 motile sperm per oocyte in men with normal fertility.
      • 0.5 to 1.0 million motile sperm per oocyte in men with infertility.
   b. Micromanipulation—microscopic manipulation of the gametes to induce fertilization. This is the most common form is ICSI.
      i. Intracytoplasmic sperm injection (ICSI)—injecting a single live sperm directly into an oocyte using a micropipette. *ICSI bypasses the process of sperm penetration through the outer layers of the oocyte.* ICSI requires only one live sperm per oocyte (a motile sperm is preferred). For details on ICSI and its indications, see page 288.
      ii. Other—subzonal insemination and partial zonal dissection. These techniques have been supplanted by ICSI.

Embryo Transfer (ET)
1. ET is the transfer of fertilized oocytes into the female reproductive tract. ET can be accomplished by
   a. Intrauterine (transcervical) transfer—after a catheter is inserted into the cervical os, embryos are injected *though the catheter and into the uterus.* This approach does not require patent fallopian tubes. Transcervical transfer is often referred to as "conventional IVF."
   b. Intrafallopian transfer—embryos are transferred *into the fallopian tube using laparoscopy.* It requires at least one patent fallopian tube. Zygote intrafallopian transfer (ZIFT) is an example of this technique.
2. Multiple embryos are usually transferred to the female. However, transferring multiple embryos increases the risk of multifetal gestations.

Assisted Reproductive Technologies (ARTs)

Assisted reproductive technologies (ARTs) manipulate male and female gametes to induce pregnancy. Examples include ICSI, IVF, ZIFT, and GIFT.

ART or Surgical Correction of Male Factor Infertility?
1. In cases when surgical correction of male factor infertility is possible (varicocele or obstructive azoospermia), ART may still be the preferred option. Important factors to consider when deciding whether to perform ART or surgical repair include
   a. Number of children desired—if only one pregnancy is desired, ART may be best. Surgical repair often cures infertility permanently, permitting the couple to have multiple children by intercourse.
   b. Cost—currently, ICSI is more expensive than surgical repair.
   c. Maternal age—if the female is > 37 years old, ICSI may be better. Since advanced maternal age (especially age > 40) reduces the success of ICSI, it may be inadvisable to delay ART while waiting to see if surgical treatment of the male's infertility is successful.
   d. Maternal infertility—some causes of female infertility may require ART.
   e. Preference of couple
   f. Time since vasectomy—vasectomy reversal $\geq$ 15 years after vasectomy achieves a low rate of pregnancy (30%) and ICSI may be preferable.
   g. When varicocele is present, not undergoing varicocele repair can cause a progressive deterioration in semen parameters and may impair the man's fertility in the future.
   h. Risks of ART and ICSI compared to risks of surgical repair.
2. Surgical repair of male infertility can be combined with ART, which may permit retrieval of more sperm and better quality sperm for ART.

Intrauterine Insemination (IUI)
1. By strict definition, IUI is not an ART because the female gametes are not manipulated. IUI is included in the section for organizational purposes.
2. Raw semen should not be placed directly into the uterus. Concentrated sperm (semen without seminal plasma) can be placed in the uterus.
3. IUI is performed during ovulation by inserting a catheter into the cervical os and injecting concentrated sperm though the catheter into the uterus. *The cervical mucus barrier is bypassed* and *fertilization occurs in vivo.*
4. IUI is most effective for infertility caused by
   a. Conditions that impair semen deposition into the vagina (e.g. hypospadias, penile curvature, and retrograde ejaculation).
   b. Abnormal cervical mucus or abnormal sperm-cervical mucus interaction.
5. For IUI, a minimum of 5 million motile sperm/ml are needed for best results. Higher pregnancy rates are achieved with better quality sperm and with ovarian stimulation. For pregnancy rates with IUI, see page 289.
6. With suboptimal sperm, IUI is less effective than IVF+ET.
7. IUI is the least expensive form of the assisted reproduction.
8. Risks are minimal. Ovarian stimulation increases the risks (see page 285).

Gamete Intrafallopian Transfer (GIFT)
1. The female usually undergoes ovarian stimulation.
2. Oocytes and semen are retrieved. The semen is processed into concentrated sperm. Then, the gametes (concentrated sperm and oocytes) are transferred into the fallopian tube by laparoscopy.
3. GIFT requires at least one patent functional fallopian tube.
4. Fertilization occurs *in vivo*; therefore, it cannot be directly observed.
5. For pregnancy rates in male factor infertility, see page 289.

In Vitro Fertilization and Embryo Transfer (IVF+ET)
1. IVF+ET consists of in vitro fertilization (by micromanipulation or incubation) and embryo transfer (into the uterus or fallopian tube).
2. "Conventional IVF" refers to transcervical transfer of embryos *into the uterus*, and often implies that fertilization occurs by incubation of gametes.
3. The female usually undergoes ovarian stimulation.
4. As maternal age increases, the success rate of IVF+ET decreases.
5. Pregnancy rate with IVF+ET for male factor infertility—see page 289.
6. Risks
   a. Complications of ovarian stimulation—see page 285.
   b. Complications of oocyte retrieval—see page 285.
   c. Increased risk of multifetal pregnancy when multiple embryos are used.
   d. When used with ICSI, see risks of ICSI below.

Intracytoplasmic Sperm Injection (ICSI)
1. Indications
   a. Severe oligospermia or azoospermia (obstructive or non-obstructive)
   b. Immotile or poorly motile sperm.
   c. Prior failure of IVF+ET using incubation of gametes.
2. Requires only a single live sperm per oocyte (motile sperm are preferred). A single sperm is injected directly into the ova using a micropipette. Thus, *ICSI bypasses sperm penetration through the outer layers of the ova.*
3. Important factors that determine the success of ICSI
   a. Maternal age—as maternal age increases, the success of ICSI decreases. *Maternal age seems to be the most important predictor of ICSI success.*
   b. The experience of the infertility team.
   c. Sperm motility and morphology are probably not important, but the sperm must be alive.
4. Risks
   a. Complications of ovarian stimulation—see page 285.
   b. Offspring have a *4-fold increase in sex chromosome abnormalities.* Couples undergoing ICSI may have a high rate of sex chromosome abnormalities (which can cause their infertility); therefore, their children may inherit these genetic defects. Thus, it is not clear if the higher rate of sex chromosome abnormalities is caused by ICSI or by transmission of these abnormalities from the parents.
   c. There appears to be *no difference in autosomal chromosome defects and congenital malformations* when comparing ICSI and intercourse.
   d. Increased risk of spontaneous abortion and ectopic pregnancy—it is not clear if this is caused by ICSI or the underlying fertility problem.
   e. Increased risk of multifetal pregnancy when multiple embryos are used.
5. ICSI pregnancy rates for male factor infertility—see page 289.

Treatments for Male Factor Infertility

| | Transfer to Female | | Ovarian Stimulation | Type of Fertilization | Minimum # of Sperm Required | Motile Sperm Required? | Pregnancy Rate* |
	Substance	Site	Method					
IUI	Sperm	Uterus	Transcervical	Yes or No	In vivo	≥ 5 million/ml	Yes	7-19% per cycle**
GIFT	Oocytes & Sperm	Fallopian Tube	Laparoscopic	Usually	In vivo	?	Yes	28% per cycle
IVF	Embryo(s)	Uterus	Transcervical	Incubation (in vitro)	Usually	25-50,000/oocyte for normal men 0.5-1.0 million/oocyte for infertile men	Yes	32% per cycle
				ICSI (in vitro)		1 sperm/oocyte	No	
ZIFT	Zygote(s)	Fallopian Tube	Laparoscopic	Usually	Incubation (in vitro)	Probably similar to Conventional IVF	Yes	32% per cycle
				ICSI (in vitro)		1 sperm/oocyte	No	
VV	Semen	Vagina	Intercourse	No	In vivo	88% achieve sperm in the ejaculate		61%
VE	Semen	Vagina	Intercourse	No	In vivo	58% achieve sperm in the ejaculate		27%
TURED	Semen	Vagina	Intercourse	No	In vivo	52% achieve sperm in the ejaculate		29%
Varicocelectomy	Semen	Vagina	Intercourse	No	In vivo	70% have improved semen quality		40-50%

IUI = intrauterine insemination; GIFT = gamete intrafallopian transfer; IVF = in vitro fertilization; ZIFT = zygote intrafallopian transfer; ICSI = intracytoplasmic sperm injection; TURED = transurethral resection of the ejaculatory ducts; VV = vasovasostomy; VE = vasoepididymostomy

* Pregnancy rate is for couples with male factor infertility. Pregnancy rate varies considerably and depends on many factors, including maternal age. As maternal age increases (especially > 35), pregnancy rates decline. Some pregnancies do not result in delivery of a live child (live birth). Pregnancy rate is less when it is not performed.

** Pregnancy rate is approximately 7-19% when ovarian stimulation is performed.

REFERENCES

General

Acosta AA, Irianni F: Office Evaluation of the male factor for assisted reproduction. AUA Update Series, Vol. 14, Lesson 18, 1995.

Jarow JP, Sigman M: Office Evaluation of the Subfertile Male. AUA Update Series, Vol. 18, Lesson 23, 1999.

McClure RD: Office Evaluation of the Infertile Man. Male Infertility and Sexual Dysfunction. Ed. WJG Hellstrom. New York: Springer-Verlag New York, Inc., 1997, pp 22-38.

Ohl DA, Sonksen J: Penile vibratory stimulation and electroejaculation. Male Infertility and Sexual Dysfunction. Ed. WJG Hellstrom. New York: Springer-Verlag New York, Inc., 1997, pp 219-229.

Report on optimal evaluation of the infertile male. AUA Best Practice Policy and ASRM Practice Committee Report, Volume 1, 2001 (http://www.auanet.org).

Report on evaluation of the azoospermic male. AUA Best Practice Policy and ASRM Practice Committee Report, Volume 2, 2001 (http://www.auanet.org).

Report on management of obstructive azoospermia. AUA Best Practice Policy and ASRM Practice Committee Report, Volume 3, 2001 (http://www.auanet.org).

Sigman M, Howards SS: Male infertility. Campbell's Urology. 7th Edition. Ed. PC Walsh, AB Retik, TA Vaughan, et al. Philadelphia: W. B. Sanders Company, 1998, pp 1287-1330.

Sikka SC: Gonadotoxicity. Male Infertility and Sexual Dysfunction. Ed. WJG Hellstrom. New York: Springer-Verlag New York, Inc., 1997, pp 292-306.

World Health Organization: WHO laboratory manual for the examination of human semen and sperm-cervical mucus interaction. 4th Edition. Cambridge, United Kingdom: Cambridge University Press, 1999.

Testis Biopsy

Kim ED, Lipshultz LI: Testis Biopsy: indications and interpretation in male infertility. AUA Update Series, Vol. 17, Lesson 40, 1998.

Sharlip ID, Chan SL: Testicular biopsy and vasography. Male Infertility and Sexual Dysfunction. Ed. WJG Hellstrom. New York: Springer-Verlag New York, Inc., 1997, pp 174-188.

Vasectomy and Vasectomy Reversal

Attar KH, et al: Clearance after vasectomy: Has the time come to modify current practice? J Urol, 177(4): 642 (abstract 1935), 2007.

Belker AM: Vasovasostomy. Male Infertility and Sexual Dysfunction. Ed. WJG Hellstrom. New York: Springer-Verlag New York, Inc., 1997, pp 230-243.

Belker AM, Thomas AJ, et al: Results of 1,469 microsurgical vasectomy reversals by the Vasovasostomy Study Group. J Urol, 145: 505, 1991.

Cook LA, et al: Vasectomy occlusion techniques for male sterilization. Cochrane Database Syst Rev, Issue 2: CD003991, 2007.

Costabile RA, Goldstein M, Belker AL, et al: Technique of vasovasostomy and vasoepididymostomy: shortening the learning curve. AUA Update Series, Vol. 18, Lesson 36, 1999.

Cox B, Sneyd MJ, et al: Vasectomy and risk of prostate cancer. JAMA, 287(23): 3110, 2002.

Griffin T, et al: How little is enough? The evidence for post-vasectomy testing. J Urol, 174(1): 29, 2005.

Hancock P, et al: British Andrology Society guidelines for the assessment of post vasectomy semen samples (2002). J Clin Pathol, 55: 812, 2002.

Thomas Jr AJ, Padron OF: Obstructive azoospermia and vasoepididymostomy. Male Infertility and Sexual Dysfunction. Ed. WJG Hellstrom. New York: Springer-Verlag New York, Inc., 1997, pp 244-257.

Varicocele

Report on varicocele and infertility. AUA Best Practice Policy and ASRM Practice Committee Report, Volume 4, 2001 (http://www.auanet.org).

Turek PJ, Lipshultz LI: The varicocele controversies, Part I. AUA Update Series, Vol. 14, Lesson 13, 1995.

Turek PJ, Lipshultz LI: The varicocele controversies, Part II. AUA Update Series, Vol. 14, Lesson 14, 1995.

Zini A, Girardi SK, Goldstein M: Varicocele. Male Infertility and Sexual Dysfunction. Ed. WJG Hellstrom. New York: Springer-Verlag New York, Inc., 1997, pp 201-218.

Assisted Reproductive Technology

Carbone Jr DJ: Male reproductive physiology and assisted reproductive technology. AUA Update Series, Vol. 18, Lesson 21, 1999.

Centers for Disease Control and Prevention: 2004 Assisted Reproductive Technology Success Rates. National Summary and Fertility Clinic Reports. (http://www.cdc.gov/art/ART2004/download.htm)

Girardi SK, Schlegel PN: Micromanipulation of the male gamete. Male Infertility and Sexual Dysfunction. Ed. WJG Hellstrom. New York: Springer-Verlag New York, Inc., 1997, pp 258-275.

Society for Assisted Reproductive Technology (SART) and the American Society for Reproductive Medicine (ASRM): Assisted reproductive technology in the United States: 2000 results generated from the ASRM/SART registry. Fertil Steril 81(5): 1207, 2004.

EMERGENT UROLOGIC CONDITIONS

Testicular Torsion
1. Types of torsion
   a. Intravaginal—torsion of the spermatic cord within the tunica vaginalis.
   b. Extravaginal—in newborns the tunica vaginalis is not adherent to the dartos (i.e. the gubernaculum attachments are not mature); therefore, the spermatic cord and the tunica vaginalis can torse as a unit.
2. Predisposing factors for testicular torsion
   a. Undescended testis (cryptorchidism)
   b. "Bell-clapper" deformity
3. Presentation
   a. Torsion is most common in males 12-18 years of age, but it can occur at any age.
   b. The patient complains of *acute onset of severe testicular pain* with or without swelling. Some males may have a history of intermittent torsion (acute episodes of torsion that spontaneously resolve).
   c. Physical findings may include a tender firm testicle, high-riding testicle, horizontal lie of testicle, absent cremasteric reflex, no pain relief with elevation of the testis, thick or knotted spermatic cord, and epididymis not posterior to the testis.
4. Diagnosis
   a. *The diagnosis of testicular torsion is mainly by clinical suspicion.* The differential diagnosis includes acute epididymitis/orchitis. Torsion is more likely when the onset of pain is acute and extremely intense. Epididymitis is more likely when the onset of pain is gradual and progresses from mild to more intense.
   b. *If testicular torsion is suspected, do not delay surgical exploration in order to perform imaging tests.*
      i. Torsion—Doppler ultrasound of the torsed testis shows minimal flow compared to the contralateral testis. Nuclear testicular scan shows decreased radiotracer activity on the torsed side.
      ii. Acute epididymitis—Doppler ultrasound of the affected testis shows increased flow compared to the contralateral testis. Nuclear testicular scan shows increased radiotracer activity on the affected side.
5. Treatment
   a. *If testicular torsion is suspected, immediate surgical exploration is mandatory* because delay may result in death of the testicle (waiting for imaging tests is contraindicated).
   b. During scrotal exploration, the affected testis is detorsed. If it is not viable, orchiectomy is performed. If it is viable, orchiopexy is performed. *Always perform a bilateral orchiopexy because the contralateral testis may be at risk for torsion.*
   c. Most testicles remain viable when they are detorsed within 6 hours. Few testicles remain viable when they are explored > 24 hours after torsion.
   d. An attempt at manual detorsion can be attempted for intravaginal torsion if an operating facility is not immediately accessible. This is done by attempting to externally rotate the testicle. Even if the testicle is detorsed, a bilateral orchiopexy should be performed to prevent further episodes of torsion.

Testicular Rupture/Testis Fracture—see page 319.

Testicular Dislocation—see page 320.

Penile Fracture—see page 320.

Priapism
1. Ischemic (low flow) priapism is a medical emergency and needs to be treated immediately because delay in treatment can result in destruction of the erectile tissue and erectile dysfunction.
2. See Priapism, page 297.

Paraphimosis
1. Paraphimosis occurs when the foreskin becomes stuck behind the glans.
2. Paraphimosis should be reduced immediately to prevent penile necrosis.
3. Topical anesthetic, penile block, pain medication, and/or sedation may help relieve the pain associated with reducing the paraphimosis. If the paraphimosis cannot be reduced manually, an emergency dorsal slit or circumcision may need to be performed.
4. To reduce the paraphimosis, you must first squeeze the edema out of penis. This is accomplished by applying a firm grip on the edematous tissue and squeezing. Once the edema has been removed, place the index and middle finger of both hands on opposite sides of the constricting skin (a gauze pad between the fingers and penis may help prevent the fingers from slipping during reduction). The thumbs of both hands are placed on the glans. As the thumbs push on the glans, the index and middle fingers pull the foreskin over the glans (a motion similar to injecting with a syringe).
5. In immunocompromised patients, diabetics, and alcoholics, dermal injury sustained while reducing a paraphimosis may be a nidus for Fournier's gangrene. Close observation is recommended if cutaneous compromise exists after reducing the phimosis.

Ambiguous Genitalia
1. This is an emergency primarily because some conditions that cause ambiguous genitalia can cause life-threatening fluid and electrolyte abnormalities.
2. See Evaluation of Ambiguous Genitalia, page 294.

Fournier's Gangrene—see page 393

Urinary Obstruction
1. Ureteral obstruction with sepsis
   a. Drain the infected urine with a nephrostomy tube and administer antibiotics. The cause of the obstruction can be treated after the infection has resolved.
   b. See Urolithiasis, Acute Ureteral Obstruction, page 142.
2. High grade ureteral obstruction
   a. Place a ureteral stent or nephrostomy tube or remove the cause of the obstruction. This will prevent progression of renal failure and kidney damage.
   b. See Urolithiasis, Acute Ureteral Obstruction, page 142.
3. Urinary retention—urinary retention should be treated immediately by placing a urethral catheter or suprapubic tube.

EVALUATION OF AMBIGUOUS GENITALIA

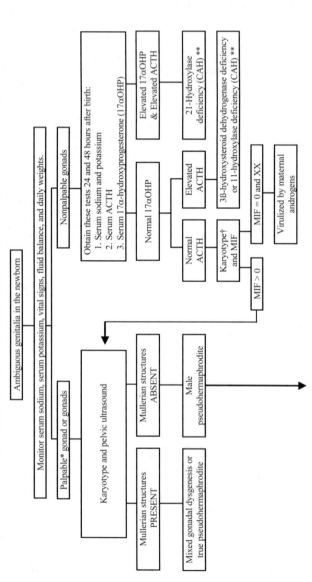

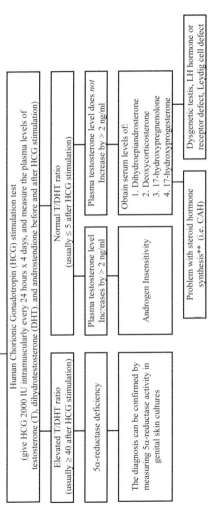

Human Chorionic Gonadotropin (HCG) stimulation test
(give HCG 2000 IU intramuscularly every 24 hours x 4 days, and measure the plasma levels of testosterone (T), dihydrotestosterone (DHT), and androstendione before and after HCG stimulation)

Elevated T/DHT ratio
(usually ≥ 40 after HCG stimulation)

5α-reductase deficiency

The diagnosis can be confirmed by measuring 5α-reductase activity in genital skin cultures

Normal T/DHT ratio
(usually ≤ 5 after HCG stimulation)

Plasma testosterone level
Increases by > 2 ng/ml

Androgen Insensitivity

Plasma testosterone level does *not*
Increase by > 2 ng/ml

Obtain serum levels of:
1. Dihydroepiandrosterone
2. Deoxycorticosterone
3. 17-hydroxypregnenolone
4. 17-hydroxyprogesterone

Problem with steroid hormone synthesis** (i.e. CAH)

Dysgenetic testis, LH hormone or receptor defect, Leydig cell defect

CAH = congenital adrenal hyperplasia; ACTH = adrenocorticotropic hormone; MIF = Mullerian inhibiting factor; LH = luteinizing hormone

* Virtually all palpable gonads are testis.
** Monitor electrolytes closely, if salt wasting is present give hydrocortisone and fludrocortisone.
† Buccal smear for Barr body may be helpful if karyotype is not available or is still pending.

References

Blyth B, Churchill BM: Intersex. Adult and Pediatric Urology. 3rd Ed. Ed. JY Gillenwater, et al. Saint Louis: Mosby-Year Book, Inc., 1996, pp 2591-2622.
Donahoe PK, Schnitzer JJ: Evaluation of the infant who has ambiguous genitalia, and principles of operative management. Semin Pediatr Surg, 5(1): 30, 1996.
Migeon CJ: Diagnosis and treatment of adrenogenital disorders. Endocrinology. 2nd Ed. Ed. LJ Degroot. Philadelphia: W. B. Sanders Co., 1989,pp 1676-1704.

Post-obstructive Diuresis

1. Post-obstructive diuresis refers to the prominent polyuria and natiuresis that occurs after relief of ureteral obstruction in a solitary kidney, bilateral ureteral obstruction, or bladder outlet obstruction.

2. The physiology of diuresis may include
   a. Osmotic diuresis—*this is the most common form of diuresis*. It is caused by accumulation of non-absorbable solutes, especially urea.
   b. Physiologic diuresis–release of fluid and sodium that has accumulated.
   c. Nephrogenic diabetes insipidus—impaired tubular concentrating.
   d. Impaired proximal tubular sodium reabsorption.
   e. Circulating hormones (e.g. elevated atrial natriuretic peptide).

3. The diuresis is usually self-limiting and lasts < 48 hours.

4. In rare cases, the diuresis lasts > 48 hours because *impaired proximal tubular reabsorption of sodium* causes salt diuresis, which can result in hypovolemia, hyponatremia, hypokalemia, and hypomagnesemia.

5. Treatment
   a. Obtain serum BUN, creatinine, & electrolytes (including magnesium).
   b. If the patient meets all of the following criteria, the patient may be discharged.
      • The duration of obstruction is relatively short.
      • No marked elevation of BUN or creatinine.
      • No major electrolyte abnormality.
      • The patient's mental status is not changed from baseline.
      • The patient can drink fluids in response to thirst.
      • Stable condition and stable vital signs.
   c. If the patient does not meet the above criteria, admit the patient.
   d. Closely monitor serum BUN, creatinine, electrolytes, blood pressure, pulse, urine output, and daily weights.
   e. If the patient cannot tolerate oral fluids or oral fluid intake is not keeping up with the urine output, start 1/2 NS to replace urine output cc per cc. If the patient is at risk for pulmonary edema or congestive heart failure, replace the urine output at a lower rate. If the patient has pulmonary edema, consider withholding IV fluids until the pulmonary edema resolves. Over zealous administration of IV fluids can prolong the diuresis.
   f. Replace sodium, potassium, magnesium, and bicarbonate as needed.

Acute spinal cord compression from cancer metastasis

For spinal compression from prostate cancer—See Acute Spinal Cord Compression From Metastasis, page 95.

REFERENCES

Fowler Jr. JE: Necrotizing fasciitis of the male genitalia. Monographs in Urology, 17 (1): 3, 1996.

Gulmi FA, Felsen D, Vaughan Jr. ED: Management of post-obstructive diuresis. AUA Update Series, Vol. 17, Lesson 23, 1998.

Hahn SM, Russo A: Oncologic emergencies. Cecil Textbook of Medicine. 19th Edition. Ed. JB Wyngaarden, LH Smith Jr., JC Bennett. Philadelphia: W. B. Sanders Company, 1992, pp 1067-1071.

Rajfer J: Congenital anomalies of the testis. Campbell's Urology. 6th Edition. Ed. PC Walsh, AB Retik, TA Stamey, et al. Philadelphia: W. B. Sanders Company, 1992, pp 1543-1562.

Weiner DM, Lowe FC: Gangrene of the male genitalia. AUA Update Series, Vol. 17, Lesson 6, 1998.

PRIAPISM

General Information
1. The AUA guideline panel defines priapism as "...a persistent penile erection that continues hours beyond, or is unrelated to, sexual stimulation" and lasts "...greater than 4 hours duration."
2. Management of priapism is aimed at detumescence, preservation of erectile function, and prevention of further episodes.
3. Types of priapism
   a. Ischemic priapism—*ischemic priapism is the most common type of priapism*. Stuttering priapism is a rare form of ischemic priapism.
   b. Non-ischemic priapism

Ischemic Priapism (Low Flow, Veno-occlusive Priapism)
1. Physiology—decreased venous outflow causes increased intracavernosal pressure. Increased intracavernosal pressure leads to erection, decreased arterial inflow, stasis of blood, local hypoxia, and local acidosis. This ultimately results in a *prolonged, painful, fully rigid erection*.
2. Exam—the penis is fully erect. The corpora cavernosa are rigid and tender, but the glans and corpus spongiosum are soft.
3. Causes
   a. Sickle cell trait and disease
   b. Malignant infiltration of the corpora—especially leukemia.
   c. Total parenteral nutrition—especially after 20% lipid infusion. The risk of priapism may be reduced by giving 10% lipids and extending administration over 24 hours.
   d. Medications—e.g. trazodone, phenothiazines (especially chlorpromazine), and cocaine (topical and systemic).
   e. Treatments for erectile dysfunction
   f. Hyperosmolar IV contrast
   g. Spinal cord injury ⎤ Treatment is usually not required in these
   h. Spinal or general anesthesia ⎦ cases because priapism is self-limiting.
4. *Ischemic priapism is an emergency and it requires immediate treatment.*
   a. Ischemic priapism is associated with progressive cavernosal fibrosis and erectile dysfunction.
   b. The longer the priapism duration, the higher the rate of impotence. 90% of men with priapism > 24 hours develop severe erectile dysfunction. Even with early intervention, impotence occurs in up to 50% of cases.
   c. See Work Up and Treatment, page 299.

Stuttering Priapism (Intermittent Priapism)
1. Stuttering priapism is recurrent priapism that occurs over an extended period of time (not rapid recurrence of a single episode).
2. Each episode of priapism should be managed in the usual fashion.
3. After the acute episode of priapism has resolved, further management is aimed at prevention. Prevention strategies include
   a. LHRH agonists or anti-androgens may be tried in patients with adult stature and full sexual maturation.
   b. Intracavernosal self-injection of phenylephrine may be considered in men that fail or decline hormone therapy.
   c. For patients with sickle cell, also see Sickle Cell and Ischemic Priapism, page 298.

Non-ischemic Priapism (High Flow, Arterial Priapism)
1. Physiology—increased arterial inflow without decreased venous outflow, resulting in high inflow and high outflow. This produces a *prolonged, non-painful, partially rigid erection* without local hypoxia or acidosis.
2. Exam—the penis is partially erect. The corpora cavernosa are partially rigid and non-tender, but the glans and corpus spongiosum are soft.
3. Cause—perineal or penile trauma that causes a fistula between the cavernous artery and the corporal tissue. Priapism can occur immediately or several days after the trauma.
4. Doppler ultrasound can identify a cavernosal artery fistula. However, arteriogram is the gold standard for diagnosis.
5. Treatment is *not* an emergency
   a. Non-ischemic priapism is treated expectantly. Approximately 62% of cases will resolve without intervention. Of the cases that spontaneously resolve, 60% recover normal erections. Potency has been restored even after months of sustained non-ischemic priapism.
   b. If non-ischemic priapism does not resolve spontaneously or if the patient wishes treatment, arterial embolization with autologous clot or absorbable gelatin is performed. If embolization fails, open surgical fistula ligation may be performed.
   c. During embolization, absorbable materials (e.g. autologous blood clot, absorbable gelatin) are preferred over permanent materials (e.g. coils, alcohol, glue) because they are less likely to result in permanent erectile dysfunction (5% versus 39%, respectively).
   d. Embolization eliminates non-ischemic priapism in 75% of cases.
   e. See Work Up and Treatment, page 299.

Sickle Cell and Ischemic Priapism
1. Initial management is simultaneous initiation of
   a. The usual management of ischemic priapism (beginning with cavernosal aspiration/irrigation and/or intracavernosal injection of phenylephrine).
   b. IV hydration
   c. Alkalization with bicarbonate in IV fluids.
   d. Analgesia—pain control often requires an opioid.
   e. Oxygen administered by nasal cannula or facemask.
2. If the above measures fail, begin packed red blood cell transfusion until hemoglobin > 10 g/dl (which should reduce the hemoglobin S to < 30%)
   a. If anemic, then perform a simple transfusion.
   b. If not anemic, then perform an exchange transfusion.
3. Prevention of recurrent or stuttering priapism may include
   a. Transfusion to keep hemoglobin > 10 g/dl.
   b. Avoid factors that precipitate sickling (e.g. dehydration, cold, hypoxia).

Other Medical Conditions and Priapism
1. Non-ischemic priapism from malignant penile infiltration (e.g. leukemia)–surveillance is the usual management. Treatment of the primary malignancy should be instituted if feasible.
2. Priapism from anesthesia or spinal cord injury—usually no treatment is required because priapism is often self-limiting in these cases. Observe the patient. If the erection does not resolve within 4 hours, work up and treat priapism in the usual manner.

Work Up

1. *The physician must differentiate ischemic from non-ischemic priapism.*
2. History—including duration of erection, degree of pain, prior episodes of priapism and how they were treated, sickle cell, cancer, trauma, drugs, medications, TPN with lipids, IV contrast, and cardiovascular disease.
3. Physical exam—includes genitals, perineum, pelvis, abdomen, nodes.
4. Labs—include CBC and sickle prep/hemoglobin electrophoresis. Reticulocyte count and urine toxicology (drug screen) may be useful.
5. Methods to differentiate ischemic from non-ischemic priapism
   a. Cavernosal blood gas
   b. Color Doppler ultrasonography—performed in the lithotomy or frog-leg position with scanning of the perineum and the entire penile shaft.

| | Cavernosal Blood Gas | | | Doppler Ultrasound |
	PO_2 (mm Hg)	PCO_2 (mm Hg)	pH	Cavernosal Artery Blood Flow Velocity
Ischemic Priapism	< 30	> 60	< 7.25	Zero or Minimal
Non-ischemic Priapism*	> 90	< 40	7.40	Normal or High
Normal Flaccid Penis†	40	50	7.35	—

* Similar to normal arterial blood
† Similar to normal mixed venous blood

Treatment (based on 2003 AUA Guideline Panel)

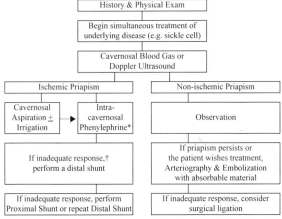

* Monitor the patient's blood pressure and pulse. In patients with cardiovascular disease, electrocardiogram monitoring is recommended.
† Resolution of priapism may be confirmed by repeat cavernosal blood gas or Doppler ultrasonography.

Therapies That Are Not Recommended

1. Oral systemic therapies, such as Sudafed (pseudoephedrine), are not recommended by the guideline panel.
2. Prostate massage, ice packs to penis, and enemas are usually not effective and were not recommended by the AUA guideline.

Corporal Aspiration & Irrigation

1. An 18 or 19 gauge needle is inserted at 9 o'clock and/or 3 o'clock at the base of the penis and blood is aspirated from the corpora.
2. Irrigate normal saline into the corpora.
3. Repeat this process as indicated.
4. Phenylephrine may be administered during corporal irrigation.

Phenylephrine (Alpha-1 Adrenergic Agonist)

1. A solution is created by mixing phenylephrine in normal saline.
   a. To obtain 500 mcg phenylephrine/ml solution—mix 0.5 cc of 1% phenylephrine (10 mg/cc) in 9.5 cc of normal saline.
   b. To obtain 200 mcg phenylephrine/ml solution—mix 0.2 cc of 1% phenylephrine (10 mg/cc) in 9.8 cc of normal saline.
2. For healthy adults, a solution of 100-500 mcg phenylephrine/ml is used. 1 ml of solution is injected into the cavernosa every 3-5 minutes until detumescence is achieved. If detumescence is not achieved after approximately one hour, proceed with a shunt.
3. For patients with cardiovascular disease and for children, a lower concentration of phenylephrine is used and a smaller volume is injected.
4. Monitor the patient's blood pressure and pulse because hypertension, tachycardia, reflex bradycardia, and arrhythmia can occur if phenylephrine enters the systemic circulation. In patients with cardiovascular disease, electrocardiogram monitoring is recommended. In general, phenylephrine has minimal side effects.
5. The longer the duration of priapism, the less likely the priapism will respond to phenylephrine.

Shunts

1. If priapism fails to respond to corporal irrigation and/or phenylephrine within one hour, a distal shunt is performed. If this does not work, consider performing a proximal shunt or another distal shunt.
2. Distal shunts (corporal-glandular shunts)
   a. Winter shunt—a Tru-cut biopsy needle is inserted into the glans penis to excise multiple cores between the distal corpora cavernosa and the glans. If this does not work, an open surgical shunt is required.
   b. Ebbehoj shunt—make a stab incision in the glans, and rotate the blade to create a communication between the corpora cavernosa and the glans.
   c. Al-Ghorab shunt—a 2 cm transverse incision is made in the dorsal glans penis 1 cm distal to the coronal sulcus. Through this incision, the distal portion of tunica albuginea is excised from each corpus.
3. Proximal shunts
   a. Quackel's shunt (corporal-spongiosum shunt)—through a perineal or penile shaft incision, the corpus spongiosum and corpus cavernosum are incised and anastomosed on one side. The more proximal the shunt, the less likely a urethral fistula will occur because the thickness of the spongiosum covering the urethra is greater in the proximal urethra.
   b. Grayhack shunt (corporal-saphenous shunt)—the saphenous vein is anastomosed to the corpus cavernosum at the base of the penis.
   c. Proximal shunts have a higher rate of erectile dysfunction than distal shunts.

REFERENCES

Pryor J, et al for the Second International Consultation on Erectile Dysfunction: Priapism. J Sex Med, 1: 116, 2004.

The management of priapism. AUA Erectile Dysfunction Guideline Update Panel, 2003. (http://www.auanet.org)

GENITOURINARY TRAUMA

Traumatic Hematuria
1. Traumatic hematuria is defined as blood in voided or catheterized urine shortly after trauma.
2. Traumatic hematuria requires evaluation when any of the following criteria are present.
    a. Gross hematuria.
    b. Penetrating trauma.
    c. Pediatric patient (age ≤ 16) and urinalysis shows > 50 RBC/HPF.
    d. Blunt trauma with microscopic hematuria and shock (SBP < 90 at anytime since the injury).
3. *Significant urinary injury may be present in the absence of hematuria.* Evaluation for genitourinary trauma should be performed (even in the absence of hematuria) when either of the following criteria are present.
    a. The mechanism of injury suggests genitourinary trauma (e.g. rapid deceleration, flank trauma).
    b. Clinical findings suggest genitourinary injury (e.g. flank ecchymosis, flank pain, posterior lower rib fractures, transverse process fractures near kidney, pelvic fracture, and injuries close to genitourinary organs).

Urethral Injury

Presentation and Diagnosis
1. Urethral injury rarely occurs in females.
2. Clinical findings that suggest urethral injury include blood at the urethral meatus, penile hematoma, scrotal hematoma, perineal hematoma, penetrating penile injury, high-riding prostate, pubic ramus fracture, penile fracture, difficulty voiding, and distended bladder.
3. *All patients with a suspected urethral injury should undergo a retrograde urethrogram (RUG).*

Contraindications to Catheter Placement
1. A urethral catheter should not be placed without a RUG when any of the following findings are present.
    a. Blood at the urethral meatus
    b. High-riding prostate on rectal exam
    c. Perineal hematoma
    d. If you suspect a urethral injury (e.g. the patient has pelvic fracture, "sleeve" ecchymosis of the penis, perineal "butterfly" hematoma, scrotal hematoma, penetrating penile injury, or penile fracture).
2. See page 312: GU Trauma, Part 1a.

Classification of Urethral Injury
1. Classification based on the extent of injury
    a. No urethral tear (no extravasation)—stretched urethra or urethral contusion.
    b. Partial urethral tear
    c. Complete urethral transection
2. Classification based on location
    a. Anterior urethral injury
    b. Posterior urethral injury

Treatment of Urethral Injury—General Principles
1. Urethral contusion (no extravasation)—urethral catheter for 10-14 days.
2. Minor partial tear (minimal extravasation)—bladder drainage for 2-3 weeks.
3. Major partial tear or complete urethral transection (major extravasation)
    a. Anterior urethra—bladder drainage for at least 4-6 weeks.
    b. Posterior urethra—bladder drainage for at least 3 months.
4. See page 312 and page 313: GU Trauma, Parts 1a and 1b.

Posterior Urethral Injury
1. *Almost all posterior urethral injuries are caused by pelvic fracture from blunt trauma.* Urethral injury occurs in 10% of men with pelvic fractures.
2. When a pelvic fracture causes a urethral tear, the membranous urethra is sheared from the prostatic apex, resulting in a high-riding prostate, "pie in the sky" bladder on cystogram (bladder is displaced cephalad), and extravasation of contrast from the urethra.
3. Immediate urethral repair
    a. *Immediate open surgical repair of the urethra has a higher rate of impotence and incontinence compared to deferred repair; therefore, deferred repair is preferred (unless the patient has an associated rectal or bladder neck injury).*
    b. When posterior urethral injury is associated with a rectal injury or bladder neck injury and the patient is stable enough for surgery, immediate repair is recommended.
4. Deferred urethral repair (with or without urethral realignment)
    a. *When rectal and bladder neck injury are absent, posterior urethral injury is treated by bladder drainage followed by deferred repair in 3-6 months.* Bladder drainage is accomplished by urethral realignment over a catheter or by suprapubic tube.
        i. Suprapubic tube—these patients almost always develop a urethral stricture.
        ii. Urethral realignment—realignment over a catheter (also called urethral stenting) within a few days after injury is achieved by fluoroscopic and/or endoscopic guidance. Realignment should not be performed by open surgery. Approximately 50% of these patients will heal without significant urethral stricture.
    b. After deferred urethral repair, impotence and urinary incontinence rates are the same whether the patient is initially managed by suprapubic tube or by urethral realignment.
5. See page 312 and page 313: GU Trauma, Parts 1a and 1b.

Anterior Urethral Injury
1. Anterior urethral injuries are usually caused by blunt trauma (e.g. straddle injury) or penetrating trauma (e.g. stab or gunshot wound).
2. Bulbous urethral injury
    a. Usually caused by a straddle injury or a direct blow to the perineum in which the urethra is crushed against the pubic bone.
    b. May present with "butterfly" shaped hematoma on perineum and scrotal hematoma (blood confined to Colles' fascia attachments).
3. Pendulous urethra
    a. May be caused by a straddle injury or a direct blow to the penis.
    b. May present with a "sleeve" hematoma of the penile shaft *without* scrotal hematoma (blood confined to Buck's fascia attachments). If Buck's fascia is ruptured, the hematoma may also be seen in the perineum and scrotum.

4. *Anterior urethral injuries are usually managed by bladder drainage and deferred repair.* When the patient is stable enough for surgery, immediate surgical repair may be considered in the following circumstances.
   a. Penile fracture
   b. Low velocity penetrating trauma—injuries from low velocity projectiles (stab wounds, handguns) cause minimal surrounding blast injury and may be repaired immediately. High velocity gunshot wounds (such as from assault rifles) may develop surrounding blast injury that can become evident well after the initial trauma; therefore, high velocity wounds should be managed by bladder drainage and deferred repair.
5. Extensive debridement of the urethra and corpus spongiosum is not advised. In the acute trauma setting, bruised tissue may look ischemic and overzealous debridement may lead to unnecessary tissue loss.

Bladder Injury

General Information
1. Bladder injury is usually caused by pelvic fracture or by blunt trauma to the lower abdomen when the bladder is distended.
2. Most bladder injuries are caused by motor vehicle accidents. A lap belt may cause blunt lower abdominal trauma. Ejection from the vehicle can cause pelvic fracture.
3. Bladder injury occurs in approximately 5% of patients with pelvic fracture.
4. Classification of bladder injuries
   a. Bladder contusion—hematuria without extravasation.
   b. Extraperitoneal bladder rupture
   c. Intraperitoneal bladder rupture
   d. Combined intraperitoneal and extraperitoneal rupture—these are managed as intraperitoneal bladder ruptures.

Presentation
1. Signs and symptoms of bladder rupture are often nonspecific.
2. Suspect a bladder rupture when any of the following criteria are present.
   a. Gross hematuria—present in 95% of bladder ruptures.
   b. Pelvic fracture
   c. Suprapubic discomfort and/or tenderness
   d. Motor vehicle accident (especially when wearing a lap belt).
   e. Delayed diagnosis of an intraperitoneal bladder rupture may be associated with ileus, urinary ascites, and increased BUN and creatinine.
3. *Bladder rupture should be highly suspected when gross hematuria occurs with pelvic fracture.* These patients must undergo cystogram.

Diagnosis
1. The hallmark of bladder rupture is extravasation from the bladder.
2. The diagnosis is made by cystogram (plain films, fluoroscopy, or CT cystogram). A scout image is obtained, then the bladder is filled with dilute contrast though a catheter. *The bladder must be filled to capacity to avoid a false negative test.* Post-drainage films should be obtained.
3. Bladder rupture may be diagnosed intraoperatively using the following methods.
   a. Direct inspection of the bladder
   b. Fill the bladder with colored dye (e.g. indigo carmine or methylene blue)
   c. Cystoscopy
   d. Intentional cystotomy for direct internal inspection of the bladder
   e. Cystogram

Treatment

1. Intraperitoneal rupture—requires exploratory laparotomy, open cystotomy, watertight closure of the bladder in 2 or 3 layers with absorbable suture, and placement of suprapubic tube.
2. Extraperitoneal rupture
   a. When extraperitoneal bladder rupture occurs with any of the following scenarios, open surgical repair (as described for intraperitoneal bladder rupture) may be indicated.
      i. Failure of the catheter to adequately drain the bladder
      ii. Bladder neck injury
      iii. Vaginal or rectal injury—if these injuries are near the bladder rupture, tissue interposition (e.g. omental flap) is recommended.
      iv. The patient will be undergoing internal fixation of a pelvic fracture—bladder repair is required in these patients to prevent urine and infection from contacting the orthopedic hardware.
   b. When the above criteria are absent, extraperitoneal bladder rupture is managed with catheter drainage only.
3. After a bladder injury or bladder surgery, a cystogram is often performed 10-14 days later. If extravasation is still present, wait another week and repeat the cystogram. If no urinary extravasation exists, the catheter may be removed. If both a suprapubic tube and a urethral catheter are in place, the urethral catheter is removed and the suprapubic tube is clamped. If the patient can void, then the suprapubic tube is removed.

Renal Trauma

General Information

1. *The kidney is the most common genitourinary organ injured by trauma.*
2. Most traumatic renal injuries are caused by *blunt* trauma.
3. Penetrating renal trauma is usually associated with other internal injuries.
4. Hematuria is often present; however, hematuria may be absent even when significant renal injury exists.
5. Pre-existing renal lesions (such as tumors and cysts) increase the risk of renal injury from blunt trauma.
6. When severe renal injuries are observed (e.g. grade 4 or 5), delayed complications include hematoma, hematuria, urinoma, infection, hypertension, and pain. Hypertension can develop years later; therefore, the blood pressure of these patients should be checked over the long-term.

Imaging of Renal Trauma

1. Renal trauma is evaluated using CT scan with IV and po contrast.
2. A hematoma medial to the kidney suggests vascular injury of the renal pedicle. Urinary extravasation medial to the kidney suggests injury to the renal pelvis or ureteropelvic junction (UPJ).

Grade	Description of Renal Trauma
\multicolumn{2}{c}{**Grading of Renal Trauma (AAST Classification)**}	
I	Non-expanding subcapsular hematoma or renal contusion (no laceration)
II	Non-expanding perirenal hematoma or laceration into cortex < 1 cm in depth (no urinary extravasation)
III	Laceration into cortex > 1 cm in depth (no urinary extravasation)
IV	Non-vascular—laceration into renal medulla or collecting system Vascular—main renal artery or vein injury with contained hemorrhage
V	Shattered kidney or pedicle avulsion

Treatment

1. Grade 5 and vascular grade 4 renal injuries should be explored.
2. Grade 1 and grade 2 renal injuries can be observed.
3. Grade 3 and nonvascular grade 4 injuries may be observed if there are no intraperitoneal injuries. When these injuries are observed, approximately 20% will develop delayed bleeding; however, most of these cases can be managed by arteriographic embolization.
4. Absolute indications for renal exploration include persistent life-threatening hemorrhage believed to arise from renal injury, renal pedicle avulsion, or expanding or pulsatile retroperitoneal hematoma.
5. Urinary extravasation from renal injury (and not from ureter or ureteropelvic junction injury) is not an absolute indication for renal exploration and it resolves without intervention in > 75% of cases.
6. Renal exploration is usually performed by a transperitoneal approach with early vascular control of the kidney. *Controlling the renal vessels before opening Gerota's fascia reduces the risk of nephrectomy.*
7. Options for surgical treatment of renal injury include suture ligation of renal bleeding, partial nephrectomy, and simple nephrectomy. Nonviable tissue should be debrided and violation of the collecting system should be closed with absorbable suture in a watertight fashion.

Renal Artery Injury

1. The absence of renal enhancement on CT scan strongly suggests thrombosis of the main renal artery.
2. An expanding pulsatile hematoma medial to the kidney suggests a renal pedicle avulsion. Renal pedicle avulsion is an absolute indication for surgical exploration.
3. Arterial revascularization is seldom indicated in patients with a normal contralateral kidney. However, reconstruction of the renal artery should be attempted when simple arterial repairs are possible, in patients with a solitary kidney, or in the presence of bilateral renal injury.

Ureteral Injury

General Information

1. Iatrogenic trauma is the most common cause of ureteral injury.
   a. Most iatrogenic ureteral injuries involve the pelvic ureter.
   b. Preoperative ureteral stent placement does not prevent intraoperative ureteral injury, but it does help identify an intraoperative ureteral injury when it does occur.
   c. Ureteral injury can occur with abdominal, pelvic, or retroperitoneal surgery. It can also occur during urologic endoscopy (e.g. ureteroscopy).
2. Penetrating trauma accounts for most non-iatrogenic ureteral injuries. Most penetrating ureteral injuries arise from gunshot wounds (GSWs); therefore, associated intra-abdominal injuries are common.
3. Ureteral injuries are classified based on the location of the injury:
   a. Ureteral pelvic junction (UPJ)
   b. Abdominal ureter (from the UPJ to the iliac vessels)
   c. Pelvic ureter (inferior to the iliac vessels)
4. Ureteral injuries are also classified based on when the diagnosis is made.
   a. Immediate diagnosis (diagnosed shortly after the injury)
   b. Delayed diagnosis (diagnosed long after the injury)
5. *Delayed diagnosis of ureteral injury results in more complications, including urinoma, infection, fistula, renal loss, and death.*

Presentation
1. The prompt identification of ureteral injury is often difficult; therefore, a high index of suspicion is required to diagnose ureteral injury.
2. Hematuria may be present, but *absence of hematuria does not exclude a ureteral injury.*
3. The following scenarios should raise the suspicion of a ureteral injury.
   a. Penetrating wounds in proximity to the ureter (especially GSWs).
   b. Sudden deceleration injury (especially in children)—UPJ avulsion is more common in children because their spine is more mobile, allowing the spine hyperextension that causes UPJ avulsion.
   c. Recent surgery in proximity to the ureter—especially abdominal perineal resection, pelvic surgery during which profuse pelvic bleeding was encountered, and hysterectomy (the ureter is usually injured during ligation of the uterine or ovarian vessels).
4. Delayed diagnosis may present with any of the following signs.
   a. Persistent flank or abdominal pain
   b. Flank mass
   c. Prolonged ileus
   d. Upper urinary tract obstruction or hydronephrosis
   e. Elevated serum creatinine and blood urea nitrogen (BUN)
   f. Prolonged high output from surgical drains—the drainage can be sent for spot creatinine. Spot creatinine will usually be 25-450 mg/dl when the fluid is urine, but it will be similar to serum creatinine when it is not urine (0.5-1.5 mg/dl for normal kidney function).

Diagnosis
1. Extravasation of urine from the ureter is diagnostic of ureteral injury.
2. Reliable methods to diagnose ureteral injury
   a. Complete IVP—one shot IVP is unreliable for diagnosing ureter injury.
   b. Retrograde pyelogram (RPG)—*RPG is the most accurate imaging test to evaluate the location and extent of ureteral injury.* Antegrade pyelogram may also be useful.
   c. CT abdomen and pelvis with IV contrast and delayed images—there is insufficient data on CT, but it appears to be accurate for diagnosing ureteral injury when delayed images are obtained.
   d. CT urogram—there is insufficient data on CT urogram, but it is probably accurate for diagnosing ureteral injury.
   e. Surgical exploration—extravasation of urine, dye, or contrast confirms the presence of a ureteral injury. The following techniques may be used to identify ureteral injury intraoperatively.
      i. Ureteral inspection—contusions and lacerations are often visible. The viability of the ureter may be compromised when the ureter is dusky, discolored, lacking capillary refill, or the ureteral edge does not bleed.
      ii. Dye study—colored dye (indigo carmine or methylene blue) can be administered by intravenous infusion, by direct injection into the renal pelvis, or by retrograde injection during cystoscopic ureteral catheterization.
      iii. Pyelogram—contrast can be administered by intravenous infusion ("on the table IVP"), by direct injection into the renal pelvis, or by retrograde injection during cystoscopic ureteral catheterization (RPG). One shot IVP is unreliable for diagnosing ureteral injury. However, intraoperative IVP may be helpful when multiple images are obtained (approximating complete IVP). For an on the table IVP, give an IV bolus of contrast (1ml/lb or 2.2ml/kg with a maximum of 150 ml) followed by serial KUBs over the next 2-10 minutes.

3. Findings on imaging studies that suggest a ureteral injury.
   a. Ureter dilation
   b. Ureter deviation
   c. Incomplete visualization of the entire ureter
   d. Delayed or absent nephrogram
   e. Urine extravasation
4. *When CT or IVP are inconclusive and a ureteral injury is suspected, perform a RPG.*
5. Complete imaging of the ureter is usually required. This may include a combination of the following tests.
   a. CT urogram or abdominal/pelvic CT scan with IV contrast and delayed images—reveals the ureteral anatomy and identifies urinoma.
   b. Retrograde pyelogram
   c. Antegrade pyelogram

Treatment—General Principles of Open Surgical Repair

1. Ureteral repair may be performed in the presence of bowel injury, fecal contamination, and vascular injury (these associated injuries do not compromise the ureteral repair). However, it may be prudent to isolate the ureteral repair with a tissue interposition (e.g. an omental flap) to prevent fistula.
2. When the urine is sterile, ureteral injuries during vascular graft surgery can be safely managed by immediate ureteral repair over a stent, tissue interposition (e.g. omental flap between the ureteral repair and the graft), and placement of a retroperitoneal drain away from the graft. When the urine is sterile, ureteral repair does not appear to increase the infection rate or failure rate of the vascular graft.
3. Principles for a successful surgical ureteral repair
   a. Adequate ureteral debridement to remove devitalized tissue. Debride until the tissue edges bleed (healthy tissue bleeds).
   b. Sufficient ureteral mobilization to permit a tension-free anastomosis. Preserve the ureteral adventitia and vasculature to ensure adequate ureteral blood supply. In some cases, nephropexy may help mobilize the proximal ureter when more ureteral length is needed.
   c. The ureteral ends should be spatulated.
   d. Watertight, tension-free, mucosa-to-mucosa anastomosis over a ureteral stent using absorbable suture.
   e. When applicable, isolate the ureteral repair from associated injuries with a tissue interposition (e.g. omental flap). *An omental flap should be based on the right gastroepiploic pedicle* (i.e. this pedicle is preserved) because this is the most reliable blood supply to the omentum.
   f. Place a retroperitoneal drain.
   g. Proximal urinary diversion (e.g. nephrostomy tube) is usually unnecessary.
4. Postoperative management
   a. If the retroperitoneal drain is removed before the urethral catheter, urine may reflux up the stent, leak through the ureteral repair, and create a urinoma. Therefore, the urethral catheter is usually removed first.
   b. The urethral catheter is usually left in place for at least 24-48 hours and then removed. If the retroperitoneal drain output remains minimal over the next 24 hours, then the retroperitoneal drain may be removed.
   c. The ureteral stent can be removed in 4-6 weeks. An IVP, CT urogram, or renal scan should be obtained 4-8 weeks after the stent is removed to rule out ureteral stricture and obstruction.

Treatment—Types of Surgical Repairs

1. Ureteral reimplant
   a. Pelvic trauma and distal ureteral mobilization may impair blood flow to the distal ureter. Thus, pelvic ureter injury (below the iliac vessels) is usually repaired by distal ureter ligation and ureteral reimplantation into the bladder. Psoas hitch or Boari flap may be required.
   b. Psoas hitch—the contralateral superior vascular pedicle of the bladder is ligated and divided, which permits bladder mobilization toward the ureteral injury. The bladder dome is pulled cephalad and sutured to the ipsilateral psoas tendon. Then, the ureter is reimplanted into the bladder dome. *When placing sutures in the psoas tendon, avoid injury to the genitofemoral nerve.* Psoas hitch is contraindicated when the bladder is too small to permit sufficient mobilization.
   c. Boari flap—a flap of bladder is rotated cephalad and tubularized. The ureter is reimplanted into the tubularized flap. Psoas hitch is often used in combination with a Boari flap. Boari flap is contraindicated in patients with a small bladder or a history of pelvic radiation.
   d. *When the entire lower one or two thirds of the ureter is damaged, the preferred repair is reimplant with psoas hitch (and Boari flap if needed).*
2. Ureteroureterostomy (UU)—primary anastomosis of the injured ureter. When possible, UU is the preferred repair for the abdominal ureter.
3. Transureteroureterostomy (TUU)
   a. TUU is useful when ureteral reimplant with psoas hitch and Boari flap cannot be utilized. It is especially useful when there is extensive damage to the distal ureter and the bladder is small or radiated.
   b. The injured ureter is brought through a window in the colonic mesentery *above the inferior mesenteric artery* (kinking of the ureter can occur when it is brought below the inferior mesenteric artery). Then, it is anastomosed to the contralateral ureter in an end-to-side fashion.
   c. Relative contraindications—upper urinary tract disease (nephrolithiasis, urothelial cancer, tuberculosis, chronic pyelonephritis), abdominal radiation, and retroperitoneal fibrosis.
   d. There are anecdotal reports of transureteropyelostomy (ureter is anastomosed to the contralateral renal pelvis).
4. Ureteropyelostomy—the ureter is anastomosed to the renal pelvis (similar to a dismembered pyeloplasty). It is used to repair UPJ injuries.
5. Ureterocalycostomy
   a. The lower pole of the kidney is amputated to expose an infundibulum, then the ureter is anastomosed to the infundibulum. The UPJ is ligated.
   b. Adequate lower pole resection is required to prevent stenosis of the anastomosis; nonetheless, the stenosis rate is high.
   c. This procedure is usually reserved for patients who have an intrarenal pelvis, where the renal pelvis cannot be exposed enough to perform a ureteropyelostomy. It may also be used for patients with extensive damage to the renal pelvis and proximal ureter.
6. Ileal ureter
   a. A segment of ileum is placed posterior to the colon and interposed in an iso-peristaltic fashion between the kidney and the bladder.
   b. Ileal ureter is not used for acute trauma. It is useful when a long segment of ureter is damaged and cannot be repaired by other means.
   c. Contraindications—creatinine > 2 mg/dl, inflammatory bowel disease, radiation damage of ileum, and high bladder pressures.
   d. When bladder pressure is normal, bacteriuria and reflux in the ileal ureter do not appear to cause deterioration of renal function.
7. See page 316: GU Trauma, Parts 4a.

Treatment—Immediate Diagnosis

1. Ureteral perforation during endoscopic procedures—these can usually be managed by placement of a ureteral stent for 4-6 weeks (unless there is associated intraabdominal organ injury. See page 147).

2. Intraoperative ureteral crush injury
   a. Remove the item that caused the crush injury (i.e. remove the clamp, suture, staple, clip, etc.)
   b. If the crush injury is minimal and the ureter appears viable, place a ureteral stent.
   c. If the crush injury is large or the viability of the ureter is in question, perform a surgical repair (e.g. ureteral debridement, anastomosis over a stent, and placement of a retroperitoneal drain).

3. Ureteral contusions
   a. If the contusion is minimal and the ureter appears viable, place a ureteral stent.
   b. If the contusion is large or the viability of the ureter is in question, perform a surgical repair (e.g. ureteral debridement, anastomosis over a stent, and placement of a retroperitoneal drain).

4. Partial lacerations of the ureter caused by stab wounds or by iatrogenic injury (open or laparoscopic)—when local ureteral tissue appears viable, the laceration may be debrided and closed primarily over a stent. When the injury is associated with blast effect (e.g. GSW) or the viability of the ureteral tissue is in question, the injured tissue should be resected and the ureter is repaired based on injury extent and location (see below).

5. Unstable patients with significant ureteral injury—patients that are not stable enough to undergo formal ureteral repair may require immediate "damage control" followed by definitive reconstruction when the patient is stable. Options for "damage control" include
   a. Ligate the ureter with a non-absorbable suture just above the injury. Place a percutaneous nephrostomy tube when the patient is more stable.
   b. Ureteric exteriorization—a ureteral catheter is placed into the ureter, secured, and brought out through the skin.
   c. Nephrectomy

6. Pelvic ureter injury—repaired by distal ureter ligation and ureteral reimplantation. Psoas hitch or Boari flap may be required.

7. Abdominal ureter injury—repaired by one of the following methods.
   a. Ureteroureterostomy (UU)—the preferred repair when possible.
   b. Transureteroureterostomy (TUU)
   c. Ureteral reimplantation with psoas hitch and Boari flap—this technique may be required when the entire lower one-third or two thirds of the ureter is damaged and a tension-free UU cannot bridge the gap.

8. UPJ injury
   a. Incomplete (partial) UPJ laceration caused by blunt trauma can be managed by one of the following methods.
      i. Placement of ureteral stent (with or without nephrostomy tube)
      ii. Ureteropyelostomy over a stent (with or without nephrostomy tube)
   b. All other UPJ injuries (e.g. complete UPJ transection and penetrating UPJ injury) can be repaired by one of the following methods.
      i. Ureteropyelostomy
      ii. Ureterocalycostomy

9. Laceration of the renal pelvis with intact UPJ—the laceration edges can be debrided and closed primarily over a ureteral stent.

Treatment—Delayed Diagnosis

1. Delayed ureter injuries are managed by placement of a percutaneous nephrostomy tube, and when possible, antegrade placement of a ureteral stent. Retrograde ureteral stenting is usually unsuccessful. Urinomas (when present) are managed by placement of a percutaneous drain.

2. Complete imaging of the ureteral defect is required before treatment. This may include a combination CT (CT urogram or abdominal and pelvic CT scan with IV contrast and delayed images), retrograde pyelogram, and antegrade pyelogram

3. Minor extravasation from ureter—this may be managed by placing a ureteral stent for 4-6 weeks. Follow up imaging studies should be performed after stent removal to evaluate for stenosis.

4. Minor ureteral stricture—treated with endoureterotomy and/or balloon dilation. Endoureterotomy (+ balloon dilation) has a higher success rate than balloon dilation alone. Higher success rates occur when strictures are non-ischemic, short (< 1 cm), duration < 6 months, located in the proximal or distal ureter (not mid ureter), and good ipsilateral renal function.

5. Major ureteral injury
   a. Pelvic ureter injury—repaired by distal ureter ligation and ureteral reimplantation. Psoas hitch or Boari flap may be required.
   b. Abdominal ureter injury—repaired by one of the following methods.
      i. Ureteroureterostomy (UU)—the preferred repair when possible.
      ii. Transureteroureterostomy (TUU)
      iii. Ureteral reimplantation with psoas hitch and Boari flap—may be required when the entire lower one-third or two thirds of the ureter is damaged and a tension-free UU cannot bridge the gap.
   c. UPJ injury—repaired by one of the following methods.
      i. Ureteropyelostomy
      ii. Ureterocalycostomy
   d. Loss of entire ureter or almost entire ureter—repaired by one of the following methods.
      i. Autotransplant
      ii. Ileal ureter
      iii. Nephrectomy

6. Nephrectomy may also be considered when the kidney on the injured side is non-functioning or poorly functioning.

Penetrating Penile or Scrotal Trauma

1. Penetrating trauma of the scrotum or penis requires surgical exploration and repair.

2. When a penile gunshot wound causes urethral injury, the management of the urethral injury depends on the velocity of the bullet. See Anterior Urethral Injury, page 302.

3. Management of penetrating injuries of the corpus cavernosum is similar to the management of penile fracture. See Penile Fracture, page 320.

4. Management of penetrating injuries to the testicle is similar to the management of testis rupture. See Testis Rupture, page 319.

5. Bleeding spermatic cord vessels can be ligated. Transection of the spermatic cord may require microvascular re-anastomosis.

6. Try to preserve as much viable tissue as possible.

7. Lacerations and minor skin loss can be debrided and closed primarily. When major skin loss is present, treatment consists of debridement followed by deferred repair. Deferred repair often requires skin grafting.

8. See page 318: GU Trauma, Part 5.

Blunt Scrotal Trauma

Cutaneous Scrotal Hematoma (Extrascrotal Hematoma)

1. Cutaneous scrotal hematomas are confined to the scrotal skin and do not extend into the space between the tunica albuginea and tunica vaginalis.
2. Cutaneous scrotal hematomas can arise from the following processes.
   a. Direct trauma to the scrotum
   b. Urethral trauma
   c. Blood tracking subcutaneously from nearby bleeding.

Hematocele (Intrascrotal Hematoma)

1. A hematocele is an accumulation of blood in the space between the tunica albuginea and the tunica vaginalis.
2. Hematocele can arise from any of the following processes.
   a. Trauma to scrotum, testis, epididymis, or spermatic cord. *Most traumatic hematoceles are caused by testis rupture.*
   b. After scrotal surgery (e.g. vasectomy, hydrocelectomy)
   c. Blood flowing from the peritoneal cavity through a patent process vaginalis—blood from an intra-abdominal source can accumulate in the scrotum when the process vaginalis is patent.

Evaluation of Scrotal Hematoma

1. History and physical examination—note the presence of perineal hematoma, penile hematoma, and blood at the urethral meatus (which are often seen with urethral injury).
2. Scrotal ultrasound with Doppler—used primarily to evaluate the integrity and vascularity of the testicles.
   a. Examine the integrity of the tunica albuginea (when a testis fracture is present, the fracture site can be seen in approximately 20% of cases).
   b. Examine the echogenicity of the testis—heterogeneous echotexture of the testis after trauma is diagnostic of testicular rupture.
   c. Check testicular blood flow with Doppler.
3. Urinalysis—blood in the urine suggests a urethral injury.
4. Retrograde urethrogram—when urethral injury is suspected.
5. When intra-abdominal bleeding is suspected, obtain a CT scan with po and IV contrast.

Treatment of Scrotal Hematoma

1. When scrotal hematoma is caused by an associated injury (urethral injury, testis rupture, intra-abdominal injury, etc.), the associated injury should be treated. See GU Trauma - Part 5, page 318.
2. Cutaneous scrotal hematomas usually resolve without intervention and are managed conservatively with scrotal support, scrotal elevation, and intermittent application of ice packs.
3. Hematoceles from scrotal surgery or from an intra-abdominal source
   a. Small stable hematoceles (no active bleeding) may be managed conservatively with scrotal support, scrotal elevation, and intermittent application of ice packs.
   b. Large hematoceles—prompt drainage is recommended to prevent infection, prolonged pain, extended disability, and testicular ischemia from compression.
4. Hematoceles from trauma
   a. *Most traumatic hematoceles are caused by testis rupture.*
   b. *When the mechanism of injury suggests significant testicular injury and testicular rupture is suspected, prompt surgical intervention is indicated.*

GU Trauma - Part 1a (Urethral Trauma)

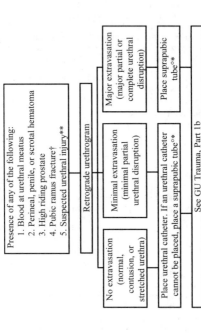

Presence of any of the following:
1. Blood at urethral meatus
2. Perineal, penile, or scrotal hematoma
3. High riding prostate
4. Pubic ramus fracture†
5. Suspected urethral injury**

↓

Retrograde urethrogram

No extravasation (normal, contusion, or stretched urethra)	Minimal extravasation (minimal partial urethral disruption)	Major extravasation (major partial or complete urethral disruption)
Place urethral catheter. If an urethral catheter cannot be placed, place a suprapubic tube°	Place urethral catheter. If an urethral catheter cannot be placed, place a suprapubic tube°*	Place suprapubic tube**

See GU Trauma, Part 1b

† With a Malgaigne pelvic fracture (a vertical fracture of the ileum with one or more pubic rami fractures), urethral injury should be highly suspected.
° Transabdominal ultrasound may be helpful to guide suprapubic tube placement. If pelvic fracture exists, the suprapubic tube may need to be placed by open cystostomy.
* In infants, a suprapubic tube may be placed initially; however, a vesicostomy is preferred for long-term management.
** Other clinical findings that suggest urethral injury include penile fracture, penetrating penile injury, inability to void, and distended bladder.

GU Trauma - Part 1b (Urethral Trauma)

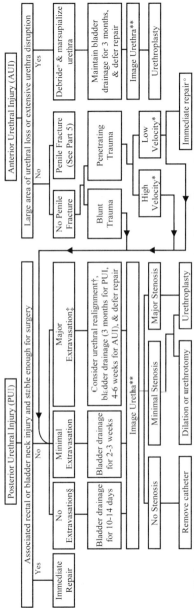

† Realignment of the urethra over a catheter may be achieved using fluoroscopic and/or endoscopic guidance. Realignment should not be performed by open surgery.
‡ Major partial urethral tear or complete urethral transection.
§ Normal urethra, contusion of the urethra, or stretched urethra.
* High velocity wounds (e.g. gunshot wounds from an assault rifle) should probably be managed by bladder drainage and deferred urethral repair. Low velocity wounds
  (e.g. gunshot wounds from a hand gun, stab wounds) may be managed by immediate urethral repair (usually preferred) or urinary diversion with delayed repair.
** Urethral imaging may include retrograde urethrogram, antegrade endoscopy, antegrade urethrogram, antegrade endoscopy, or voiding cystourethrogram.
° Extensive debridement of the urethra is not advised. Bruised viable tissue may look ischemic and overzealous debridement may lead to unnecessary tissue loss.

GU Trauma - Part 2

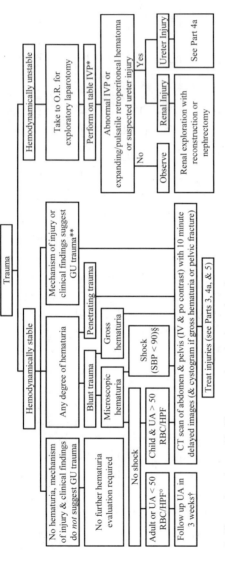

† If hematuria persists, consider CT urogram and complete hematuria work up.

° If microhematuria and pelvic fracture occur together, some suggest getting a cystogram.

* On table IVP is performed by giving an IV bolus of contrast (1 ml/lb or 2.2 ml/kg with a maximum of 150 ml) followed by KUB in 10 minutes. Does the patient have two kidneys? Are the kidneys functioning? If the nephrogram is absent, is there a renal shadow? Is there any extravasation?

** Mechanisms of injury that suggest GU trauma include rapid deceleration injury and flank trauma. Clinical findings that suggest GU trauma include flank ecchymosis, posterior lower rib fractures, transverse process fractures near the kidney, pelvic fracture, and injuries close to the GU organs.

§ Systolic blood pressure (SBP) < 90 at any time since the injury (i.e. including in the field).

GU Trauma - Part 3

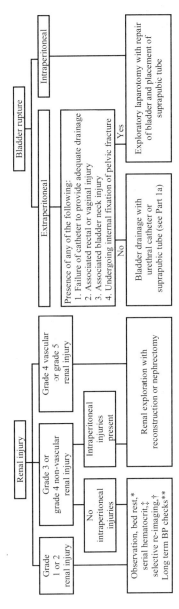

* Bed rest until gross hematuria clears.
† Follow up imaging is usually unnecessary for grade 1, 2, and 3 renal injuries with stable hematocrit. Patients with declining hematocrit or grade 4 renal injury should undergo repeat CT abdomen and pelvis (with IV contrast and 10 minute delayed images) within 36-72 hours after the previous imaging study.
‡ Patients with declining hematocrit from renal injury can often be managed by embolization.
** Long-term follow up of blood pressure is recommended in severe renal injuries (especially grade 4 or 5) that are observed. These patients are at risk for developing hypertension.

GU Trauma - Part 4a (Ureteral Trauma)

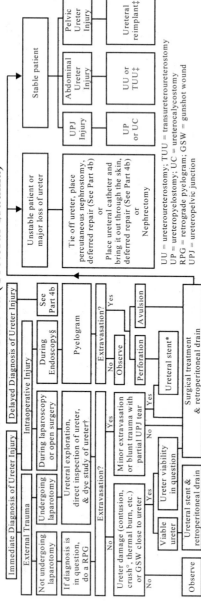

UU = ureteroureterostomy; TUU = transureteroureterostomy
UP = ureteropyelostomy; UC = ureterocalycostomy
RPG = retrograde pyelogram; GSW = gunshot wound
UPJ = ureteropelvic junction

* When the patient is undergoing open surgery, a retroperitoneal drain should be placed.
† Intravenous dye (indigo carmine or methylene blue), retrograde or antegrade dye injection, RPG, or on the table IVP with multiple delayed films. Check for extravasation.
‡ When the entire lower one-third or two-thirds of the ureter is damaged, the preferred management is ureteral reimplant with psoas hitch (with or without Boari flap).
° Nephropexy can be utilized to mobilize the proximal ureter and help bridge the gap.
° Crush injuries include those caused by staplers, sutures, clips, and clamps. Remove sutures, clips, staples and clamps from the ureter and then assess ureter viability.
§ Including any procedures during which instruments are passed into the ureteral lumen (e.g. ureteroscopy, ureteral stent placement, ureteral dilation).

GU Trauma - Part 4b (Ureteral Trauma)

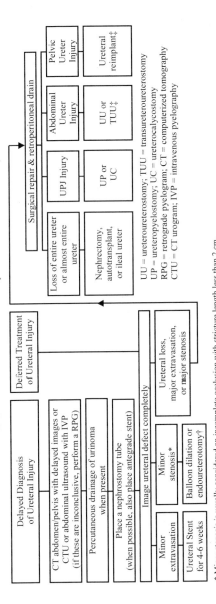

Delayed Diagnosis of Ureteral Injury

CT abdomen/pelvis with delayed images or CTU or abdominal ultrasound with IVP (if these are inconclusive, perform a RPG)

Percutaneous drainage of urinoma when present

Place a nephrostomy tube (when possible, also place antegrade stent)

Image ureteral defect completely

- Minor stenosis*
  - Balloon dilation or endoureterotomy†
- Minor extravasation
  - Ureteral Stent for 4-6 weeks
- Ureteral loss, major extravasation, or major stenosis

Deferred Treatment of Ureteral Injury

Surgical repair & retroperitoneal drain

- **Loss of entire ureter or almost entire ureter**
  - Nephrectomy, autotransplant, or ileal ureter
- **UPJ Injury**
  - UP or UC
- **Abdominal Ureter Injury**
  - UU or TUU‡
- **Pelvic Ureter Injury**
  - Ureteral reimplant‡

UU = ureteroureterostomy; TUU = transureteroureterostomy;
UP = ureteropyelostomy; UC = ureterocalycostomy
RPG = retrograde pyelogram; CT = computerized tomography
CTU = CT urogram; IVP = intravenous pyelography

* Minor stenosis is usually considered an incomplete occlusion with stricture length less than 2 cm.
† Endoureterotomy (with or without balloon dilation) has a higher success rate than balloon dilation alone. Higher success rates occur for strictures with the following characteristics: non-ischemic, short (< 1 cm), stricture duration < 6 months, proximal or distal ureter location (not mid ureter), and good ipsilateral renal function.
‡ When the entire lower one-third or two-thirds of the ureter is damaged, the preferred management is ureteral reimplant with psoas hitch (with or without Boari flap). Nephropexy can be utilized to help mobilize the proximal ureter and help bridge the gap.

GU Trauma - Part 5 (Genital Trauma)

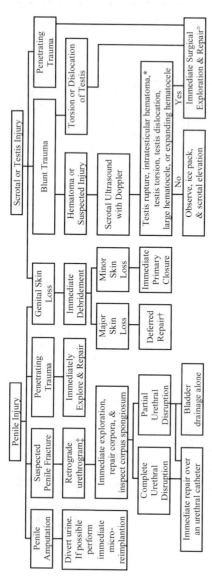

* Imaging and physical exam cannot distinguish between intratesticular hematoma and testis rupture; thus, these men are assumed to have testis rupture. If exploration shows no testis rupture, obtain a follow up ultrasound to demonstrate resolution of the hematoma and to rule out an incidental testis tumor.

† Deferred repair of penile skin loss may include primary closure or skin grafting.

° Preserve viable testis tissue to maintain fertility and endocrine function. When massive testis damage is sustained, orchiectomy may be required.

‡ Retrograde urethrogram is generally recommended (especially if there is blood at the urethral meatus, hematuria, difficulty voiding, bilateral corporal rupture, or suspected urethral injury).

Testicular Trauma

General Information

1. Most testicular injuries are caused by blunt trauma from athletic activity.
2. Testicular trauma can affect fertility and endocrine function.

Intratesticular Hematoma Without Rupture

1. Intratesticular hematoma appears as a hypoechoic or heterogeneous area on ultrasound.
2. Imaging and physical examination cannot reliably distinguish between intratesticular hematoma and testicular rupture. Therefore, men with intratesticular hematoma are assumed to have testicular rupture and surgical exploration is recommended.
3. *When the mechanism of injury suggests significant testicular injury and testicular rupture is suspected, prompt surgical intervention is indicated even when scrotal ultrasound is inconclusive.*
4. In some cases, an intratesticular hematoma is suggested on ultrasound, but surgical exploration reveals no testicular rupture. In this case, the differential diagnosis includes intratesticular hematoma (without testis rupture) and incidental testis tumor. A follow up ultrasound should be obtained several weeks later to demonstrate resolution of a suspected intratesticular hematoma. If the intratesticular lesion does not resolve, the possibility of a testis tumor must be considered.

Testicular Rupture (Testicular Fracture)

1. Testicular rupture is a tear in the tunica albuginea, often resulting in extrusion of seminiferous tubules and hematocele (bleeding into the space between the tunica albuginea and the tunica vaginalis).
2. Scrotal ultrasound usually shows a heterogeneous testicular echotexture. The fracture site in the tunica albuginea can be seen on ultrasound in 20% of cases. Extruding seminiferous tubules may also be identified.
3. Diagnosis is based mainly on clinical suspicion. *When the mechanism of injury suggests significant testicular injury and testicular rupture is suspected, prompt surgical intervention is indicated even when the scrotal ultrasound is inconclusive.*
4. *Testicular rupture is an emergency that requires prompt surgical repair.* 80-90% of testicles are salvaged when surgery is performed within 72 hours after blunt trauma, whereas only 32-45% are salvaged when surgery is delayed beyond 72 hours. Prompt surgery is required to avoid testicular loss, infection, infertility, and chronic pain.
   a. The scrotum is explored and the hematocele is evacuated.
   b. Extruding seminiferous tubules and necrotic tissue are debrided.
   c. The tunica albuginea is closed with running 4-0 absorbable sutures.
   d. Repair epididymal injuries.
   e. Place a penrose drain in the peri-testicular space and bring it out through a separate incision. Maintain the drain for 24-36 hours after surgery.
   f. A 7 day course of broad spectrum antibiotics is recommended.
   g. When there is minimal viable testis tissue, orchiectomy should probably be performed.

Testicular Torsion

1. Traumatic testicular torsion requires immediate surgical exploration, detorsion, and bilateral testis fixation.
2. See Testicular Torsion, page 292.

Testicular Dislocation

1. Traumatic testis dislocation is displacement of the testis to a position other than in the scrotum. It usually occurs from blunt trauma to the scrotum or perineum, especially high speed motorcycle accidents when the rider's scrotum and perineum impact the fuel tank.
2. Testis dislocation may be unilateral or bilateral.
3. The testis may dislocate to the following sites: abdomen, pubis, inguinal canal, femoral canal, penis, and perineum.
4. Testis torsion and testis rupture may occur in a dislocated testis.
5. Patients present with testicular pain and an empty ipsilateral hemiscrotum. When dislocation is suspected and the testis cannot be found, ultrasound or CT may help localize the testis. Ultrasound with Doppler may help identify associated testis torsion or rupture.
6. Management requires prompt surgical exploration and orchiopexy to prevent testis atrophy, infertility, and loss of endocrine function. An inguinal incision is recommended to avoid blind manipulation of the spermatic vessels. Manual closed reduction under sedation has been reported, but it is generally unsuccessful.

Penile Fracture

General Information

1. Penile fracture is a rupture or tear of the tunica albuginea of the corpus cavernosum, which typically occurs when an excessive bending force is applied to the erect penis.
2. Penile fracture usually occurs during aggressive intercourse in which the penis slips out of the vagina and impacts the perineum or pubic symphysis.
3. Penile fracture almost always occurs during an erection. The tear almost always occurs distal to the suspensory ligament and is usually transverse.
4. The long-term risks of penile fracture include erectile dysfunction and Peyronie's disease (plaque, curvature, pain with erection). When urethral injury is repaired, long-term risks include urethral stricture and penile shortening.

Presentation

1. At the time of injury, the patient usually experiences a "pop" or "snap" of the penis immediately followed by penile pain and detumescence.
2. Bleeding from the rupture usually fills the subcutaneous tissues, creating a hematoma with swelling and ecchymosis confined by Buck's fascia (this penile shaft hematoma is called the "eggplant deformity"). When Buck's fascia is disrupted, the hematoma may extend to the perineum, scrotum, or pubic area. The penis often deviates away from the side of the fracture. Occasionally, a clot forms at the rupture site, which can minimize bleeding into the surrounding tissue and make the physical findings unimpressive.
3. In 10-20% of cases, the tear in the corpus cavernosa extends into urethra, causing urethral injury. Urethral injury usually presents with blood at the urethral meatus and difficulty voiding. When the patient can void, hematuria may be present. However, urethral injury can occur in the absence of these signs. Urethral injuries are more likely to occur with bilateral corporal ruptures than with unilateral corporal ruptures.
4. Conditions that mimic penile fracture include rupture of the dorsal penile artery, rupture of penile veins, and rupture of the suspensory ligament of the penis.

Diagnosis

1. Penile fracture is a clinical diagnosis. *When the clinical presentation is consistent with penile fracture, diagnostic studies are unnecessary.*
2. When the clinical presentation is unclear, surgical exploration is often recommended because testing is generally unreliable; nonetheless, some urologists utilize additional testing.
   a. Cavernosography—usually performed by injecting 30-50 cc of half strength contrast into the corpora during fluoroscopy. Images should probably be performed in the anterior-posterior direction and in both oblique directions. Another image is obtained 10 minutes later to detect delayed extravasation. False negative studies (minimal or no extravasation) may occur with small tears or when a clot has "plugged" the tear. False positive studies can occur when the normal venous drainage of the corpora is misinterpreted as extravasation.
   b. Ultrasound—negative results cannot exclude a penile fracture because a clot may fill the fracture site and small tears in the tunica may be missed.
   c. MRI—may be more accurate for detecting penile fracture than ultrasound or cavernosography.
3. The SIU consensus 2004 suggests preforming a retrograde urethrogram (RUG) to diagnose urethral injury in all cases of penile fracture. RUG should definitely be performed when any of the following criteria exist: blood at the urethral meatus, hematuria, difficulty voiding, bilateral corporal rupture, or suspected urethral injury.

Treatment

1. *Penile fracture is an emergency and requires immediate surgical intervention.* Patients managed by immediate surgical repair have a lower risk of penile curvature, erectile dysfunction, and prolonged hospital stay.
2. Surgical repair
   a. In most cases, a circumferential distal penile shaft incision ("circumcision incision") with degloving of the penile skin provides adequate exposure of the corpus cavernosum and urethra.
   b. Inspect the corpus cavernosum and corpus spongiosum and identify areas of injury
   c. Hematoma is evacuated and hemorrhage is controlled.
   d. Debridement should be minimized.
   e. The defect in the tunica albuginea is closed primarily (the SIU guideline recommends absorbable sutures such as Vicryl). Suturing of the erectile tissue within the corpora should be avoided.
3. Associated urethral injury
   a. Complete urethral transection—the urethra should be mobilized and debrided to permit a tension free anastomosis. The urethra is repaired primarily with absorbable suture over a urethral catheter. Extensive debridement of the urethra and corpus spongiosum is not advised. In the acute trauma setting, bruised corporal tissue may look ischemic and overzealous debridement may lead to unnecessary tissue loss.
   b. Partial urethral disruptions—these may be managed by any of the following methods.
      i. Placing a urethral catheter
      ii. Placing a suprapubic tube
      iii. Primary urethral repair over a catheter
4. Postoperatively, erections may be suppressed with benzodiazepines, amyl nitrate, or ketoconazole.
5. See page 318: GU Trauma, Part 5.

Pediatric Trauma

1. Pediatric is defined as age ≤ 16.
2. Two *unique* injuries are associated with sudden deceleration injury (occur in all age groups but are more common in children):
   a. UPJ avulsion—more common in children because their spine is more mobile, allowing the hyperextension that causes this injury.
   b. Arterial intimal tear—more common in children because of they have less perirenal fat and greater mobility of the renal pedicle.
3. Pediatric males may have bladder neck disruption with a pelvic fracture. (although a membranous urethra disruption is more common).

REFERENCES

General

Brandes S and the SIU Consensus Group: Diagnosis and management of ureteric injury: an evidence based analysis. BJU Int, 94: 277, 2004.

Gomez RG, and the SIU Consensus Group: Consensus statement on bladder injuries. BJU Int, 94: 27, 2004.

Moore EE, et al: Organ injury scaling: spleen, liver, and kidney. J Trauma, 29: 1664, 1989. [AAST grading system]

McAninch JW, Santucci RA: Genitourinary trauma. Campbell's Urology. 8th Edition. Ed. PC Walsh, AB Retik, TA Vaughan, et al. Philadelphia: W. B. Sanders Company, 2002, pp 3707-3744.

Renal Trauma

Miller KS, McAninch JW: Radiographic assessment of renal trauma: our 15-year experience. J Urol, 154: 352, 1995.

Morey A, Bruce JE, McAninch JW: Efficacy of radiographic imaging in pediatric blunt renal trauma. J Urol, 156: 2014, 1996.

Santucci RA and the SIU Consensus Group: Evaluation and management of renal injuries: consensus statement of the renal trauma subcommittee. BJU Int, 93: 937, 2004.

Urethral Trauma

Chapple C and the SIU Consensus Group: Consensus on urethral trauma. BJU Int, 93: 1195, 2004.

Krambeck AE, Elliott DS: Primary realignment of traumatic urethral distraction. AUA Update Series, Vol. 24, Lesson 30, 2005.

Genital Trauma

Blake SM, Bowley DM: Traumatic dislocation of the testis: a rare sequel of perineal injury. Emerg Med J, 20: 567, 2003.

Jabren GW, Hellstrom WJG: Trauma to the external genitalia. Urologic Emergencies. Ed. H Wessells, JW McAninch. Totowa, NJ: Humana Press, 2005, pp 71-93.

Jack GS, Garraway I, et al: Current treatment options for penile fractures. Reviews in Urology, 6(3): 114, 2004.

Morey AF and the SIU Consensus Group: Consensus on genitourinary trauma: external genitalia. BJU Int, 94: 507, 2004.

Vijayan P: Traumatic dislocation of testis. Indian J Urol, 22: 71, 2006.

GENITOURINARY INFECTIONS: GENERAL CONCEPTS

Complicated Versus Uncomplicated Infections

1. Urinary tract infection (UTI) refers to an infection of the urinary system.
2. Complicated UTI—a UTI in a patient with any of the following criteria.
   a. Immunosuppressed (e.g. diabetes mellitus, HIV, on immunosuppressants such as steroids or chemotherapy)
   b. Pregnant
   c. Male
   d. Pediatric
   e. Indwelling urinary catheter, stent, or drain.
   f. Structural abnormality of the urinary tract (e.g. vesicoureteral reflux, calyceal diverticulum, ureteropelvic junction obstruction).
   g. Urinary obstruction
   h. Renal insufficiency
   i. Presence of urolithiasis
3. Uncomplicated UTI—a non-complicated UTI in a female.

Evaluation of Pediatric UTI—see page 231.

Diagnosis of UTI

1. A presumptive diagnosis of UTI can be made when symptoms of UTI are present and urine reveals pyuria. *Pyuria alone is not sufficient to diagnose UTI. A definitive diagnosis of UTI requires urine culture.*
2. Urinalysis findings that support the diagnosis of UTI
   a. Leukocyte esterase—white blood cells (WBCs) release this enzyme into the urine. When WBCs are present in the urine, this test is positive.
   b. Pyuria—usually defined as > 5 WBCs/high power field (x400) in centrifuged urine.
   c. Bacteria
   d. Nitrite positive—urine contains nitrate from protein metabolism. Some bacteria have reductase enzymes that convert the urinary nitrate to nitrite. *A positive nitrite test (Greiss test) indicates that bacteria are present in the urine.* False negatives do occur.
      i. Bacteria that reduce nitrate to nitrite (i.e. cause positive nitrite)— E. coli, Klebsiella, Enterobacter, Serratia, Proteus, Staphylococcus, Pseudomonas.
      ii. Bacteria that do not reduce nitrate to nitrite—streptococcus.
3. *E. coli is the most common bacterial pathogen causing UTI.*
   a. E. coli can adhere to human epithelial cells using small hair-like appendages (called pili or fimbriae). Bacterial adhesion is important for colonization and infection.
   b. Pathogenic E. coli usually have one of the following pili.
      i. Mannose sensitive pili (type 1 pili)—d-mannose inhibits the binding capacity of these pili.
      ii. Mannose resistant pili (P pili)—d-mannose does not affect the binding capacity of these pili. *E. coli causing pyelonephritis typically have P pili.*

General Risk Factors for Infection
1. Immunocompromised
   a. Disease states—e.g. diabetes mellitus, HIV, malignancy, malnutrition.
   b. Immunosuppressant medications—e.g. steroids, chemotherapy.
2. Urine stasis and/or obstruction (e.g. urine retention, ureter obstruction, vesicoureteral reflux, diverticulum, etc.)
3. Broad spectrum antibiotics increase the risk of fungal infections.

Antibiotics
1. Fluoroquinolones (FQ)
   a. Mechanism of action—inhibition of bacterial DNA gyrase.
   b. Examples—levofloxacin, ciprofloxacin, ofloxacin.
   c. Moxifloxacin and gemifloxacin should not be used for UTI because they achieve low urine concentrations.
   d. FQ are not approved for use in age < 16 years.
   e. FQ can cause a false positive result on urinary opiate tests.
   f. Side effects include
      i. CNS toxicity—symptoms may range from mild (dizzy, "feeling foggy") to severe (confusion, seizures).
      ii. Photosensitivity
      iii. Tendon ruptures—FQ have rarely been associated with Achilles tendon ruptures. The risk is higher in patients with renal insufficiency and patients on steroids.
2. Beta-lactams
   a. These antibiotics have a beta-lactam ring as part of their molecular structure. *An intact beta-lactam ring is essential for the antimicrobial activity of these drugs.*
   b. Mechanism of action—inhibition of bacterial cell wall synthesis.
   c. Examples—penicillins, cephalosporins, aztreonam.
   d. One mechanism of bacterial resistance is beta-lactamase (also called penicillinase), an enzyme that inactivates many beta-lactam antibiotics by cleaving their beta-lactam ring.
   e. Methicillin, nafcillin, dicloxacillin are resistant to beta-lactamase.
   f. Ampicillin and amoxicillin are among the few antibiotics that cover both Enterococcus faecalis and Enterococcus faecium. Therefore, *clinicians often use either ampicillin or amoxicillin when coverage for Enterococcus is required.*
   g. Beta-lactams commonly cause yeast infections (e.g. vaginitis, balanitis).
3. Trimethoprim and sulfamethoxazole (TMP-SMZ)
   a. Mechanism of action—inhibition of bacterial folate metabolism.
   b. Contraindicated in age < 2 months because it may cause kernicterus.
   c. Side effects—gastrointestinal symptoms (nausea, vomiting, anorexia), skin reactions, thrombocytopenia, increase in serum potassium, and hemolytic anemia in G6PD deficiency.
4. Nitrofurantoin
   a. Mechanism of action—inhibition of multiple bacterial enzymes.
   b. Antimicrobial activity is impaired in alkaline urine.
   c. Contraindicated in children < 1 month old because of the risk of hemolytic anemia from immature erythrocyte enzyme systems.
   d. Side effects—pulmonary fibrosis with chronic use, hemolytic anemia in G6PD deficiency, peripheral neuropathy, hepatitis, and cholestasis.
5. Aminoglycosides
   a. Mechanism of action—inhibition of bacterial protein synthesis.
   b. Side effects—ototoxicity (deafness and vertigo), acute tubular necrosis, renal failure, and neuromuscular blockade.

Unresolved and Recurrent Infection

Unresolved UTI
1. Unresolved UTI is an infection that is not completely eradicated (urine culture remains positive). The causes of unresolved UTI include
   a. Bacteria resistant to the antibiotic
   b. Renal dysfunction—antibiotic excretion may be hindered by renal dysfunction, leading to a sub-therapeutic urinary concentration.
   c. Non-compliance with antibiotic therapy
   d. Fistula—fistula may cause continuous inoculation of the urine, making eradication of the bacteria impossible.
2. Treatment of unresolved UTI
   a. Ensure that the antibiotic is appropriate and that the patient is compliant.
   b. When fistula is suspected, perform CT of the abdomen and pelvis and cystoscopy.
   c. In patients with renal failure, it may be necessary to irrigate the urinary tract with antibiotic to attain adequate antimicrobial levels. Antibiotic irrigation by urethral catheter and/or nephrostomy tube may be needed.

Recurrent (Relapsing) UTI
1. Recurrent UTI occurs when an infection is eradicated from the urine (culture turns negative), but the culture becomes positive again. Recurrent UTI can arise from persistent bacteria within the genitourinary (GU) tract (bacterial persistence) or from bacteria outside the GU tract (re-infection).
2. Bacterial persistence—in some cases, antibiotics eradicate bacteria in the urine, but do not eradicate bacteria from all regions of the GU tract. These persistent bacteria spread into the urine again. These UTIs are usually caused by the same organism with the same sensitivity profile and often recur within 1-3 weeks of the previous infection.
   a. Urolithiasis—antibiotics may eradicate bacteria from the urine, but they may not eradicate bacteria from the stone.
   b. Foreign bodies—examples include catheter fragments, indwelling ureteral stents, and non-absorbable surgical material (e.g. sutures, clips, staples, slings). Antibiotics may eradicate bacteria from the urine, but they may not eradicate bacteria from the foreign body.
   c. Poorly draining area of the urinary system—inefficient drainage of infected urine may prevent complete bacterial eradication. Causes of poor drainage include
      i. Urinary obstruction
      ii. Urine retention
      iii. Diverticulum—calyceal, bladder, or urethral diverticulum.
   d. Bacterial prostatitis—a short course of antibiotics may eradicate bacteria from the urine, but it may not eradicate bacteria from the prostate. *Chronic bacterial prostatitis is the most common cause of recurrent UTIs in adult males.*
3. Re-infection—in this case, antibiotics eradicate bacteria in the urine, but bacteria from outside the GU tract invade and re-infect the urine. These recurrent UTIs may be caused by different organisms and can occur anytime after the previous infection. Causes of re-infection include
   a. Fistula to the urinary tract
   b. Urine retention
   c. Vesicoureteral reflux
   d. Immunosuppression (especially poorly controlled diabetes mellitus)
   e. Sexual activity—in females, sexual activity can cause frequent UTIs.

Evaluation of Recurrent UTI
1. For females with recurrent uncomplicated acute cystitis (especially when UTI occurs only a few times a year), see page 338.
2. Evaluation may include
   a. Physical exam—check for urethral diverticulum, cystocele, vesico-vaginal fistula, prostatitis, etc.
   b. Creatinine—poor renal function limits urinary excretion of antibiotics.
   c. Urine culture and sensitivity (catheterized sample if necessary).
   d. Post void residual measurement
   e. Consider imaging of the urinary tract with CT urogram and cystoscopy.
   f. Bacterial localization studies may be useful
      i. In men, evaluate for bacterial prostatitis (see page 365).
      ii. Bladder and bilateral ureteral catheterization for culture.
   g. Minimize immunosuppression
      i. In diabetics, maintain control of blood sugar.
      ii. Correct malnutrition.

UTI with Clean Intermittent Catheterization

General Information
1. In general, *clean intermittent catheterization (CIC) has a lower risk of UTI than indwelling catheterization.* However, patients with high intravesical pressure (such as with DSD) may be at higher risk for UTI and renal deterioration with CIC than with an indwelling catheter.
2. Compared to indwelling catheters, CIC has a lower risk of epididymitis, orchitis, peno-scrotal abscess, urethral strictures, fistula, and urolithiasis.

Prevention of Recurrent Infection in Patients Using CIC
1. Ensure the patient is complying with the techniques of CIC: cleaning catheters appropriately, washing hands before catheterizing, cleaning the meatus before catheterizing, etc.
2. The NIDRR consensus 1992 and the English national evidence based guidelines 2001 indicate that sterile and clean intermittent catheterization have a similar rate of UTI. However, more recent evidence suggests that sterile intermittent catheterization does have a lower risk of UTI than CIC. The 2006 Consortium for Spinal Cord Medicine states "Lower infection rates can be achieved with sterile techniques..." and recommends "Consider sterile catheterization for individuals with recurrent symptomatic infections occurring with clean intermittent catheterization."
3. Prophylactic antibiotics
   a. Daily antibiotics—there is insufficient data to determine if daily antibiotics reduce UTI; however, they do increase resistant organisms.
   b. Antibiotic cycling—a study in patients with neurogenic bladder on CIC showed that cycling 2 oral antibiotics reduced the rate of symptomatic UTI and the number of hospitalizations, but did not appear to increase antibiotic resistance (J Antimicrob Chemother, 57: 784, 2006). Each cycle consisted of one dose of the first antibiotic during week one, followed by one dose of the second antibiotic during week two. Then, the cycle was repeated. Antibiotics were selected from the following list and were chosen to be effective against previous infections.
      i. For a history of gram negative UTI—two double strength tablets of TMP-SMX, nitrofurantoin 300 mg, cefixime 400 mg, amoxicillin 3000 mg, or fosfomycin trometamol 6000 mg.
      ii. For a history of gram positive UTI—amoxicillin 3000 mg or fosfomycin trometamol 6000 mg.

4. Intravesical antibiotics—can be used to treat and prevent UTI in patients using CIC. The antibiotic may be absorbed and cause systemic side effects (e.g. ototoxicity has been reported after intravesical administration of aminoglycosides, primarily in patients with end stage renal disease). The following regimen was used successfully in patients with neurogenic bladder or augmentation cystoplasty.
   a. Mix 480 mg gentamicin sulfate into 1 liter of sterile normal saline. Keep the solution refrigerated. The solution should probably be discarded after 30 days, although it may retain its potency for up 2 months. Rapid infusion or infusion of cold fluid into the bladder can cause autonomic dysreflexia; thus, each dose should be removed from the refrigerator and warmed to room temperature before it is gently infused.
   b. Catheterize the patient and completely empty the bladder.
   c. Gentamicin solution (480mg/1000 ml normal saline) is gently infused through the catheter into the bladder. The infused volume may vary, but 30 cc is often used in adults with normal bladder capacity.
   d. The catheter is removed and the solution is left in the bladder until the next scheduled catheterization.
   e. Instillations may be performed once per day (for UTI prophylaxis) or twice per day (for UTI treatment).
   f. Avoid intravesical infusion when there is a risk of systemic absorption (e.g. gross hematuria, traumatic catheterization).
   g. It may be prudent to check serum gentamicin levels; however, using this protocol, serum gentamicin levels were very low and serum creatinine remained stable in patients with normal renal function.
   h. Approximately 25% can have breakthrough UTIs, some of which are gentamicin resistant.
5. Intravesical antiseptics—it is unknown if this helps prevent UTI in patients using CIC. Examples of antiseptics include acetic acid, chlorhexidine, and povidone-iodine.
6. There is insufficient evidence to determine if they following therapies decrease the risk of UTI in patients using CIC.
   a. Oral cranberry supplement—limited evidence suggests no benefit.
   b. Oral vitamin C supplement—limited evidence suggests no benefit.
   c. Methenamine—limited evidence suggests no benefit (see page 339).
7. Control diabetes.

UTI with Indwelling Catheter

General Information
1. The risk of bacteriuria with an indwelling catheter is 5% per day; thus, almost all patients have bacteriuria by 20 days after catheter insertion.
2. *The longer a urinary catheter is left indwelling, the higher the risk of UTI.*
3. *The most important factor for preventing UTI with an indwelling catheter is a closed drainage system.* Drainage systems should remain closed with as few disconnections as possible.

Catheter Type And Risk of UTI
1. Latex and silicone catheters have a similar risk of UTI.
2. Silver alloy catheters (not silver oxide catheters) delay the onset of asymptomatic bacteriuria compared to standard catheters and may reduce symptomatic UTI in patients catheterized for less than 7-10 days. There is no evidence that silver alloy catheters are beneficial for catheterization longer than 30 days. The risk of argyria (silver toxicity) is not well defined, but it is probably minimal (especially with short-term catheterization).

3. Antibiotic impregnated catheters delay the onset of asymptomatic bacteriuria and reduce the rate of symptomatic UTI in patients catheterized for less than one week.

4. Suprapubic tube—limited data suggests that suprapubic tubes may have a lower risk of UTI than urethral catheters, especially for short-term catheterization (< 2 weeks). Theoretically, there are fewer bacteria on the abdominal wall than on the genitals, which may decrease the risk of infection. Prostatitis, epididymo-orchitis, urethritis, and urethral strictures occur less often with suprapubic tubes than with urethral catheters. Some patients prefer a suprapubic tube because it allows them to engage in sexual activity.

Drainage Bag And Risk of UTI

1. A catheter plug or valve (permits intermittent emptying of the catheter) has the same risk of UTI as a drainage bag.

2. Changing the drainage bag regularly does not prevent UTI.

3. Adding antiseptic agents (such as hydrogen peroxide or chlorhexidine) to the drainage bag does not decrease the risk of UTI.

4. Prevent back flow of urine—reflux of urine from the drainage bag into the bladder increases the risk of UTI.
   a. Keep the drainage bag below the level of the bladder.
   b. Empty the drainage bag frequently enough to prevent backflow.

5. Expert opinion recommends that the contact between the drainage bag and the floor should be avoided.

Biofilms

1. A biofilm is a sheet of bacteria encased in an extracellular matrix.

2. Biofilms can form on the inner and on the outer surface of a catheter.

3. Biofilm bacteria are rarely eradicated by antibiotics because
   a. The biofilm bacteria create an extracellular matrix. This extracellular matrix acts as a barrier that protects the bacteria from antibiotics.
   b. Biofilm bacteria are less susceptible to antibiotics because they grow more slowly than free-floating bacteria. Thus, even when antibiotics penetrate the extracellular matrix, they may not eradicate the bacteria.

4. *Antibiotics alone do not eradicate the bacteria in biofilms. Removal of the biofilm is required.* In a prospective, randomized, controlled trial of patients with an indwelling catheter and UTI, Raz et al (2000) compared patients whose catheter was changed to patients whose catheter was not changed. This study showed that changing to a new catheter before starting antibiotics resulted in a faster eradication of bacteria, a faster resolution of fever, a faster clinical improvement, and a lower rate of symptomatic UTI recurrence. *When a patient with an indwelling catheter has a UTI, the catheter should be replaced with a new catheter, preferably before starting antibiotics.* Obtain a urine culture when the new catheter is placed.

5. When a biofilm contains urease producing organisms, the catheter can become encrusted with struvite and apatite (see How UTI Increases Stone Risk, page 130). These encrustations may obstruct the catheter.

No Proven Benefit for Preventing UTI with an Indwelling Catheter

1. Changing the catheter and/or drainage bag regularly—does not reduce the risk of UTI. The interval for changing the bag and catheter should be based on the manufacturer's recommendations and on the patient's clinical needs. Catheters can become encrusted and clogged over time. Assess the rate of encrustation and change the catheter before it becomes obstructed.

2. Vigorous meatal cleansing—scrubbing is not necessary. Daily washing of the meatus (and under the foreskin) with soap and water is sufficient.

3. Application of antiseptic or antimicrobial agents to the meatus—these agents do not reduce bacteriuria compared to washing with soap and water.

4. Adding antiseptic to drainage bags—does not decrease the risk of UTI.

5. Intravesical agents—in patients with an indwelling catheter, irrigation (continuous flushing), instillation (infusion followed by holding the agent in the bladder for a while), and washout (infusion followed by immediate drainage) do not reduce the risk of UTI, may cause resistant organisms, and may introduce bacteria by breaching the closed catheter system. However, some urologists use intravesical antiseptics or antibiotics when standard methods of UTI prevention have failed. Avoid intravesical irrigation when there is a risk of systemic absorption (e.g. gross hematuria, traumatic catheterization).

   a. Intravesical gentamicin—usually used for instillation or washout. For dosing, see page 327.

   b. Intravesical GU irrigant (neomycin and polymyxin)—1 ampule is mixed in 1 liter of normal saline. This solution is used for continuous bladder irrigation at a rate of 1 liter per 24 hours for up to 10 days. Absorption into the bloodstream can cause systemic side effects (e.g. ototoxicity).

   c. Intravesical acetic acid—0.25% acetic acid is infused into the bladder and immediately drained (washout). The infused volume may vary, but 30 cc is often used in adults with normal bladder capacity. Mix 10 teaspoons (50 cc) of plain white vinegar in 1 quart (approximately 1 liter) of water. Use tap water that is boiled and cooled, distilled water, or sterile water. Keep the solution refrigerated. The solution should probably be discarded after 2-3 weeks. Rapid infusion or infusion of cold fluid into the bladder can cause autonomic dysreflexia; thus, each dose should be removed from the refrigerator and warmed to room temperature before it is gently infused. Acetic acid does not seem to reduce bacteriuria or UTI, but may reduce catheter encrustation.

6. Prophylactic antibiotics during catheter change—*non-traumatic replacement an indwelling catheter is associated with a low risk of bacteremia; therefore, antimicrobial therapy for a non-traumatic catheter change is not beneficial.* When a catheter change is traumatic (e.g. causes bleeding), when the patient is at risk for endocarditis, or the patient has a history of catheter related infections (especially with catheter changes), then prophylactic antibiotics should be considered.

7. There is insufficient evidence to determine if the following therapies decrease the risk of UTI in patients with indwelling catheters.

   a. Daily prophylactic antibiotics—may increase resistant organisms.

   b. Oral cranberry supplement

   c. Oral vitamin C supplement—limited evidence suggests no benefit.

   d. Methenamine—does not reduce the risk of UTI in patients with an indwelling catheter (see page 339).

Prevention of UTI with an Indwelling Catheter

1. Remove a temporary catheter as soon as possible—removing a catheter sooner will decrease the risk of UTI.

2. Drainage systems should remain closed. Minimize disconnections.

3. Consider using antibacterial catheters (for details, see Catheter Type and Risk of UTI, page 327)

   a. Silver alloy catheters delay the onset of asymptomatic bacteriuria and may reduce symptomatic UTI in patients catheterized for < 7-10 days.

   b. Antibiotic impregnated catheters delay the onset of asymptomatic bacteriuria and reduce the rate of symptomatic UTI in patients catheterized for < 7 days.

4. Prevent back flow of urine—reflux of urine from the drainage bag into the bladder increases the risk of UTI.
   a. Keep the drainage bag below the level of the bladder.
   b. Empty the drainage bag frequently enough to prevent backflow.
5. Expert opinion recommends that the contact between the urinary drainage bag and the floor should be avoided.
6. Expert opinion recommends hand washing immediately before and after manipulation of the catheter or its components.
7. Suprapubic tube—limited data suggests that indwelling suprapubic tubes may have a lower risk of UTI than urethral catheters. Theoretically, there are fewer bacteria on the abdominal wall than on the genitals, which may decrease the risk of infection. Some patients prefer a suprapubic tube because it allows them to engage in sexual activity.
8. Control diabetes.

Treatment of UTI with an Indwelling Catheter

1. This is minimal data on the treatment for catheter related UTI. Duration of therapy should probably be 7-21 days, depending on the clinical scenario.
2. *Remove the catheter if possible. If the catheter cannot be removed, then the catheter should be replaced with a new catheter, preferably before starting antibiotics (this eliminates the bacterial biofilm).* Ideally, a urine culture should be obtained when the new catheter is placed.

Purple Bag Syndrome/Blue Bag Syndrome

1. This syndrome is uncommon and occurs with indwelling urinary catheters in which the drainage bag and tubing turn blue or purple (the color can be subtle or intense). The color of the urine remains normal.
2. Indoxyl sulfate (a metabolite of tryptophan) is excreted in the urine. In alkaline urine, bacteria that possess the phosphatase-sulfatase enzyme metabolize indoxyl sulfate into indigo (blue) and/or indirubin (red). The indigo and indirubin concentrate in the plastic of the bag and tubing.
3. Bacteria that may be associated with these syndromes include Providencia stuartii, Klebsiella pneumoniae, Enterobacter agglomerans, E. Coli, Morganella morganii, and Proteus. Bacterial strains that contain the phosphatase-sulfatase enzyme are rare; therefore, this syndrome is rare.
4. This syndrome is more common in constipated and elderly patients.
5. This syndrome is benign. However, the presence of bacteria may be associated with UTI. In addition, this syndrome occurs in alkaline urine, which may be associated with struvite and apatite encrustation.
6. Treatment is indicated when there is symptomatic UTI or problematic encrustations. Administer oral antibiotics and change the catheter and drainage bag. With treatment, the discoloration usually resolves.

UTI in Patients with Spinal Cord Injury (SCI)

(Based on the 1992 NIDRR consensus and the CSCM 2006 consensus)

General Information

1. Risk factors for UTI in patients with SCI
   a. Bladder over-distention
   b. Vesicoureteral reflux
   c. High pressure voiding—patients with a high detrusor leak point pressure (DLPP > 40 cm water) are at higher risk for not only UTI, but also for deterioration of renal function. See Leak Point Pressure, page 172.
   d. Urolithiasis
   e. Urinary obstruction—detrusor sphincter dyssynergia (DSD), urethral stricture, prostate enlargement, etc.

2. Persistent bacteriuria is common in patients with a condom catheter, indwelling catheter, urinary diversion, and intermittent catheterization.

3. Screening and treatment of asymptomatic bacteriuria is not recommended in patients with SCI or in patients with indwelling catheters. However, treatment of asymptomatic bacteriuria may be considered when urease producing organisms occur in a patient with urolithiasis or problematic catheter encrustations. Urease producing organisms may contribute to stone formation (See How UTI Increases Stone Risk, page 130).

4. *By definition, a UTI in a person with SCI is a complicated UTI and should be treated with 7-14 days of antibiotics.* Longer courses of antibiotics have not been beneficial.

5. People with SCI often do not present with the classic signs and symptoms of UTI because of altered sensation. UTI may present with cloudy urine, foul smelling urine, fatigue, lethargy, vague abdominal/flank discomfort, spastic limbs, autonomic dysreflexia, or urine incontinence (leak between CIC or leak around indwelling catheter). Fever may or may not be present.

Methods of Bladder Drainage and Risk of UTI

1. The NIDRR consensus 1992 indicates that clean intermittent catheterization (CIC) has a similar risk of UTI as sterile intermittent catheterization. However, recent evidence suggests that sterile intermittent catheterization may have lower the risk of UTI than CIC. The 2006 Consortium for Spinal Cord Medicine (CSCM) guidelines state "Lower infection rates can be achieved with sterile techniques..." and recommends "Consider sterile catheterization for individuals with recurrent symptomatic infections occurring with clean intermittent catheterization."

2. *CIC has a lower risk of UTI than indwelling catheterization.* However, patients with high intravesical pressure (such as with DSD) may have a higher risk for UTI and renal deterioration with CIC than with an indwelling catheter.

3. *Condom catheters cause less bacteriuria and UTI than indwelling catheters.* However, patients with high intravesical pressure (such as with DSD) and urine retention may be at higher risk for UTI and renal deterioration with a condom catheter than with an indwelling catheter.

4. Compared to CIC, indwelling catheters have a higher risk of epididymo-orchitis, peno-scrotal abscess, urethral strictures, fistula, and urolithiasis (bladder and renal).

5. Suprapubic tube—limited data suggests that indwelling and temporary suprapubic tubes may have a lower risk of UTI than urethral catheters. Theoretically, there are less bacteria on the abdominal wall than on the genitals, which may decrease the risk of infection. Some patients prefer a suprapubic tube because it allows them to engage in sexual activity.

Evaluation for Febrile UTI or Recurrent Afebrile UTI

1. Invasive testing should be deferred until UTI treatment is complete.

2. Image the upper tracts—renal ultrasound, CT scan, or IVP may be considered; however, CT urogram or CT scan may be the most informative. Check for urolithiasis and hydronephrosis.

3. Image the bladder—check for bladder stones. In patients who void or who use a condom catheter, check a post void residual.

4. Urodynamics—check for elevated intravesical pressure, poor bladder compliance, detrusor sphincter dyssynergia, and bladder outlet obstruction.

5. Cystogram—check for vesicoureteral reflux.

6. Cystoscopy—check for urethral stricture, bladder stones, bladder lesion, diverticula, etc.

Sterile Pyuria

1. "Sterile pyuria" refers to the presence of WBCs in the urine when a standard urine culture shows no bacterial growth (the standard culture media does not support growth of mycobacteria, fungus, viruses, etc.).
2. Causes—mycobacteria (sterile pyuria is a classic finding in genitourinary tuberculosis), Chlamydia, Ureaplasma, virus (e.g. adenovirus), fungus, protozoa (e.g. Trichomonas vaginalis), parasite (e.g. Schistosomiasis), inflammatory (prostatitis, cystitis, nephritis, papillary necrosis), or tumor (benign or malignant).
3. Evaluation of sterile pyuria may include
   a. BUN, creatinine, CBC with differential.
   b. Formal urinalysis (eosinophils in the urine may indicate a parasite infection or interstitial nephritis).
   c. Urine culture for bacteria, fungus, and mycobacteria. Obtain at least 3 consecutive early morning urine samples for acid fast staining and mycobacterial culture with sensitivity.
   d. Urethral swab for Chlamydia, Ureaplasma, and Mycoplasma.
   e. Urine cytology or other urothelial tumor marker.
   f. CT urogram
   g Cystoscopy
4. Treatment depends of the underlying cause.

REFERENCES

General

Clark SA, et al: Are prophylactic antibiotics necessary with clean intermittent catheterization? A randomized controlled trial. J Pediatr Surg, 40: 568, 2005.

CSCM - Consortium for Spinal Cord Medicine: Bladder management for adults with spinal cord injury: a clinical practice guideline for health care providers. August 2006.

NIDRR - National Institute on Disability and Rehabilitation Research: The prevention and management of urinary tract infections among people with spinal cord injuries. J Am Paraplegia Soc, 15: 194, 1992.

Pellowe CM, et al: Updating the evidence base for national evidence based guidelines for preventing health care associated infection in NHS hospital in England: a report with recommendations. British Journal of Infection Control, 5(6): 10, 2004 [Update of J Hosp Infect, 47 (suppl): S39, 2001].

Rubenstein JN, Schaeffer AJ: Managing complicated urinary tract infections - the urologic view. Infect Dis Clin N Am, 17: 333, 2003.

Salomon J, et al: Prevention of urinary tract infection in spinal cord injured patients: safety and efficacy of a weekly oral cyclic antibiotic program with a 2 year follow up. J Antimicrob Chemother, 57: 784, 2006.

Vainrub B, Musher DM: Lack of effect of methenamine in suppression of, or prophylaxis against, chronic urinary infection. Antimicrob Agents Chemother, 12(5): 625, 1977.

Purple Bag Syndrome/Blue Bag Syndrome

Dealler SF, et al: Enzymatic degradation of urinary indoxyl sulfate by Providencia stuartii and Klebsiella pneumoniae causes the purple urine bag syndrome. J Clin Microbiol, 26(10): 2152, 1988.

Dealler SF, et al: Purple urine bags. J Urol, 142: 769, 1989.

Wang IK, et al: Purple urine bag syndrome in a hemodialysis patient. Intern Med, 44: 859, 2005.

Indwelling Catheter and UTI

Centers for Disease Control and Prevention: Guideline for the prevention of catheter associated urinary tract infections, 1981. (http://www.cdc.gov/ncidod/dhqp/gl_catheter_assoc.html).

Harding GK, et al: How long should catheter acquired urinary infection in women be treated? A randomized controlled study. Ann Intern Med, 114: 713, 1991.

Niel-Weise BS, et al: Urinary catheter policies for long term bladder drainage. Cochrane Database Syst Rev, Issue 1: CD004201, 2005.

Raz R, et al: Chronic indwelling catheter replacement before antimicrobial therapy for symptomatic urinary tract infection. J Urol, 164(4): 1254, 2000.

Saint S, Chenoweth CE: Biofilms and catheter associated urinary tract infections. Infect Dis Clin N Am, 17: 411, 2003.

Catheter Type and UTI

Brosnahan J, et al: Types of catheters for management of short term voiding problems in hospitalized adults. Cochrane Database Syst Rev, Issue 1: CD004013, 2004.

Horgan AF, et al: Acute urinary retention: comparison of suprapubic and urethral catheterisation. Br J Urol, 70:149, 1992.

Ichsan J, Hunt DR: Suprapubic catheters: a comparison of suprapubic versus urethral catheters in the treatment of acute urinary retention. Aust N Z J Surg, 57(1): 33, 1987.

Johnson JR, et al: Systematic review: antimicrobial urinary catheters to prevent catheter associated urinary tract infection in hospitalized patients. Ann Inten Med, 144: 116, 2006.

Saint S, et al: Condom versus indwelling urinary catheters: a randomized trial. J Am Geriatr Soc, 54(7): 1055, 2006.

Saint S, et al: The potential clinical and economic benefits of silver alloy urinary catheters in preventing urinary tract infection. Arch Intern Med, 160: 2670, 2000.

Sethia KK, et al: Prospective randomized controlled trial of urethral versus suprapubic catheterization. Br J Surg, 74(7): 624, 1987.

Cranberry In Patients on CIC, Indwelling Catheter, or Condom Catheter

Schlager TA, et al: Effect of cranberry juice on bacteriuria in children with neurogenic bladder receiving intermittent catheterization. J Pediatr, 135: 698, 1999.

Foda MM, et al: Efficacy of cranberry in prevention of urinary tract infections in a susceptible pediatric population. Can J Urol, 2: 98, 1995.

Waites KB, et al: Effect of cranberry extract on bacteriuria and pyuria in persons with neurogenic bladder secondary to spinal cord injury. J Spinal Cord Med, 27(1): 35, 2004.

Intravesical Irrigations

Arap M, Petrou SP: Efficacy of intermittent gentamicin sulfate solution for recalcitrant recurrent cystitis in women. Infections in Urology, July/August 2003: 45, 2003.

Defoor W, et al: Safety of gentamicin bladder irrigation in complex urologic cases. J Urol, 175(5): 1861, 2006.

de Jong, et al: Neomycin toxicity in bladder irrigation. J Urol, 150(4): 1199, 1993.

Gerharz EW, et al: Neomycin induced perception deafness following bladder irrigation in patients with end stage renal disease. Br J Urol, 76(4): 479, 1995.

Waites KB, et al: Evaluation of 3 methods of bladder irrigations to treat bacteriuria in persons with neurogenic bladder. J Spinal Cord Med, 29: 217, 2006.

LOWER URINARY TRACT INFECTIONS

Evaluation of Pediatric UTI—see page 231.

Urethritis in the Male—see page 357.

Sexually Transmitted Diseases—see page 373.

Prostate Infections—see page 365.

Asymptomatic Bacteriuria in Adults

General Information

1. The Infectious Diseases Society of America (ISDA) defines asymptomatic bacteriuria as "...isolation of a specific quantitative count of bacteria in an appropriately collected urine specimen obtained from a person without symptoms or signs referable to urinary infection."
2. Organisms causing asymptomatic bacteriuria
   a. In women without an indwelling catheter, E. coli is the most common cause of asymptomatic bacteriuria.
   b. When an indwelling catheter or condom catheter is in place, polymicrobial colonization is the most common cause of asymptomatic bacteriuria.
3. Examples of conditions that cause asymptomatic bacteriuria
   a. Bowel incorporated into urinary tract—ileal conduit, augmentation cystoplasty, ileal chimney, ileal ureter.
   b. Cutaneous ostomy—vesicostomy, ureterostomy, pyelostomy.
   c. Indwelling catheter—urethral, suprapubic, or nephrostomy tube.
   d. Intermittent catheter use
   e. Condom catheter
4. *Antibiotic therapy for asymptomatic bacteriuria often leads to resistant organisms.*

Diagnosis

1. *Diagnosis of asymptomatic bacteria is based on urine culture*, and is defined by the following criteria.
   a. Voided specimen
      i. For women—2 consecutive voided urine specimens with isolation of the same bacterial strain and a count of $\geq$ 100,000 cfu/ml.
      ii. For men—a single clean-catch voided urine specimen with one bacterial strain isolated and a count of $\geq$ 100,000 cfu/ml.
   b. Catheterized specimen—a single catheterized urine specimen with one bacterial species and a count of $\geq$ 100 cfu/ml (men or women).
2. Pyuria is not sufficient to diagnose bacteriuria.

Screening and Treatment (based on the IDSA 2005 guidelines)

1. *In most circumstances, screening and treatment for asymptomatic bacteriuria is not recommended.* The IDSA specifically recommended against screening and treatment of asymptomatic bacteriuria in non-pregnant women, elderly people residing in the community or in a long-term care facility, diabetic women, patients with spinal cord injury, and patients with indwelling catheters.

2. *Screening and treatment for asymptomatic bacteriuria is recommended in pregnant women* (see page 215).
3. *Screening and treatment for asymptomatic bacteriuria is recommended prior to traumatic genitourinary procedures associated with mucosal bleeding (e.g. TURP, urethral dilation, traumatic catheterization)* because these patients have a high rate of post-procedure bacteremia and sepsis.
    a. When possible, urine culture should be obtained so that the results are available before the procedure.
    b. Antimicrobial therapy should be started shortly before the procedure (e.g. the night before or immediately before the procedure).
    c. When a catheter is left in place after the procedure, the antibiotics should be continued (duration of therapy was not specified by the guidelines).
4. Screening for bacteriuria in patients with an indwelling catheter is not recommended unless they will be undergoing a traumatic genitourinary procedure.
5. When a patient with urolithiasis has a urease producing organism in the urine, treatment of asymptomatic bacteriuria may be considered to prevent formation and growth of the stones (See How UTI Increases Stone Risk, page 130).
6. *Non-traumatic replacement an indwelling catheter is associated with a low risk of bacteremia; therefore, antimicrobial therapy for a non-traumatic catheter change is not beneficial.*

Acute Bacterial Cystitis (ABC) in Women

Factors that Increase the Risk of ABC in Women
1. Sexual activity
2. New sexual partner within the past year
3. Additional risk factors for premenopausal women
    a. First UTI at age ≤ 15 years
    b. Family history of UTI in the mother
    c. Spermicide use (with or without a condom) for birth control
    d. Diaphragm use for birth control
4. Additional risk factors in postmenopausal women
    a. Postmenopausal status
    b. History of UTIs when premenopausal
    c. Urine incontinence
    d. Cystocele
    e. Elevated post void residual

Factors that Do *NOT* Change the Risk of ABC in Women
Although the following factors have been advocated to reduce UTI in women, the available evidence indicates that these factors do not prevent infection.
1. Void after intercourse.
2. Wipe the vagina from front to back after voiding.
3. Avoid tight fitting clothes and panty hose.
4. Drink a lot of water.
5. Void soon after the urge arises (do not hold the urine).
6. Avoid hot tub use.
7. Avoid douching.
8. Avoid tampon use.

Presentation

1. Symptoms may include dysuria, frequency, urgency, fever, and suprapubic discomfort. The patient may have hematuria, cloudy urine, or foul smelling urine.
2. In the elderly, the first sign may be mental status changes such as confusion or lethargy.

Work Up

1. A presumptive diagnosis of ABC can be made when a patient has symptoms of ABC and urinalysis (clean catch or catheterized urine) is consistent with infection. Findings on dipstick may include nitrite positive, leukocyte esterase positive, and heme positive. Microscopic exam may show RBCs, WBCs, and bacteria.
2. Urine culture and sensitivity—in women with signs and symptoms of uncomplicated acute bacterial cystitis, an initial urine culture is often unnecessary. However, a urine culture should always be obtained when a complicated infection is suspected.
3. If a patient fails to respond to antibiotics, a urine culture should be performed. See Evaluation of Recurrent ABC, page 338.

Treatment of Uncomplicated ABC (Based on the IDSA 1999 Guidelines)

1. Basic concepts of treatment
   a. A single dose of antibiotics is not adequate to treat ABC.
   b. *For trimethoprim-sulfamethoxazole (TMP-SMZ) and most fluoroquinolones (FQ), three days of therapy is recommended (longer regimens are not more effective).*
   c. *For nitrofurantoin, at least 7 days of therapy should be administered.*
   d. Beta-lactam penicillins are less effective for acute bacterial cystitis than trimethoprim (TMP), TMP-SMZ, and FQ.
   e. Bacterial cystitis is eradicated in 90% of appropriately treated patients after the initial course of antibiotics.
2. Initial empirical treatment (culture not done or still pending)
   a. *TMP or TMP-SMZ for 3 days*—recommended as first line empirical therapy in areas where E. coli resistance to TMP-SMZ or TMP is low (e.g. < 20%). Check local hospitals and labs for resistance levels in your area. The NAUTICA study on outpatient urine cultures revealed regions where E. coli resistance to TMP-SMZ is < 20%:
      i. U.S.—IA, IL, MN, MO, NE, OH, and WI.
      ii. Canada—Alberta, British Columbia, New Brunswick, Nova Scotia, Ontario, Quebec, Saskatchewan.
   b. *FQ for 3 days*—recommended as first line empirical therapy in areas where E. coli resistance to TMP-SMZ or TMP is high (e.g. > 20%). Moxifloxacin and gemifloxacin should not be used because of inadequate urine levels. Check local hospitals and labs for resistance levels in your area. The NAUTICA study on outpatient urine cultures revealed regions where E. coli resistance to TMP-SMZ is > 20%:
      i. U.S.—AZ, CA, CO, GA, FL, NC, NY, OR, PA, TX, and UT.
      ii. Canada—Manitoba.
   c. *Another option is nitrofurantoin for 7 days.*
   d. There is some evidence that UTIs in older women or UTIs caused by Staphylococcus saprophyticus may require more than 3 days of antibiotics, and a 7 day regimen may be more appropriate.
3. Adjust the antibiotic regimen based on urine culture.

4. Alternative/complementary treatments
   a. d-mannose—in vitro, d-mannose inhibits mannose sensitive pili in some strains of E. coli. After an oral dose, d-mannose appears to be excreted in the urine (probably in very small amounts) and may prevent E. coli adherence to the urothelium by inhibiting mannose sensitive pili. It is purported that this action prevents and treats UTI caused by certain strains of E. coli (anecdotal evidence).
   b. Cranberry juice—there is insufficient evidence to determine if cranberry effectively treats UTI. Because cranberry is acidic, it can make cystitis symptoms worse.

Treatment of Complicated ABC

1. The duration of antibiotics for complicated ABC depends on the clinical scenario, but therapy should probably be at least 7-10 days.
2. Treatment of complicated ABC in special circumstances
   a. Spinal cord injury—see page 330.
   b. Indwelling catheter—see page 327.
   c. Clean intermittent catheterization—see page 326.

Persistent Symptoms After Treatment of ABC (Chronic Cystitis)

1. When symptoms persist after an appropriate course of antibiotics, the initial evaluation may include the following tests.
   a. Ensure that the patient was compliant with therapy.
   b. Urine culture and sensitivity—rule out unresolved or recurrent ABC.
   c. Post void residual—make sure symptoms are not from urinary retention.
   d. Pelvic examination—vaginitis may mimic the symptoms of cystitis. Oral antibiotics increase the risk of yeast vaginitis.
   e. Consider performing cystoscopy and urine cytology.
2. In some cases, antibiotics eradicate bacteria from the urine, but bladder inflammation persists, causing symptoms to continue (even though the urine culture is negative). Symptoms may take several months to resolve.
3. There is no standard protocol for persistent symptoms after a bacterial infection is eradicated. The author recommends treating the symptoms and preventing recurrence while the inflammation subsides. I use the following regimen for 3-6 months.
   a. Prevent re-infection—administer a daily prophylactic antibiotic.
   b. Oral medications for symptom relief—anticholinergic drugs for urgency and frequency, urinary analgesics (such as Pyridium®) for dysuria, and NSAIDs for pelvic pain.
   c. Dietary changes—avoid urinary irritants such as caffeine, alcohol, spicy foods, artificial sweeteners (e.g. saccharin, Nutrasweet), carbonated drinks, and acidic foods (such as cranberry juice and vitamin C).
   d. Quercetin 500 mg po BID—an herbal anti-inflammatory bioflavonoid.
   e. Avoid constipation
   f. Physical and emotional stress reduction
4. If symptoms get worse during therapy or do not resolve within 3-6 months, I perform urine culture, urine cytology, physical exam (including pelvic exam), cystoscopy, and CT urogram. Pelvic ultrasound may be performed to more thoroughly assess the reproductive organs.
5. The differential diagnosis includes distal ureteral calculus, bladder cancer, vaginitis, interstitial cystitis, endometriosis, colitis, diverticulitis, etc.

Evaluation of Recurrent ABC
1. For recurrent uncomplicated ABC caused by re-infection in adult women, formal evaluation of the urinary tract is usually unnecessary. However, some evaluate the urinary tract when ABC occurs frequently or when symptoms persist long after the infection is eradicated.
2. See Unresolved and Recurrent Infections, page 325.

Preventing Re-infection
1. Avoid use of spermicides and diaphragm for birth control.
2. Topical estrogen therapy in postmenopausal women—*topical vaginal application of estrogen decreases vaginal pH, normalizes vaginal flora (by restoring Lactobacilli colonization), decreases contamination with fecal bacterial pathogens (Enterobacteriaceae), and decreases the risk of UTI.* The optimal type of estrogen and the optimal dose are unknown; however, vaginal creams and vaginal rings appear to be effective. *Oral estrogen therapy does not appear to be effective in preventing UTIs.*
   a. Contraindications—history of venous thrombosis or pulmonary embolus, recent stroke or myocardial infarction, estrogen dependant cancer (such as breast cancer), undiagnosed abnormal genital bleeding, and liver dysfunction.
   b. Side effects—embolic (pulmonary embolism, deep venous thrombosis, stroke), cardiac (myocardial infarction), increased risk of female cancers (breast, endometrial, and ovarian cancer), slightly increased risk of dementia, gallbladder disease, and visual disturbances.
3. Prophylactic antibiotics—prophylaxis with oral antibiotics has been proven to reduce the recurrence of UTIs by up to 95%.
   a. Daily—women who have frequent infections may take a daily low dose of antibiotic for 6-12 months. If re-infection occurs after cessation of prophylactic therapy, resume prophylaxis.
   b. After intercourse—those who engage in intercourse several times a day should not exceed the maximum dose or frequency of the antibiotic.
4. Self treatment (self-start therapy)—this is not a method of preventing UTI; it is a method of rapidly treating a developing UTI. Patients are given a prescription for antibiotics (with refills). When they feel the onset of UTI symptoms, they treat themselves with a course of antibiotics. Some physicians also request that patients have a urine culture done before starting the antibiotics.
5. Cranberry juice—data suggests that cranberry may *prevent* UTI in sexually active women. There is insufficient evidence to determine if cranberry is effective for *treating* UTIs. The optimal dose and form (juice or tablets) is unknown.
   a. Mechanism of action—consumption of cranberry causes urinary excretion of hippuric acid (a bacteriostatic agent) and lowers urinary pH. However, these effects are usually insufficient to confer significant antibacterial activity (even when a very high dose of cranberry is ingested). The antibacterial activity of cranberry probably arises from 2 compounds that prevent bacterial adhesion by inhibiting the pili of E. coli: fructose inhibits the mannose sensitive pili and proanthocyanidin inhibits the mannose resistant pili.
   b. Side effects—occasionally diarrhea. Cranberry can increase urinary oxalate, which may increase the risk of urolithiasis.
   c. Drug interaction—there are rare reports of cranberry interacting with coumadin and increasing risk of hemorrhage.
6. d-mannose—it is purported that d-mannose prevents and treats UTI caused by certain strains of E. coli (anecdotal evidence). See page 337.

7. Methenamine—in acidic urine, methenamine is hydrolyzed to formaldehyde (a urinary antiseptic). To be effective, urine pH must be less than 5.5. Achieving pH < 5.5 usually requires oral intake of an acidifying agent, such as potassium acid phosphate (K-Phos® original) or vitamin C. Methenamine is not effective in patients with an indwelling catheter, and is probably not beneficial in patients using intermittent catheterization. It should be used to prevent UTI, but not to treat UTI.
   a. Dose (adult)
      i. Methenamine hippurate 1 gram po BID [Tabs: 1 gm] with an acidifying agent if urine pH > 5.5.
      ii Methenamine mandelate 1 gram po QID [Tabs: 0.5, 1 gm; Suspension 0.5 gm/5ml] with an acidifying agent if urine pH > 5.5.
      iii. Uroqid-acid® (No. 2) two tablets po BID to QID with a full glass of water [Tabs: each tablets contains 500 mg methenamine mandelate with 500 mg of the acidifying agent sodium acid phosphate].
      iv. Acidifying agents include K-Phos® original 2-4 tabs dissolved in 6-8 oz. water po QID or vitamin C 1-2 grams po QID. Adjust the acidifying agent to keep urine pH < 5.5.
   b. Recommended laboratory tests during therapy: liver function tests when using methenamine hippurate, potassium and phosphate when using K-Phos® original, and sodium and phosphate when using Uroqid-acid®.
   c. Drink a moderate amount of fluids. Consuming too much fluid can dilute the methenamine.
   d. Carbonic anhydrase inhibitors (such as acetazolamide), thiazides, calcium carbonate, and sodium bicarbonate can produce alkaline urine, which negates the antiseptic effect of methenamine. Patients should avoid foods and medicines that alkalinize the urine.
   e. Do not take methenamine with sulfonamides because sulfonamides may form an insoluble precipitate with formaldehyde in the urine.
   f. Side effects—methenamine may cause nausea, vomiting, rash, and dysuria. Vitamin C can increase the risk of urolithiasis (see Medications That May Induce Urolithiasis, page 131).
8. Intravesical antibiotics—may be used when the organism is resistant to oral antibiotics or when the patient cannot tolerate the standard antibiotic regimen. Intravesical gentamicin may eradicate recurrent cystitis caused by a gentamicin sensitive organism. Example regimen:
   a. Mix 480 mg gentamicin sulfate into a 1000 cc bottle of sterile normal saline. Keep the solution refrigerated. The solution should be discarded after 30 days, although it may retain its potency for up 2 months.
   b. The patient is catheterized and the bladder is completely emptied.
   c. Gentamicin (480 mg/1000 ml normal saline) is gently instilled through the catheter and into the bladder using a catheter tip syringe. The instilled volume may vary; however, 30 cc is often used in adults with normal bladder capacity.
   d. The catheter is removed and the solution is left in the bladder until the patients voids.
   e. An instillation is performed each day for one week. Some urologists continue the regimen as follows: 4 times a week for the second week, then 3 times a week for the next 6 weeks.
   f. Avoid intravesical instillation when there is a risk of systemic absorption (e.g. gross hematuria, traumatic catheterization)
   g. It may be prudent to check serum gentamicin levels; however, using this protocol, serum creatinine did not appear to be altered.
   h. Approximately 30% can have breakthrough UTIs, some of which are gentamicin resistant.

9. These behaviors have been advocated to help prevent UTIs, but current evidence suggests that they do not help.
    a. Void after intercourse.
    b. Wipe the vagina from front to back after voiding.
    c. Avoid tight fitting clothes and panty hose.
    d. Drink a lot of water.
    e. Void soon after the urge arises (not holding the urine).
    f. Avoid hot tub use.
    g. Avoid douching.
    h. Avoid tampon use.

Emphysematous Cystitis—see page 395

Pyocystis

1. Pyocystis is a pus-filled bladder. It usually occurs in a defunctionalized bladder (a bladder in which no urine collects because of renal failure or because of a supravesical urinary diversion). Pyocystis probably occurs in defunctionalized bladders because urothelial cells are shed into the bladder, where they degenerate and liquefy. This liquefied cellular material accumulates in the bladder and may serve as a media for infection.
2. Presentation—purulent, bloody, or malodorous urethral discharge. The patient is often febrile and may have suprapubic pain. Some patients have no symptoms referable to the urinary tract.
3. The initial management usually consists of
    a. Place a catheter—drain the purulent fluid from the bladder and send the fluid for culture and sensitivity.
    b. Antibiotics—ill patients should be started on IV antibiotics. Oral antibiotics may be sufficient in minimally ill patients.
    c. Intravesical antibiotic or antiseptic—initially administered by instillation twice a day or by continuous bladder irrigation. After clinical signs of infection have resolved, instillation is often continued twice a week for 2-4 weeks. Repeat this cycle as needed. Antiseptics that have been used include acetic acid, chlorhexidine, and povidone-iodine. For doses of antiseptics and antibiotics, see page 327 and page 329.
4. If bladder irrigations fail to sufficiently control pyocystis, more aggressive treatment may be required.
    a. Chemical sclerosis of the bladder—sclerosing agents (e.g. 6% acetic acid left in the bladder for 1 hour) have been used to induce fibrosis of the bladder urothelium, which seems to prevent shedding of urothelial cells. After sclerosis, it may take as long as 9 months before the scarring reduces the incidence of pyocystis.
    b. Cystectomy—removing the bladder removes it as a source of infection.
    c. Surgically created fistula—these fistulas prevent accumulation of the cellular secretions by allowing them to drain spontaneously from the bladder.
        i. Vaginal vesicostomy (for females)—a fistula is created from the bladder to the vagina.
        ii. Perineal vesicostomy (for males)—a fistula is created from the bladder to the perineum.

REFERENCES

General

Arap M, Petrou SP: Efficacy of intermittent gentamicin sulfate solution for recalcitrant recurrent cystitis in women. Infections in Urology, July/August 2003: 45, 2003.

Krieger J: Urinary tract infections: what's new? J Urol, 168: 2351, 2002.

Schaeffer AJ: Infections of the urinary tract. Campbell's Urology. 8th Edition. Ed. PC Walsh, AB Retik, et al. Philadelphia: W. B. Sanders Company, 2002, pp 515-602.

Warren JW, et al for the Infectious Diseases Society of America: Guidelines for the antimicrobial treatment of uncomplicated acute bacterial cystitis and acute pyelonephritis is women. Clin Infect Dis, 29: 745, 1999.

Zhanel GG, et al: Antibiotic resistance in outpatient urinary isolates: final results from the North American Urinary Tract Infection Collaborative Alliance (NAUTICA). Int J Antimicrob Agents, 26: 380, 2005.

Asymptomatic Bacteriuria

Nicolle LE, et al: Infectious Diseases Society of America (ISDA) guidelines for the diagnosis and treatment of asymptomatic bacteriuria in adults. Clin Infect Dis, 40: 643, 2005.

U.S. Preventative Services Task Force: Screening for asymptomatic bacteriuria: recommendation statement. Rockville, MD: Agency for Health care Research and Quality; Feb. 2004. (http://www.ahrq.gov/clinic/3rduspstf/asymbac/asymbacrs.htm)

Estrogens and UTI

Brown JS, et al: Urinary tract infections in postmenopausal women: effect of hormone therapy and risk factors. Obstet Gynecol, 98: 1045, 2001.

Cardozo L, et al: A systematic review of estrogens for recurrent urinary tract infections: third report of the Hormones and Urogenital Therapy Committee. Int Urogynecol J Pelvic Floor Dysfunct, 12(1): 15, 2001.

Rozenberg S, et al: Estrogen therapy in older patients with recurrent urinary tract infections: a review. Int J Fertil, 49: 71, 2004.

Cranberry and UTI

Aston JL, et al: Interaction between warfarin and cranberry juice. Pharmacotherapy, 26: 1314, 2006.

Jepson RG, et al: Cranberries for preventing urinary tract infection. Cochrane Database Syst Rev, 2: CD001321, 2004.

Raz R, et al: Cranberry juice and urinary tract infection. Clin Infect Dis, 38: 1413, 2004.

Rindone JP, Murphy TW: Warfarin-cranberry juice interaction resulting in profound hypoprothrombinemia and bleeding. Am J Ther, 13: 283, 2006.

Pyocystis

Guerrier K, et al: Experiences with pyocystis. Arch Surg, 103: 63, 1971.

Lees JA, et al: Pyocystis, pyonephrosis and perinephric abscess in end stage renal disease. J Urol, 134: 716, 1985.

Ray P, et al: The pyocystis syndrome. Br J Urol, 43: 583, 1971.

Stevens PS, Eckstein HB: The management of pyocystis following ileal conduit urinary diversion in children. Br J Urol, 47: 631, 1975.

Weinberg RW: Pyocystis. J Urol, 117: 798, 1977.

UPPER URINARY TRACT INFECTIONS

Acute Renal Infections

1. Acute renal infections
   a. Acute pyelonephritis
   b. Acute bacterial nephritis (ABN)
   c. Renal abscess
   d. Perirenal (perinephric) abscess
   e. Emphysematous pyelonephritis
   f. Emphysematous pyelitis
   g. Pyonephrosis/infected hydronephrosis
2. *Acute renal infections usually occur by ascending infection from the bladder; therefore, signs and symptoms of acute cystitis are often present.* Urine culture is usually positive, but may be negative if the patient has recently been taking antibiotics. *E. coli is the most common causative organism of both acute cystitis and acute renal infections.*
3. Occasionally, hematogenous spread (usually of gram positive organisms such as Staphylococcus aureus) can cause acute renal infections. Suspect hematogenous spread in intravenous drug abusers and patients with cutaneous infections. In cases of hematogenous spread, signs and symptoms of cystitis may be absent (e.g. no pyuria, no bacteriuria, no growth on urine culture).
4. When an acute renal infection progresses, it appears to advance along a continuum from pyelonephritis to ABN to renal/perirenal abscess. Therefore, pyelonephritis precedes the formation of an abscess.
5. Presentation
   a. *Patients with severe renal infections may present with signs and symptoms similar to pyelonephritis.*
   b. The clinical presentation of acute renal infection includes fever, chills, flank or abdominal pain, and gastrointestinal symptoms (nausea, vomiting, anorexia). Symptoms of acute cystitis may be present.
   c. Physical exam usually reveals fever and costovertebral angle tenderness (CVAT) on the affected side. A flank mass may be palpable when a renal or perineal abscess is present.
   d. Blood tests usually reveal an elevated WBC count with elevated neutrophils (left shift on differential).
   e. Pyelonephritis rarely presents with a positive blood culture. Positive blood cultures are found in 40-50% of patients with renal abscess, perinephric abscess, pyonephrosis, and ABN. Almost 100% of patients with emphysematous pyelonephritis have a positive blood culture.
   f. *After starting antibiotics, patients with pyelonephritis are usually afebrile within 72 hours, whereas patients with a more serious renal infection are usually febrile for more than 72 hours.*
6. When placing a percutaneous drain into a retroperitoneal abscess (renal, perirenal, pararenal) or an infected collecting system (pyonephrosis, emphysematous pyelitis), a subcostal puncture is preferred because this avoids violation of the pleura and prevents spread of infection into the pleural space (empyema). Transperitoneal drainage should be avoided to prevent peritonitis.

Chronic Renal Infections
1. Chronic renal infections
   a. Chronic pyelonephritis
   b. Xanthogranulomatous pyelonephritis (XGP)
   c. Malacoplakia
   d. Tuberculosis
   e. Echinococcus
2. Presentation of chronic renal infection is highly variable and nonspecific.
3. E. coli is the most common cause of chronic pyelonephritis and malacoplakia; however, *proteus is the most common cause of XGP.*

Acute Pyelonephritis in Women

General Information
1. Pyelonephritis is infection of the renal parenchyma without an inflammatory mass and without abscess.
2. *E. coli is the most common causative organism.*
3. Pyelonephritis usually occurs by ascending infection from the bladder, but can also occur by hematogenous spread to the kidney. Suspect hematogenous spread (usually of gram positive organisms) in intravenous drug abusers and patients with cutaneous infections. In cases of hematogenous spread, signs and symptoms of cystitis may be absent (e.g. no pyuria, no bacteriuria, no growth on urine culture).

Presentation
1. Most cases of pyelonephritis occur in women. Approximately 75% of patients have a previous history of cystitis.
2. The clinical presentation can range from mild cystitis with flank ache to sepsis; however, most patients are not severely ill.
3. The diagnosis is made by clinical findings, which often include fever, chills, abdominal or flank pain, gastrointestinal symptoms (nausea, vomiting, anorexia), and symptoms of acute cystitis.
4. Physical exam usually reveals fever and costovertebral angle tenderness (CVAT) on the affected side.
5. Urinalysis typically shows WBCs and WBC casts.
6. Blood tests usually reveal an elevated WBC count and elevated neutrophils (left shift on differential). Blood cultures are usually negative.
7. *Intravenous urogram (IVU) is normal in 75% of patients with pyelonephritis.* Findings on IVU suggestive of pyelonephritis include renal enlargement, decreased nephrogram, and dilation of the collecting system without obstruction. CT may show similar findings. On CT, fat stranding may be seen around the affected kidney.
8. Renal ultrasound usually shows renal enlargement and abnormal renal echogenicity.

Work Up

1. After history and physical exam, testing should include complete blood count with differential, urinalysis, and urine culture with sensitivity.
2. Blood cultures should be obtained in moderately/severely ill patients and in patients with prominent fever or leukocytosis.
3. Renal imaging by CT or ultrasound should be considered in patients with any of the following characteristics.
   a. Severely ill, unstable, or septic.
   b. Diabetes mellitus—diabetics with a clinical diagnosis of pyelonephritis should undergo renal imaging because they have a higher risk of renal abscess and emphysematous pyelonephritis.
   c. Immunocompromised (e.g. diabetes mellitus, HIV, taking steroids, or on chemotherapy).
   d. Known structural abnormality of the urinary tract (e.g. calyceal diverticulum, hydronephrosis, vesicoureteral reflux, etc.).
   e. Urinary obstruction
   f. Urolithiasis
   g. Failure to respond to antibiotics (e.g. febrile > 72 hours on antibiotics)

Treatment (Based on the 1999 ISDA Guidelines)

1. Mildly ill—compliant women with mild acute uncomplicated pyelonephritis (low grade fever, normal or slightly elevated WBC, no nausea or vomiting) can be treated with oral antibiotics as an outpatient.
   a. The recommended empiric therapy is an oral fluoroquinolone (FQ). Moxifloxacin and gemifloxacin should not be used for pyelonephritis because they achieve low urine levels.
   b. Adjust antibiotics based on urine culture and treat for 7 days if a FQ is used and for 14 days if a non-FQ is used.
   c. *After starting antibiotics, patients with pyelonephritis are usually afebrile within 72 hours, whereas patients with a more serious renal infection are usually febrile for more than 72 hours.*
   d. If the patient does not respond adequately after initiating antibiotics (fever > 72 hours, insufficient decline in blood WBC, or little clinical improvement), then consider admitting the patient for intravenous antibiotics, blood cultures, renal imaging, and repeat urine culture.
2. Moderately or severely ill—women with high fever, high blood WBC, vomiting, dehydration, or sepsis.
   a. Admit the patient to the hospital, obtain urine and blood cultures, and start intravenous antibiotics. If the patient is severely ill, renal imaging should be performed.
   b. The recommended initial empiric therapy consists of one of the following *intravenous* regimens:
      i. A fluoroquinolone (FQ)
      ii. An aminoglycoside with or without ampicillin.
      iii. An extended spectrum cephalosporin with or without an aminoglycoside.
   c. Treat with intravenous antibiotics until the patient is afebrile for 24-48 hours, then change to oral antibiotics and continue oral antibiotics for 2 weeks. Adjust the antibiotics based on culture results.
   d. If the patient does not respond adequately after initiating antibiotics (fever > 72 hours, insufficient decline in blood WBC, or little clinical improvement), then consider re-imaging the kidneys and repeating the urine and blood cultures.
3. 10-30% of patients will relapse after an initial 14 day course of antibiotics. A second 14 day course of antibiotics usually eradicates the infection, but if it does not, a 6 week course of antibiotics may be necessary.

Chronic Pyelonephritis

1. Chronic pyelonephritis generally refers to a scarred, atrophic, and poorly functioning kidney from previous episodes of acute pyelonephritis.
2. Acute pyelonephritis is diagnosed by clinical criteria, whereas chronic pyelonephritis is diagnosed by radiographic or pathologic findings.
3. The clinical presentation is usually nonspecific. Patients are often asymptomatic. They may have proteinuria, hypertension, anemia of chronic disease, or renal insufficiency. Hypertension may be caused by renin secretion from the scarred kidney.
4. Imaging may reveal atrophy and scarring of the kidney. Clubbing of the calyces may also be seen.
5. Treatment
   a. Reduce risk factors for UTI (e.g. treat vesicoureteral reflux).
   b. Control hypertension and other diseases that may affect renal function.
   c. When the contralateral kidney is normal, nephrectomy of the affected kidney may be considered when it is nonfunctioning and causing chronic pain, recurrent infections, or renin mediated hypertension.

Emphysematous Pyelonephritis—see page 396.

Acute Bacterial Nephritis (Acute Lobar Nephronia)

General Information

1. Acute bacterial nephritis (ABN) is an uncommon interstitial nephritis caused by bacterial infection of the renal cortex, which results in an inflammatory mass or masses without liquefaction.
2. ABN may be focal or multifocal. Acute focal bacterial nephritis (AFBN) is present when there is a single inflammatory mass within the kidney. Acute multifocal bacterial nephritis (AMBN) is present when there is multiple inflammatory masses within the kidney.
3. *E. coli is the most common causative organism.*
4. ABN usually occurs by ascending infection from the bladder, but can also occur by hematogenous spread to the kidney. Suspect hematogenous spread (usually of gram positive organisms) in intravenous drug abusers and patients with cutaneous infections. In cases of hematogenous spread, signs and symptoms of cystitis may be absent (e.g. no pyuria, no bacteriuria, no growth on urine culture).
5. ABN probably represents a middle ground between uncomplicated pyelonephritis and renal abscess. In other words, renal infection tends to progress from uncomplicated pyelonephritis to ABN to renal or perirenal abscess. 25% of patients progress to abscess.
6. Up to 50% of patients with ABN have vesicoureteral reflux.

Presentation

1. Clinical and laboratory manifestations are similar to pyelonephritis except patients with ABN are more severely ill than patients with pyelonephritis and 50% have positive blood cultures.
2. Imaging—the affected kidney is usually enlarged (nephromegally). *The affected area within the kidney is solid and shows no liquefaction.*
   a. CT is the best study for diagnosing ABN. CT shows nephromegally, diminished nephrogram, and *a solid, poorly defined, enhancing mass (focal) or masses (multifocal) that may be misinterpreted as neoplasm.* Enhancement of the affected area is often patchy and/or striated.
   b. Ultrasound shows nephromegally and a poorly marginated sonolucent mass with internal echoes that disrupt the corticomedullary junction.

Work Up

1. In most cases, these patients are initially diagnosed with pyelonephritis. The severity of their condition or inadequate response to antibiotics (febrile > 72 hours) prompts renal imaging, which reveals ABN.
2. If ultrasound raises the suspicion of ABN, CT with and without intravenous contrast should be performed.
3. Consider obtaining a voiding cystourethrogram (VCUG) after the infection has been completely treated (up to 50% of patients with ABN have reflux).

Treatment

1. Admit the patient to the hospital, obtain blood and urine cultures, and start intravenous fluids.
2. Start broad spectrum intravenous antibiotics. Treat with intravenous antibiotics until the patient is afebrile for 24-48 hours, then change to oral antibiotics and continue oral antibiotics for at least 2 weeks. Adjust the antibiotics based on culture results.
3. *After starting antibiotics, patients with pyelonephritis are usually afebrile within 72 hours, whereas patients with ABN usually remain febrile for more than 72 hours.*
4. If the patient fails to respond adequately to antibiotic therapy:
   a. Re-image the patient to check for obstruction and abscess—CT scan with intravenous contrast and delayed images or CT urogram may be utilized to evaluate for abscess and for obstruction.
   b. Repeat blood and urine cultures.
5. Interval imaging may be performed to demonstrate resolution of the infection.

Renal Abscess

General Information

1. A renal abscess is a collection of purulent fluid within the renal capsule and in the renal parenchyma (cortex or medulla). A renal cortical abscess is also called a renal carbuncle.
2. *Gram negative organisms are the most common cause.*
3. Renal abscess usually arises from an ascending infection by gram-negative organisms. When hematogenous spread causes a renal abscess, the infection usually arises from a gram positive organism (such as staphylococcus aureus) and the abscess is usually located in the renal cortex (cortical abscess or carbuncle). Suspect hematogenous spread in intravenous drug abusers and patients with cutaneous infections.
4. Renal abscesses may contain gas. Sometimes the abscess appears to contain only gas and no fluid.

Presentation

1. 50% of patients have diabetes mellitus.
2. 65% of patients have a history of recurrent UTI.
3. Clinical and laboratory manifestations are similar to pyelonephritis except patients with renal abscess are more severely ill, 50% have positive blood cultures, and 50% have a flank mass.
4. A normal IVU does not exclude the presence of a renal abscess.
5. Ultrasound reveals a sonolucent mass with internal echoes.
6. *CT is the best method for diagnosing renal abscess. CT usually shows a well-defined, low-density fluid filled mass. The mass itself does not enhance, but the abscess wall may enhance (rim enhancement).*
7. Gallium scan shows increased gallium uptake in the region of the abscess.

Treatment
1. Antibiotics—start broad spectrum intravenous antibiotics and treat until the patient is afebrile for 24-48 hours, then change to oral antibiotics and continue them for at least 2 weeks. Adjust antibiotics based on the culture.
2. When placing a percutaneous drain into a retroperitoneal abscess, a subcostal puncture is preferred because this avoids violation of the pleura and prevents spread of the infection into the pleural space (empyema). Transperitoneal drainage should be avoided to prevent peritonitis.
3. Abscess < 3 cm in size
   a. If the patient is not severely ill and not immunocompromised, then an initial trial of antibiotics alone may be considered. If the patient does not respond adequately, re-image the kidney and consider percutaneous or open surgical management.
   b. When the patient is severely ill, immunocompromised, or has an abscess containing gas, percutaneous drainage should be strongly considered.
4. Abscess > 3 cm is size
   a. Initial treatment usually consists of antibiotics and percutaneous drainage. Large abscesses may require multiple percutaneous tubes to adequately drain the purulent fluid. If the patient does not improve or percutaneous tubes fail to adequately drain the abscess, open surgical management is indicated.
   b. For abscesses > 5 cm, some surgeons favor percutaneous drainage as the initial therapy, while others favor open surgical management. If percutaneous drainage fails, open surgical management is indicated.
5. Open surgical management
   a. Surgical management options include open drainage of the abscess or nephrectomy. When the contralateral kidney is normal, nephrectomy may be considered when the affected kidney is poorly functioning or associated with recurrent bouts of infection.
   b. Open surgical drainage has higher cure rate than percutaneous drainage, but it has a higher morbidity.
6. Culture the abscess fluid.
7. If urinary obstruction is present, treat it accordingly.
8. Obtain interval imaging to demonstrate resolution of the abscess.
9. Special situations
   a. Renal tuberculosis—see Genitourinary Tuberculosis, page 399.
   b. Renal abscess caused by echinococcus should not be drained percutaneously because this can cause anaphylaxis.

Pararenal (Paranephric) Abscess

1. A paranephric abscess is a collection of purulent fluid near the kidney, but outside Gerota's fascia.
2. Paranephric abscesses usually arise from a perinephric abscess or an abscess in a nearby organ that extends into the paranephric space. Nearby organs from which infection can arise include bowel (e.g. appendicitis), pancreas, and lung.
3. Management of pararenal abscess depends on the primary source of the infection. When pararenal abscess arises from a perirenal abscess, treat as a perirenal abscess.

Perirenal (Perinephric) Abscess

General Information

1. A perirenal abscess is a collection of purulent fluid within Gerota's fascia, but outside the renal capsule.
2. *E. coli is the most common causative organism.*
3. Clinical and laboratory manifestations are similar to pyelonephritis except patients with renal abscess are more severely ill and 50% have positive blood cultures, and 50% present with a flank mass.
4. Most patients present with symptoms longer than 2 weeks in duration.
5. Approximately 40% of patients have diabetes mellitus and up to 50% have renal calculi.
6. *CT is the best method for diagnosing perirenal abscess. CT usually shows a well-defined low-density fluid filled mass. The mass itself does not enhance, but the abscess wall may enhance (rim enhancement).*
7. Gallium scan shows increased gallium uptake in the region of the abscess.

Treatment

1. *Treatment of perirenal abscess is similar to treatment of renal abscess.*
2. Interval imaging should be performed to demonstrate resolution of the abscess.

Pyonephrosis & Infected Hydronephrosis

1. Infected hydronephrosis is infection of hydronephrosis. Pyonephrosis usually refers to infection of chronic hydronephrosis, in which chronic obstruction has led to loss of renal parenchyma and impaired renal function.
2. Most patients have urinary calculi and a history of UTI.
3. The most common infecting organism is E. coli.
4. Clinical and laboratory manifestations are similar to pyelonephritis except patients with pyonephrosis are more severely ill and 50% have positive blood cultures.
5. If the ureter is completely obstructed, pyuria and bacteriuria may be absent.
6. Initial treatment consists of intravenous antibiotics and drainage of the infected collecting system.
   a. In minimally ill patients, initial treatment may be accomplished by placement of a percutaneous nephrostomy tube or by cystoscopy with placement of a ureteral stent. If a ureteral stent cannot be placed or if a ureteral stent does not adequately drain the infection, a percutaneous nephrostomy tube should be placed.
   b. In moderately or severely ill patients, initial treatment is usually placement of a percutaneous nephrostomy tube.
   c. If the patient's condition does not improve with a ureteral stent or nephrostomy tube, surgical management is indicated. Surgical management usually consists of nephrectomy because the affected kidney is often poorly functioning or non-functioning.
7. When placing a percutaneous drain into an infected collecting system, a subcostal puncture is preferred because is avoids violation of the pleura and prevents spread of the infection into the pleural space (empyema). Transperitoneal drainage should be avoided to prevent peritonitis.

Xanthogranulomatous Pyelonephritis (XGP)

General Information

1. XGP is a chronic infection of the renal parenchyma that causes diffuse renal destruction.
2. The inflammatory reaction can extend into the hilum and perinephric fat. In severe cases, the inflammation can spread beyond Gerota's fascia into the retroperitoneum and adjacent organs.
3. *Proteus is the most common causative organism.*

Presentation

1. XGP is usually unilateral.
2. *The affected kidney is usually non-functioning and is often associated with renal calculi and obstruction of the collecting system.*
3. Most patients have a history of recurrent pyelonephritis.
4. Clinical and laboratory manifestations are similar to pyelonephritis except patients with XGP often have anemia. 60% have a flank mass.
5. XPG has been called "the great imitator" because it mimics the clinical presentation, imaging characteristics, and pathological appearance of renal malignancy.
6. Imaging usually reveals a renal mass, calyceal deformity, enlarged kidney, and a stone in the affected kidney. *Imaging cannot distinguish between XGP and renal malignancy.*

Diagnosis

1. *XGP cannot be diagnosed based on imaging or clinical findings. It can only be diagnosed from surgically removed tissue; therefore, XGP is a pathologic diagnosis.*
2. Microscopic examination of XGP shows inflammation, necrosis, and large lipid laden macrophages ("foamy macrophages" or "foam cells").

Treatment

1. *XGP is treated by surgical excision of all inflammatory tissue.* Drainage alone invariably fails to cure XGP. There is no effective medical therapy for XGP.
2. Intraoperative frozen sections are not reliable for diagnosis because the lipid laden macrophages of XGP can be difficult to distinguish from the clear cells of renal cell carcinoma. Furthermore, there have been reports of XGP coexisting with renal cell carcinoma and with urothelial carcinoma.
3. *Most cases are managed by nephrectomy* because the affected kidney is usually non-functioning. Partial nephrectomy may be attempted in cases of focal XGP, solitary kidney, bilateral XGP, or renal insufficiency.
4. The severe inflammatory reaction makes surgery difficult.
   a. Open surgery is preferred because laparoscopic surgery has a very high complication rate and a high rate of conversion to an open procedure.
   b. *Imaging studies may underestimate the degree of involvement.* The inflammatory reaction often extends beyond the kidney, so be prepared to remove nearby organs. Administer a preoperative bowel preparation and, in left sided XGP, administer a pneumovax vaccine (ideally as early as possible before surgery) because splenectomy may be required.
5. *An attempt should be made to excise all of the inflammatory tissue.* When the inflammatory reaction extends beyond Gerota's fascia, the inflammatory tissue should be removed from surrounding organs.

REFERENCES

General

Chen J, Koontz Jr WW: Inflammatory lesions of the kidney. AUA Update Series, Vol. 14, Lesson 26, 1995.

Renzulli JF II, Anderson KR: Non-tubercular inflammatory disease of the kidney. AUA Update Series, Vol. 24, Lesson 4, 2005.

Schaeffer AJ: Infections of the urinary tract. Campbell's Urology. 8th Edition. Ed. PC Walsh, AB Retik, et al. Philadelphia: W. B. Sanders Company, 2002, pp 515-602.

Singer AJ: Editorial Comment: Xanthogranulomatous pyelonephritis: urologist beware. Issues in Urology, 18(6): 262, 2006.

Warren JW, et al for the Infectious Diseases Society of America: Guidelines for the antimicrobial treatment of uncomplicated acute bacterial cystitis and acute pyelonephritis is women. Clin Infect Dis, 29: 745, 1999.

Renal, Perirenal, and Pararenal Abscess

Dembry L, Andriole VT: Renal and perirenal abscess. Infect Dis Clin North Am, 11: 663, 1997.

Meng M, et al: Current treatment and outcomes of perinephric abscesses. J Urol, 168: 1337, 2002.

Noble MJ: Perinephric abscess. AUA Update Series, Vol. 21, Lesson 10, 2002.

Shu T, et al: Renal and perirenal abscesses in patients with otherwise anatomically normal urinary tracts. J Urol, 172: 148, 2004.

Siegel JF, et al: Minimally invasive treatment of renal abscess. J Urol, 155: 52, 1996.

Pyonephrosis

Camunez F, et al: Percutaneous nephrostomy in pyonephrosis. Urol Radiol, 11: 77, 1989.

Lees JA, et al: Pyocystis, pyonephrosis and perinephric abscess in end stage renal disease. J Urol, 134: 716, 1985.

Ng CK, et al: Outcome of percutaneous nephrostomy for the management of pyonephrosis. Asian J Surg, 25: 215, 2002.

Watson RA, et al: Percutaneous nephrostomy as adjunct management in advanced upper urinary tract infection. Urology, 54: 234, 1999.

Renal Infections

	Presentation	Infection	Most Common Cause of Infection	Associated Conditions	Positive Blood Cx	Flank Mass	Other Findings
Acute	Fever, chills, flank/abdominal pain, GI symptoms (nausea, vomiting, anorexia), signs & symptoms of cystitis, CVAT, leukocytosis. Patients with bacterial nephritis, abscess, emphysematous pyelonephritis, or pyonephrosis are more severely ill than patients with acute pyelonephritis.	Acute Pyelonephritis	E. Coli	Ascending	70% Recurrent Cystitis	Rare	Rare	Nephromegaly, decreased nephrogram, dilated collecting system, no discrete mass
		Acute Bacterial Nephritis	E. Coli	Ascending	50% VUR	40-50%	Rare	Enhancing solid intra-renal mass that mimics malignancy
		Renal Abscess	Gram Negative	Ascending	50% DM	40-50%	50%	Non-enhancing fluid filled intra-renal mass, rim enhancement of mass often present
		Perinephric Abscess	E. Coli	Ascending	40% DM 35% Calculi	40-50%	50%	Non-enhancing fluid filled extra-renal mass, rim enhancement of mass often present
		Pyonephrosis	E. Coli	Ascending	>50% Calculi	40-50%	Rare	Hydronephrosis, poorly functioning kidney
		Emphysematous Pyelonephritis	E. Coli	Ascending	75% DM	100%	50%	Gas in the renal parenchyma
Chronic	Variable (may be asymptomatic)	Chronic Pyelonephritis	*	Ascending	50-70% Recurrent UTI	*	Rare	Atrophic and poorly functioning kidney
		XGP	Proteus	Ascending	Calculi, Obstruction	Rare	60%	Solid renal mass that mimics malignancy, non-functioning kidney, "foam" cells
		Malacoplakia	E. Coli	Ascending	40% immuno-deficient	Occasional	Often	Solid intra-renal mass, Michaelis-Gutmann bodies, von Hansemann cells

XGP = Xanthogranulomatous pyelonephritis, CVAT = costovertebral angle tenderness, DM = diabetes mellitus, Cx = culture, VUR = vesicoureteral reflux.

* Patients usually do not have positive urine or blood cultures between acute infections. For acute episodes, see acute pyelonephritis.

GENITAL INFECTIONS

Sexually Transmitted Diseases—see page 373.

Fournier's Gangrene—see page 393.

Prostatitis—see page 365.

Genital Ulcers
1. STDs that cause genital ulcers—genital herpes, chancroid, primary syphilis, lymphogranuloma venereum (LGV), and granuloma inguinale. *Ulcers caused by genital herpes and chancroid are usually painful, whereas ulcers caused by syphilis are usually painless.*
2. Non-STD causes of genital ulcers
   a. Infectious—candida balanitis, bacterial skin infection, etc.
   b. Non-infectious—Reiter's syndrome, trauma, drug reaction, Behcet's disease (painful oral and genital ulcers, uveitis, non-mucous membrane skin lesions), pyoderma gangrenosum, etc.
3. All sexually active patients that present with genital ulcers should be tested for syphilis and genital herpes. Tests for chancroid, LGV, and granuloma inguinale should be performed in areas where these STDs are prevalent.
4. Treatment is often necessary before test results are available. The clinician should treat the diagnosis considered most likely based on the clinical presentation and epidemiology.

Cellulitis
1. Cellulitis is a skin infection involving the cutaneous and subcutaneous tissue without abscess and without fasciitis.
2. *Cellulitis is usually caused by beta-hemolytic streptococcus.* Streptococcus often causes cellulitis and rarely causes abscesses, whereas Staphylococcus often causes abscesses and rarely causes cellulitis.
3. *Infections of the skin typically present with 4 specific signs: redness, warmth, swelling, and pain.* Cellulitis may have an *orange peel* appearance (edema and dimpling of the skin). Inflammation may be present in local lymph nodes. Fever and leukocytosis are often present.
4. *It is critical that the clinician distinguishes between genital cellulitis and Fournier's gangrene because Fournier's gangrene is a life-threatening emergency.* Crepitus, foul odor, bruising, cutaneous anesthesia, eschar, or necrosis suggests the presence Fournier's gangrene (see page 393).
5. *Cellulitis is diagnosed by clinical findings.* Aspiration or biopsy of the skin is usually unnecessary. Obtain blood cultures when the infection is severe.
6. Treatment
   a. Antibiotic therapy is directed toward Streptococcus and Staphylococcus.
   b. In uncomplicated cellulitis, a 5 day course of cephalexin, erythromycin, clindamycin, or dicloxacillin is usually sufficient. Other agents may be considered based on resistance profiles in your community.
   c. In severe genital cellulitis, Fournier's gangrene should be considered.
   d. Scrotal elevation (promotes drainage of edema).
   e. Control diabetes.
7. When treating genital cellulitis, close observation is warranted. Poor response to treatment may be caused by Fournier's gangrene or organisms that are resistant to the initial antibiotic, such as methicillin resistant staphylococcus aureus (MRSA).

<u>Vaginitis</u>

General Information

1. Vaginitis is an inflammation of the vaginal mucosa, and may be caused by
   a. Hormonal vaginitis—postpartum, postmenopausal (atrophic vaginitis).
   b. Irritant (chemical) vaginitis—caused by contact with irritating substances such as spermicides, soaps, douches, tampons, etc.
   c. Allergic vaginitis—caused by direct contact with an allergen (e.g. latex) or by systemic exposure to an allergen (e.g. drug eruption).
   d. Infectious vaginitis—usually caused by bacterial vaginosis, Trichomonas vaginalis, or Candida.
2. Infectious vaginitis is characterized by vaginal discharge and vulvar irritation (pruritus, pain, burning). Vaginal odor and dysuria may occur.
3. The vagina is normally colonized with lactobacilli that produce hydrogen peroxide. Hydrogen peroxide is toxic to vaginal pathogens and keeps the vaginal pH between 3.5 and 4.5 in pre-menopausal women. In postmenopausal women, the vaginal pH may be > 4.5.
4. Common methods of evaluating infectious vaginitis
   a. Saline wet mount—vaginal discharge is placed on a slide and diluted with 1 to 2 drops of normal saline. A cover slip is applied and the slide is examined under a microscope using low (x100) and high (x400) power.
   b Potassium hydroxide preparation—vaginal discharge is placed on a slide and diluted with 1 to 2 drops of 10% potassium hydroxide (KOH). A cover slip is applied. The slide is air or flame dried and examined under a microscope using low (x100) and high (x400) power. Yeast are best visualized on KOH because KOH lyses cells that obscure yeast.
   c. Whiff test—the whiff test is positive when the KOH preparation emits an amine ("fishy") odor. The fishy odor arises from amines that are liberated when KOH alkalizes the vaginal discharge.
   d. Vaginal pH—pH of the vaginal discharge is measured using pH paper.

Trichomonas Vaginalis—see page 381.

Candida

1. The most common cause of yeast vaginitis is Candida albicans.
2. Risk factors include pregnancy, immunosuppression, poorly controlled diabetes, exogenous estrogens (e.g. oral contraceptives), and antibiotic use (especially penicillins, cephalosporins, and broad spectrum antibiotics).
3. Women often have dysuria, dyspareunia, vaginal discharge, and vaginal irritation (pain, pruritus, erythema, and swelling of the vulva).
4. Physical examination may reveal vulvar edema, fissures, and excoriations. A thick curd-like vaginal discharge is usually present (looks like cottage cheese). Vaginal pH is normal (pH < 4.5).
5. Diagnosis—requires vaginitis symptoms and one of the following findings.
   a. Saline wet mount, KOH, or gram stain of vaginal discharge shows yeast or pseudohyphae (elongated budding filaments).
   b. A culture of vaginal discharge reveals Candida.
6. When microscopy of vaginal discharge is negative but candida is suspected, obtain a culture of the vaginal discharge to confirm the diagnosis. Administer empiric therapy until the culture results are available.

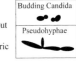

Candida

Budding Candida

Pseudohyphae

7. 95% of infections are uncomplicated. Complicated vaginitis has any of the following criteria: severe, recurrent, caused by non-albicans Candida, pregnancy, uncontrolled diabetes, or immunocompromised host.

Treatment of Uncomplicated Candida Vaginitis		
Non-pregnant	Topical OTC	Clotrimazole 1% cream 5 g intravaginally q HS x 7-14 days, or Miconazole 2% cream 5 g intravaginally q HS x 7 days, or Miconazole 100 mg vaginal suppository q HS for 7 days, or Miconazole 200 mg vaginal suppository q HS for 3 days, or Miconazole 1200 mg vaginal suppository single dose, or Tioconazole 6.5% ointment 5 g intravaginally one dose, or Butoconazole 2% cream 5 g intravaginally q HS x 3 days
	Topical Rx	Clotrimazole 100 mg vaginal tablet q HS x 7 days, or Clotrimazole 200 mg vaginal tablet q HS x 3 days, or Nystatin 100,000 unit vaginal tablet q HS x 14 days, or Terconazole 0.4% cream 5 g intravaginally q HS x 7 days, or Terconazole 0.8% cream 5 g intravaginally q HS x 3 days, or Terconazole 80 mg vaginal suppository q HS x 3 days, or Butoconazole 2% cream sustained release 5 g intravaginally one dose
	Oral Rx	Fluconazole 150 mg po one dose
Pregnant		Topical azole (avoid topical nystatin and oral fluconazole)

Rx = prescription, OTC = over the counter

8. Complicated Candida albicans infections require daily topical therapy for ≥ 7 days or 2 to 3 doses of fluconazole 150 mg po administered 72 hours apart. See the CDC recommendations for non-albicans infections.
9. If a patient does not respond as expected, culture the vaginal discharge.
10. Treat male sex partners if they have balanitis (see Balanitis, page 356).

Bacterial Vaginosis (BV)
1. *BV is the most common cause of vaginal discharge and foul odor.*
2. The cause of BV is unknown. In BV, the normal vaginal flora decrease in number and vaginal pH rises, which allows proliferation and overgrowth of Gardnerella vaginalis, mycoplasma hominis, and other organisms.
3. Risk factors—IUD, pregnancy, douching, and multiple sexual partners.
4. *More than 50% of women with BV are asymptomatic.*
5. Diagnosis—diagnosis is based on the Amsel criteria. BV is present when any 3 of these criteria are present.
   a. Homogeneous, thin, white discharge that coats the vaginal walls.
   b. Presence of *clue cells* on microscopic examination (epithelial cells with cell borders that are obscured by small bacteria).
   c. Vaginal fluid pH > 4.5
   d. *Positive whiff test* (fishy odor when KOH is added to vaginal discharge).
6. Culture for Gardnerella vaginalis is not recommended.

Treatment of Bacterial Vaginosis	

Non-pregnant	Recommended Regimens:
	  Metronidazole 500 mg po BID x 7 days, or
	  Clindamycin cream 2%, one applicator (5 g) intravaginally q HS x 7 days, or
	  Metronidazole gel 0.75%, one applicator (5 g) intravaginally q day x 5 days
	Alternative Regimens:
	  Clindamycin 300 mg po BID x 7 days, or
	  Clindamycin ovules 100 mg intravaginally q HS x 3 days

Pregnant	Metronidazole 500 mg po BID x 7 days, or Metronidazole 250 mg po TID x 7 days, or Clindamycin 300 mg po BID x 7 days

7. Follow up is unnecessary in non-pregnant women if symptoms resolve. Pregnant women should have a follow up evaluation 1 month after completing treatment to ensure that treatment was effective.
8. Routine treatment of sex partners is not recommended.

Infectious Vaginitis

| | Appearance of Vulva & Vagina | Vaginal Discharge | | | Vaginal pH | KOH Whiff Test ‡ | Saline Wet Mount | Treat Sex Partner |
		Color	Consistency	Odor				
Normal	Normal	White	Thin	No	3.5-4.5*	Negative	Lactobacilli, rare WBCs	—
Bacterial Vaginosis	Normal	Grey or white	Thin	Fishy	> 4.5	Positive	Clue cells, rare WBCs	No
Trichomonas vaginalis	Edema, erythema, cervical petechiae ("strawberry cervix")	Yellow-green	Frothy	Fishy	> 4.5	Sometimes Positive	Motile Trichomonas, > 10 WBC/HPF	Yes
Candida	Edema, erythema, fissures	White	Curd-like "cottage cheese"	No	< 4.5	Negative	Yeast, pseudohyphae†	If partner has candida balanitis

KOH = potassium hydroxide; WBC = white blood cell; HPF = high power field (x400)
* Vaginal pH may be > 4.5 in postmenopausal women.
† Yeast and pseudohyphae are more easily identified on the KOH preparation.
‡ A positive whiff test is characterized by the release of a fishy (amine) odor when KOH is added to the vaginal discharge.

Balanitis and Balanoposthitis

General Information
1. Balanitis is inflammation of the glans penis. Balanoposthitis is inflammation of the glans penis and prepuce.
2. Risk factors for balanitis
   a. Poorly controlled diabetes mellitus—this is the most common condition causing adult balanitis.
   b. Poor hygiene
   c. Broad spectrum antibiotic use—increases the risk of yeast balanitis.
3. Long-term effects of chronic balanitis
   a. Phimosis
   b. Balanitis xerotica obliterans (BXO)—see page 52.
   c. Leukoplakia—see page 52.
   d. Meatal stenosis

Causes of Balanitis
1. Irritant (chemical) balanitis—caused by contact with irritating substances such as spermicides, soaps, etc.
2. Allergic balanitis—caused by direct contact with an allergen (e.g. latex) or by systemic exposure to an allergen (e.g. drug eruption).
3. Non-infectious cutaneous disorders
   a. Reiter's syndrome—arthritis, urethritis, and conjunctivitis. Most patients with this syndrome have the HLA-B27 phenotype. They often have psoriasis like lesions on the glans (called circinate balanitis).
   b. Psoriasis
   c. Zoon's (plasma cell) balanitis—see page 51.
   d. Balanitis xerotica obliterans (BXO)—see page 52.
   e. Carcinoma in situ—see page 52.
   f. Pemphigus
   g. Lichen planus
4. Infectious balanitis
   a. Candida—*Candida is the most common cause of infectious balanitis and commonly occurs in diabetics or after broad spectrum antibiotics.*
   b. Gardnerella vaginalis
   c. Trichomonas vaginalis
   d. Genital herpes
   e. Human papilloma virus
   f. Other less common causes—Streptococcus (group A and B), Staphylococcus aureus, anaerobic bacteria, mycobacteria, and syphilis.

Presentation
1. Symptoms include rash, pain, pruritus, and foul odor.
2. Physical examination may reveal erythema, ulceration, fissures, scaling, edema, discharge, lesions, and phimosis.

Work Up
1. Some physicians treat balanitis empirically based on the likely cause.
2. Obtain cultures when the patient does not respond to empiric therapy. Swab under the prepuce for fungal and bacterial culture. Consider culture for Trichomonas vaginalis.
3. If ulceration is present, test for syphilis and herpes. See Genital Ulcers, page 352. Consider tests for other STDs.
4. Consider tests for diabetes (fasting serum glucose or hemoglobin A1c).
5. If the diagnosis is uncertain or the condition persists, consider performing a biopsy.

Treatment
1. Retract the foreskin daily, soak in warm water or saline, and clean the penis with gentle wiping. Avoid soaps, latex, and topical cleansers while inflammation is present.
2. Candida balanitis—usually presents with blotchy erythema that appears glazed or has small papules. It is usually sore and itchy.
   a. Clotrimazole cream 1% applied topically BID until symptoms resolve. [Cream: 15, 30, 45, 90 gram]
   b. Miconazole cream 2% applied topically BID until symptoms resolve [Cream: 15, 30, 90 gram]
   c. Nystatin cream 100,000 units/g topically BID until symptoms resolve. [Cream: 15, 30, 240 gram]
   d. Fluconazole 150 mg po one dose [Tabs: 150 mg]—may be used alone as initial therapy or added to topical regimens when balanitis is severe.
3. Anaerobic bacterial balanitis—often presents with foul smelling discharge. Inguinal lymphadenopathy may be present.
   a. Metronidazole 500 mg po BID for 1 week [Tabs: 500 mg].
   b. Clindamycin 10 mg/ml topically BID until symptoms resolve [Gel: 7.5, 30 g].
4. Aerobic bacterial balanitis—often caused streptococcus, or staphylococcus. Treat based on the specific organism and its sensitivities.
5. Irritant balanitis—hydrocortisone 1% topically BID until symptoms resolve.
6. For treatment of BXO, see page 52.
7. For treatment of Zoon's (plasma cell) balanitis, see page 516.
8. When balanitis does not respond to treatment (e.g. balanitis persisting for more than 6 weeks), consider performing a biopsy.

Urethritis in the Male

General Information
1. Urethritis is inflammation of the urethra.
   a. Non-infectious urethritis—causes include trauma (e.g. catheterization, cystoscopy), Reiter's syndrome, urethral stricture, urethral stone, and urethral lesions (e.g. condyloma, malignancy).
   b. Infectious urethritis—often classified as gonococcal urethritis (caused by Neisseria gonorrhoeae) or nongonococcal urethritis (not caused by Neisseria gonorrhoeae).
2. *In most cases of nongonococcal urethritis (NGU), the causative organism cannot be identified. When an organism is identified, it is usually Chlamydia trachomatis or Ureaplasma urealyticum.* Other causes of NGU include Mycoplasma hominis, Mycoplasma genitalium, Trichomonas vaginalis, and herpes simplex virus.
3. Mycoplasma and Ureaplasma are often part of the normal genital flora of healthy adults; however, these organisms may become pathogenic.
4. Prostatitis can present with signs and symptoms similar to urethritis.

Presentation
1. Symptoms may included dysuria, urethral discharge, and urethral pruritus.
2. Gonococcal urethritis typically causes *profuse* purulent urethral discharge, whereas non-gonococcal urethritis usually causes *scant* urethral discharge (that may be clear, purulent, or absent).

Diagnosis
1. The presence of any of the following criteria suggests urethritis.
   a. Purulent or mucopurulent urethral discharge.
   b. First void urine reveals positive leukocyte esterase. First void urine is the first 10-30 cc of voided urine obtained ≥ 1 hour after the last void.
   c. Centrifuged first void urine reveals ≥ 10 WBC/HPF on microscopy.
   d. Gram stain of urethral discharge shows ≥ 5 WBC/oil immersion field.
2. *All patients with urethritis should be tested for gonorrhea and chlamydia* (see page 373 and page 374). Tests for Trichomonas (page 381), herpes (page 377), mycoplasma, and ureaplasma may be considered at first presentation, but are often performed only if the initial therapy fails.
3. Routine bacterial cultures do not detect Mycoplasma and Ureaplasma; a special culture medium is required. Mycoplasma genitalium detection requires a PCR assay. Urethral specimens are obtained using a calcium alginate swab (not a cotton tip swab). Testing may also be performed on expressed prostatic secretions, semen, and calculi.

Treatment of Gonococcal Urethritis—see Gonorrhea, page 374.

Treatment of Non-gonococcal Urethritis (Based on CDC Guidelines 2006)
1. Doxycycline treats most Chlamydia, Ureaplasma, and Mycoplasma. However, doxycycline resistance is reported in up to 40% of cases.

Initial Treatment of Non-gonococcal Urethritis	
Recommended Regimens	**Alternative Regimens**
Doxycycline 100 mg PO BID x 7 days or Azithromycin 1g PO one dose	Erythromycin base 500 mg PO QID x 7 days or Erythromycin ethylsuccinate 800 mg PO QID x 7 days or Levofloxacin 500 mg PO q day x 7 days or Ofloxacin 300 mg PO BID x 7 days

2. Persistent or recurrent infections
   a. Patients who were not compliant with initial therapy or who were re-exposed may be treated again with the initial regimen. Ensure that the patient's sex partners have been evaluated and treated.
   b. Test for Trichomonas (see page 381). Consider culture and sensitivities for Ureaplasma, Mycoplasma, Chlamydia, Gonorrhea, and herpes.

Treatment of Persistent NGU (failure of initial therapy)
Metronidazole 2 g po one dose with Azithromycin 1 g po one dose* or Tinidazole 2 g po one dose with Azithromycin 1 g po one dose*
* If azithromycin was not used in the initial regimen.

   c. Azithromycin usually eradicates doxycycline resistant Chlamydia, Mycoplasma genitalium, and Ureaplasma (but does not eradicate Mycoplasma hominis). Metronidazole eradicates Trichomonas.

Organism	Usual Organism Sensitivity			
	Doxycycline	**Azithromycin**	**Erythromycin**	**Fluoroquinolone**
Chlamydia	+	+	+	+
Ureaplasma	+	+	+	+
M. genitalium	+	+	+/–	+/–
M. hominis	+	–	–	+

"+" = sensitive, "–" = resistant, "+/–" = intermediate sensitivity

3. If the patient does not respond to the initial regimen or the secondary regimen, consider the following possibilities.
   a. The patient was not compliant with therapy.
   b. The patient was re-exposed after therapy—consider treating the patient and the patient's sex partner again.
   c. The patient has a resistant organism—consider trying a quinolone (treats doxycycline resistant Mycoplasma hominis) or erythromycin (treats doxycycline and azithromycin resistant Chlamydia and Ureaplasma). If not already done, test the patient for Trichomonas, Ureaplasma, Mycoplasma, Chlamydia, Gonorrhea, and herpes.
   d. Non-infectious urethritis
   e. Alternative diagnosis—e.g. prostatitis, herpes, urethral lesion, urethral stone, bladder stone, etc. Consider performing a prostate exam, cystoscopy, and urine cytology.
4. Patients should abstain from sexual activity until 7 days after treatment is initiated.
5. Sex partners—patients with NGU should refer for evaluation and treatment all sex partners within the proceeding 60 days.
6. Follow up—patients should return if symptoms persist or recur.

Acute Epididymitis, Orchitis, & Epididymo-orchitis

General Information
1. Epididymitis is inflammation of the epididymis. Orchitis is inflammation of the testicle. Epididymo-orchitis is a combined epididymitis and orchitis.
2. Complications from epididymo-orchitis include
   a. Testis or epididymal abscess
   b. Pyocele (intrascrotal abscess)—see page 363.
   c. Chronic epididymitis or chronic orchitis—see page 361.
   d. Testicular atrophy
   e. Infertility—this is rare.

Causes of Epididymo-Orchitis
1. Non-infectious causes of epididymo-orchitis
   a. Behcet's disease—painful oral and genital ulcers, uveitis, non-mucous membrane skin lesions.
   b. Amiodarone—causes an epididymitis localized to the head of the epididymis and appears to be caused by concentration of amiodarone in this region. There is no associated urethral or urinary inflammation. It does not respond to antibiotics, but may resolve when the dose of amiodarone is reduced.
   c. Testicular or epididymal tumor
2. Infectious causes of epididymo-orchitis
   a. *In men < 35 years old, the most common causes of epididymo-orchitis are Neisseria gonorrhoeae and Chlamydia trachomatis* (i.e. sexually transmitted).
   b. *In men > 35 years old, the most common cause of epididymo-orchitis is E. coli* (i.e. not sexually transmitted).
   c. Viral—causes include mumps (see page 266) and coxsackie virus.
   d. Granulomatous—causes include tuberculosis (tuberculous epididymitis) and BCG. See Granulomatous Epididymo-orchitis, pages 362.
   e. Other rare causes—fungus, Ureaplasma, and Trichomonas.

Presentation

1. The most common symptom is *testicular pain*. The differential diagnosis includes testicular torsion. Torsion must be treated emergently (see Testicular Torsion, page 292). *Torsion is more likely when the onset of pain is sudden and extremely intense. Epididymitis is more likely when the onset of pain is gradual and progresses from mild to more intense.*

2. If epididymo-orchitis is caused by a sexually transmitted disease (STD), urethritis and urethral discharge may be present.

3. Physical examination may reveal
   a. Swelling and tenderness of the testicle, epididymis, and/or spermatic cord. Scrotal erythema and edema may be present on the affected side.
   b. Fever
   c. Hydrocele—a reaction to local inflammation. It often resolves slowly (weeks to months) after antibiotic therapy.

Work Up

1. History and physical examination—the diagnosis of epididymo-orchitis is usually made based on history and clinical findings.

2. When a STD is suspected, test for gonorrhea (see page 374), Chlamydia (see page 373), and other STDs. A gram stain of urethral discharge may make a presumptive diagnosis.

3. Midstream clean catch urine culture and sensitivity.

4. Scrotal ultrasound with Doppler is usually unnecessary, but may confirm the diagnosis.

Treatment

1. For mycobacteria, see Granulomatous Epididymo-orchitis on page 362.

2. Scrotal support (jockey type underwear rather than boxers).

3. Analgesics such as nonsteroidal anti-inflammatory medications.

4. Application of an ice pack may reduce swelling and decrease pain.

5. Empiric antibiotics should be started while the cultures are pending.

Initial Treatment for Acute Epididymo-orchitis	
If gonorrhea or chlamydia are likely (e.g. age < 35) †	**If STD is unlikely (e.g. age > 35)**
Ceftriaxone 250 mg IM single dose and	Ofloxacin 300 mg po BID x 10 days or
Doxycycline 100 mg po BID x 10 days	Levofloxacin 500 mg po q day x 10 days

† The CDC did not recommend alternative regimens. Alternative medications for treating gonorrhea or chlamydia are listed on page 376; however, their effectiveness for acute epididymo-orchitis is unclear.

6. Adjust the antibiotic based on culture results.

7. In severely ill patients (high fever, high leukocytosis, uncontrolled pain, sepsis), the patient may need to be treated with intravenous antibiotics.

8. Pain and fever usually improve within 3 days, but induration may take weeks or months to resolve.
   a. If the patient's condition does not improve after 3 days of antibiotics, consider reassessing the patient, repeating the urine culture, and obtaining a scrotal ultrasound (check for abscess, tumor, and infarction).
   b. Sometimes pain and swelling do not resolve with antibiotics. Scrotal ultrasound may show an irregular testis, raising the suspicion of malignancy. Radical inguinal orchiectomy may be required to determine a diagnosis and to relieve the pain.

9. If a STD caused epididymo-orchitis, patients and their sex partners should avoid sex until treatment is complete (see Gonorrhea, page 374).

Chronic Epididymo-orchitis, Orchalgia, & Epididymalgia

General Information
1. Chronic epididymitis is often defined as 3 or more months pain or discomfort in the scrotum, testis, and/or epididymis that is localized to the *epididymis* on clinical examination.
2. Chronic orchitis may be defined as 3 or more months pain or discomfort in the scrotum, testis, and/or epididymis that is localized to the *testis* on clinical examination.
3. The pain may be constant or intermittent. It may be unilateral or bilateral.
4. Patients with chronic epididymitis often have associated testicular pain.
5. Chronic epididymitis and chronic orchitis appear to be similar or related entities, and the diagnostic approach and treatment is often similar; therefore, they are discussed together in this section.

Classification of Chronic Testis and Epididymal Pain
1. Inflammatory
   a. Chronic active infection—evidence suggests that some cases of chronic epididymitis may be caused by chlamydia or trichomonas.
   b. Post-infective—inflammation may persist after infection is eradicated.
   c. Granulomatous—from tuberculosis, BCG, sarcoidosis, etc.
   d. Drug induced—amiodarone can cause epididymitis.
   e. Medical syndromes—Behcet's disease.
2. Obstructive—pain caused by obstruction of the epididymis or vas deferens (e.g. congenital obstruction, vasectomy)
3. Epididymalgia/orchalgia—normal epididymis and testis on exam and no identifiable cause of pain.

Differential Diagnosis
1. Testis or epididymal tumor
2. Intermittent testis torsion
3. Varicocele
4. Prostatitis
5. Tender sperm granuloma of the vas after vasectomy
6. Referred pain
   a. Stone in the mid or lower ureter—this can cause referred pain to the ipsilateral testis.
   b. Previous hernia repair—ipsilateral chronic orchalgia after inguinal hernia repair has been reported and is thought to be caused by injury to the genital branch of the genitofemoral nerve.
   c. Indirect inguinal hernia—may cause irritation to the genital branch of the genitofemoral nerve.
   d. Referred pain rarely occurs from aneurysm of the common iliac artery or aorta and degenerative spine disease (presumably of neurologic origin).

Work Up
1. History and physical (with special attention to the genitals, inguinal region, abdomen, and prostate). Check for inguinal hernia, scar from previous inguinal hernia repair, varicocele, vas granuloma, and masses.
2. Urinalysis and urine culture.
3. Culture urethral discharge when it is present.
4. Urethral swab culture for chlamydia and trichomonas.
5. Meares-Stamey type test for prostatitis (see Prostatitis, page 365).
6. Doppler scrotal ultrasound—check for testis or epididymis tumor.
7. Consider IVP, CT Urogram, or non-contrast CT to check for ureteral stones.

Treatment

1. There is little data available on the efficacy of treatment for chronic epididymis and testis pain.
2. Conservative management
   a. Pain medications—non-steroidal anti-inflammatory medications are commonly used. Referral to a pain specialist may be helpful.
   b. Scrotal support—prevents gravity from pulling on the spermatic cord.
   c. Avoid activities that exacerbate the pain.
   d. Warm compresses
   e. Spermatic cord block—this temporarily improves the pain. Rarely, long-term pain relief occurs if it "breaks the cycle of pain." It can be performed by injecting a local anesthetic (e.g. xylocaine without epinephrine) into the spermatic cord. Some urologists combine an injectable steroid (e.g. methylprednisolone) with the local anesthetic. When a cord block relieves the pain, then the pain is probably not referred.
   f. Empiric antibiotics
   g. Acupuncture
3. Surgical options—there is a reasonable chance that surgical therapy will not relieve the pain. Some urologists recommend performing a cord block before surgical intervention to confirm that the pain is neither referred nor psychological; however, it is unclear if pain relief after a cord block predicts the chance of pain relief after surgery. Several urologists report a high rate of complete pain relief (> 75%) with testicular denervation in patients who had pain relief with a cord block.
   a. If nerve injury from hernia repair is suspected, testicular denervation may relieve the pain.
   b. If a post-vasectomy sperm granuloma is thought to be the source of pain, excision of the granuloma may relieve the pain.
   c. If obstruction from vasectomy is thought to be the source of the pain, vasovasostomy or epididymectomy may relieve pain.
   d. If intermittent torsion is suspected, bilateral testis fixation may relieve the pain.
   e. Testicular denervation—transection or excision of the genital branch of the genitofemoral may relieve the pain.
   f. Epididymectomy—some patients who still have pain after epididymectomy may have pain relief when orchiectomy is performed.
   g. Orchiectomy—it appears that inguinal orchiectomy may be better at relieving pain than scrotal orchiectomy.

Granulomatous Epididymo-orchitis

1. This is a rare entity. Causes include tuberculosis and BCG.
2. BCG epididymo-orchitis
   a. Symptomatic BCG epididymitis and orchitis may be treated with INH* 300 mg po q day and rifampin 600 mg po q day for 3-6 months.
   b. Asymptomatic BCG granulomatous prostatitis requires no therapy.
3. Tuberculous epididymitis—see page 399.

* When giving isoniazid (INH), administer pyridoxine (vitamin B6) 50 mg po q day to prevent neurotoxicity and check liver function tests periodically.

Scrotal Abscess and Pyocele

Cutaneous Scrotal Abscess (Extrascrotal Abscess)

1. Cutaneous scrotal abscess is an abscess of the scrotal skin that does not extend to the tunica vaginalis. It usually arises from a cutaneous source.
2. Staphylococcus aureus is the most common organism found in cutaneous abscesses, but infections are often polymicrobial.
3. Presentation
   a. The involved area demonstrates *redness, warmth, swelling, pain, and fluctuance*. In some cases, a pustule may be seen or the abscess may extend to the skin surface, resulting in purulent discharge.
   b. Inflammation may be present in local lymph nodes.
   c. Fever and leukocytosis may be present.
4. Treatment
   a. Incision and drainage (I & D), which includes evacuation of pus and probing the abscess to break up loculations, is usually sufficient treatment. Systemic antibiotics are usually unnecessary, unless the abscess is large, the patient is immunocompromised, there is extensive surrounding cellulitis, or the patient has systemic manifestations (such as fever and chills). Consider obtaining a culture of the abscess fluid.
   b. If antibiotics are utilized, initial empiric antibiotics should be directed against Staphylococcus and Streptococcus (see Cellulitis, page 352). Adjust therapy based on culture sensitivities.
   c. Close observation is prudent in patients at risk for Fournier's gangrene.

Pyocele (Intrascrotal Abscess)

1. A pyocele is pus within the space between the tunica albuginea and the tunica vaginalis.
2. Pyocele can arise from any of the following processes.
   a. Spread from extrascrotal abscess.
   b. Complication of epididymitis or orchitis—epididymitis, orchitis, epididymal abscess, or testicular abscess can spread into the tunica vaginalis.
   c. Flow of pus from the peritoneal cavity through a patent process vaginalis—appendicitis, intraabdominal abscess, bacterial peritonitis.
   d. Direct inoculation—from scrotal surgery or penetrating trauma.
3. Scrotal ultrasound may reveal the extent of the abscess and determine if intrascrotal involvement is present. Abdominal imaging (CT or ultrasound) may be considered when the infection is thought to arise from an intraabdominal source.
4. For pyoceles that arise from an intra-abdominal infection, treat the primary infectious source. Purulent fluid in the scrotum may need to be drained.
5. For pyoceles that arise from epididymitis or orchitis, treatment consists of incision and drainage (I & D) of the scrotal sac. Initial antibiotics should be broad spectrum and include coverage for the likely causative organisms (chlamydia and gonorrhea for age < 35 and E. coli for age > 35). Adjust antibiotics based on cultures. Orchiectomy may be necessary when the testis is necrotic or infarcted. If the testis is not removed during the initial surgical drainage and the patient's infection does not resolve, consider orchiectomy (the testis and epididymis may be harboring infection).
6. For pyoceles that arise from spread of extrascrotal abscess or from scrotal surgery, treatment consists of I & D of the scrotal sac. Initial antibiotics should be broad spectrum and include coverage for the likely causative organisms (Streptococcus and Staphylococcus). Adjust antibiotics based on cultures.

REFERENCES

General

Centers for Disease Control and Prevention: Sexually transmitted diseases treatment guidelines 2006. Morbidity and Mortality Weekly Report, 55 (No. RR-11): 1-94, 2006. [Update in Morbidity and Mortality Weekly Report, 56 (14): 332-6, 2007].

Edwards S: 2001 National guideline on the management of balanitis. London: Association for Genitourinary Medicine and Medical Society for the Study of Venereal Disease, 2001. (http://www.bashh.org/guidelines/2002/balanitis_0901b.pdf)

Schaeffer AJ: Infections of the urinary tract. Campbell's Urology. 8th Edition. Ed. PC Walsh, AB Retik, et al. Philadelphia: W. B. Sanders Company, 2002, pp 515-602.

Walker P, Wilson J: 2001 National guideline for the management of epididymo-orchitis. London: Association for Genitourinary Medicine and Medical Society for the Study of Venereal Disease, 2001. (http://www.bashh.org/guidelines/2002/epididymoorchitis_0601.pdf)

Vaginitis

Amsel R, et al: Nonspecific vaginitis. Diagnostic criteria and microbial and epidemiologic associations. Am J Med, 74: 14, 1983.

Papppas PG, et al: ISDA guidelines for treatment of Candidiasis. Clin Infect Dis, 38: 161, 2004.

Urethritis

Deguchi T, Maeda S: Mycoplasma Genitalium: another important pathogen of nongonococcal urethritis. J Urol, 167: 1210, 2002.

Horner PJ, Shahmanesh M: National guideline on the management of nongonococcal urethritis. London: Association for Genitourinary Medicine and Medical Society for the Study of Venereal Disease, 2002. (http://www.bashh.org/guidelines/2002/NGU_0901c.pdf)

Chronic Epididymitis and Chronic Orchalgia

Davis BE, Noble MJ: Analysis and management of chronic orchalgia. AUA Update Series, Vol. 11, Lesson 2, 1992.

Ducic I, Dellon AL: Testicular pain after inguinal hernia repair: an approach to resection of the genital branch of genitofemoral nerve. J Am Coll Surg, 198: 181, 2004.

Kursh ED, Schover LR: The dilemma of chronic genital pain. AUA Update Series, Vol. 16, Lesson 37, 1997.

Levine LA, Matkov TG: Microsurgical denervation of the spermatic cord as primary treatment of chronic orchalgia. J Urol, 165: 1927, 2001.

Nickel JC, et al: The patient with chronic epididymitis: characterization of an enigmatic syndrome. J Urol, 167: 1701, 2002.

Nickel JC: Chronic epididymitis: a practical approach to understanding and managing a difficult urologic enigma. Reviews in Urology 5(4): 209, 2003.

West AF, et al: Epididymectomy is an effective treatment for scrotal pain after vasectomy. BJU Int, 85: 1097, 2000.

Cellulitis, Scrotal Abscess, and Pyocele

Santucci RA, Krieger JN: Pyocele of the scrotum: a consequence of spontaneous bacterial peritonitis. J Urol, 153: 745, 1995.

Satchithananda K, et al: Acute appendicitis presenting with a scrotal mass: ultrasound appearance. Br J Radiol, 73: 780, 2000.

Slavis SA, et al: Pyocele of the scrotum: consequence of spontaneous rupture of testicular abscess. Urology, 33: 313, 1989.

Stevens DL, et al: IDSA Practice guidelines for the diagnosis and management of skin and soft tissue infections. Clin Infect Dis, 41: 1373, 2005.

PROSTATITIS & PROSTATE INFECTIONS

Prostatitis

General Concepts
1. For the nomenclature and classification of prostatitis, see page 367.
2. Prostatitis can increase PSA. Treatment can normalize PSA.
3. The most common type of prostatitis is *nonbacterial*.
4. *The hallmark of chronic prostate syndromes is pain.* These syndromes may present with genitourinary pain, back pain, suprapubic pain, perineal pain, dysuria, frequency, urgency, painful ejaculation, and rarely erectile dysfunction. The prostate may be tender.
5. White blood cells (WBCs) and lipid-laden macrophages in the prostate fluid are rarely seen in normal prostates, but are often seen when prostate inflammation is present.
6. Consider alternative diagnoses in men with chronic "prostate" symptoms.
   a. Cystitis or urethritis—urine culture (and, if necessary, urethral culture).
   b. Genitourinary tumor—obtain a urine cytology and PSA.
   c. Herpes—genital herpes can cause prostate pain several days prior to the cutaneous eruption. Determine if the patient has or is at risk for herpes.
   d. Hematuria—work up significant hematuria (see Hematuria, page 122).
   e. Bladder stone—especially in older men with obstructive voiding.
   f. Urethral stricture—perform retrograde urethrogram and/or cystoscopy if urethral stricture is suspected.
   g. Other—inflammatory bowel disease, peri-rectal inflammation, interstitial cystitis, peri-vesical inflammation.

Work Up
1. History and physical examination
2. Urinalysis and urine culture
3. Meares Stamey 4 glass test
   a. Retract the foreskin and clean the penile meatus. The initial 5-10 ml of voided urine is collected and labeled VB1 (Voided Bladder 1). After 100-200 ml of urine is voided, 10 ml of "midstream" urine is collected and labeled VB2. While keeping the foreskin retracted, the prostate is massaged and the expressed fluid is collected and labeled EPS (Expressed Prostatic Secretions). After prostate massage, the initial 5-10 ml of voided urine is collected and labeled VB3. VB1-3 and EPS are sent for culture. The EPS and VB2 are examined under the microscope for WBCs.
   b. VB1—initial 5-10 ml of voided urine—represents urethral flora.
   c. VB2—10 ml of midstream voided urine—represents bladder flora.
   d. EPS—expressed prostatic secretions—represents prostatic flora.
   e. VB3—post-EPS voided urine—represents bladder and prostatic flora.
   f. When EPS or VB3 colony counts are at least 10 fold higher than VB1 and VB2, bacterial prostatitis is present.
   g. More than 10 WBCs per high power field in the EPS suggests prostatic inflammation, but does not confirm prostate infection. A positive EPS culture confirms bacterial prostate infection. Lipid-laden macrophages are also indicative of prostate inflammation.
   h. Avoid this test in acute bacterial prostatitis because it may cause sepsis.

4. Modified Meares Stamey test
   a. A midstream, clean catch urine specimen is obtained and labeled
     pre-massage. After the prostate is massaged, the initial 5-10 ml of
     voided urine is collected and labeled post-massage. These specimens are
     sent for culture and sensitivity. The post-massage urine is also examined
     under the microscope for WBCs. The pre-massage urine is examined
     (e.g. dipstick urinalysis) to determine if cystitis is present.
   b. Pre-massage urine—represents bladder flora.
   c. Post-massage urine—represents mixture of bladder and prostate flora.
   d. When post-massage urine colony counts are at least 10 fold higher than
     pre-massage urine, bacterial prostatitis is present.
   e. Avoid this test in acute bacterial prostatitis because it may cause sepsis.

Specimen	Represents Flora and WBC from this Location	Chronic Bacterial Prostatitis (NIH II)	Chronic Pelvic Pain Syndrome Inflammatory (NIH IIIa)	Chronic Pelvic Pain Syndrome Noninflammatory (NIH IIIb)	Urethritis or Urethral Colonization	Bacterial Cystitis*
VB1 Culture	Urethra	-	-	-	+	+
VB2 Culture	Bladder	-	-	-	-	+
EPS Culture	Prostate	+	-	-	-	+
EPS WBC	Prostate	+	+	-	-	+
VB3 Culture	Bladder & Prostate	+	-	-	-	+
Pre-massage Culture	Bladder	-	-	-	-	+
Post-massage Culture	Bladder & Prostate	+—	-	-	-	+
Post-massage WBC	Bladder & Prostate	+	+	-	-	+

    * Treat cystitis and repeat studies (see 5 below).

5. Bacterial cystitis may mask the presence of coexisting prostatitis. Patients
  who present with bacterial cystitis may be treated with amoxicillin or
  nitrofurantoin for 5 days. These antibiotics will concentrate in the urine but
  not in the prostate. Once the cystitis is eradicated, the tests described above
  may be more reliable in diagnosing prostatitis.
6. Consider the following additional tests (If bacterial cystitis or bacterial
  prostatitis is present, perform these tests after it is adequately treated).
   a. PSA
   b. Urine cytology or other urothelial tumor markers
   c. Post void residual
   d. Urine flow rate
   e. Symptom index—symptom severity and impact on quality of life can be
     measured using the NIH Chronic Prostatitis Symptom Index
     (NIH-CPSI; J Urol 162: 369, 1999). This score can be followed over
     time to determine the effects of intervention.
   f. Urodynamics—this may be helpful in men whose prostate syndrome is
     characterized by severe voiding symptoms or abnormal flow rates.
   g. Prostate ultrasound—for persistent symptoms, this may help identify
     prostatic calculi, abscess, ejaculatory duct obstruction, etc.

Classification of Prostatitis

NIH Category	NIH Classification†	Classification by Drach, Fair, Meares, & Stamey‡	Description	Symptomatic*	Bacteria Cultured From Prostatic Fluid	WBC in Prostatic Fluid
I	Acute bacterial prostatitis	Acute bacteria prostatitis	Acute prostate infection	+ (local & systemic)	**	**
II	Chronic bacterial prostatitis	Chronic bacter al prostatitis	Recurrent prostate infection	+ (local only)	+	+
IIIa	Chronic pelvic pain syndrome: Inflammatory	Chronic nonbacterial prostatitis	Prostate inflammation without infection	+ (local only)	–	+
IIIb	Chronic pelvic pain syndrome: Noninflammatory	Prostadynia	Prostate/pelvic symptoms without infection and without inflammation	+ (local only)	–	–
IV	Asymptomatic inflammatory prostatitis	—	Incidentally detected on prostate biopsy or other test	–	+/–	+/–

+ = Yes, – = no, WBC = white blood cell
† See Urology, 54: 229, 1999.
‡ See J Urol, 120: 266, 1978.
* Systemic symptoms include fever and chills. Local symptoms include suprapubic pain, perineal pain, dysuria, urinary frequency, urinary urgency, etc.
** Prostate massage is contraindicated in acute bacterial prostatitis. However, voided urine shows WBCs and positive bacterial culture.

Bacterial Prostatitis

1. Bacterial prostatitis is a symptomatic bacterial infection of the prostate.
2. *The most common cause of bacterial prostatitis is E. coli* (for acute and chronic bacterial prostatitis).
3. The prostatic epithelial cell lipid membrane prevents non-lipid soluble drugs from reaching the acini. The inflamed prostate has an alkaline pH. Thus, the ideal antibiotic for prostatitis is lipid soluble, weakly basic, and concentrated in the prostate. These characteristics are found in fluoroquinolones (FQs), trimethoprim-sulfamethoxazole (TMP-SMX), clindamycin, erythromycin, and to a lesser degree doxycycline. However, *FQs are the first choice for prostatitis because their cure rate is highest.*
4. Most of the infection in bacterial prostatitis is in the *peripheral* zone.

Acute Bacterial Prostatitis

1. This infection is characterized by fever, irritative and/or obstructive voiding symptoms, and an extremely tender, warm, boggy prostate. It is usually diagnosed in *young* men. The most common cause is *E. coli.*
2. *Avoid prostate massage*, aggressive prostate exam, and urethral instrumentation because these may cause pain and sepsis.
3. Work up and treatment
   a. Acute bacterial prostatitis is diagnosed by clinical findings. Prostate massage is contraindicated.
   b. Urine culture, CBC with differential, and blood cultures.
   c. Place a suprapubic tube in patients with urinary retention (avoid urethral catheterization).
   d. If high fever, prominent leukocytosis, or sepsis are present, admit the patient to the hospital and treat with an intravenous (IV) fluoroquinolone or a combination of IV ampicillin and an aminoglycoside. When the acute toxicity resolves, the patient may be switched to oral antibiotics.
   e. If admission is not indicated, broad spectrum oral antibiotics are started. FQs are the antibiotic of choice.
   f. Antibiotics should be adjusted based on the urine culture and should be continued for 4-6 weeks. This extended course of antibiotics is recommended to prevent chronic prostatitis.
   g. Antipyretics, stool softeners, and analgesics may be helpful.
   h. If fevers persist despite appropriate antibiotic therapy, obtain a pelvic CT scan to look for a prostate abscess. See Prostate Abscess, page 371 and Emphysematous Prostatitis, page 394.

Chronic Bacterial Prostatitis

1. This syndrome is characterized by recurrent symptomatic infection of the prostate and may present with genitourinary pain, back pain, suprapubic pain, perineal pain, dysuria, urinary frequency, urinary urgency, painful ejaculation, and rarely erectile dysfunction. This infection is lower grade than acute bacterial prostatitis and is usually diagnosed in *older* men.
2. *E. Coli is the most common cause of chronic bacterial prostatitis.* Other causative organisms include Klebsiella, Pseudomonas, Proteus, Enterococcus, Staphylococcus epidermidis, Staphylococcus saprophyticus, Chlamydia trachomatis, Ureaplasma urealyticum, and Mycoplasma hominis. See page 357 for antibiotic sensitivities to the rare organisms.
3. Recurrent urinary tract infections (UTIs) are common. *Chronic bacterial prostatitis is the most common cause of recurrent UTIs in adult males.*
4. These patients have an increased incidence of prostatic calculi, which may be a nidus for recurrent infections.
5. Zinc (an antibacterial agent) is lower in the prostatic fluid of men with chronic prostatitis.

6. Chronic prostatitis can cause infertility.
7. Prostate exam may be tender and boggy.
8. Treatment
   a. Start empiric therapy with a FQ (therapeutic dose) or TMP-SMX (one double strength tablet po BID). Adjust the antibiotics based on EPS or post-massage culture results. Consider 8-16 weeks of antibiotic therapy as the initial treatment (with a 4 week course, relapses occur more frequently). When the first course of antibiotics is almost complete, the EPS may be examined for WBCs. If WBCs are still present, consider extending the course of antibiotics for another few weeks.
   b. If an infection recurs or persists, re-culture and consider a longer course of antibiotics (up to 4 months). If infection still recurs, consider a 6 month course of suppressive antibiotics, such as TMP-SMX (one double strength tablet po q day) or a FQ (prophylactic dose).
   c. Non-steroidal anti-inflammatory drugs (NSAIDS), anticholinergics, and alpha blockers may help reduce symptoms.
   d. For additional therapies that may be helpful, see page 370.
   e. TURP—this should only be considered in men with prostatic calculi and recurrent/persistent culture proven bacterial prostatitis. The goal is removal of infected tissue and prostatic calculi (a nidus for recurrent infection). However, TURP may not be successful because the peripheral zone (which often remains after TURP) has the highest concentration of infection. TURP should be used as a last resort.

Inflammatory Chronic Pelvic Pain Syndrome (Nonbacterial Prostatitis)
1. Nonbacterial prostatitis is more common than bacterial prostatitis.
2. This is characterized by prostate inflammation (WBCs in the prostatic fluid) but *no* identifiable prostate infection. Symptoms may be similar to those seen with chronic bacterial prostatitis. The prostate may be tender.
3. The etiology is unclear, but may involve one of the following:
   a. Reflux of urine into the prostatic ducts ("chemical prostatitis")
   b. Unidentified infectious agents (e.g. Trichomonas vaginalis)
   c. Autoimmune disorder
4. Treatment
   a. Consider an empiric 6-8 week course of TMP-SMX or a FQ. If there is no response to TMP-SMX or FQs, consider doxycycline 100 mg po BID for 4-6 weeks (doxycycline and FQ typically cover Ureaplasma, Chlamydia, and mycoplasma; however, TMP-SMZ does not cover any of these organisms). If this is not effective, further antibiotic therapy is not recommended.
   b. For additional therapies that may be helpful, see page 370.

Noninflammatory Chronic Pelvic Pain Syndrome (Prostadynia)
1. This entity is characterized by *absence* of prostate inflammation (no WBCs in the prostatic fluid) and *no* prostatic bacterial infection. It may present with symptoms similar to chronic bacterial prostatitis.
2. These patients are often middle age adults that have voiding complaints and pelvic pain.
3. On urodynamics, these patients often demonstrate decreased urine flow with incomplete relaxation of the bladder neck during voiding (although the striated sphincter relaxes normally) and abnormally high urethral closing pressure at rest.
4. The etiology of prostadynia is unclear, but may include pelvic floor muscle tension and bladder neck/urethral spasm.
5. Treatment—same as Inflammatory Chronic Pelvic Pain Syndrome.

Therapies That May Be Helpful in Treating Chronic Prostate Syndromes
1. Non-steroidal anti-inflammatory drugs (NSAIDS)
2. Anticholinergics may reduce urinary urgency.
3. Alpha blockers—a recent meta-analysis indicated that α-blockers may improve urinary symptoms, but they do not relieve pain.
4. Frequent ejaculation helps eliminate congested prostatic fluid; therefore, it may help relieve symptoms. However, ejaculation is painful in some patients (these patients may be served best by avoiding ejaculation).
5. Sitz baths
6. Stress reduction
7. Prostate massage (up to 3 times per week), especially in men with infrequent ejaculation (removes congested prostatic fluid and may improve antibiotic penetration).
8. Diet, vitamins, and supplements
   a. Avoid caffeine, alcohol, saccharin, spicy foods, and acidic foods.
   b. Oral zinc supplements
   c. Oral nickel supplements
   d. Quercetin 500 po BID—a bioflavonoid which improved symptom scores and quality of life in a prospective randomized double blind placebo controlled trial of patients with category III prostatitis.
   e. Saw palmetto
   f. Prosta-Q™ is a dietary supplement with ingredients that include quercetin, zinc, and saw palmetto.
9. 5α-reductase inhibitors (finasteride or dutasteride)
10. Allopurinol 300 mg po q day [Tabs: 100, 300 mg]
11. Diazepam to relax the pelvic floor muscles
12. "Triple therapy"—consists of a pain medicine, a muscle relaxant, and an α-blocker and is used to try to break the cycle of pain. Patients should avoid alcohol. They will likely be unable to work and should not drive during therapy. Therapy consists of a strong pain medicine (e.g. Tylenol with codeine) for not more than 1-2 weeks, with NSAIDs for pain thereafter. The α-blocker should be advanced to the maximum dose before the triple therapy is instituted. A potent muscle relaxant (e.g. diazepam) may be given for up to 2 weeks and is then tapered off.
13. Tricyclic antidepressants have been used to treat chronic prostate pain.
14. Referral to pain specialist
15. Biofeedback
16. Supportive counseling
17. Transurethral microwave thermotherapy (TUMT)—probably should be used as a last resort.

Asymptomatic Inflammatory Prostatitis
1. This asymptomatic entity is incidentally discovered during tests for other genitourinary problems (e.g. prostate biopsy, fertility work up, etc.)
2. Treatment is probably not necessary. However, a trial of antibiotics may be useful if infertility is present or if the PSA is elevated.

Granulomatous Prostatitis
1. This entity is rare. Causes include intravesical BCG and tuberculosis.
2. Symptomatic BCG prostatitis can be treated with INH* 300 mg po q day and rifampin 600 mg po q day for 3-6 months. Asymptomatic BCG granulomatous prostatitis requires no therapy.

* When giving isoniazid (INH), administer pyridoxine (vitamin B6) 50 mg po q day to prevent neurotoxicity and check liver function tests periodically.

Prostate Abscess

General Information

1. Prostate abscesses arise from the following mechanisms.
   a. Reflux of infected urine into the prostate—this is the most common mechanism leading to prostate abscess. E. coli is the most common causative organism. Intravesical BCG has also been implicated.
   b. Hematogenous spread—Staphylococcus aureus is the most common organism found in prostate abscesses caused by hematogenous spread.
   c. Direct inoculation—rarely, prostate abscess can be caused by transrectal prostate biopsy and procedures for BPH (such as TUNA or TUMT).

Presentation

1. Prostate abscess can occur in any age group, including newborns.
2. Most prostatic abscesses occur in men with diabetes mellitus. Other risk factors include chronic bacterial prostatitis, bladder outlet obstruction, and immunocompromise (e.g. HIV, transplant).
3. The symptoms of prostatic abscess are often non-specific and may include symptoms that mimic prostatitis, cystitis, or urethritis. Therefore, a high index of suspicion is necessary to diagnose prostatic abscess. *Suspect prostate abscess in men with acute prostatitis who do not respond to antibiotics within 48 hours (especially men with diabetes or HIV).*
4. Patients may present with irritative voiding symptoms, perineal pain, fever, or urinary retention. When the abscess erodes into the urethra, urethral discharge may be present. Digital rectal examination may be normal or it may reveal tenderness, fluctuance, or induration of the prostate.

Diagnosis

1. A high index of suspicion is necessary to diagnose prostatic abscess.
2. Diagnosis is made by pelvic CT, pelvic MRI, or transrectal ultrasound.
   a. Ultrasound—the abscess usually appears hypoechoic.
   b. CT scan—the abscess usually appears as an area of low attenuation. Rim enhancement is seen when IV contrast is administered.
   c. MRI—high intensity on T2 images. Rim enhancement is seen when gadolinium is administered.

Treatment

1. Consider placing a suprapubic tube in men with urinary retention.
2. Microabscesses or small focal abscess (e.g. < 1 cm) in patients who are not severely ill and not septic—intravenous antibiotics and catheter drainage of the bladder may be adequate.
3. Large abscesses—intravenous antibiotics and abscess drainage is usually required. Drainage can be achieved by the following procedures.
   a. Needle aspiration—when a drain is not left in place, the purulent fluid may reaccumulate, making multiple aspirations necessary.
      i. Transperineal percutaneous drainage—performed using ultrasound guidance (transrectal or transabdominal) under local anesthesia.
      ii. Transrectal drainage—performed using transrectal ultrasound guidance under local anesthesia.
   b. Transurethral drainage—this procedure is more suitable for abscesses that are close to the urethra or abscesses that do not respond to needle aspiration. These procedures are contraindicated in men who cannot tolerate general or spinal anesthesia.
      i. Transurethral incision or unroofing of the abscess
      ii. Transurethral resection of the prostate (TURP)—may be associated with a higher risk of sepsis than incision and unroofing.

   c. Open surgical drainage—may be necessary if transurethral drainage and
      needle aspiration are insufficient or when the abscess extends outside the
      prostate. Open prostatectomy and transperineal incision and drainage
      have been utilized.
4. An attempt should be made to culture the abscess fluid for aerobes,
   anaerobes, fungus, and mycobacteria.
5. Consider testing patients for HIV.

Emphysematous Prostatitis—see page 394.

REFERENCES

Prostatitis
Britton JJ Jr, Carson CC: Prostatitis. AUA Update Series, Vol. 17, Lesson 20,
    1998.
Carson CC, Childs SJ, Krieger JN: Symposium - current management of
    prostatitis. Contemporary Urology, December (suppl.): 5, 1999.
Drach GW, et al: Classification of benign diseases associated with prostatic pain:
    prostatitis or prostadynia. J Urol, 120: 266, 1978.
Leskinen M, Lukkarinen O, Marttila T: Effects of finasteride in patients with
    inflammatory chronic pelvic pain syndrome: a double blind, placebo
    controlled, pilot study. Urology, 53: 502, 1999.
Litwin MS, et al: The National Institutes of Health chronic prostatitis symptom
    index: development and validation of a new outcome measure. Chronic
    Prostatitis Collaborative Research Network. J Urol, 162: 369, 1999.
Meares E Jr, Stamey T: Bacteriologic localization patterns in bacterial prostatitis
    and urethritis. Invest Urol, 5: 492, 1968.
Nickel JC: Treatment of chronic prostatitis: new role for old friends. Urology
    Times, 27 (suppl. 2): S9, 1999.
**Nickel JC, Nyberg LM, Hennenfent M: Research guidelines for chronic
    prostatitis: consensus report from the first National Institutes of Health
    International Prostatitis Collaborative Network. Urology, 54: 229, 1999.**
Persson BE, et al: Ameliorative effect of allopurinol on nonbacterial prostatitis: a
    parallel double blind controlled study. J Urol, 155: 961, 1996.
Roberts RO, Lieber MM, Bostwick DG, et al: A review of clinical and
    pathological prostatitis syndromes. Urology, 49: 809, 1997.
Shoskes DA, Zeitlin SI, Shahed A, et al: Quercetin in men with category III
    chronic prostatitis: a preliminary prospective, double blind, placebo
    controlled trial. Urology, 54: 960, 1999.
Yang G, et al: The effect of α-adrenergic antagonists in chronic prostatitis/
    chronic pelvic pain syndrome: a meta-analysis of randomized controlled
    trials. J Androl, 27:847, 2006.

Prostate Abscess
Collado A, et al: Ultrasound guided needle aspiration in prostatic abscess.
    Urology, 53: 548, 1999.
Collins SM, et al: Prostatic abscess in the newborn: an unrecognized source of
    urosepsis. Urology, 57: 554vi, 2001.
Ludwig M, et al: Diagnosis and therapeutic management of 18 patients with
    prostatic abscess. Urology, 53: 340, 1999.
Matlaga BR, et al: Prostate abscess following bacillus Calmette Guerin
    treatment. J Urol, 167: 251, 2002.
Oliveira P, et al: Diagnosis and treatment of prostatic abscess. Int Braz J Urol,
    29: 30, 2003.
Wosnitzer MS, Weiss RE: Diagnosing and managing prostatic abscess: views
    from the literature. Issues in Urology, 19(3): 108, 2007.

SEXUALLY TRANSMITTED DISEASES (STDs)

General Information

1. STDs are acquired by sexual contact (genital, oral, or anal contact). Examples include

Trichomonas vaginalis	Treponema palladium (syphilis)
Phthirus pubis (pubic lice)	Klebsiella granulomatis (Granuloma Inguinale)
Sarcoptes scabiei (scabies)	Lymphogranuloma venereum
Neisseria gonorrhoeae (GC)	Haemophilus ducreyi (chancroid)
Hepatitis B virus	Herpes simplex virus (HSV)
Chlamydia trachomatis	Human papilloma virus (HPV)
Molluscum contagiosum	Human immunodeficiency virus (HIV)

2. Syphilis, chancroid, HIV, gonorrhea, and chlamydia are reportable in every state. Reporting for other STDs depends on state and local requirements.
3. A "bubo" is an inflamed lymph node. This term is often used for enlarged lymph nodes caused by STDs.
4. The incubation period is the time interval between exposure to the disease and clinical signs and symptoms of the disease.

The Asymptomatic Patient with Recent STD Exposure

1. Patients with a possible STD exposure often request STD screening.
2. There is no standard evaluation; however, the following screening tests may be used for the asymptomatic patient with STD exposure.
   a. Physical examination—check for genital lesions and discharge.
   b. HIV enzyme immunoassay or a rapid test—follow-up testing is necessary if the initial test is negative. Consider repeating the HIV test 3 and 6 months after the initial test. A positive immunoassay or rapid test must be confirmed by a western blot or immunofluorescence test.
   c. Hepatitis B blood tests—anti-Hbc, anti-Hbs, HBsAg.
   d. RPR or VDRL—may turn positive 1 week after the chancre appears, but may take 4-6 weeks to become positive after exposure. Therefore, a repeat test may be considered 1-3 months after the initial exposure.
   e. HSV I and II IgG and IgM blood tests—test should be performed at least one week after exposure.
   f. Tests for GC and Chlamydia—urethral swab or first void urine.

<u>Genital Ulcers</u>—see page 352.

<u>Chlamydia</u>

General information

1. Cause—Chlamydia trachomatis (an intracellular organism).
2. Strains L1, L2, and L3 cause lymphogranuloma venereum. Strains D through K cause urethritis, epididymo-orchitis, cervicitis, and pelvic inflammatory disease (PID).
3. Incubation period = 3-21 days.
4. Chlamydia trachomatis infection often coexists with gonorrhea; therefore, treatment for both organisms is usually administered.

Diagnosis
1. Definitive diagnostic test—culture. Culture is the only test that provides antibiotic sensitivities.
2. Non-amplified tests—these tests are performed on urethral or cervical swabs, but fail to detect a substantial proportion of infections.
   a. Enzyme immunoassays (EIA)—detects bacterial antigens.
   b. Direct fluorescent antibody (DFA)—detects bacterial antigens.
   c. Nucleic acid hybridization (NAH)—detects bacterial DNA or RNA.
3. Nucleic acid amplified test (NAAT)—amplifies and detects bacterial DNA or RNA. NAAT is more sensitive than non-amplified tests and can be performed on urethral swabs, cervical swabs, and urine. Tests using polymerase chain reaction (PCR) are examples of NAATs.
4. Serologic tests (i.e. blood tests) are not recommended.
5. *The preferred diagnostic test for Chlamydia is either nucleic acid amplified test or culture.* When sensitivities are needed, culture is required.
6. Urethral swab—obtain specimens preferably ≥ 1 hour after voiding. For chlamydia testing, an intraurethral specimen is required. Insert the swab into the urethra for a distance of 2-4 cm in males and 1-2 cm in females, rotate the swab 1 or more times, and withdraw.
7. Urine samples for NAAT—the first 10-30 cc of voided urine should be used for testing ("first void" specimen). Obtain specimens preferably ≥ 1 hour after the last void.

Clinical Manifestations
1. Asymptomatic infection is common in males and females.
2. Strains L1, L2, and L3 cause lymphogranuloma venereum; however, strains D through K cause most of the manifestations listed below.
3. In males
   a. Urethritis—*Chlamydia is one of the most common causes of non-gonococcal urethritis.* When symptomatic, urethral discharge, dysuria, and urethral pruritus may be present. Urethral discharge is often scant, and may be clear or purulent. See Urethritis in the Male, page 357.
   b. Epididymitis/orchitis—*Chlamydia and gonorrhea are the most common causes of epididymitis and orchitis in males less than 35 years old.*
   c. Prostatitis—rare.
   d. Reiter's syndrome—arthritis, urethritis, and conjunctivitis. Most patients with this syndrome have the HLA-B27 phenotype.
4. In females—urethritis, cervicitis, and pelvic inflammatory disease (PID).
5. In males and females—proctitis, conjunctivitis (rare), endocarditis (rare).

Treatment
1. Since gonorrhea often coexists with Chlamydia trachomatis, treatment for both organisms is usually administered.
2. See Gonorrhea, Treatment, Follow Up, and Sex Partners, page 376.
3. For treatment of disseminated, conjunctival, pulmonary, and pediatric Chlamydia infections, see the complete CDC recommendations.

Gonorrhea

General Information
1. Cause—Neisseria gonorrhoeae (a gram negative diplococcus).
2. Incubation period = 2-6 days.
3. Also called "the clap", "the strain", and "GC" (short for GonoCoccus).
4. Without therapy, the infection often resolves spontaneously in 2-3 months.
5. Chlamydia trachomatis infection often coexists with gonorrhea.

Diagnosis

1. Definitive diagnostic test—culture (Thayer-Martin or chocolate agars are often used). Culture is the only test that provides antibiotic sensitivities.
2. Gram stain of urethral discharge—the presence *intracellular gram negative diplococci* inside WBCs provides a presumptive diagnosis in males. A negative gram stain does not rule out a gonorrhea infection.
3. Non-amplified tests—these tests are performed on urethral or cervical swabs, but fail to detect a substantial proportion of infections.
4. Nucleic acid amplified tests (NAAT)—more sensitive than non-amplified tests and can be performed on urethral swabs, cervical swabs, and urine. (For details on non-amplified tests and NAAT, see Chlamydia, page 373).
5. Serologic tests (i.e. blood tests) are not recommended.
6. *The preferred diagnostic test for gonorrhea is either nucleic acid amplified test or culture*. When sensitivities are needed, culture is required.
7. Urethral swab—obtain specimens preferably ≥ 1 hour after voiding. For gonorrhea testing, collection of discharge at the meatus is sufficient. When discharge is absent or when testing for chlamydia, an intraurethral swab is required. Insert the swab into the urethra for a distance of 2-4 cm in males and 1-2 cm in females, rotate the swab 1 or more times, and withdraw.
8. Urine samples for NAAT—the first 10-30 cc of voided urine should be used for testing ("first void" specimen). Obtain specimens preferably ≥ 1 hour after the last void.

Clinical Manifestations

1. Manifestations in females—most females are *asymptomatic*.
   a. Urethritis—may mimic cystitis.
   b. Cervicitis—this may cause purulent vaginal discharge.
   c. Pelvic inflammatory disease (PID)—PID is also called salpingitis. Patients present with cervical motion tenderness and adnexal tenderness. The risk of PID is higher in women with an intrauterine device (IUD) or a history of PID. PID can lead to late manifestations, including
      i. Infertility—caused by fallopian tube scarring. The more times a women has PID, the greater the likelihood of infertility.
      ii. Increased risk of ectopic pregnancy—from fallopian tube scarring.
      iii. Chronic pelvic pain—may be caused by adhesions of the adnexa.
   d. Fitz-Hugh-Curtis syndrome—peri-hepatic spread of adnexal gonorrhea, often causing right upper abdominal pain. It resolves with antibiotics, but painful intraperitoneal adhesions may remain.
2. Manifestations in males—most males are *symptomatic*.
   a. Urethritis—characterized by irritative voiding symptoms and profuse purulent urethral discharge. *Urethritis is the most common manifestation in males*. Urethral stricture may be a late manifestation of urethritis.
   b. Epididymitis—*Chlamydia and gonorrhea are the most common causes of epididymitis in males less than 35 years old.*
   c. Prostatitis—rare.
3. Manifestations in men or women—pharyngitis (from oral-genital contact), proctitis (from anal-genital contact), and disseminated gonorrhea.
4. Disseminated gonorrhea—occurs in 1% and may ultimately lead to endocarditis, meningitis, or hepatitis. Symptoms include
   a. Migratory asymmetric polyarthralgia usually in one joint at a time.
   b. Rash—papules or pustules on an erythematous base, usually on the extremities.
   c. Fever
   d. Tenosynovitis—typically involving the flexor tendon sheaths in the wrist or the Achilles tendon (referred to as "lover's heel").

Treatment (Adults)
1. *Chlamydia often coexists with gonorrhea; therefore, treatment for both organisms is administered* (unless the chlamydia test is negative).
2. Patients and their partners must avoid sex until treatment is complete (for single dose regimens, treatment is complete 7 days after the single dose).
3. For treatment of disseminated, conjunctival, pharyngeal, neonatal, and pediatric gonorrhea, see the complete CDC recommendations.

		Treatment of Adults with Uncomplicated Urethritis, Cervicitis, or Proctitis Caused by Gonorrhea & Chlamydia	
		To cover Neisseria gonorrhoeae†	To cover chlamydia trachomatis (when chlamydia infection is not ruled out)
Non-pregnant Adults	Recommended Regimen	Ceftriaxone 125 mg IM one dose or Cefixime 400 mg PO one dose§	Doxycycline 100 mg PO BID x 7 days or Azithromycin 1g PO one dose
	Alternative Regimens	Spectinomycin 2 g IM one dose* or Single dose cephalosporin‡	Erythromycin base 500 mg PO QID x 7 days or Erythromycin ethylsuccinate 800 mg PO QID x 7 days or Levofloxacin 500 mg PO q day x 7 days or Ofloxacin 300 mg PO BID x 7 days
Pregnant Adults	Recommended Regimen	Ceftriaxone 125 mg IM one dose or Cefixime 400 mg PO one dose§ (if penicillin allergy use Spectinomycin 2 g IM one dose*)	Azithromycin 1 g po one dose or Amoxicillin 500 mg po TID x 7 days

PO = by mouth; IM = intramuscular

§ Cefixime tablets are not available in the United States; however, cefixime oral suspension (100 mg/5 ml) is available. For alternatives to cefixime, see ‡.

‡ Single dose cephalosporin regimens include cefpodoxime 400 mg po, cefuroxime 1 gram po, cefoxitin 2 g IM with probenecid 1g po, ceftizoxime 500 mg IM, or cefotaxime 500 mg IM.

† Quinolones should no longer be used for gonorrhea infections.

* Spectinomycin is no longer available in the United States. Currently, there is no alternative antibiotic available.

Follow Up
1. For uncomplicated gonorrhea infections, a test of cure is not necessary in patients who respond to therapy. For chlamydia infections, a test of cure should be performed in pregnant women 3 weeks after treatment is complete. Patients who remain symptomatic require culture and sensitivity for gonorrhea and chlamydia.
2. If infection is present after response to antibiotics, re-infection is more likely than persistent infection.

Sex Partners
1. Patients should refer their sex partners for evaluation.
2. Treat all sex partners who have had sexual contact with the patient within 60 days from the onset of the patient's symptoms.
3. If the patient has *not* had sexual contact for > 60 days prior to the onset of symptoms, treat the patient's last sex partner.

Genital Herpes

General Information

1. Cause—herpes simplex virus (HSV), a double-stranded DNA virus. There are two serotypes: HSV-1 and HSV-2.
2. *HSV-1 causes most cases of oral herpes, while HSV-2 causes most cases of genital herpes.* Clinical recurrences are more common with HSV-2.
3. Incubation period = 4-6 days.
4. *Transmission of HSV may occur in the absence of cutaneous lesions and symptoms.*
5. Genital herpes is a life long infection that cannot be cured.
6. *Most people do not know they are infected with HSV.*

Diagnosis

1. Definitive diagnostic test—viral culture of fluid isolated from a lesion.
2. Tests on lesions
   a. Viral culture of fluid isolated from a lesion—the sensitivity of this test is low and false negatives are common.
   b. Tzanck smear—microscopic examination of fluid or scraping from the lesion shows *multinucleated giant cells* and/or Cowdry intranuclear inclusion bodies (eosinophilic ovoid bodies in the nucleus that are surrounded by a clear halo). This suggests herpes but is *not* diagnostic.
   c. PCR and HSV DNA tests are not FDA approved for testing genital lesions.
3. Serologic tests
   a. Request IgM and IgG antibody assays for HSV-1 and HSV-2.
   b. IgM appears within one week and is gone by 3-6 months after infection. IgG appears within 1-3 months of infection and remains detectable indefinitely.
   c. These tests cannot determine whether an infection was oral, anogenital, or both. However, HSV-1 causes most cases of oral herpes, while HSV-2 causes most cases of genital herpes.

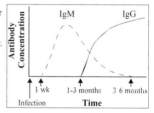

   d. Serologic tests may be used to
      i. Confirm a clinical diagnosis of genital herpes (especially when viral culture is negative).
      ii. Diagnose patients with unrecognized infection (including sex partners of patients with HSV).

IgM	IgG	General Interpretation
+	−	Recent infection (within 3 months)
+	+	Recent infection or reactivation of previous infection
−	+	Previous infection (longer than 3-6 months prior)
−	−	No infection or no antibodies formed

Clinical Manifestations

1. *Most people with HSV do not know they have HSV (they did not manifest symptoms or did not recognize the symptoms).*
2. *Herpes is characterized by painful vesicles or ulcerations on an erythematous base that follow a neural distribution.* Vesicles are usually 1-2 mm in diameter and may be accompanied by fever, malaise, and tender inguinal lymphadenopathy.

3. Herpes lesions and symptoms usually resolve spontaneously in 7-14 days.
4. *Recurrences are often preceded by a prodrome,* which consists of pain or altered sensation in the region of an impending outbreak. Approximately 60% of patients have a local recurrence. The signs and symptoms of recurrence are less severe than the initial episode.
5. Less common manifestations—nongonococcal urethritis, meningitis, encephalitis, and radiculomyelitis (which can cause urinary retention).
6. Neonatal infection can occur if the mother has HSV.

Preventing Transmission of HSV
1. The risk of HSV-2 transmission can be decreased by valacyclovir 500 mg po q day (suppressive dose). Transmission prevention has been confirmed in heterosexual couples, but probably occurs with other sexual interactions.
2. Transmission of HSV may be reduced by proper use of latex condoms.

Treatment for Non-pregnant Adults
1. *Treatment of genital herpes does not eradicate the virus and does not stop viral shedding.* Oral (systemic) therapy speeds healing of ulcers and reduces the duration of symptoms and viral shedding. Topical therapy is not recommended because it is less effective than systemic therapy.
2. Episodic therapy—best for infrequent recurrences (< 6 per year). The patient begins self treatment when the prodrome or lesions start.
3. Suppressive therapy—best for frequent recurrences (≥ 6 per year). *Suppressive therapy decreases recurrence.* Medication is taken daily. After one year, consider stopping therapy to see if recurrences diminish (safety data is limited for daily dosing longer than 1 year).
4. First episode—if healing is incomplete after the initial course of therapy, extend therapy until the lesions heal. Recommended regimens—
   a. Acyclovir 400 mg PO TID x 7-10 days, or
   b. Acyclovir 200 mg PO five times a day x 7-10 days, or
   c. Famciclovir 250 mg PO TID x 7-10 days, or
   d. Valacyclovir 1000 mg PO BID x 7-10 days
5. Recurrent episodes < 6 times per year—start episodic therapy.
   a. Acyclovir 400 mg PO TID x 5 days, or
   b. Acyclovir 800 mg PO BID x 5 days, or
   c. Acyclovir 800 mg PO TID x 2 days, or
   d. Famciclovir 125 mg PO BID x 5 days, or
   e. Famciclovir 1000 mg PO BID x 1 day, or
   f. Valacyclovir 500 mg PO BID x 3 days, or
   g. Valacyclovir 1000 mg PO q day x 5 days
6. Recurrent episodes ≥ 6 times per year—start suppression.
   a. Acyclovir 400 mg PO BID, or
   b. Famciclovir 250 mg PO BID, or
   c. Valacyclovir 500 mg PO q day, or
   d. Valacyclovir 1000 mg PO q day

> Acyclovir [Caps: 200 mg; Tabs: 400, 800 mg; Suspension 200 mg/ 5 ml]
> Famciclovir [Tabs: 125, 250, 500 mg]
> Valacyclovir [Tabs: 500, 1000 mg]

7. Pregnant females—there is insufficient information regarding the safety of acyclovir, famciclovir and valacyclovir during pregnancy.
8. For herpes that is systemic, complicated, pediatric, neonatal, non-genital, during pregnancy, or in patients with HIV, see the CDC recommendations.

Follow Up
Consider following the patient until signs and symptoms resolve.

Sex Partners
1. Evaluation and counseling of sex partners is recommended.
2. Treat partners with symptomatic infections.
3. Asymptomatic partners may be offered serologic testing.

Lymphogranuloma Venereum (LGV)

General Information
1. Cause—Chlamydia trachomatis serotypes L1, L2, and L3 (an intracellular organism).
2. Incubation period = days to weeks.

Diagnosis
1. Definitive diagnostic test—culture of purulent fluid isolated from the rectum or lymph nodes.
2. Tests on purulent fluid—culture, nucleic acid amplification tests, and direct immunofluorescence are available.
3. Serologic tests—complement fixation, although not definitive, is the most common method used to diagnose LGV. An immunofluorescent antibody test may be used, but is not widely available.
4. Frei test—an intradermal delayed hypersensitivity test which is no longer used because it is neither sensitive nor specific for LGV.

Clinical Manifestations
1. In most patients, the primary lesion is not noticed. If a lesion is evident, it is often a small painless transient papule or pustule. 2 to 6 weeks after exposure, tender inguinal lymphadenopathy develops.
2. *In most STDs, regional lymphadenopathy occurs simultaneously with the primary genital lesion. In LGV, regional lymphadenopathy occurs in the absence of a primary lesion* (the primary lesion healed or was not evident).
3. In 10-20% of cases, lymph nodes above and below the inguinal ligament become enlarged, creating the *"groove sign"* (the inguinal ligament creates a groove between the enlarged nodes).
4. Over the next 2-8 weeks, the skin overlying the lymphadenopathy becomes erythematous, indurated, and wrinkled. The infection in the nodes progress to abscesses that may erode to the skin, causing sinus tracts.
5. Skin rashes may accompany this infection.
6. Chronic rectal infection can cause rectal abscesses, fistulas, and strictures.

Treatment
1. Recommended regimen for non-pregnant adults—Doxycycline 100 mg PO BID x 21 days.
2. Alternative regimen for non-pregnant adults—Erythromycin base 500 mg PO QID x 21 days.
3. Recommended regimen for pregnant and breast feeding females—Erythromycin base 500 mg PO QID x 21 days.

Follow Up
Follow patients until the signs and symptoms have resolved completely.

Sex Partners
1. Treat all sex partners who have had sexual contact with the patient within 30 days from the onset of the patient's symptoms.
2. Treat all sex partners that have signs or symptoms of the disease.

Granuloma Inguinale (Donovanosis)

General Information
1. Cause—Klebsiella granulomatis (formerly known as Calymmatobacterium granulomatis), an intracellular gram negative organism.
2. Repeated exposure is probably necessary for transmission.
3. Incubation period = 2-3 months.
4. Granuloma inguinale is rare in the United States, but is common in India, Papua New Guinea, central Australia, and southern Africa.

Diagnosis
1. Definitive diagnostic test—identification of *Donovan bodies* in a scraping or biopsy of the cutaneous lesions. Donovan bodies are intracellular organisms that and look like "safety pins" or "dumbbells."
2. The causative organism is very difficult to culture.

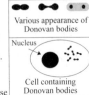

Various appearance of Donovan bodies

Nucleus

Cell containing Donovan bodies

Clinical Manifestations
1. A papule erodes through the skin, causing a nonpurulent *"beefy red"* painless ulceration. These lesions are vascular and bleed easily. Spontaneous healing is rare. Lesions can grow very large if left untreated.
2. The lesions are usually *painless* unless superinfection is present.
3. Regional lymphadenopathy is uncommon. Primary lesions can extend into the groin, giving the appearance of a swollen lymph nodes (*"pseudobubo"*).

Treatment
1. The patient is treated for a minimum of 3 weeks. If the lesions have not completely healed after 3 weeks of therapy, then antibiotics are continued until the lesions have healed completely.
2. Recommended regimen for non-pregnant adults—Doxycycline 100 mg po BID for a minimum of 3 weeks
3. Alternative regimens for non-pregnant adults
   a. Azithromycin 1 g po q week for a minimum of 3 weeks, or
   b. Ciprofloxacin 750 mg po BID for a minimum of 3 weeks, or
   c. Erythromycin base 500 mg po QID for a minimum of 3 weeks, or
   d. Trimethoprim-sulfamethoxazole one double strength tablet po BID for a minimum of 3 weeks.
4. Regimen for pregnant and breast feeding females—erythromycin base 500 mg po QID for a minimum of 3 weeks and consider adding a parenteral aminoglycoside.

Follow Up
Follow patients until the signs and symptoms have resolved completely.

Sex Partners
1. Offer evaluation and treatment to asymptomatic sex partners who have had sexual contact with the patient within 60 days from the onset of the patient's symptoms.
2. Treat all sex partners that have signs or symptoms of the disease.

Trichomonas

Diagnosis

1. Cause—Trichomonas vaginalis (a flagellated protozoa).
2. Definitive diagnostic test—culture or identification of
   T. vaginalis on a saline wet mount of the vaginal discharge.
3. *Culture is the most sensitive and specific test for T. vaginalis.*
4. Tests for females
   a. Culture of vaginal discharge.
   b. Saline wet mount—vaginal discharge is placed on a slide
      and diluted with 1 to 2 drops of normal saline. A cover slip is applied
      and the slide is examined under a microscope using low (x100) and high
      (x400) power. *When T. vaginalis infection is present, the wet mount
      usually shows more than 10 WBC/HPF and motile T. vaginalis
      organisms* (they are larger than WBCs, but smaller than epithelial cells).
      Saline wet mount detects only 50% of infections (its sensitivity is low).
   c. Point of care tests—these tests are FDA approved for women and are
      performed on vaginal secretions. They are more sensitive than saline wet
      mount, but less sensitive than culture. False positives do occur.
      i. OSOM Trichomonas Rapid Test—results are available in 10 minutes.
      ii. Affirm™ VP III—checks for Trichomonas vaginalis, Gardnerella
          vaginalis, and Candida albicans. Results are available in 45 minutes.
5. Test for males
   a. Culture of urethral swab, first void urine, or semen. First void urine is
      the first 10-30 cc of voided urine obtained $\geq$ 1 hour after the last void.
   b. Saline wet mount is not sensitive in males and is not recommended.

Clinical Manifestations

1. Males—*usually asymptomatic*; however, it may cause urethritis (see
   Urethritis in the Male, page 357) and prostatitis (rare).
2. Females—*usually symptomatic*; the most common manifestation is
   vaginitis (see Vaginitis, page 353 and page 355).
   a. Malodorous green frothy vaginal discharge—discharge has pH > 4.5 and
      may have "fishy" odor.
   b. Erythema and irritation of the vulva, vagina, and cervix. Punctate
      hemorrhages (petechiae) of the vagina and cervix ("strawberry cervix").

Treatment

1. Recommended regimen for non-pregnant adults
   a. Metronidazole 2 g PO single dose, or
   b. Tinidazole 2 g PO single dose
2. Alternative regimen for non-pregnant adults—metronidazole 500 mg PO
   BID x 7 days.
3. Pregnant females—metronidazole 2 g PO single dose (avoid breast feeding
   for 12-24 hours after the dose).
4. Patients and their sex partners must avoid sex until therapy is complete *and*
   symptoms have resolved.

Follow Up

1. Patients who respond to therapy do not need a follow up test of cure.
2. Recurrence after response to antibiotics usually indicates re-infection
   rather than persistent infection.
3. Patients who remain symptomatic may require another course of
   metronidazole. Consider culture for Trichomonas to confirm diagnosis.
4. For treatment failure, see the complete CDC recommendations.

Sex Partners

Treat current sex partners.

Syphilis

General Information

1. Cause—Treponema pallidum (spirochete).
2. Infection occurs by intimate contact with a person that has chancres or condyloma latum. Transmission does not occur when lesions are absent.
3. Immune response to syphilis includes
   a. Non-specific antibody response that produces anti-cardiolipin antibodies (cardiolipin is a normal component of many tissues). Anti-cardiolipin antibodies may be found in conditions other than syphilis.
   b. Specific antibody response that produces anti-treponemal antibodies.
4. Incubation period = 2-4 weeks (i.e. dermal lesions appear 2-4 weeks after inoculation).

Diagnosis

1. Definitive diagnostic tests—tissue or exudate that yields a positive *direct fluorescent antibody* (DFA) test or spirochetes on *darkfield microscopy.*
2. Tests on exudate
   a. Direct fluorescent antibody (DFA)—antibody that binds to syphilis.
   b. Dark field microscopy—permits visualization of spirochetes.
3. Serologic tests—a presumptive diagnosis can be made by a non-treponemal serologic test, but the diagnosis must be confirmed by a treponemal serologic test.
   a. Non-treponemal serologic tests—these tests detect anti-cardiolipin antibodies, which are not specific to syphilis. Since false positives may occur, a positive non-treponemal test must be confirmed by a treponemal serologic test. VDRL and RPR usually turn positive within 1 week after the chancre appears. *VDRL and RPR may be used to measure response to treatment* because they usually revert to negative after adequate treatment.
      i. VDRL (Venereal Disease Research Laboratory)
      ii. RPR (Rapid Plasma Reagin)
   b. Treponemal serologic tests—these tests detect anti-treponemal antibodies. They usually remain positive for life (in spite of treatment); therefore, these tests cannot distinguish an active infection from a previously treated infection and are *not used to measure response to treatment.*
      i. FTA-ABS (Fluorescent Treponemal Antibody absorbed)
      ii. TP-PA (Treponema Palladium Particle Agglutination)
4. Non-treponemal serologic tests are always positive in secondary syphilis, but may be negative in primary, tertiary or latent syphilis.

Primary Syphilis

1. Consists of the initial infection which typically begins with 1-2 cm papules that ulcerate after a few days. These *painless* ulcers (also called chancres) have raised, indurated edges ("punched out" lesions) and are often nonpurulent.
2. Nontender regional lymphadenopathy is often present.
3. Condyloma latum—white or grey raised papules on the skin (these may look similar to condyloma acuminata, but are a distinct entity). In primary syphilis, they develop by direct local extension of spirochetes from the chancre. Condyloma latum may also be present in secondary syphilis.
4. Chancres usually heal (even if untreated) in 3-8 weeks. Thus, primary syphilis regresses spontaneously, leaving the patient without symptoms and without lesions.

Secondary Syphilis (Disseminated Syphilis)

1. Secondary syphilis is caused by hematogenous dissemination of spirochetes. It often appears 4-10 weeks after the initial chancre appears and is characterized by
   a. Macular-papular rash on the trunk and extremities, classically involving the *palms of the hands and the soles of the feet.*
   b. Generalized lymphadenopathy
   c. Condyloma latum—in secondary syphilis, these develop by hematogenous dissemination of spirochetes and usually develop in moist areas of the skin (e.g. axilla and groin).
   d. Systemic symptoms including fever, malaise, muscle aches, headaches, and sore throat.
   e. Rare manifestations include uveitis, iritis, periostitis, arthritis, glomerulonephritis, and hepatitis.
2. Secondary syphilis regresses spontaneously after 1-3 months, leaving the patient without symptoms and without lesions.
3. Serologic tests are always positive in secondary syphilis. Thus, a negative serologic test excludes syphilis in a patient with rash, lymphadenopathy, fever, etc.

Latent Syphilis

Latent syphilis begins after secondary syphilis regresses. During this period, the patient has neither symptoms nor lesions, and usually has positive serologic syphilis tests.
   a. Early latent syphilis—latent syphilis < 1 year duration.
   b. Late latent syphilis—latent syphilis > 1 year duration.

Tertiary Syphilis

1. After a variable duration of latent syphilis, tertiary syphilis may develop.
2. Tertiary syphilis is characterized by 3 entities, which may occur separately or in combination: late benign (gummatous) syphilis, neurosyphilis, and cardiovascular syphilis.
   a. Late benign (gummatous) syphilis–characterized by granulomas (called gummas) that can occur anywhere in the body. They can be destructive to local tissue. With antibiotic therapy, gummas heal promptly.
   b. Neurosyphilis—which may include any of the following:
      i. Tabes dorsalis—progressive degeneration of the dorsal spinal cord columns, resulting in impaired vibration sense, proprioception (the ability to determine the position and location one's own limb without looking at the limb) and stereogenesis (the ability to recognized an object by touching it, but without looking it). These deficits may cause ataxia and a traumatic arthropathy called *Charcot's joints.* The posterior nerve roots and ganglia may be affected, resulting in *loss of deep tendon reflexes* and pain in the distribution of the nerve root. The cause of tabes dorsalis is unknown. Spirochetes are *not* present in the dorsal column or in the posterior nerve roots.
      ii. Argyll Robertson pupil—a pupil that "accommodates but does not react." In other words, the pupil constricts when the eyes are focused on a close object (accommodates) but does not constrict when light is flashed in the eye (nonreactive).
      iii. "Lightening" pains—sudden severe pains, often in the extremities, of unclear etiology (perhaps caused by posterior nerve root irritation).
      iv. Mental status changes—psychosis, dementia, confusion, etc.
      v. General paresis—a syphilitic syndrome characterized by mental status changes, paralysis, and aphasia.
      vi. Other—meningitis, encephalitis, stroke.

    c. Cardiovascular syphilis—which may include
        i. Syphilitic aortitis—spirochetes occlude the vasa vasorum of the
            aorta (obliterative endarteritis), causing necrosis and inflammation of
            the aorta. It usually occurs in the ascending aorta. Radiographic
            evidence of this process may be seen as linear calcifications in the
            wall of the ascending aorta.
        ii. Aortic valve insufficiency—aortitis may cause dilation of the
            ascending aorta, which moves the valve cusps apart, resulting in
            aortic valve insufficiency.
        iii.Aortic aneurysm—aortitis may cause progressive aortic dilation,
            ultimately leading to aortic aneurysm.

Treatment (Adults)
1. Primary syphilis
    a. No penicillin allergy (pregnant or not)—benzathine penicillin G 2.4
       million units IM single dose.
    b. Penicillin allergy
        i. Not pregnant—doxycycline 100 mg po BID x 14 days or tetracycline
            500 mg po QID x 14 days.
        ii. Pregnant—desensitize to penicillin then treat accordingly.
2. Secondary syphilis—treat same as primary syphilis.
3. Early latent syphilis—treat same as primary syphilis.
4. Late latent syphilis or latent syphilis of unknown duration
    a. No penicillin allergy (pregnant or not)—benzathine penicillin G 2.4
       million units IM q week x 3 weeks.
    b. Penicillin allergy
        i. Not pregnant—doxycycline 100 mg po BID x 28 days or tetracycline
            500 mg po QID x 28 days.
        ii. Pregnant—desensitize to penicillin then treat accordingly.
5. Tertiary syphilis without neurosyphilis—treat same as late latent syphilis.
6. Neurosyphilis
    a. No penicillin allergy (pregnant or not)—recommended regimen is
       aqueous crystalline penicillin G 3-4 million units IV q 4 hours or
       continuous infusion x 10-14 days. An alternative regimen is 10-14 days
       of both procaine penicillin 2.4 million units IM q day and probenecid
       500 mg po QID.
    b. Penicillin allergy—desensitize to penicillin then treat accordingly.
7. Jarisch-Herxheimer reaction—begins a few hours after antibiotics are
   started and resolves within 12-24 hours. Patients have may have low grade
   fever, muscle aches, headache, malaise, and exacerbation of skin lesions.
   This reaction is probably an inflammatory response triggered by the rapid
   lysis of spirochetes. This reaction is usually not dangerous (although it
   may induce premature labor or fetal distress during pregnancy). There is
   no way to prevent this reaction. It is often treated with antipyretics.
8. For treatment of neonatal syphilis, pediatric syphilis, and syphilis that did
   not respond to treatment, see the complete CDC recommendations.

Follow Up
1. Criteria for treatment failure and for cure have not been established.
2. Primary and secondary syphilis
    a. Follow up evaluation (clinical and non-treponemal serologic evaluation)
       is recommended at 6 and 12 months after treatment.
    b. Treatment failure is probably present when non-treponemal serologic
       titers do not decrease 4 fold within 6 months. These patients should be
       evaluated for HIV.
3. For follow up of latent, tertiary (with or without neurosyphilis), neonatal,
   and pediatric syphilis, see the complete CDC recommendations.

Sex Partners

1. Transmission of syphilis does not occur when lesions are absent. However, anybody exposed to a person with syphilis should be evaluated clinically and serologically and treated if syphilis is suspected.
2. Patients with primary, secondary, and early latent syphilis
   a. Treat all sex partners who have had sexual contact with the patient within 90 days from the patient's diagnosis (even if the partner is seronegative).
   b. Treat all sex partners who had sexual contact with the patient > 90 days from the patient's diagnosis if the partner's serologic test is not available immediately or the partner's compliance with follow up is uncertain.
3. Patients with latent or tertiary syphilis—long-term sex partners of these patients should be evaluated and treated if syphilis is suspected.

Condyloma Acuminatum (Genital Warts)

General Information

1. Cause—human papillomavirus (HPV), a double stranded DNA virus.
2. Infection usually occurs by direct skin-to-skin sexual contact. HPV is not transmitted by blood or body fluid.
3. Risk factors for HPV infection in women
   a. Sexually active
   b. Age < 25
   c. Higher number of sex partners
   d. Early age of first sexual intercourse (16 years or younger)
   e. Male partner who has had multiple sexual partners.
4. Most HPV infections are transient and asymptomatic. Some of these infections persist and cause lesions.
5. HPV rarely leads to cervical carcinoma, penile carcinoma, anal cancer, and Buschke-Lowenstein tumor. HPV types that have a high oncogenic potential: 16, 18, 31, 33, 35, 39, 45, 51, 52, 56, 58, 59, 68, and 82. *The most common oncogenic types are 16 and 18 (responsible for 70% of cervical cancers).*
6. *90% of visible genital warts are caused by HPV types 6 and 11, which have an extremely low oncogenic potential.* Currently, there is no evidence that genital warts are associated with developing cervical cancer.
7. Incubation period—the incubation period is variable, but warts often appear 3-12 months after exposure. Latency periods as long as several decades have been reported.
8. *HPV infection may exist in the absence of visible lesions.*

Prevention of HPV Transmission

1. Gardasil® is a vaccine that protects against HPV types 6, 11, 16, 18 (and thus, protects against the most common causes of genital warts and cervical cancer). It is FDA approved for non-pregnant females age 9 to 26, and is ideally administered before the onset of sexual activity. It is not FDA approved for use in males. Gardasil® is administered as 3 intramuscular injections: an initial injection followed by an injection 2 months and 6 months later.
2. Barrier methods (such as condoms) may decrease transmission to and from areas covered by the barrier, but transmission can occur to and from areas that are not covered.
3. There is minimal evidence that treatment of genital warts prevents transmission.

Clinical Manifestations
1. Painless wart-like lesions. They often have a cauliflower-like appearance.
2. The lesions may be flat, papular, or pedunculated.
3. Intraurethral warts may present with hematuria, dysuria, or blood spotting at the meatus. Bladder warts are very rare and are usually associated with urethral warts.

Diagnosis
1. Definitive diagnostic test—biopsy.
2. In males, examination should include the anus, scrotum, pubic region, penis, and penile meatus (evert the meatus to identify distal urethral and meatal warts). In females, examination should include the anus, pubic region, urethral meatus, external genitals, vagina, and cervix. If urethral warts are suspected, perform urethroscopy.
3. Genital warts have a typical gross appearance and *clinical inspection is sufficient to diagnose most cases of external genital warts* (i.e. there is a good correlation between gross appearance and histological findings).
4. Consider biopsy if any of the following criteria exist.
   a. The diagnosis is in doubt.
   b. Lesions do not respond to therapy.
   c. Lesions are atypical (pigmented, indurated, fixed, bleeding, ulcerated).
   d. The patient is immunocompromised.
5. Biopsy shows squamous cells with a *perinuclear halo* (koilocytosis). Microscopic appearance is sufficient to diagnose most cases of genital warts. *HPV detection and typing is not recommended for genital warts.*
6. Application of 3% to 5% acetic acid ("acetowhitening")—areas infected with HPV may turn white when acetic acid is applied. False positives and false negatives are common. When a patient wishes to be tested for HPV but has no visible lesions, some urologists utilize this test to select a biopsy site. However, the CDC does not recommend acetowhitening for HPV screening because it is not specific for HPV.
7. Blood tests cannot reliably diagnose a past or present HPV infection.
8. HPV does not grow in tissue culture, so viral culture is not an option.
9. Virus detection and typing can be performed by polymerase chain reaction (PCR) on urine, urethral swab, or tissue sample. *Routine virus detection and typing for genital warts is not recommended because it has no proven benefit in diagnosis or management.*

Treatment of External Genital Warts
1. If left untreated, genital warts may resolve spontaneously, remain unchanged, or increase in size or number.
2. *The primary goal of treatment is to eliminate visible warts.*
3. Treatment may lead to a wart-free state, but the viral infection may still persist because normal skin and internal sites may also contain HPV. Therefore, *elimination of visible warts may not decrease infectivity nor transmission.* Recurrences are frequent despite treatment.
4. There is no evidence that using more than one treatment at a time will improve outcome. Most patients will require a course of therapy rather than a single treatment.
5. When using topical therapy, warts usually respond within 3 months.
6. Treatment may cause permanent scarring, hyperpigmentation, or hypopigmentation. Topical therapy can cause pain, local irritation, and rash (especially if too much is applied or it is left on too long).

7. Patient applied (nonpregnant adults)—recommended therapy:
    a. Podofilox (Condylox®) 0.5% solution or gel topically to warts BID x 3 days, followed by 4 days without therapy [0.5% gel: 3.5 grams; 0.5% solution: 3.5 ml]. This 7 day cycle may be repeated 3 more times (a total of 4 cycles) as needed. The daily dose should not exceed 0.5 cc and the application area should not exceed 10 cm^2, or
    b. Imiquimod (Aldara™) 5% cream topically to warts qHS three times per week for up to 16 weeks [5% cream: 250 mg single use packets]. Wash the treatment area with soap and water 6-10 hours after application.
8. Health provider applied (for nonpregnant adults)—recommended therapy:
    a. Cryotherapy every 1-2 weeks as needed, or
    b. Podophyllin 10%-25% resin in tincture of benzoin topically to each wart. Wash the treated area with soap and water 1-4 hours after application. Application may be repeated once a week. The daily dose should not exceed 0.5 cc and the application area should not exceed 10 cm^2. Avoid use on open lesions or wounds, or
    c. Trichloroacetic acid or bichloroacetic acid 80%-90% topically to warts and let it dry (it causes a white coating to appear). If excess acid was used, apply talc, sodium bicarbonate (baking soda), or liquid soap to remove the unreacted acid. Application may be repeated once a week, or
    d. Surgical removal (excision, curettage, or electrosurgery)
9. Alternative therapy, health provider applied (for nonpregnant adults)
    a. Laser ablation, or
    b. Intralesional interferon
10. For treatment of HPV during pregnancy or warts in locations other than the external genitals or urethra, see the CDC guidelines.

Treatment of Urethral Meatal Warts

Recommended therapy (nonpregnant adults)
    a. Cryotherapy with liquid nitrogen.
    b. Podophyllin 10%-25% resin in tincture of benzoin topically to warts. The treated lesions must dry before they are permitted to contact moist tissue. Application may be repeated once a week.

Treatment of Intraurethral Warts

1. Excision—urethral warts can be removed by cystoscopic excision using cold cup biopsy forceps. The biopsy site (base of the wart) can be lightly cauterized to stop the bleeding.
2. Laser fulguration—urethral warts can be removed by cystoscopic fulguration using the Nd:YAG laser.
3. Intraurethral instillation of 5-fluorouracil (5-FU)—has been used to eradicate lesions or to prevent recurrence after lesion removal. Complications include dysuria, meatal stenosis, meatitis, scrotal irritation, and urethral ulceration.
    a. To eradicate existing urethral warts—5% 5-FU cream instilled intraurethral through a funnel shaped applicator after each void for 3-8 days [5% cream: 25 grams]. Another regimen is 5-FU solution (500 mg in 50 cc normal saline) instilled intraurethral once a week for 7 weeks, and then each month thereafter until lesions resolve.
    b. To prevent recurrence after urethral wart removal—5% 5-FU cream instilled intraurethral through a funnel shaped applicator once a week for 6 weeks.
4. After treatment, surveillance urethroscopy in 3-6 months is recommended. Long-term surveillance may be prudent.

Follow Up
1. Follow patients while lesions persist and for complications of therapy.
2. Consider a follow up visit 3 months after treatment (recurrence usually occurs within 3 months). Patients with intraurethral warts should undergo urethroscopy during follow up.
3. If the lesions do not respond to therapy, biopsy them.
4. Women should have a routine gynecologic exam and pap smear (even when they have been vaccinated with Gardasil®).

Sex Partners
1. Examination of sex partners is not necessary for the management of genital warts because no data indicate that reinfection plays a role in recurrence.
2. Examination and counseling of sex partners may be offered.

Chancroid

General Information
1. Cause—Haemophilus ducreyi (a gram negative organism)
2. Infection usually occurs by sexual contact.
3. Incubation period = 2-14 days

Diagnosis
1. Definitive diagnostic test—culture. Culture is approximately 80% sensitive, but the culture media is not widely available.
2. A presumptive diagnosis may be made if all of the following criteria exist:
   a. *Painful* genital ulcer or ulcers.
   b. The clinical presentation is typical for chancroid.
   c. HSV absent—tests for herpes simplex virus are negative.
   d. Syphilis absent—ulcer exudate shows no spirochetes or a serologic test for syphilis is negative at least 7 days after onset of the ulcers.

Clinical Manifestations
1. A cutaneous lesion that progresses from a papule to a *painful* ulcer with undermined ragged edges, often covered with grey purulent exudate.
2. Tender regional lymphadenopathy may be present.

Treatment
1. Recommended regimens for non-pregnant adults
   a. Azithromycin 1 g PO single dose, or
   b. Ceftriaxone 250 mg IM single dose, or
   c. Ciprofloxacin 500 mg PO BID x 3 days, or
   d. Erythromycin base 500 mg PO TID x 7 days
2. Recommended regimen for pregnant females
   a. Ceftriaxone 250 mg IM single dose, or
   b. Erythromycin base 500 mg PO QID x 7 days.

Follow Up
1. Re-examine the patient 3-7 days after therapy is initiated. Symptoms usually improve in 3 days and ulcers begin healing in 7 days. Larger lesions may take several weeks to heal completely. Men with HIV and uncircumcised men may heal more slowly.
2. If no improvement is seen in 3-7 days, possible reasons include
   a. Noncompliance with therapy.
   b. The chancroid strain is resistant to the antibiotic that was administered.
   c. Incorrect diagnosis.
   d. Simultaneous infection with another STD (such as HIV).

Sex Partners
1. Treat all sex partners who have had sexual contact with the patient within 10 days from the onset of the patient's symptoms.
2. Treat all sex partners that have signs or symptoms of the disease.

Scabies

General Information
1. Cause—Sarcoptes scabiei (a parasitic mite).
2. Infection occurs by contact with infested people, clothes, or bedding.
3. The female mite burrows into the skin to lay eggs, leaving an indistinct tract along the skin. New mites hatch in 4-5 weeks. Scabies can occur anywhere, but commonly infect the hands, feet, axilla, groin, and penis.
4. Scabies rarely survive more than 24 hours without a host.

Diagnosis
Definitive diagnostic test—identification of mites on scrapings of the affected area (this usually requires magnification).

Clinical Manifestations
1. Pruritus, especially at night or when the infested individual is warm. Pruritus is caused by an allergic reaction to the mites.
2. An erythematous nodule, excoriation from itching, and bacterial superinfection may be present.
3. With the first infection, it may take up to 3 months for pruritus and rash to develop because it can take this long for sensitization. With subsequent infections, sensitization has already occurred, and pruritus often develops within hours.

Treatment
1. Recommended regimen for nonpregnant adults
   a. Permethrin cream (5%) applied topically from the neck down, then wash off 8-14 hours later.
   b. Ivermectin 200 ug/kg orally single dose, which is repeated in 2 weeks.
2. Alternative regimens for nonpregnant adults—Lindane lotion (1%) 1 oz. or Lindane cream (1%) 30 g applied topically in a thin layer from the neck down, then wash off 8 hours later. Do not use lindane when extensive dermatitis is present or after taking a bath or shower (it has caused seizures in this setting), in children < 2 years old, pregnancy, or lactating women.
3. Recommended regimen for pregnant females—permethrin cream (5%) applied topically from the neck down, then washed off 8-14 hours later.
4. Bedding, clothes, and towels should not be shared. They should be laundered with hot water or isolated from body contact for at least 72 hours. Avoid sharing of brushes and combs and wash them in hot water. Fumigation is not necessary.
5. Pruritus and rash may persist for 2 weeks after adequate treatment of scabies. Topical medicines may reduce the pruritus.
6. For treatment of children, persistent infections, or persistent symptoms, see the complete CDC recommendations.

Follow Up
Consider following the patient until symptoms have resolved. If symptoms persist > 2 weeks after treatment, reevaluate the patient. If infection persists, consider treating with a different regimen.

Sex Partners
Treat all sex partners and household members who have had contact with the patient within 30 days from the onset of the patient's symptoms.

Pubic Lice (Crabs)

General Information
1. Cause—Pediculosis Pubis (a wingless insect).
2. Infection occurs by contact with infested people, clothes, or bedding.
3. Lice look like small crabs and usually attach on a hair shaft close to the skin. They feed off the hosts blood.
4. Lice lay eggs on the hair shaft close to the skin. These eggs, which are called nits, hatch in 7-10 days.
5. Lice rarely survive more than 24 hours without a host.

Diagnosis
Definitive diagnostic test—identification of lice or nits on the hair shaft (usually visible to the naked eye).

Clinical Manifestations
1. Pruritus, especially at night or when the infested individual is warm (this is caused by an allergic reaction to the lice). This usually begins approximately 1-2 weeks after the infection.
2. Erythematous rash, excoriation from itching, and bacterial superinfection may be present.

Treatment
1. Recommended regimen for pregnant or nonpregnant adults
   a. Permethrin cream (1%) applied topically to affected areas, then washed off 10 minutes later, or
   b. Pyrethrins with piperonyl butoxide applied to the affected area, then washed off 10 minutes later.
2. Alternative regimen for nonpregnant adults
   a. Malathion 0.5% lotion applied to the affected area and then washed off 8-18 hours later, or
   b. Ivermectin 200 ug/kg orally single dose, which is repeated in 2 weeks.
3. Do not apply the topical regimens to the eyes or eyelashes.
4. Fine toothed combs can be used to comb out the nits.
5. Bedding, clothes, and towels should not be shared. They should be laundered with hot water or isolated from body contact for at least 72 hours. Avoid sharing of brushes and combs and wash them in hot water. Fumigation is not necessary.
6. For treatment of children, eyelash involvement, persistent infections, or persistent symptoms, see the complete CDC recommendations.

Follow Up
If symptoms persist 1 week after treatment, reevaluate the patient. If infection persists, consider treating with a different regimen.

Sex Partners
Treat all sex partners and household members who have had contact with the patient within 30 days from the onset of the patient's symptoms. Avoid sexual contact until treatment is completed and medical evaluation reveals cure.

SEXUALLY TRANSMITTED DISEASES

Disease	Causative Agent Name	Classification	Primary Genital Manifestations	Regional Adenopathy*	Syndromes	Incubation Period	Definitive Diagnostic Test
Gonorrhea	Neisseria gonorrhoeae	Gram negative diplococcus	Female usually asymptomatic, profuse purulent urethral/vaginal d/c	–/+	Urethritis, cervicitis, PID, proctitis, epididymitis, *Fitz-Hugh-Curtis*	2-6 days	Culture
Chlamydia	Chlamydia trachomatis (strains D-K)	Intracellular organism	Male & female often asymptomatic, scant urethral d/c	–/+	Urethritis, cervicitis, PID, proctitis, epididymitis, *Fitz-Hugh-Curtis*, *Reiter's syndrome*	3-21 days	Culture
Trichomonas	Trichomonas vaginalis	Flagellated protozoa	Male usually asymptomatic, green frothy vaginal d/c, vaginal & cervical petechiae	–	Urethritis, vaginitis, cervicitis ("strawberry cervix")	few days?	Wet mount, culture
Chancroid	Haemophilus ducreyi	Gram negative bacillus	Painful ulcer	+	Painful genital lesion	2-14 days	Culture
Genital Herpes	Herpes Simplex Virus (strains I & II)	Double stranded DNA virus	Painful vesicles or ulcers	–/+	Recurrent painful genital lesions	2-6 days	Culture
Syphilis	Treponema pallidum	Spirochete	Painless ulcer with raised edges (chancre)	+	Condyloma latum, gummas, lightning pains, tabes dorsalis, Argyll-Robertson pupil, aortitis, rash on hands and feet	14-28 days	Dark field microscopy, fluorescent antibody
Granuloma Inguinale	Klebsiella granulomatis	Intracellular gram negative organism	Painless "beefy red" ulcer	–	Lesion extension to groin mimics adenopathy (pseudobubo)	60-90 days	Donovan body on biopsy
Lymphogranuloma Vereceum	Chlamydia trachomatis (serotypes L1-L3)	Intracellular organism	Usually not noticed (small painless papule)	+ (Not with primary lesion)	*Groove sign*, sinus, fistula, abscess, rectal stricture	days-weeks	Culture
Genital Warts (Condyloma)	Human Papilloma Virus (HPV)	Double stranded DNA virus	Painless "warts" or papillary lesions	–	Condyloma acuminatum ("genital warts")	3-12 months	Clinical exam ± biopsy

* Regional adenopathy occurs simultaneously with the primary lesion unless specified otherwise; "+" = present; "–" = absent; PID = pelvic inflammatory disease, d/c = discharge.

Human Immunodeficiency Virus (HIV)

1. Cause—HIV-1 and HIV-2 (retroviruses containing 2 strands of RNA). Most cases of HIV in the U.S. are caused by HIV-1.
2. Urologic manifestations of HIV include
   a. Higher risk of renal cancer, penile cancer, and testis cancer (seminoma, nonseminoma, and lymphoma).
   b. Neurologic bladder dysfunction (usually urine retention).
   c. Hypogonadism—often treated with testosterone.
   d. Protease inhibitors can cause urinary calculi (see page 131).
3. Diagnosis—the initial test is an enzyme immunoassay or a rapid test, which can give false positive results. Therefore, *a positive immunoassay or rapid test must be confirmed by a western blot or immunofluorescence test.*
4. *A negative HIV test does not rule out a recent infection (e.g. an infection within the previous 3 months).* 95% of patients will test positive within 3 months of infection. If the initial test is negative and exposure occurred within 6 months, follow up tests are necessary to confirm a negative test (consider testing 3 and 6 months after the initial test).

Hepatitis B

1. Cause—hepatitis B virus (HBV), a double-stranded DNA virus.
2. Hepatitis B is prevented by vaccination.
3. There are no known urologic manifestations of hepatitis B.
4. Serology tests
   a. HBV surface antigen (HBsAg)—present in acute and chronic infection. During acute infection, it may be present for a few days to 2-3 months.
   b. Antibody to HBsAg (Anti-HBs, HBsAb)—present after vaccination or after previous infection. It becomes positive 5-6 months after infection.
   c. Antibody to HBV core antigen (Anti-HBc, HBcAb)—Anti-HBc IgM is present for 2-12 months after the acute infection.
5. Which tests do I order?—the initial tests include HBsAg, Anti-Hbc IgM, Anti-HBs, and liver function tests.

REFERENCES

Centers for Disease Control and Prevention: Sexually transmitted diseases treatment guidelines 2006. Morbidity and Mortality Weekly Report, 55 (11): 1-94, 2006.

Centers for Disease Control and Prevention: Update to CDC's sexually transmitted diseases treatment guidelines 2006: fluoroquinolones no longer recommended for treatment of gonococcal infections. Morbidity and Mortality Weekly Report, 56 (14): 332-6, 2007.

Centers for Disease Control and Prevention: Human papillomavirus: HPV information for clinicians. November 2006. (http://www.cdc.gov/std/HPV/common-infection/CDC_HPV_ClinicianBro_HR.pdf)

Centers for Disease Control and Prevention: Oral alternatives to cefixime for the treatment of uncomplicated Neisseria gonorrhoeae urogenital infections. April 2004. (http://www.cdc.gov/std/treatment/Cefixime.htm)

Centers for Disease Control and Prevention: Discontinuation of spectinomycin. Morbidity and Mortality Weekly Report, 55 (13): 370, 2006.

Centers for Disease Control and Prevention: Screening tests to detect Chlamydia trachomatis and Neisseria gonorrhoeae infections—2002. Morbidity and Mortality Weekly Report, 51 (15): 1-37, 2002.

Corey L, et al: Once daily valacyclovir to reduce the risk of transmission of genital herpes. N Engl J Med, 350: 11, 2004.

Pinto PA, Mellinger BC: HPV in the male patient. Urol Clin North Am, 26(4): 797, 1999.

GAS FORMING INFECTIONS

Causes of Gas in the Genitourinary System
1. Recent invasion into the urinary tract (endoscopic, open, or percutaneous)
   a. Bladder—catheterization, cystoscopy, incision into bladder.
   b. Renal pelvis or ureter—ureteroscopy, retrograde pyelogram, nephrostomy tube placement, nephrostogram, incision into upper tract.
2. Fistula to bowel, vagina, or skin
3. Urinary diversion—patients with a conduit or ureterosigmoidostomy may have reflux of gas into the collecting system.
4. Trauma—gas may be introduced by a penetrating wound.
5. Infarction of renal tumor—can cause gas in the kidney (see page 396).
   a. Spontaneous infarction of renal tumor
   b. Iatrogenic infarction of renal tumor (embolization)
6. Infection with gas forming organisms
   a. *Gas is formed by fermentation*, which metabolizes sugars into carbon dioxide and hydrogen. Uncontrolled diabetes mellitus provides abundant glucose substrate for this pathway.
   b. Organisms that can produce gas include E. coli, Klebsiella, Proteus, Clostridium perfringens, and Candida albicans.
7. Scrotal gas may be identified on imaging studies when bowel herniates into the scrotal sac.

Fournier's Gangrene

General Information
1. Fournier's gangrene is a *necrotizing fasciitis* of the male genitalia and perineum that involves mainly subcutaneous tissues.
2. Mortality varies, but probably approaches 30%.
3. It may be rapidly progressing (sometimes you can see the infection advancing over the course of minutes).
4. The most common sources of infection are the lower genitourinary tract, colon, rectum, or cutaneous infections of the genitals, perineum, or anus.
5. Risk factors for developing Fournier's gangrene
   a. Diabetes mellitus
   b. Alcohol abuse
   c. Other immunocompromised states including HIV, cancer, etc.
6. The infection often spreads along dartos fascia, Colles' fascia, and Scarpa's fascia because these layers are contiguous. It can spread along other fascial planes including Buck's fascia. It rarely involves deep fascial planes and muscle. It rarely forms purulent collections.
7. It may be caused by aerobes and anaerobes. However, *the most commonly cultured organism is E. coli.* Other commonly cultured organisms include enterococcus, staphylococcus, streptococcus, Bacteroides fragilis, and Pseudomonas aeruginosa.

Presentation
1. *The most prominent sign is painful swelling and induration of the penis, scrotum, or perineum.*
2. Cellulitis, eschar, necrosis, ecchymosis, crepitus, or cutaneous anesthesia may be present on the genitals, perineum, anus, or anterior abdominal wall. Edema tends to extend beyond the area of erythema.
3. Foul odor
4. Fever—may be absent in patients with significant immunocompromise.
5. Imaging may show gas in the subcutaneous tissues.
6. *Diagnosis is based on clinical suspicion.*

Treatment
1. Broad spectrum empiric IV antibiotics to cover gram negative, gram positive, aerobic, and anaerobic bacteria (e.g. ampicillin-sulbactam and clindamycin and ciprofloxacin)
2. Immediate aggressive surgical debridement
   a. Debride all necrotic, ischemic, and infected tissue (debride all tissue that does not bleed). Removal of threatened tissue is controversial. Try to preserve the thigh tissue so that a subcutaneous pocket for the testicles can be made if necessary. A suprapubic tube should be placed, especially if there is urethral stricture, urinary extravasation, or involvement of the penis or urethra (a cystoscopy or retrograde urethrogram may be performed intraoperatively). If anorectal or colonic involvement is suspected, proctoscopy should be performed under anesthesia prior to surgical intervention. If there is rectal or colonic involvement, a diverting colostomy may be indicated. Place subcutaneous Penrose drains at the periphery of the debrided areas to prevent fluid accumulation. Irrigate the wound copiously with antibiotic solution.
   b. Send *at least 1 cubic centimeter of tissue* for quantitative tissue culture and sensitivity for aerobes and anaerobes.
   c. Some advocate returning to the operating room in 24 hours to reassess the tissue and perform additional debridement as needed.
3. Post-operative management
   a. Wet to dry dressings using normal saline or Dakin's solution should be applied three times a day. If the patient's condition permits, daily whirlpool therapy may be instituted to assist in mechanical debridement. Hyperbaric oxygen therapy may be of benefit (see pages 125).
   b. Strict control of diabetes and adequate nutrition are essential to wound healing.
   c. Aggressive hydration is often required because weeping from the wound can cause significant fluid loss.
   d. Adjust antibiotics based on tissue culture.
   e. Skin grafts or flaps may be necessary to cover bare areas after the infection has been treated.

Emphysematous Prostatitis
1. This condition is rare and usually arises from either prostate abscess or Fournier's gangrene.
2. Emphysematous prostatic abscess—for evaluation and treatment, see Prostate Abscess, page 371.
3. Fournier's gangrene extension into prostate—see Fournier's gangrene, page 393

Emphysematous Cystitis

1. Emphysematous cystitis is an infection of the bladder characterized by *gas in the bladder wall* (gas only in the bladder lumen is not emphysematous cystitis). In severe cases, the infection and gas can spread to surrounding tissue or to the upper urinary tracts.
2. It usually occurs in diabetics or immunocompromised patients.
3. Presentation varies from relatively asymptomatic to severely ill.
4. Symptoms include lower abdominal pain, hematuria, and fever. Patients usually have pyuria and bacteriuria.
5. Imaging studies reveal gas in the bladder wall.
6. Evaluation includes urine culture and sensitivity, blood cultures, and CT scan of the abdomen and pelvis (to check for spread outside the bladder and spread to the upper tracts).
7. Most patients have a mild to moderate form of the disease. In these patients, treatment includes intravenous broad spectrum antibiotics, control of diabetes, bladder drainage with a catheter, and hydration. Surgical debridement or cystectomy is utilized in patients who do not respond adequately to conservative measures.

Emphysematous Pyelitis

1. Emphysematous pyelitis is characterized by gas only in the collecting system (no gas in the renal parenchyma or in the perinephric space).
2. Patients usually present with signs and symptoms of acute pyelonephritis; however, they tend to be more ill than patients with acute pyelonephritis and less ill than patients with emphysematous pyelonephritis.
3. Diabetes mellitus is present in 50% of cases.
4. *E. coli is the most common causative organism.*
5. CT is the most accurate study to diagnose emphysematous pyelitis. On CT, gas and gas-fluid levels are present in the collecting system. *On sonogram, gas in the calyces and renal pelvis appears as highly echogenic regions with posterior acoustic shadowing that may be mistaken for calculi.*
6. Most patients respond to conservative therapy. When ureteral obstruction is absent, intravenous antibiotics are the treatment of choice. If obstruction is present, treat with intravenous antibiotics and place a ureteral stent or nephrostomy tube (nephrostomy tube is preferred in moderately or severely ill patients).
7. When placing a percutaneous drain into an infected collecting system, a subcostal puncture is preferred because this precludes violation of the pleura and prevents spread of the infection into the pleural space (empyema).
8. Emphysematous pyelonephritis has a much worse prognosis and a higher mortality than emphysematous pyelitis.

Renal Abscess Containing Gas

1. A renal abscess is a *focal* renal infection characterized by a mass that may contain pus and/or gas, whereas emphysematous pyelonephritis is a *diffuse* renal infection with gas in the renal parenchyma (usually without abscess formation).
2. Renal abscess containing gas may be a less serious condition than emphysematous pyelonephritis. Satisfactory outcomes have been achieved with antibiotic therapy alone; however, these abscesses should probably be treated like non-gas containing abscesses (see Renal Abscess, page 346).

Emphysematous Pyelonephritis

General Information
1. Emphysematous pyelonephritis is a severe, diffuse acute pyelonephritis that is *characterized by gas in the renal parenchyma*. Occasionally, infection and gas may extend into the collecting system, perinephric tissue, or paranephric tissue.
2. *E. coli is the most common causative organism.*
3. If the diagnosis is not made promptly, it may progress rapidly to sepsis and renal failure. Mortality ranges from 20-80%.
4. *Diabetics presenting with pyelonephritis should undergo renal imaging to check for emphysematous pyelonephritis and urinary obstruction.*

Presentation
1. Most cases (90%) occur *in middle age or elderly diabetics*. Non-diabetics often have urinary obstruction.
2. *Presenting symptoms are similar to pyelonephritis*: flank pain, fever, and chills. Patients are often extremely ill with lethargy, confusion, and shock. Costovertebral angle tenderness is usually present. A flank mass is occasionally be palpable.
3. Urinalysis usually shows pyuria and bacteriuria. *Urine culture usually reveals E. coli.* Klebsiella, Proteus, Pseudomonas, and Candida are also seen, but *Clostridium is rarely found*. Urine culture may be negative in up to 25% of cases.
4. Emphysematous pyelonephritis is usually unilateral.
5. Imaging
   a. *CT scan is the imaging study of choice.* CT shows gas in the renal parenchyma. Gas may also be present in the perinephric space and in the collecting system.
   b. On ultrasound, the renal parenchyma shows highly echogenic regions with posterior acoustic shadowing. Extensive perinephric gas may completely obscure visualization of the kidney.

Treatment
1. Start broad spectrum parenteral antibiotics immediately.
2. Control blood glucose.
3. *Emphysematous pyelonephritis is usually managed by nephrectomy.* Conservative management without nephrectomy appears to have a higher mortality and it often fails to salvage function of the affected kidney.
4. In stable patients with either limited emphysematous pyelonephritis or gas in a focal renal abscess, conservative management may be attempted.
   a. Relieve urinary obstruction when present (stent or nephrostomy tube).
   b. Percutaneous drainage of fluid and gas collections.
   c. If the patient does not improve promptly, nephrectomy is indicated.

Renal Gas After Infarction & Post-infarction Syndrome

Renal Gas After Infarction
1. Gas in the kidney can arise after spontaneous or therapeutic infarction of the kidney and is generally considered a self-limiting process.
2. The gas appears within a few days after infarction and can last as long as 6 months.
3. The cause of gas formation may be anaerobic metabolism and formation of carbon dioxide gas.

Post Infarction Syndrome

1. Post-infarction syndrome occurs in 90% of patients undergoing therapeutic renal embolization and may include
   a. Flank pain—usually beginning 30-60 minutes after infarction and often lasting 24-48 hours.
   b. Leukocytosis—often with elevated neutrophils (left shift).
   c. Fever—may be as high as 104° F (40° C) and last 3-4 days.
   d. Nausea and vomiting
   e. Ileus
2. Patients with post-infarction syndrome (fever, leukocytosis, flank pain) may appear to have acute bacterial pyelonephritis.
3. *When renal gas occurs with post-infarction syndrome, the patient may appear to have emphysematous pyelonephritis. Post-infarction syndrome should be managed conservatively, whereas emphysematous pyelonephritis is usually managed by nephrectomy.*

REFERENCES

General

Amendola MA, Rossi PG: Abnormal gas in the genitourinary tract. Contemporary Urology, November, 2000: 31, 2000.

Joseph RC, et al: Genitourinary tract gas: imaging evaluation. Radiographics, 16: 295, 1996.

Stevens DL, et al: IDSA Practice guidelines for diagnosis and management of skin and soft tissue infections. Clin Infect Dis, 41: 1373, 2005.

Emphysematous Renal Infections

Best CD, et al: Clinical and radiological findings in patients with gas forming renal abscess treated conservatively. J Urol, 162: 1273, 1999.

Evanoff GV, et al: Spectrum of gas within the kidney: emphysematous pyelonephritis and emphysematous pyelitis. Am J Med, 83: 149, 1987.

Roy, C et al: Emphysematous pyelitis: findings in five patients. Radiology, 218: 647, 2001.

Shokeir AA, et al: Emphysematous pyelonephritis: 15-year experience with 20 cases. Urology, 49: 343, 1997.

Wan YL, et al: Predictors of outcome in emphysematous pyelonephritis. J Urol, 159: 369, 1998.

Emphysematous Prostatitis

Lu DC, et al: Emphysematous prostatic abscess due to Klebsiella pneumoniae. Diagn Microbiol Infect Dis, 31: 559, 1998.

Mariani AJ, et al: Emphysematous prostatic abscess: diagnosis and treatment. J Urol, 129: 385, 1983.

Renal Infarction

Jafri SZ, et al: Therapeutic angioinfarction of renal cell carcinoma: CT follow up. J Comput Assist Tomogr, 13: 443, 1989.

Ward JF, et al: The use of percutaneous transcatheter embolization in urology. AUA Update Series, Vol. 22, Lesson 39, 2003.

Wolf S, Markowitz SK: Spontaneous gas formation in a sterile renal cell carcinoma. Urol Radiol, 9: 222, 1988.

MALACOPLAKIA & TUBERCULOSIS

<u>Malacoplakia</u>

General Information
1. Malacoplakia means "soft plaque" in greek.
2. The monocyte lysosome helps fight infection by phagocytosis, killing, and degradation of bacteria. Microtubule assembly is essential for proper lysosome function.
3. The current theory suggests that malacoplakia is caused by abnormal microtubule assembly. This impairs the function of monocyte lysosomes, which leads to inefficient killing and degradation of bacteria. Thus, *malacoplakia arises from incomplete eradication of a bacterial infection.*
4. Mortality is 50% when multifocal disease is present. Mortality approaches 100% within 6 months of diagnosis when both kidneys are involved.

Presentation and Diagnosis
1. Malacoplakia is rare. It usually presents at age > 50 years.
2. Most patients with malacoplakia have chronic genitourinary infection, usually with E. coli. Urine culture is positive in 90% of patients.
3. *Malacoplakia can occur in any part of the genitourinary tract, but it occurs most commonly in the bladder.*
4. Malacoplakia often presents as a solid mass; therefore, it is often treated as malignancy (i.e. surgical removal).
5. Signs and symptoms depend on the organ involved.
   a. Bladder malacoplakia—often presents with irritative voiding symptoms and hematuria. Cystoscopy may show a soft yellow or brown plaque.
   b. Renal malacoplakia—often presents with fever, flank pain, or flank mass. Imaging usually reveals a solid mass, but it may be cystic if necrosis is present. Multifocal or diffuse renal involvement may enlarge the kidney and impair renal function. Additional imaging characteristics:
      i. Renal ultrasound—hypoechoic or hyperechoic lesion.
      ii. IVP—mass effect which may displace the calyces.
      iii. CT scan—low attenuation lesion.
      iv. Arteriography—hypovascular lesion with peripheral neovascularity.
6. Gross appearance—soft yellow or brown plaques may be present.
7. Histological appearance
   a. *Michaelis-Gutmann bodies are pathognomonic for malacoplakia.* These lesions may range in appearance from a dot to a *targetoid "owl's eye"* and may be intracellular or extracellular. The exact etiology of these lesions is unclear; however, they may represent mineralized residual bacterial fragments.

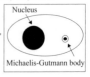

   b. von Hansemann cells—large mononuclear cells with foamy cytoplasm.
8. Diagnosis requires biopsy (malacoplakia is a pathologic diagnosis).

Treatment

1. *Upper tract malacoplakia is often persistent or progressive and is associated with significant morbidity and mortality*; therefore, it is usually treated surgically. Unilateral renal involvement often requires nephrectomy, especially if the patient is immunocompromised or has multifocal lesions.

2. *Lower urinary tract malacoplakia is usually benign and self-limiting.* Bladder malacoplakia has been treated with transurethral resection and medical therapy.

3. Medical therapy

    a. Long-term antibiotics—fluoroquinolones, rifampin, or trimethoprim-sulfamethoxazole are preferred because they retain their antibacterial activity inside the lysosome.

    b. Bethanechol—increases cyclic GMP, which enhances microtubule assembly, ultimately leading to improved lysosome function and bacterial digestion.

    c. Vitamin C—reduces cyclic AMP, which enhances microtubule assembly, ultimately leading to improved lysosome function and bacterial digestion.

    d. Stop immunosuppressants if possible (e.g. steroids).

4. Gallium scan may be used to determine response to medical therapy because uptake of the tracer is reduced after successful treatment.

Genitourinary Tuberculosis (GU TB)

General Information

1. Tuberculosis (TB) is caused by Mycobacterium tuberculosis, an intracellular aerobe that multiplies slowly. It is contracted by inhalation.

2. After exposure, the immune response is primarily cellular. This cellular response, which causes the characteristic caseating granulomas and the purified protein derivative (PPD) skin reaction, can subdue TB for years. TB may reactivate or remain dormant. Reactivation is usually precipitated by immunosuppression or biological stress (e.g. trauma, illness).

Presentation

1. Most cases of tuberculosis are confined to the lungs, but 15% of patients have extrapulmonary TB. *The genitourinary tract is the most common site of extrapulmonary TB.*

2. *Genitourinary TB can occur in the absence of active pulmonary TB.*

3. Symptoms of GU TB include flank pain, suprapubic pain, and irritative voiding symptoms. Fevers, weight loss, and night sweats are unusual.

4. *The classic finding of genitourinary TB is "sterile pyuria"* (pyuria is present, but standard culture shows no bacterial growth). Hematuria may be present.

5. Renal TB

    a. *The kidneys are the most common site of genitourinary TB.*

    b. Renal TB is caused by hematogenous spread of TB to the kidney.

    c. Renal TB may cause papillary necrosis and infundibular stenosis.

    d. Infundibular stenosis can lead to calyceal dilation. The calyceal walls can calcify, which appear as calcified "balls" on plain x-ray and as fluid collections with calcified walls on CT. A "putty" kidney occurs when the dilated calyces fill with putty-like caseous material.

    e. Renal granulomas form and erode into the collecting system, releasing mycobacteria into the urine (bacilluria). Bacilluria can lead to "downstream" infection of the ureters and lower urinary tract.

6. Ureteral TB
   a. Ureteral TB occurs from mycobacteria flowing down from the kidney.
   b. The most common finding is ureteral stricture with hydronephrosis. *The distal ureter (ureterovesical junction) is the most common site of ureteral strictures caused by TB.*
   c. *The concomitant presence of infundibular stenosis and ureteral stricture is highly suggestive of urinary tuberculosis.*
7. Bladder TB
   a. Bladder TB occurs from mycobacteria flowing down from the kidney.
   b. The ureteral orifice is the most common part of the bladder that is affected by TB. The ureteral orifice may appear edematous in the early stages of infection. Later, scarring and fibrosis leads to a "golf hole" ureteral orifice.
   c. Chronic bladder infection can cause a contracted bladder (called a "thimble bladder").
8. Genital TB
   a. Genital TB typically arises from hematogenous spread.
   b. The most common site of genital TB is the epididymis. TB may cause the epididymis to feel like a "string of beads." TB of the testis, prostate, penis, and urethra are rare.
   c. TB of the genitals can cause infertility.

Diagnosis

1. *To confirm the diagnosis of urinary TB, obtain at least 3 consecutive early morning urine samples for acid-fast staining and mycobacterial culture with sensitivities.* This method of diagnosis comes from a study by Teklu and Ostrow (1975) in which 97% of patients with urinary TB had at least one positive culture out of three consecutive early morning urinary mycobacterial cultures.
2. A positive PPD test supports the diagnosis of tuberculosis, but a negative skin test does not exclude tuberculosis. PPD can produce false negative results in immunosuppressed patients (such as patients with HIV, steroid use, malnutrition, overwhelming infection, malignancy, etc.).
3. Patients should have a chest x-ray and mycobacterial cultures of the blood and sputum.

Initial Treatment (Based on the 2003 CDC Guidelines)

1. *The initial treatment for genitourinary TB is 6 months of anti-tuberculosis medications.* The following regimen is recommended by the CDC, unless the organisms are known or suspected to be resistant to these agents. For dosing, see the CDC guidelines.
   a. First 2 months: isoniazid (INH), rifampin, pyrazinamide, and ethambutol (ethambutol may be stopped if the culture shows a TB strain that is sensitive to the other medications).
   b. Next 4 months: INH and rifampin.
2. Proximal or mid ureteral stenosis—when significant ureteral obstruction is present, the CDC recommends placement of a ureteral stent or a nephrostomy tube. Definitive management of the stenosis may be performed after eradication of TB.
3. Distal ureteral stenosis
   a. Some distal ureteral strictures are caused by edema and they may resolve with anti-tuberculosis medications.
   b. When minimal partial obstruction of the distal ureter is present, the patient may be monitored during anti-tuberculosis therapy to see if the stenosis resolves.

    c. When significant distal ureteral obstruction is present, the CDC recommends placement of a ureteral stent or a nephrostomy tube. After several weeks, a retrograde pyelogram may be performed to see of the stenosis has resolved. Definitive management of the stenosis may be performed after eradication of TB.

    d. The CDC does not recommend the use of corticosteroids for treating TB induced ureteral stenosis; however, some urologic literature suggests using corticosteroids. The following protocol is sited in the literature.

      i. Start anti-TB therapy and monitor the patient with weekly imaging (IVU, CT urogram, or renal scan).

      ii. If the stenosis does not improve within 3 weeks, administer corticosteroids with the anti-TB therapy.

      iii. If the stenosis does not improve within the next 6 weeks, place a ureteral stent. Definitive management of the stenosis may be performed after eradication of TB.

Surgical Treatment

1. When elective open or laparoscopic surgery is required for TB treatment, it should be performed after at least 6 weeks anti-TB therapy.

2. Nephrectomy is indicated in the following circumstances.

    a. Non-functioning or poorly functioning kidney causing hypertension, chronic pain, or persistent infection.

    b. Infected kidneys that do not respond to anti-TB drugs.

    c. Renal malignancy in an infected kidney.

3. When ureteral strictures persist after anti-TB drugs, definitive treatment may be necessary. Management is similar to ureteral strictures arising from other causes.

4. When the bladder is small and contracted, an augmentation cystoplasty may be required.

REFERENCES

Malacoplakia

Chen J, Koontz Jr WW: Inflammatory lesions of the kidney. AUA Update Series, Vol. 14, Lesson 26, 1995

Dasgupta P, et al: Malacoplakia: von Hansemann's disease. BJU Int, 84: 464, 1999.

Renzulli JF II, Anderson KR: Non-tubercular inflammatory disease of the kidney. AUA Update Series, Vol. 24, Lesson 4, 2005.

Tuberculosis

Centers for Disease Control and Prevention: Treatment of Tuberculosis. Morbidity and Mortality Weekly Report, 52 (No. RR-11): 1-88, 2003.

Johnson Jr. WD, et al: Tuberculosis and parasitic diseases of the genitourinary system. Campbell's Urology. 8th Edition. Ed. PC Walsh, AB Retik, et al. Philadelphia: W. B. Sanders Company, 2002, pp 743-795.

Teklu B, Ostrow JH: Urinary tuberculosis: a review of 44 cases treated since 1963. J Urol, 115: 507, 1975.

SURGICAL PRINCIPLES

Postoperative Myocardial Infarction

1. The mortality of postoperative myocardial infarction (MI) is > 50%.
2. *Myocardial ischemia and MI are most common 1-2 days postoperatively.*
3. Prevention of postoperative MI
   a. Preoperative cardiac assessment
   b. Minimize cardiac stress—for example, control pain adequately, avoid fluid overload, avoid hypertension, and avoid hypotension.

Postoperative Fever

1. The most common causes of postoperative fever are the "5 W's."
   a. "Wind"—refers to atelectasis, which usually presents with low grade fever, but no other systemic signs (e.g. absence of tachycardia, chills, rigors, tachypnea, etc.). *Atelectasis is the most common cause of fever within 24 hours of surgery. Atelectasis increases the risk of pneumonia.*
   b. "Water"—refers to urinary tract infection (UTI), and is usually caused by a urethral catheter. A higher risk of UTI is associated with a longer duration of catheterization. Remove the catheter as soon as possible.
   c. "Wound"—surgical site infection (SSI).
   d. "Walk"—this refers to deep venous thrombosis (which is usually prevented by walking).
   e. "Wonder Drugs"—some drugs can cause fever (especially sulfonamides and beta-lactams). Allergic reactions to drugs can also cause fever.

Mnemonic ("5 W's")	Description	Typical Time of Presentation (# days postop)	Prevention Strategy
Wind	Atelectasis	0-3	Incentive spirometer
Water	UTI (catheter related)	3-5	Remove catheter ASAP
Wound	Surgical site infection	5-7	Prophylactic antibiotics
Walk	VTE	14	VTE prophylaxis
Wonder drugs	Medications	Anytime	Stop unnecessary drugs

UTI = urinary tract infection; VTE = venous thromboembolism

2. Other causes of postoperative fever include phlebitis (at the IV site), central line infection, pneumonia (e.g. from atelectasis or aspiration), abscess, anastomotic leak, Clostridium difficile colitis, gout, appendicitis, cholecystitis, and pancreatitis.
3. Causes of fever intraoperatively or immediately (< 6 hours) postoperative
   a. Malignant hyperthermia—usually associated with succinylcholine or inhalational anesthetics such as halothane.
   b. Manipulation of infected focus intraoperatively (e.g. abscess drainage)
   c. Transfusion reaction
   d. Endocrine (e.g. thyroid storm, Addisonian crisis)
4. Causes of fever within 24 hours of surgery
   a. Atelectasis
   b. Clostridium or Streptococcus wound infections
   c. Aspiration pneumonia (from aspiration during surgery)
   d. Transfusion reaction
   e. Endocrine (e.g. thyroid storm, Addisonian crisis)

Surgical Site Infections (SSI)

Incision/Wound Classification

1. Classification based on the depth of infection
   a. Superficial SSI—involves only the skin and subcutaneous tissue.
   b. Deep SSI—involves fascia, muscle, or other deep soft tissues.
   c. Organ/space SSI—involves organs or spaces (other than the incision) that were opened or manipulated during surgery.
2. Classification based on contamination of incision.

Classification	Description	Risk of Infection*
Clean	Incision is closed primarily, and No infection/inflammation in the operative field, and No break in sterile technique, and Drains (when placed) have a closed system, and No transection of the GU, GI, or respiratory tracts.	≤ 5%
Clean Contaminated	No infection in the operative field, and No break in sterile technique, and Controlled transection of the GU, GI, biliary, or respiratory tracts without unusual contamination (e.g. surgery on appendix, vagina, or oropharynx).	3-11%
Contaminated	Non-purulent inflammation present, or Major break in sterile technique, or Gross spillage from GI tract, or Penetrating traumatic wounds < 4 hours old.	10-17%
Dirty-infected	Purulent inflammation present, or Preoperative perforation of viscera, or Penetrating traumatic wounds > 4 hours old.	> 27%

GU = genitourinary; GI = gastrointestinal
* When no antibiotics are administered.

Diagnosis of Surgical Site Infection

1. *Surgical site infections (SSI) usually present 5-7 days postoperatively with warmth, redness, swelling/induration, and tenderness.* Discharge, fever, and leukocytosis may also be present.
2. Send discharge for gram stain and culture with sensitivity. If discharge is absent, swab inside the incision to obtain a sample.
3. Profuse watery discharge (serous or serosanguinous) is often a sign of incision dehiscence. Dehiscence usually occurs on postoperative days 5-7.
4. If a deep infection or organ/space infection is suspected, imaging (such as a CT scan) may be needed to determine the extent of the infection and to evaluate for abscess.

Causes of Surgical Site Infection

1. SSI usually arises 5-7 days postoperatively. *The most common organism causing superficial SSI is Staphylococcus aureus.* Staphylococcus is also the most common organism causing penile prosthesis infection.
2. *SSI within 24 hours postoperatively is usually caused by Clostridium or Streptococcus.* On gram stain, Clostridium shows gram positive rods, whereas Streptococcus shows gram positive cocci in clusters. Clostridium tends to produce a red-brown (blood tinged) discharge.
3. When surgery invades the intestinal tract, female genital tract, or urinary tract, SSI is more likely to be caused by a mixture of organisms, which often includes gram negative organisms.
4. Pseudomonas aeruginosa infections may cause a green discharge and a "fruity" odor.

Treatment of Superficial Surgical Site Infection (Based on ISDA 2005)

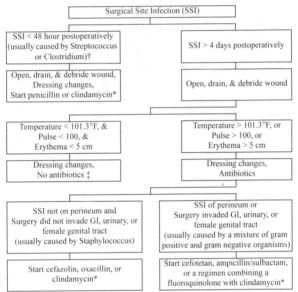

† Streptococcus and Clostridium are usually sensitive to penicillin, vancomycin, and clindamycin.

‡ Consider administering antibiotics in immunocompromised patients.

* Clindamycin is usually used for patients with penicillin allergy. Vancomycin may be used where MRSA infection rates are high.

Prevention of Surgical Site Infection
1. Preoperative prevention
   a. Encourage tobacco cessation at least 30 days prior to surgery (tobacco use delays wound healing and may increase the risk of SSI).
   b. Patients with asymptomatic bacteriuria who undergo traumatic genitourinary procedures associated with mucosal bleeding have a high rate of post-procedure bacteremia and sepsis. Therefore, *screening and treatment is recommended prior to traumatic genitourinary procedures associated with mucosal bleeding (e.g. TURP, urethral dilation, traumatic catheterization)*.
      i. When possible, urine culture should be obtained so that the results are available before the procedure.
      ii. Antimicrobial therapy should be started shortly before the procedure (e.g. the night before or immediately before the procedure).
      iii. Antimicrobial therapy should continued after the procedure when an indwelling catheter remains in place (duration was not specified by the guidelines).
   c. Even though preoperative antiseptic showers reduce the number of bacteria on the body, they have not been shown to reduce the risk of SSI.

2. Intraoperative prevention
   a. Removing hair before surgery (based on CDC recommendations)—do not remove hair preoperatively unless it will interfere with surgery. If hair removal is needed, *remove the hair with clippers (preferably electric clippers) immediately before surgery.*
      i. Clipping hair results in less SSI than shaving.
      ii. Trimming hair immediately before surgery appears to result in less SSI than trimming hair earlier before surgery.
      iii. No hair removal may result in less SSI than hair removal (data inconclusive).
   b. Administer prophylactic antibiotics when indicated.
   c. Monofilament sutures have a lower rate of SSI than braided sutures.
   d. Drains placed through the operative incision increase the risk of SSI. Many surgeons recommend placing a drain through a separate incision (away from the operative incision) to reduce the risk of SSI.
   e. Closed suction drains (e.g. JP) appear to cause less SSI than open drains (e.g. Penrose). The longer a drain remains in place, the higher the degree of bacterial colonization.
3. Postoperative prevention
   a. After primary closures, protect the incision with a sterile dressing for 24 to 48 hours (the incision is usually epithelialized in 24-48 hours).
   b. Wash your hands before and after dressing changes.
   c. Remove drains and catheters as soon as possible.
4. Perioperative—control diabetes.

Antibiotic Prophylaxis for Surgery

Guidelines (Based on CDC, SIP, IDSA, and ASHP guidelines)

1. Antibiotics are not indicated for "clean" surgical procedures (unless a prosthesis is placed).
2. *Most urologic and vaginal procedures are "clean contaminated" and antibiotic prophylaxis is usually indicated.*
3. Antibiotic prophylaxis is recommend for patients who have a high risk of postoperative bacteriuria (e.g. patients with an indwelling catheter postoperatively or who have a positive urine culture).
4. *The first dose of intravenous antibiotic should be infused within 60 minutes before incision.* However, when a fluoroquinolone or vancomycin is indicated, the infusion should begin within 120 minutes before incision to prevent antibiotic associated reactions.
5. Administration of the antibiotic at the time of anesthesia induction is safe and results in adequate drug concentration in the serum and tissue at the time of the incision. There was no consensus whether the infusion must be completed before incision.
6. Antibiotic prophylaxis should be discontinued within 24 hours after the end of surgery (unless there is a reason to continue them longer).
7. The antibiotic dose should be repeated intraoperatively if surgery is still in progress 2 half-lives after the first antibiotic dose. This ensures adequate drug levels in the tissue until the wound is closed.
8. Choose an antibiotic that is active against the pathogens most likely to colonize the operative site and most likely to cause wound infection.
9. Recommended prophylactic regimens
   a. Urologic procedures (without entry into bowel)—cefazolin IV
   b. Kidney transplant—cefazolin IV.
   c. Hysterectomy—cefazolin or cefotetan IV.
   d. Colorectal surgery—see page 406.

Antibiotic Prophylaxis: Special Circumstances
1. For patients colonized with methicillin resistant staphylococcus aureus (MRSA), vancomycin should be utilized for prophylaxis.
2. For patients at risk for endocarditis, see the American Heart Association guidelines. These guidelines were updated in 2007 (a copy can be obtained at http://dx.doi.org/10.1161/CIRCULATIONAHA.106.183095).
3. Patients with a prosthetic joint replacement (Based on AUA Advisory)
   a. Patients with a prosthetic joint replacement should receive antibiotic prophylaxis when they meet both of the following criteria:
      i. Any of the following characteristics are present: their joint placement was placed within the last 2 years, immunosuppressed (e.g. diabetes mellitus, malnutrition, HIV, autoimmune disease), or malignancy.
      ii. Any of the following procedures are performed: stone manipulation (including ESWL), transmural incision into the urinary tract, endoscopic procedure of the upper urinary tract, incision into bowel, transrectal prostate biopsy, endoscopy or catheterization in patients at risk for bacteriuria (urinary diversion, indwelling stent, indwelling catheter, intermittent catheterization, urinary retention, recent UTI).
   b. The recommended adult antibiotic regimens include
      i. One oral dose of fluoroquinolone 1-2 hours preoperatively, or
      ii. Ampicillin 2 gm IV (or vancomycin 1 gm IV if allergic to ampicillin) and gentamicin 1.5 mg/kg 30-60 minutes preoperatively.

Colorectal Surgery
1. Antibiotic prophylaxis for colorectal surgery may consist of intravenous (IV) antibiotics, oral antibiotics, or a combination of both. Most colorectal surgeons in the United States use a combination of oral and IV antibiotics. Furthermore, a recent study (Can J Surg 45: 173, 2002) indicates that a combination of IV and oral antibiotics may reduce surgical infections.
2. Oral antibiotics may be omitted in the presence of bowel obstruction.
3. An example of an oral antibiotic regimen is "Nichols' prep." This regimen is usually administered after a mechanical bowel preparation.
   a. Adult dose—neomycin 1 gram po and erythromycin base 1 gram po at 19 hours, 18 hours, and 9 hours before surgery (if surgery is at 8 AM, the doses are given at 1 PM, 2 PM, and 11 PM the evening before surgery).
   b. Pediatric dose—neomycin 20 mg/kg/dose po and erythromycin base 10 mg/kg/dose po gram po at 19 hours, 18 hours, and 9 hours before surgery.

	Antibiotic Prophylaxis for Colorectal Surgery (ASHP 1999)	
	Intravenous Antibiotic	Oral Antibiotics†
Recommended Regimens	cefoxitin or cefotetan or cefazolin & metronidazole	neomycin & erythromycin base* or neomycin & metronidazole
PCN Allergy	clindamycin & ciprofloxacin or clindamycin & gentamicin or clindamycin & aztreonam or metronidazole & gentamicin or metronidazole & ciprofloxacin	† Administered no more than 18-24 hours before surgery. * An example is Nichols' prep: neomycin 1 gram po and erythromycin base 1 gram po at 19 hours, 18 hours, and 9 hours before surgery (adult dose).

4. Mechanical bowel preparation
   a. Mechanical bowel preparation is contraindicated in the presence of bowel obstruction.
   b. Historically, mechanical bowel preparation was given preoperatively for colorectal surgery; however, recent evidence (meta-analysis and Cochrane review) suggests that mechanical bowel preparation does not reduce the risk of surgical site infection, anastomotic leakage, or other complications. In fact, it may increase the risk of these complications (although the data do not reach statistical significance).
   c. Bowel preparation may include dietary restrictions (e.g. clear liquids), cathartics (e.g. polyethylene glycol or sodium phosphate), and enemas. Example mechanical bowel preparation:
      i. Adult—the day before surgery start clear liquids and administer 1 gallon polyethylene glycol po over 4 hours starting at 8 AM (one large glass po every 15 minutes).
      ii. Pediatric—the day before surgery start clear liquids and administer polyethylene glycol electrolyte lavage solution given orally or by nasogastric tube at 25-40 ml/kg/hr until rectal effluent is clear.
      iii. Consider oral anti-nausea medication prior to polyethylene glycol.

Venous Thromboembolism (VTE)

General Information

1. Venous thromboembolism (VTE) includes deep venous thrombosis (DVT) and pulmonary embolism (PE).
2. *PE is the most common preventable cause of postoperative death.*
3. Virchow's triad—these are the 3 basic risk factors for VTE
   a. Venous stasis
   b. Intimal injury—injury to the inner surface of a blood vessel induces clot.
   c. Hypercoagulable state
4. Clinical risk factors for VTE—see table.
5. Risk factors specific to urologic surgery
   a. Lithotomy position
   b. Pelvic surgery
6. A greater number of risk factors increases the risk of VTE.

Risk Factors for VTE
Age ≥ 40
Obesity
History of VTE
Malignancy
Prolonged immobilization (especially ≥ 4 days)
Long surgical duration (especially > 2 hours)
Lithotomy position
Pelvic surgery
Congestive heart failure
Varicose veins
Fracture of hip or leg
Estrogen use
Pregnant or postpartum

DVT: Presentation and Diagnosis

1. DVT is usually asymptomatic.
2. *Signs and symptoms of DVT and PE are neither sensitive nor specific for diagnosis.* Only 25% of patients with signs and symptoms of DVT will actually have a DVT.
3. *The mean time of presentation for DVT is 2 weeks postoperatively*; however, 60% present less than 3 weeks and 40% present more than 3 weeks postoperatively. Some DVTs present > 30 days after surgery.
4. Signs and symptoms of DVT—include leg swelling, calf pain, low grade fever, and Homan's sign (with the knee flexed about 30 degrees, rapid passive dorsiflexion by the physician induces pain in the calf).
5. Diagnosis is usually made by Doppler ultrasound of the lower extremity.

PE: Presentation and Diagnosis
1. Most fatal PEs occur without a previous diagnosis of VTE.
2. Symptoms of PE—most patients have dyspnea and pleuritic chest pain. Other less common symptoms include cough, hemoptysis, palpitations, and wheezing.
3. Signs of PE—include tachypnea, crackles on pulmonary exam, low grade fever, and hypoxemia.
4. Diagnosis is usually made by CT angiography (CTA) of the lungs. V/Q scan and chest x-ray may be considered when intravenous iodine contrast is contraindicated or when CTA is inconclusive.
5. Arterial blood gas (ABG) is usually not useful for diagnosing PE because it can be normal up to 20% of cases. However, it may provide information regarding the need for supplemental oxygen. When ABG is abnormal, it usually shows reduced PaO_2 (hypoxemia) and reduced $PaCO_2$.
6. The "classic" electrocardiogram findings are S wave in lead I, Q wave in lead III, and inverted T wave in lead III (S_I, Q_{III}, T_{III}). However, it is not always present and is not sensitive nor specific for PE.

Prevention of Postoperative Venous Thromboembolism

General Information
1. *PE is the most common preventable cause of postoperative death.*
2. *Based on overwhelming evidence that prophylaxis reduces adverse outcomes and is cost effective, the AHRQ ranked "appropriate use of prophylaxis to prevent venous thromboembolism in patients at risk" as the most important safety practice to optimize patient care.*
3. Possible strategies for addressing postoperative VTE
   a. Early diagnosis—not effective. Diagnosis based on signs and symptoms is unreliable. Furthermore, death may be the first sign of PE.
   b. Routine screening—not effective. Screening for asymptomatic DVT does not prevent clinically significant VTE and is not cost effective.
   c. Prophylaxis—*prophylaxis in patients at risk for VTE is the preferred strategy to address postoperative DVT and PE.* It has been proven to be practical and effective.
4. Methods of preventing postoperative VTE
   a. Ambulation and dorsiflexion exercises
   b. Mechanical prophylaxis
   c. Pharmacological prophylaxis

Ambulation and Dorsiflexion
1. Ambulation and dorsiflexion exercises are considered prophylaxis strategies, but neither have been well studied.
2. Early, aggressive, persistent ambulation and dorsiflexion exercises are usually recommended as part of any prevention strategy.

Mechanical Prophylaxis
1. Mechanical prophylaxis works by compression of the leg veins.
2. Examples include graduated compression stockings (GCS) and intermittent pneumatic compression devices (IPC).
3. GCS and IPC have been shown to decrease DVT, but *no mechanical prophylaxis strategy has been shown to reduce the risk of PE or death.*
4. The major advantage of mechanical prophylaxis is the lack of bleeding potential.
5. The ACCP 2004 recommend "the use of mechanical prophylaxis primarily in patients who are at high risk of bleeding or as an adjunct to anticoagulation based prophylaxis."

Graduated Compression Stockings (GCS)
1. Graduated compression stockings are also called T.E.D. hose (ThromboEmbolism Deterrent hose).
2. GCS have been shown to decrease DVT in low risk patients, but not in high risk patients. *No mechanical prophylaxis strategy has been shown to reduce the risk of PE or death.*
3. Proper use
   a. Graduated compression stocking must fit appropriately to be effective. Stockings that are too tight or that roll down on the leg can cause a tourniquet effect, impair venous flow, and increase the risk of VTE. Stockings that are too loose may be ineffective.
   b. Align the toe hole under the toe.
   c. Do not fold or roll the stocking down on the leg.
   d. GCS should be removed for no longer than 30 minutes a day.
   e. GCS should be used until the patient is fully ambulatory.
   f. Contraindications include severe peripheral vascular disease, pulmonary edema, severe peripheral neuropathy, local skin conditions (e.g. severe dermatitis, recent skin graft), and major leg deformity.

Intermittent Pneumatic Compression (IPC) Devices
1. These devices intermittently squeeze the leg, causing the following effects.
   a. Prevents venous stasis—leg compression pumps blood through the veins and promotes venous return.
   b. Stimulates local fibrinolytic activity—compression of the vascular endothelial cells increases local fibrinolytic activity, which dissolves microthrombi.
2. A meta-analysis of randomized trials showed that the use of IPC devices in postoperative patients reduces the risk of DVT by 60% compared to no prophylaxis. *No mechanical prophylaxis strategy has been shown to reduce the risk of PE or death.*
3. In patients undergoing urologic surgery, both thigh length and calf length intermittent compression devices appear to be effective for preventing DVT (i.e. they reduce the risk of DVT by a similar amount).
4. *The major problem with these devices is poor compliance.* Nurses often fail to reapply the devices after the patient has finished ambulating. To be effective, IPC should be used at all times except when the patient is ambulating.
5. Proper use
   a. IPC must fit appropriately to be effective. If they are too loose, they may be ineffective.
   b. IPC should be used at all times except when the patient is ambulating. IPC should be used until the patient is fully ambulatory.
   c. Contraindications include severe peripheral vascular disease, patients with DVT, pulmonary edema, and major leg deformity.

Pharmacologic Prophylaxis

1. Currently recommended options for prophylaxis include low dose unfractionated heparin (LDUH), low molecular weight heparin (LMWH), warfarin, and fondaparinux.
2. *Aspirin alone is not recommended for prevention of VTE.*
3. Dextran has been used for VTE prophylaxis, but its use is no longer recommended because of the unacceptably high rate of bleeding, anaphylaxis, and pulmonary edema.
4. *Pharmacologic prophylaxis (specifically warfarin and heparin), has been shown to reduce the risk of DVT, PE, and fatal PE.*
5. The risks of pharmacologic anticoagulation include bleeding, hematoma, and lymphocele. Some studies find an increased risk of these complications, while other studies find no increased risk.

ACCP 2004 Recommendations for VTE prophylaxis in Urologic Surgery

1. The risk assignment and prevention recommendations presented herein may not be appropriate for every patient. The clinician should decide on a prophylaxis strategy for each individual patient based on that patient's risk factors and specific clinical circumstance.
2. "In patients undergoing transurethral or other low risk urologic procedures, we recommend against the use of specific prophylaxis other than early and persistent mobilization." Consider prophylaxis in patients who have multiple risk factors for VTE.
3. "For patients undergoing major, open urologic procedures [such as radical prostatectomy, cystectomy, or nephrectomy], we recommend routine prophylaxis with LDUH twice daily or three times daily. Acceptable alternatives include IPC and/or GCS or LMWH."
4. "For urology patients who are at particularly high risk [i.e. multiple risk factors], commencing prophylaxis with GCS with or without IPC just prior to surgery and then adding LDUH or LMWH postoperatively should be considered, even though this approach has not been formally evaluated in this patient population."
5. "For urologic surgery patients who are actively bleeding, or are at very high risk for bleeding, we recommend the use of mechanical prophylaxis with CGS and/or IPC at least until the bleeding risk decreases."
6. "For patients undergoing laparoscopic procedures, and who have additional thromboembolic risk factors, we recommend the use of thromboprophylaxis with one or more of the following: LDUH, LMWH, IPC, or GCS."
7. "The optimal duration of prophylaxis is uncertain. Patients who are believed to be at high risk for thromboembolism... or patients who have limited mobility at hospital discharge, should be considered for post-hospital discharge thromboprophylaxis." A recent study suggests that prophylaxis should be continued for at least 4 weeks postoperatively. In patients undergoing curative open abdominal surgery for pelvic or abdominal cancer, patients receiving 4 weeks of LMWH had a lower rate of VTE than patients receiving 6-10 days of LMWH postoperatively.
8. Consider stopping estrogens at least 4-6 weeks before surgery. When estrogens are not stopped before surgery, consider VTE prophylaxis.

VTE Risk Stratification and Prophylaxis for Patients Undergoing Surgery
(The following charts are based on ACCP 2004 and ICS 2001)

Based on the first chart, determine which type of surgery the patient will be undergoing. On the second chart, determine the level of risk. Based on the level of risk, the third chart reveals the recommended VTE prophylaxis regimen and the chance of VTE.

Surgery Type	Description	Examples
Minor	< 30-45 minutes and non-abdominal	Outpatient surgery, Transurethral surgery
Non-major	45 minutes - 2 hours	Uncomplicated abdominal or pelvic surgery
Major	> 2 hours	Complicated abdominal or pelvic surgery, Abdominal or pelvic surgery for malignancy

Surgery Type	Additional Risk Factors*	Risk Level for Postoperative VTE		
		Age < 40	Age 40-60	Age >60
Minor	No	Low	Moderate	Moderate
	Yes	Moderate	Moderate	Moderate
Non-major	No	Low/Mod	Moderate	High
	Yes	High	High	High
Major	No	Moderate	High	High
	Yes	High	Highest	Highest

VTE = venous thromboembolism

* When the patient has multiple risk factors, the physician may elect to increase the level of risk. Additional risk factors include history of VTE, malignancy, prolonged immobilization, obesity, congestive heart failure, varicose veins, estrogen use, pregnant, postpartum, and recent hip or leg fracture.

Risk Level	Risk Without Prophylaxis			Recommended VTE Prevention ‡
	Calf DVT	PE	Fatal PE	
Low	2%	0.2%	<0.1%	Early, Aggressive, and Persistent Ambulation
Moderate	10-20%	1-2%	0.1-0.4%	LDUH (q 12 hours) or LMWH or GCS or IPC
High	20-40%	2-4%	0.4-1.0%	LDUH (q 8 hours) or LMWH or IPC
Highest†	40-80%	4-10%	1-5%	LMWH or fondaparinux or warfarin (keep INR = 2-3) or a combination of mechanical compression (GCS and/or IPC) and heparin (LDUH or LMWH)

GCS = graduated compression stockings; IPC = intermittent pneumatic compression
LMWH = low molecular weight heparin; LDUH = low dose unfractionated heparin
DVT = deep venous thrombosis; PE = pulmonary embolism;
† All patients with spinal cord injury or major trauma are considered highest risk.
‡ GCS and IPC should be applied before inducing anesthesia. Anticoagulants may be started postoperatively when the bleeding risk decreases.

REFERENCES

Surgical Site Infection

ISDA—Stevens DL, et al: Practice guidelines for the management of skin and soft tissue infections. Clin Infect Dis, 41: 1373, 2005.

Antibiotic Prophylaxis for Surgery

ASHP—American Society of Health System Pharmacists therapeutic guidelines on antimicrobial prophylaxis in surgery. Am J Health Syst Pharm, 56: 1839, 1999.

CDC—Mangram AJ, et al: Guideline for the prevention of surgical site infection, 1999. Infect Control Hosp Epidemiol, 20, 250, 1999.

Holtom PD, et al: Antibiotic prophylaxis for urological patients with total joint replacement. AUA and AAOS advisory statement. J Urol, 169: 1796, 2003.

IDSA—Dellinger EP, et al for the Infectious Diseases Society of America: Quality standard for antimicrobial prophylaxis in surgical procedures. Clin Infect Dis, 18: 422, 1994.

Lewis RT: Oral versus systemic antibiotic prophylaxis in elective colon surgery: a randomized study and meta-analysis send a message from 1990s. Can J Surg, 45: 173, 2002.

SIP—Bratzler DW, et al: Antimicrobial prophylaxis for surgery: an advisory statement from the national surgical infection prevention project. Clin Infect Dis, 38: 1706, 2004.

Bowel Preparation

Guenaga KF, et al: Mechanical bowel preparation for elective colorectal surgery. Cochrane Database Syst Rev, 1: CD001544, 2005.

Nichols RL, et al: Efficacy of preoperative antimicrobial preparation of the bowel. Ann Surg, 176: 227, 1972.

Slim K, et al: Meta-analysis of randomized clinical trials of colorectal surgery with or without mechanical bowel preparation. Br J Surg, 91(9): 1125, 2004.

Hair Removal Before Surgery

CDC—Mangram AJ, et al: Guideline for the prevention of surgical site infection, 1999. Infect Control Hosp Epidemiol, 20, 250, 1999.

Tanner J et al: Preoperative hair removal to reduce surgical site infection. Cochrane Database Syst Rev, 2: CD004122, 2006.

Venous Thromboembolism

ACCP—Geerts WH, et al: Prevention of venous thromboembolism: The Seventh ACCP Conference on Antithrombotic and Thrombolytic Therapy. Chest, 126: 338S, 2004.

AHRQ—Making health care safer: A critical analysis of patient safety practices. Summary. July, 2001. AHRQ publication No. 01-E057. Agency for Healthcare Research and Quality, Rockville, MD.

Agnelli G, et al: A clinical outcome based prospective study on venous thromboembolism after cancer surgery. Ann Surg, 243: 89, 2006.

ICS—Nicolaides AN, et al: Prevention of thromboembolism. International Consensus Statement. Guidelines compiled in accordance with the scientific evidence. Int Angiol, 20(1): 1, 2001.

Kibel AS, Loughlin KR: Pathogenesis and prophylaxis of postoperative thromboembolic disease in urological pelvic surgery. J Urol, 153: 1763, 1995.

Soderdahl DW, et al: A comparison of intermittent pneumatic compression of the calf and whole leg in preventing deep venous thrombosis in urologic surgery. J Urol, 157: 1774, 1997.

Urbankova J, et al: Intermittent pneumatic compression and deep vein thrombosis prevention: a meta-analysis in postoperative patients. Thromb Haemost, 94(6): 1181, 2005.

URETERAL STENTS

General Information
1. Stent length is measured along the straight portion of the stent.
2. Outer diameter is measured in French (3 French = 1 mm).
3. The curls/coils help prevent stent migration.
4. Flow through the stent depends on
   a. Inner diameter—the larger the inner diameter, the higher the flow.
   b. Side holes—flow through stents with side holes is approximately two times greater than the flow through stents without side holes.
5. Flow goes through as well as around the stent.
6. Flow can be antegrade and retrograde (reflux). Side holes allow the reflux pressure to dissipate along the ureter so it is not transmitted to the kidney.

Methods to Select the Appropriate Stent Size
1. Stent length in cm = patient height in inches – 42 (adults only).
2. Stent length in cm = 0.9 x (ureteral length on IVP in cm). This approximation can be used only with the standard 17 x 14 inch KUB.
3. Place a calibrated ureteral catheter up the ureter to the renal pelvis. Then, through the cystoscope, look at the measurement at the ureteral orifice.

Management Tips
1. Prevent stent migration by using a long enough stent and by generating ≥ 180° curl on the ends.
2. In patients with high intravesical pressures (e.g. contracted or neurogenic bladder), consider avoiding ureteral stents because high pressure reflux through the stent may cause renal damage.
3. ESWL may be needed to knock stones off a calcified stent.
4. Consider stent removal in the O.R. if there is excessive resistance during attempted stent removal in the office or if the stent is knotted/twisted.
5. Stents indwelling ≥ 6 months are more likely to fracture.
6. If a stent is difficult to remove in the O.R., try the following:
   a. Watch the proximal curl unfurl with fluoroscopy during stent removal.
   b. Pass a guidewire through the stent to unfurl the proximal curl.
7. If a stent is difficult to pass, try one of the following:
   a. Use a hydrophilic stent. If a hydrophilic stent is not available, you can dip a regular stent in sterile mineral oil.
   b. Try a smaller diameter stent.
   c. Use a stiffer guide wire.

REFERENCES
Mardis HK, Kroeger RM, Hepperlen TW, et al: Polyethylene double-pigtail ureteral stents. Urol Clin North Am, 9(1): 95, 1982.

Mardis HK: Self-retained internal ureteral stents: use and complications. AUA Update Series, Vol. 26, Lesson 29, 1997.

Saltzman B: Ureteral stents, indications, variations, and complications. Urol Clin North Am, 15(3): 481, 1988.

Smith MJV, Chir B: Ureteral stents: their use and misuse. Monographs in Urology, Volume 14: 1, 1993.

USE OF INTESTINE IN
THE URINARY TRACT

Urinary Diversions and Neobladders
1. Cutaneous urinary diversion—*non-continent* diversion in which urine flows out an ostomy into a collection bag. Examples include cutaneous ureterostomy and conduits (ileal, ileocecal, colonic, etc.).
2. Catheterizable urinary diversion—*continent* catheterizable reservoir.
   a. Continence mechanisms include pressure equilibration (e.g. intussuscepted bowel) and flap valve (e.g. tunnelled implant).
   b. Catheterizable diversion types—ileal (e.g. Kock pouch), ileocolonic (e.g. Mainz pouch), and right colon (e.g. UCLA pouch, Miami pouch).
3. Orthotopic bladder replacement (neobladder)—*continent* reservoir that allows voiding per urethra.
   a. The *urethral sphincter* is the continence mechanism.
   b. Neobladder types—ileal (e.g. Hautmann, Studer), ileocolonic (e.g. Mainz pouch), colonic (e.g. sigmoid neobladder).
4. Ureterosigmoidostomy and variations—*continent* diversions that divert the urine to the gastrointestinal tract.
   a. The *anal sphincter* as the continence mechanism.
   b. Examples—ureterosigmoidostomy, ileocecal sigmoidostomy, rectal bladder urinary diversion, augmented valved rectum.

Complications Associated With Urinary Diversions and Neobladders
1. Electrolyte abnormalities
   a. The type and severity of the metabolic disturbance depends on
      • The segment of intestine used (i.e. ileum, jejunum, colon, etc.)
      • The length of intestine used (reflects the surface area exposed to urine).
      • The duration of urine contact with the intestine—with a conduit, the urine flows rapidly out of the intestinal segment. With a continent reservoir, the urine stays in contact with the intestine for long periods.
      • The patient's renal function.
   b. It is unknown if patients with intestine incorporated into the urinary tract should be treated prophylactically for electrolyte disturbances. Patients who have electrolyte abnormalities should be treated.
   c. Colon and/or ileum—causes hypokalemic, hyperchloremic acidosis.
      • Hyperchloremic acidosis arises from active transport of ammonium chloride from the urine and into the blood stream. Increased ammonia absorption may induce encephalopathy in patients with liver disease.
      • Ammonium excretion is the main mechanism by which the kidneys eliminate acid. When colon and/or ileum is incorporated into the urinary tract, acid elimination is impaired. The body compensates by titrating acid using bone buffers, resulting in bone demineralization.
      • Acidosis and hypokalemia can be treated with *potassium citrate*. In severe cases, blockers of chloride transport (chlorpromazine 25 mg po TID or nicotinic acid 400 mg po TID or QID) may be used to decrease the absorption of ammonium chloride.
   d. Stomach—causes hypokalemic, hypochloremic metabolic alkalosis.
      • Hypochloremic alkalosis occurs because of hydrochloric acid (HCl) secretion by the stomach. Potassium is also lost in gastric secretions.
      • Treatment may require *H2 blockers or hydrogen pump blockers*.

e. Jejunum—causes hyperkalemic, hypochloremic, hyponatremic, acidosis.
  • Sodium and chloride are secreted, while potassium and hydrogen are absorbed. Sodium loss results in water loss. Dehydration increases aldosterone secretion, resulting in urine that has lower sodium and higher potassium. When this urine reaches the jejunum, the concentration gradients favor sodium secretion and potassium absorption, causing worse hyperkalemia and hyponatremia.
  • Total parenteral nutrition (TPN) can exacerbate these electrolyte disturbances (the mechanism is unknown). The more proximal the jejunal segment used, the more likely the exacerbation with TPN.
  • Treatment of the acute episode consists of hydration with sodium chloride solution, correction of the acidosis with bicarbonate, and correction of hyperkalemia. Long-term prophylactic therapy consists of *oral sodium chloride* supplement.
2. Bone demineralization—acidosis reduces vitamin D production; therefore, intestinal calcium absorption and bone mineralization are impaired. Furthermore, chronic acidosis causes bone demineralization (excess protons bind to bone and displace calcium). Bone demineralization may retard bone growth in children and increase bone loss in those at risk for osteoporosis (e.g. postmenopausal women, steroid use). Treatment consists of correcting the acidosis. If this does not result in bone remineralization, administer dietary calcium and vitamin D supplements.
3. Impaired linear growth—occurs in children who have long-standing diversions. Growth retardation is likely caused by metabolic abnormalities.
4. Infection—patients with intestine incorporated into the urinary tract have a higher incidence of urinary tract infection. Reasons for this may include chronic bacterial colonization of the intestinal segment and inability of the intestine to inhibit bacterial proliferation.
5. Mucus production—mucus production of segments incorporated into the urinary tract (from most abundant to least abundant): colon, ileum, stomach. Mucus may occlude catheters and cause inadequate emptying. Mucus may also be a nidus for stone formation. In catheterizable urinary reservoirs, irrigation with normal saline is recommended to clear the mucus. *Oral intake of dairy products can increase mucus production.*
6. Diarrhea—can occur following the resection of the ileum, colon, or ileocecal valve. Patients with myelomeningocele depend on constipation for their fecal continence; thus, removal of the ileocecal valve should be avoided in these patients. Causes of diarrhea after diversion include
  • Decreased transit time of intestinal contents—occurs after resection of ileum, colon, or ileocecal valve.
  • Fat and bile acid malabsorption—occurs after ileal resection.
  • Overgrowth of small bowel bacteria—occurs after ileocecal valve resection.
7. Urolithiasis—increased risk of urinary calculi may occur from
  a. Urinary infection or colonization with urease producing bacteria (see How Urinary Tract Infection Increases Stone Risk, page 130).
  b. Enteric hyperoxaluria after ileal resection (see Hyperoxaluria, page 138).
  c. Mucous production (mucous can be a nidus for stone formation).
  d. Acidosis and hypokalemia may increase stone risk (see How Acidosis Increases Stone Risk, page 130).
  e. Dehydration from diarrhea.
8. Increased risk of cancer (see Risk of Cancer at the Entero-Urothelial Anastomosis, page 416)

9. Vitamin B_{12} (cobalamin) deficiency—B_{12} is absorbed in the distal ileum; thus, removal of the distal ileum (especially > 50 cm) can cause B_{12} deficiency. B_{12} deficiency may cause megaloblastic anemia, neurologic manifestations, psychiatric disorders, orthostatic hypotension, infertility, hyperpigmentation, gastrointestinal symptoms, and inflammation of the tongue or mouth. *Megaloblastic anemia* presents with mean red blood cell volume (MCV) > 100 fl and hypersegmented neutrophils. The neurologic sequela are variable and result from *loss of myelin*. Demyelination often occurs in the dorsal and lateral columns of the spinal cord (*combined degeneration*). Screening for B_{12} deficiency includes a history, physical exam, and serum B_{12} level. It usually takes 5 years to manifest B_{12} deficiency; therefore, obtain B_{12} levels starting no later than 5 years after surgery. Normal B_{12} levels do not exclude deficiency. A symptomatic patient should receive vitamin B_{12} even when the serum level is normal.

10. Abnormal drug kinetics—toxicity can occur when drugs are excreted in the urine, then reabsorbed through the urinary diversion. This toxicity has occurred with *phenytoin* and *methotrexate*. When administering toxic drugs such as chemotherapy, consider draining the diversion/conduit with a catheter to minimize drug contact with the intestinal segment.

11. Hematuria-dysuria syndrome—this symptom complex occurs only in gastrocystoplasty and consists of hematuria, dysuria, and suprapubic pain. The dysuria may be particularly severe in those who have bladder and urethra sensation. Treatment consists of H2 blockers or hydrogen pump blockers. Irrigation of the bladder with bicarbonate may be helpful.

12. Hypergastrinemia—when the antrum of the stomach is used in the urinary tract, exposure to alkaline urine can stimulate the antral G cells to secrete gastrin. Gastrin induces gastric acid secretion, and may increase the risk of gastric and duodenal ulcers.

Risk of Cancer at the Entero-Urothelial Anastomosis

1. There is an increased risk of cancer and benign polyps in the intestinal segment of certain urinary diversions (this does *not* include recurrences of the tumor for which the urinary diversion was done).

2. These tumors are usually adenocarcinoma, usually of intestinal origin, and usually occur at or near the urothelial-intestinal anastomosis. Even when the urinary stream has been diverted away from the intestine, a urothelial remnant left on the bowel may still induce a tumor.

3. Most data on these tumors comes from ureterosigmoidostomy. 5-13% of patients develop malignant tumors at or near the urothelial-intestinal anastomosis after a ureterosigmoidostomy, with a latency period of approximately 16 years (range: 3 to 53 years). Up to 40% of patients develop benign polyps after a ureterosigmoidostomy. Patients must be followed each year with IVP or CT urogram, stool occult blood, colonoscopy, and, if possible, urine cytology. Barium enema is avoided. The optimum time to start these tests is unknown; however, surveillance should probably begin no later than 5-10 years after urinary diversion.

4. There are rare reports of tumors in augmented bladders and conduits. The latency periods that have been reported are 5 to 29 years for tumors in augmented bladders (ileocystoplasties, cecocystoplasties, and colocystoplasties), 20 years for tumors in ileal conduits, and 1 to 26 years for tumors in colon conduits. In humans, no malignancy has been reported when stomach was used for urologic reconstruction. However, tumors have been identified in animal models using gastrocystoplasty. It is unclear if surveillance is required in patients with augmentations or conduits.

Selecting an Intestinal Segment for the Urinary Tract

1. Pelvic radiation—consider using transverse colon or stomach because these are furthest away from the radiation field.
2. Myelomeningocele—avoid using the ileocecal valve because removal of this segment may cause intractable diarrhea.
3. Ulcerative colitis—avoid using colon.
4. Peptic ulcer disease—avoid using stomach.
5. Short bowel syndrome—consider using stomach to prevent further shortening of the intestine.
6. Acidosis–consider using stomach (other segments can exacerbate acidosis)
7. Renal insufficiency—consider using stomach when creatinine > 2 because other intestinal segments may exacerbate acidosis.
8. Diverticulosis—consider avoiding colon.
9. Hepatic dysfunction—consider using stomach because other intestinal segments may cause excessive ammonia levels.

Summary of Intestinal Segments

1. Stomach
   a. Advantages—useful in patients with pelvic radiation, acidosis, renal failure, or hepatic failure. Acid secretion may inhibit bacterial growth and reduce infection. Least mucus production of intestinal segments.
   b. Disadvantages—hypokalemic hypochloremic metabolic alkalosis, hematuria dysuria syndrome, hypergastrinemia when the antrum is used.
2. Jejunum
   a. Advantages—hyperkalemic hypochloremic metabolic acidosis, hyponatremia, bone demineralization.
3. Ileum
   a. Advantages—familiar to urologists.
   b. Disadvantages—hypokalemic hyperchloremic acidosis, fat and bile malabsorption, diarrhea, vitamin B12 deficiency, bone demineralization, not ideal after pelvic radiation.
4. Ileocecal region
   a. Disadvantages—hypokalemic hyperchloremic acidosis, fat and bile malabsorption, diarrhea (especially with myelomeningocele), vitamin B12 deficiency, bone demineralization, not ideal after pelvic radiation.
5. Colon
   a. Advantages—transverse colon useful in those who had pelvic radiation.
   b. Disadvantages—hypokalemic hyperchloremic metabolic acidosis, most mucus production of intestinal segments, bone demineralization.

REFERENCES

Adams MC, Bihrle R, Rink RC: The use of stomach in urologic reconstruction. AUA Update Series, Vol. 14, Lesson 27, 1995.

Bowyer GW, Davies TW: Methotrexate toxicity associated with an ileal conduit. Br J Urol, 60: 592, 1987.

DeMarco RT, Koch MO: Metabolic complications of continent urinary diversion. AUA Update Series, Vol. 22, Lesson 15, 2003.

Fossa SD, Heilo A, Bormer O: Unexpectedly high serum methotrexate levels in cystectomized bladder cancer patients with an ileal conduit treated with intermediate doses of the drug. J Urol, 143: 498, 1990.

McDougal WS: Use of intestinal segments in the urinary tract: basic principles. Campbell's Urology. 6th Edition. Ed. PC Walsh, AB Retik, TA Stamey, et al. Philadelphia: W. B. Sanders Company, 1992, pp 2595-2629.

Rink RC, Hollensbe D, Adams MC: Complications of bladder augmentation in children and comparison of gastrointestinal segments. AUA Update Series, Vol. 14, Lesson 15, 1995.

DOSES OF COMMONLY USED MEDICATIONS

ADULT DOSES

Acetohydroxamic acid (Lithostat®)–250 mg po TID or QID [Tabs: 250 mg].

Acyclovir—see Genital Herpes, page 378.

Aldara™ (imiquimod)—see Condyloma Acuminatum, page 386.

Alfuzosin (Uroxatral®)—10 mg po q day (after meal) [Tabs: 10 mg].

Allopurinol—300 mg po q day (for uric acid lithiasis) [Tabs: 100, 300 mg].

Alprostadil—see page 249 and page 250.

Alum—see Treatment of Gross Hematuria, page 126.

Amicar® (aminocaproic acid)—see Treatment of Gross Hematuria, page 124.

Aminobenzoate potassium (Potaba®)—3 g po q 6 hours or 2 g po q 4 hours for at least 2-3 months [Tabs/Caps: 0.5 grams].

Aminocaproic acid (Amicar®)—see Treatment of Gross Hematuria, page 124.

Anafranil (clomipramine)—see Premature Ejaculation, page 258.

Androderm® (testosterone)—2.5 to 7.5 mg topically q 24 hours at night [Patches: 2.5, 5 mg]. Starting dose is 5 mg q 24 hours (adjust dose based on testosterone levels). Apply the patch to clean, dry, intact, non-irritated skin on the back, abdomen, upper arms, or thighs. Do *not* apply to bony prominences, scrotum, genitals, injured skin, or areas subject to prolonged pressure. Change the application site each day. Rash at the application site develops in up to 50%. If a rash develops, start triamcinolone acetonide 0.1% cream (*not ointment*) topically to the patch site prior to application.

AndroGel™ (testosterone)—AndroGel™ 1% 5 to 10 grams applied topically every 24 hours. [Gel packages: 2.5, 5 grams] or [Pump bottle: 88 grams (1.25 grams per pump)]. Staring dose is 5 grams q 24 hours, which may be increased in 2.5 gram increments to 10 grams as needed. Squeeze the contents of the package into the palm of the hand and immediately apply it to clean, dry, intact skin of the shoulders, upper arms, and/or abdomen. Let the application sites dry before dressing. Wash hands thoroughly after applying AndroGel™. Do *not* apply to scrotum or genitals. Wait at least 5-6 hours before showering or swimming. Avoid skin contact with other people at sites where AndroGel™ is applied.

Avodart™ (dutasteride)—0.5 mg po q day [Caps: 0.5 mg].

B & O supprettes® (belladonna & opium rectal suppositories)—one suppository pr q 6-24 hours. [B & O No. 15A (opium 30 mg, belladonna 16.2 mg) or B & O No. 16A (opium 60 mg, belladonna 16.2 mg)].

BCG—1 vial Tice® BCG in 50 cc NS or 1 vial Theracys® BCG in 50 cc NS intravesically (see page 39).

Belladonna and Opium suppository—See B & O supprettes®.

Bethanechol chloride—see Urecholine®.

Bicalutamide (Casodex®)—50 mg po q day (for combined androgen deprivation for prostate cancer) [Tabs: 50 mg].

Bicitra® (sodium citrate)—10-30 meq po BID to QID (each ml of solution yields 1 meq sodium and 1 meq bicarbonate) [240 ml bottle: 500 mg sodium citrate dihydrate and 334 mg citric acid monohydrate per 5 ml]

Cardura® (immediate release doxazosin)—start 1 mg po q day and slowly titrate up as needed to a maximum dose of 8 mg po q day. [Tabs: 1, 2, 4, 8 mg].

Cardura® XL (extended release doxazosin)—start 4 mg po q day with breakfast. Increase dose to 8 mg as needed. [Tabs: 4, 8 mg].

Casodex® (bicalutamide)—50 mg po q day (for combined androgen deprivation for prostate cancer) [Tabs: 50 mg].

Caverject® (alprostadil)—see Alprostadil, page 250.

Cellulose sodium phosphate—5 gm po BID or TID (for absorptive hypercalciuria)

Cholestyramine—400 mg po TID or 300 mg po QID (for hyperoxaluria).

Cialis® (tadalafil)—5-20 mg po before sexual activity.
    [Tabs: 5, 10, 20 mg]. Maximum dosing frequency is once per day.

Clomipramine (Anafranil)—see Premature Ejaculation, page 258.

Colchicine—0.6 mg po TID or 1.2 mg po BID after meals [Tabs: 0.5, 0.6 mg] (for Peyronie's).

Condylox® (podofilox)—see Condyloma Acuminatum, page 386.

D-penicillamine—250-1000 mg po QID [Caps: 125, 250 mg] (for cystinuria) and give with pyridoxine 25-50 mg po q day [Tabs: 25, 50, 100 mg].

Darifenacin (Enablex®)—7.5-15 mg po q day [Tabs: 7.5, 15 mg].

Detrol® (tolterodine)—1-2 mg po BID [Tabs: 1, 2 mg].

Detrol® LA (tolterodine)—2-4 mg po q day [Extended release caps: 2, 4 mg].

Ditropan® (oxybutynin)—2.5 mg or 5 mg po BID or TID [Tabs: 5 mg].

Ditropan® XL (oxybutynin)—5-30 mg po q day, start at 5 mg q day & titrate dose up in 5 mg increments once per week as indicated [Tabs: 5, 10, 15 mg].

Doxazosin immediate release (Cardura®)–start 1 mg po q day and slowly titrate up as needed to a maximum dose of 8 mg po q day. [Tabs: 1, 2, 4, 8 mg].

Doxazosin extended release (Cardura® XL)—start 4 mg po q day with breakfast. Increase dose to 8 mg as needed. [Tabs: 4, 8 mg].

Dutasteride (Avodart™)—0.5 mg po q day [Caps: 0.5 mg].

Edex® (alprostadil)—see Alprostadil, page 250.

Eligard™ (leuprolide acetate)—7.5 mg SC q month or 22.5 mg SC q 3 months or 30 mg SC q 4 months or 45 mg SC q 6 months.

Elmiron® (pentosan polysulfate)—100 mg po TID (take with water 1 hour before or 2 hours after a meal) [Caps: 100 mg].

Enablex® (darifenacin)—7.5-15 mg po q day [Tabs: 7.5, 15 mg].

Eulexin® (flutamide)—250 mg po TID [Caps: 125 mg].

Famciclovir—see Genital Herpes, page 378.

Finasteride (Proscar®)—5 mg po q day (for BPH) [Tabs: 5 mg].

Flavoxate (Urispas)—100-200 mg po TID or QID [Tabs: 100 mg].

Flomax® (tamsulosin)—0.4 or 0.8 mg po q day [Caps: 0.4 mg].

Fluorouracil (5%)—topically BID for 3-4 weeks [5% Cream: 25 grams] (for CIS of penis).

Fluoxetine (Prozac)—see Premature Ejaculation, page 258.

Flutamide (Eulexin®)—250 mg po TID [Caps: 125 mg].

Goserelin Acetate (Zoladex®)—3.6 mg SC q month or 10.8 mg SC q 3 months.

Histrelin—see Vantas™.

Hydrochlorothiazide—50 mg po q day or BID [Tabs: 25, 50, 100 mg] (for renal leak hypercalciuria or type 1 absorptive hypercalciuria).

Hyoscyamine (Levsin, Cystospaz, Anaspaz)—0.125-0.375 mg po/sl q 4 hours prn (maximum dose = 1.5 mg/day) [Tabs: 0.125 mg].

Hyoscyamine extended release (Levsinex Timecaps, Levbid)—0.375-0.750 mg po q 12 hours [Tabs/Caps: 0.375 mg].

Hytrin® (terazosin)—start at 1 mg po qHS and slowly titrate up as needed to a maximum dose of 10 mg po qHS. See page 113. [Tabs: 1, 2, 5, 10 mg].

Imiquimod (Aldara™)—see Condyloma Acuminatum, page 386.

Ketoconazole (Nizoral®)—200-400 mg po TID (for androgen deprivation for prostate cancer) [Tabs: 200 mg].

Leuprolide acetate—see Lupron® (IM injections), Eligard™ (SC injections), and Viadur™ (one year subcutaneous implant).

Levitra® (vardenafil)—5-20 mg po before sexual activity. [Tabs: 2.5, 5, 10, 20 mg]. Maximum dosing frequency is once per day.

Lithostat® (acetohydroxamic acid)—250 mg po TID or QID [Tabs: 250 mg].

Lupron® (leuprolide acetate)—7.5 mg IM q month or 22.5 mg IM q 3 months or 30 mg IM q 4 months.

Magnesium gluconate—500 mg po BID [Tabs: 500 mg] (for hypomagnesiuria)

Magnesium oxide—140 mg po QID or 400-500 mg po BID [Caps: 140, 250, 400, 420, 500 mg] (for hypomagnesiuria).

Megace®—see megestrol acetate.

Megestrol acetate (Megace®)—20 mg po bid (for hot flashes) [Tabs: 20, 40 mg].

Methenamine—see page 339.

Mitomycin C—40 mg in 20 cc sterile water intravesically (see page 39).

MUSE® (alprostadil)—see MUSE®, page 249 [urethral suppository: 125, 250, 500, 1000 mcg].

Nilandron™—see nilutamide.

Nilutamide (Nilandron™)—300 mg po q day for 30 days, then 150 mg po q day (for combined androgen deprivation for prostate cancer) [Tabs: 50 mg].

Oxybutynin—see Ditropan® (oral) and Oxytrol™ (transdermal).

Oxytrol™ (oxybutynin)—one patch applied to dry, intact skin of the abdomen, hip, or buttock every 3 to 4 days (avoid re-application to the same skin site within 7 days) [patch: 3.9 mg/day].

Papaverine—see Papaverine, page 250.

Paroxetine (Paxil)—see Premature Ejaculation, page 258.

Paxil (paroxetine)—see Premature Ejaculation, page 258.

Penicillamine—see D-penicillamine.

Pentosan polysulfate—see Elmiron®.

Phenazopyridine (Pyridium®)—200 mg po TID [Tabs: 100, 200 mg].

Podofilox (Condylox®)—see Condyloma Acuminatum, page 386.

Podophyllin—see Condyloma Acuminatum, page 386.

Potaba® (aminobenzoate potassium)—3 g po q 6 hours or 2 g po q 4 hours for at least 2-3 months [Tabs/Caps: 0.5 grams].

Potassium citrate—20 meq po TID (for stone disease).

Proscar® (finasteride)—5 mg po q day (for BPH) [Tabs: 5 mg].

Prostaglandin E1—see page 249 and page 250.

Proxeed™—one packet po BID (mixed in at least 4 ounces of juice).

Prozac (fluoxetine)—see Premature Ejaculation, page 258.

Pyridium® (phenazopyridine)—200 mg po TID [Tabs: 100, 200 mg].

Pyridium® Plus—one tablet po QID (after meals and qHS).

Sanctura® (trospium)—20 mg po BID [Tabs: 20 mg].

Sanctura® XR (trospium)—60 mg po q day [Tabs: 60 mg].

Sertraline—see Premature Ejaculation, page 258.

Sildenafil (Viagra®)—25-100 mg po before sexual activity. [Tabs: 25, 50, 100 mg]. Maximum dosing frequency is once per day.

Silver nitrate—see Treatment of Gross Hematuria, page 126.

Sodium cellulose phosphate—5 gm po BID or TID (for absorptive hypercalciuria)

Sodium citrate—see Bicitra®.

Solifenacin (Vesicare®)—5-10 mg po q day [Tabs: 5, 10 mg].

Striant™ (testosterone)—one buccal system (30 mg) applied to the gum region every 12 hours. The system should be placed in a comfortable position just above the incisor tooth (on either side of the mouth). Alternate application sites from one side of the mouth to the other. [Buccal system: 30 mg].

Tadalafil (Cialis®)—5-20 mg po before sexual activity. [Tabs: 5, 10, 20 mg]. Maximum dosing frequency is once per day.

Tamsulosin (Flomax®)—0.4 or 0.8 mg po q day [Caps: 0.4 mg].

Terazosin (Hytrin®)—start at 1 mg po qHS and slowly titrate up as needed to a maximum dose of 10 mg po qHS. See page 113. [Tabs: 1, 2, 5, 10 mg].

Testoderm® TTS (testosterone)–5 to 10 mg topically q 24 hours [Patches 5 mg]. Starting dose is 5 mg q 24 hours (adjust dose based on testosterone levels). Apply to intact skin of the arm, back, or upper buttocks. Do *not* apply to scrotum or genitals. Change application area each day.

Testosterone (buccal)—see Striant™.

Testosterone (intramuscular)—testosterone enanthate or testosterone cypionate 50-400 mg IM q 2-4 weeks [5 ml vial: 200 mg/ml].

Testosterone (transdermal gel)—see AndroGel™.

Testosterone (transdermal patch)—see Androderm® and Testoderm® TTS.

Testosterone 2% cream—apply topically BID (for symptomatic BXO).

Thiazide—see hydrochlorothiazide.

Thiola™—1-2 g per day divided QID [Tabs: 100 mg].

Thiotepa—60 mg in 30-60 cc of normal saline instilled intravesically (see page 39).

Tiopronin—see Thiola™.

Tolterodine—see Detrol®.

Trelstar® (triptorelin)—3.75 mg IM q 1 month or 11.25 mg IM q 3 months.

Triptorelin—see Trelstar®.

Trospium –see Sanctura® and Sanctura XR®.

Urecholine® (bethanechol chloride)—10-50 mg po TID or QID; take on empty stomach [Tabs: 5, 10, 25, 50 mg].

Urispas (flavoxate)—100-200 mg po TID or QID [Tabs: 100 mg].

Uroxatral® (alfuzosin)—10 mg po q day (after meal) [Tabs: 10 mg].

Valacyclovir—see Genital Herpes, page 378.

Vantas™ (histrelin)—one implant (50 mg) inserted subcutaneously in the inner aspect of the upper arm every 12 months (a previous Vantas™ implant must be removed before placing a new implant).

Vardenafil (Levitra®)—5-20 mg po before sexual activity. [Tabs: 2.5, 5, 10, 20 mg]. Maximum dosing frequency is once per day.

Vesicare® (solifenacin)—5-10 mg po q day [Tabs: 5, 10 mg].

Viadur™ (leuprolide acetate)—one implant (65 mg) inserted subcutaneously in the inner aspect of the upper arm every 12 months (a previous Viadur™ implant must be removed before placing a new implant).

Viagra® (sildenafil)—25-100 mg po before sexual activity. [Tabs: 25, 50, 100 mg]. Maximum dosing frequency is once per day.

Vitamin E—800-1200 IU po q day (for Peyronie's disease).

Yohimbine—5.4 mg po TID (for erectile dysfunction) [Tabs: 5.4 mg].

Zoladex® (goserelin acetate)—3.6 mg SC q month or 10.8 mg SC q 3 months.

Zoloft (sertraline)—see Premature Ejaculation, page 258.

PEDIATRIC DOSES

     1 teaspoon = 5 ml; 1 ounce = 30 ml

D-penicillamine—30 mg/kg/day po divided QID (for cystinuria) and give with pyridoxine 1-2 mg/kg/day po.

Ditropan®—see oxybutynin.

Hydrochlorothiazide—1 mg/kg/day po divided BID [solution: 5 mg/5 ml] (for renal leak hypercalciuria or type 1 absorptive hypercalciuria).

Nitrofurantoin [suspension: 25 mg/5 ml].
- Therapeutic dose = 5-7 mg/kg/day po divided QID.
- Prophylaxis/suppression dose = 1.5 mg/kg po q day.
- Maximum dose = 100 mg per dose.
- Contraindicated in children < 1 month old because of the risk of hemolytic anemia from immature erythrocyte enzyme systems.

Oxybutynin (Ditropan®)—0.1 mg/kg/dose po BID or TID [elixir: 5 mg/5 ml].

Phenazopyridine (Pyridium®)—12 mg/kg/day po divided TID (age >6 years only).

Pyridium®—see phenazopyridine.

Thiazide—see hydrochlorothiazide.

Thiola™—15 mg/kg/day po divided QID (for cystinuria).

Trimethoprim/Sulfamethoxazole [elixir: 40 mg trimethoprim and 200 mg sulfamethoxazole per 5 ml].
- Therapeutic dose = 0.5 ml/kg/dose po BID.
- Prophylaxis/suppression dose = 0.5 ml/kg po q day.
- Maximum dose = 20 ml per dose.
- Contraindicated in children less than 2 months old because it may cause kernicterus.

INDEX

A